EARLY DRUG DEVELOPMENT

EARLY DRUG DEVELOPMENT

Strategies and Routes to First-in-Human Trials

Edited by

MITCHELL N. CAYEN
Cayen Pharmaceutical Consulting, LLC

WILEY

A JOHN WILEY & SONS, INC., PUBLICATION

Published by John Wiley & Sons, Inc., Hoboken, New Jersey.
Published simultaneously in Canada.

Library of Congress Cataloging-in-Publication Data:

Early drug development : strategies and routes to first-in-human trials / edited by Mitchell N. Cayen.
p. ; cm.
Includes bibliographical references.
ISBN 978-0-470-17086-1 (cloth)
1. Drug development. I. Cayen, Mitchell N.
[DNLM: 1. Drug Discovery—methods. 2. Clinical Trials, Phase I as Topic. 3. Drug Approval—organization & administration. 4. Drugs, Investigational—therapeutic use. 5. Research Design. QV 744 E12 2010]
RM301.25.E27 2010
615′.19–dc22

2009045882

10 9 8 7 6 5 4 3 2 1

CONTENTS

PART IV PRE-IND DRUG DEVELOPMENT

CONTRIBUTORS

Örn Almarsson, Alkermes, Inc., Waltham, Massachusetts

Mark Ammann, United BioSource Corporation, Ann Arbor, Michigan

Laura P. Andrews, Genzyme Corporation, Framingham, Massachusetts

Judith Atkins, Paraxel International Inc., Waltham, Massachusetts

Hugh E. Black, Hugh E. Black & Associates, Inc., Sparta, New Jersey

Lorrene A. Buckley, Eli Lilly and Company, Indianapolis, Indiana

Peter L. Bullock, Paul P. Carbone Cancer Center, University of Wisconsin, Madison, Wisconsin

John Caldwell, University of Liverpool, Liverpool, United Kingdom

Mitchell N. Cayen, Cayen Pharmaceutical Consulting, LLC, Bedminster, New Jersey

Gary Eichenbaum, Johnson & Johnson Pharmaceutical Research and Development, Raritan, New Jersey

Kathryn Hackett-Fields, QualiStat, Inc., Helmetta, New Jersey

Carolyn D. Finkle, MedImmune, Gaithersburg, Maryland

Christopher J. Galli, TransForm Pharmaceuticals/ChemPharm LEX, Johnson & Johnson Pharmaceutical Research and Development, Lexington, Massachusetts

Parag Garhyan, Eli Lilly and Company, Indianapolis, Indiana

James D. Green, Biogen Idec, Inc., Cambridge, Massachusetts

Ulf B. Hillgren, Pfizer Global Research and Development, Groton, Connecticut

Anthony B. Jones, Taylor Technology, Inc., Princeton, New Jersey

Christopher Kemper, Pharmanet Development Group, Princeton, New Jersey

Kathleen J. Kovacs, Pfizer Global Research and Development, Groton, Connecticut

Duane B. Lakings, DSE Consulting, Inc., Elgin, Texas

Ronald W. Moch, Hugh E. Black & Associates, Inc., Rockville, Maryland

Stephen B. Montgomery, Hugh E. Black & Associates, Inc., Alpharetta, Georgia

Amin A. Nomeir, Schering-Plough Research Institute, Kenilworth, New Jersey

Shari L. Perlstein, Pfizer Global Research and Development, Groton, Connecticut

Rafael A. Ponce, ZymoGenetics, Seattle, Washington; presently at: Amgen Inc., Seattle, Washington

Stanley A. Roberts, CoxX Research LLC, San Diego, California

Mary M. Sommer, Pfizer Global Research and Development, Groton, Connecticut

Vangala Subrahmanyam, Sai Advantium Pharma Ltd., Hinjewadi, Pune, India

Alfred P. Tonelli, Johnson & Johnson Pharmaceutical Research and Development, Raritan, New Jersey

Keith Wilner, Pfizer Global Research and Development, La Jolla, California

FOREWORD

From 1950 to the late 1990s, the global pharmaceutical industry was responsible for a series of advances that addressed major disease areas and led to significant improvements in public health and quality of life. In no particular order, these treatments may be exemplified by drugs (a) controlling blood pressure, and latter, blood cholesterol; (b) controlling gastric acid secretion; (c) controlling female fertility; and (d) progressively addressing major cancers, so that many tumor types are now treated as chronic diseases rather than terminal illnesses. The reader will be able to add many other examples to this list. Although these years were also marked by instances of patients harmed by drug treatments, most notably thalidomide in the early 1960s, the introduction of new therapies has revolutionized medical care for many people, created new personal freedoms, and is a major factor in the increase in life expectancy achieved in many countries over the past 50 or more years.

In recent years, the ability of the pharmaceutical industry to sustain this remarkable contribution has been challenged. Although we have seen a huge growth both in scientific understanding in the biomedical sciences and in the technical feasibility of many aspects of drug research and development, these advances have not been accompanied by corresponding increases in research productivity: put very simply, the research and development pipeline of new medicines has gotten blocked, so that fewer and fewer new agents reach the market each year. The reasons for this are many and varied. Making new compounds with interesting and therapeutically relevant biological activity is a challenge, but those that are produced lack other key features of usable drugs. In recent years it has proved very difficult indeed to develop such active compounds into novel medicines. The business model used by many pharmaceutical companies is not capable of infinite replication. The development of more "blockbuster" drugs, which have underpinned much of the growth seen from the mid-1970s onward, is now less and less likely in times when science seeks to stratify drug development and medicine seeks individualized therapies. The protection of intellectual property and the maximization of marketing exclusivity are now more important than ever and come under pressure from health care providers, who emphasize the need for low-cost generic prescribing as one means to address the escalation of costs. The regulatory environment in the early twenty-first century is both sophisticated and questioning in all jurisdictions and is supported by the very high expectations of the public in terms of both the efficacy and safety of new therapies. It is to be hoped that recent developments in this area, such as the U.S. Food and Drug Administration's Critical Path and the European Union's Innovative Medicines Initiative, will bear fruit, but there have been few successes thus far.

Against this background, this new volume provides an invaluable guide to the earliest and most critical stages of drug development, getting promising new chemicals into humans quickly, effectively, and safely, to provide information of maximum benefit for critical decision making. The Editor, who has a lifetime of experience in exactly this arena, has identified a series of key topics and matched them to well-qualified authors, resulting in an extremely helpful handbook to guide the experienced investigator and novice alike through what can all too easily be a mine field.

Drug development is simultaneously an art and a science. It depends on excellent science in all of the various chemical, biological, and clinical disciplines that contribute, but at present at least the coordination of the management of all of the resources required as well as critical and fully informed decision making is best regarded as an art. It is my view that this new volume represents a substantial contribution by providing an integrated approach to an area that has suffered from excessive fragmentation.

John Caldwell

Pro-Vice-Chancellor and Dean of the Faculty of Medicine
University of Liverpool, United Kingdom
August 2009

PREFACE

During my career in the pharmaceutical industry in Canada and the United States, initially as a bench scientist and subsequently in managing departments in big pharma companies, and now as an industry consultant, I have never ceased to view the drug discovery and development paradigm with a combination of excitement, awe, wonder, and caution. There are many reasons for this mix of emotions. First, the discovery and development of successful medicines represent hugely complex challenges, with what seems to be a constantly shifting end zone. Our learning curve about the etiology and treatment of disease, coupled with the numerous changes in regulatory climate, help contribute, in my view, to make successful pharmaceutical development one of the most difficult of business enterprises. The second and probably more fundamental reason for these feelings is that the more I have learned over the years about how foreign compounds interface with living organisms, the more I realize that there is so much that I will never learn or understand. This is a sobering thought. Those of us who are in the business of developing medicines to treat human disease are doing the best we can to assure that we do not put patients at risk and that there is a high likelihood of therapeutic success. Given the complexity of the human body, the best we can hope for, based on all our advances over several millennia, is that successful therapeutics continue to morph from hit-and-miss to higher odds of positive outcomes in larger percentages of the target population. We still have a long way to go. It continues to amaze me that in most therapeutic areas, we have only reached the stage where we are merely alleviating disease symptoms rather than curing the actual disease.

It is therefore not surprising that the road to successful drug development has many twists, turns, and intersections, and that many travelers take different routes. It is critical to note that the path must eventually lead not to the submission of a new drug application (NDA), but to the attainment of an approvable NDA. The primary goal of this book is to describe those routes that have the greatest likelihood of a successful journey during the initial stages of the voyage [i.e., up to the first-in-human (FIH) trial]. The authors who provide these perspectives have had decades of experience in both big and small pharma companies, biotechnology companies, contract research organizations, regulatory affairs, and various aspects of consulting. Each chapter focuses on a specific discipline that contributes to the late discovery and early development of new candidate drugs, and is designed to describe the state-of-the-science, challenges, strategies, and "how to" regarding study designs and data interpretation. Many basic concepts are described and explained. The text can be used as a primer for new investigators as well as a resource for the experienced. It should be noted that each author is presenting the topic from his or her viewpoint and perspectives and that for the most part, no one size fits all. Indeed, given the fact that no single discipline can stand on its own, there is some overlap between chapters, and the reader may therefore obtain different viewpoints on similar topics (e.g., safety assessment of metabolites in Chapters 2, 3, 8, and 9; the TGN1412 monoclonal antibody human toxicity issue in Chapters 10 and 12). For example, approaches will vary based on such factors as:

- Small-molecule versus biotherapeutic drug
- Route of drug administration
- Frequency of drug administration
- Target disease
- Corporate resources, goals, portfolio management, and competitive landscape

We decided early where on the drug development path to end this book, and that was in the planning (but not implementation) of an FIH study. However, the more difficult decision was deciding where to begin. For various reasons, including the fact that there are numerous excellent published treatises on the discovery process, we decided arbitrarily to start at the point where a new chemical entity (NCE) has been shown to possess pharmacological activity in an initial screen (hit-to-lead), and then proceed to the next step toward the process of selection as a candidate drug (lead optimization). Accordingly, there is extensive discussion of those disciplines and activities necessary to demonstrate that the FIH trial will have a high likelihood of success; these disciplines include toxicology, safety pharmacology, CMC (chemistry, manufacturing, and controls), ADME (absorption, distribution, metabolism, and excretion), pharmacokinetics and toxicokinetics, GLPs (good laboratory practices), bioanalysis, regulatory submissions, and related activities. It is emphasized that there is no such thing as the perfect drug candidate, whether from the efficacy or safety viewpoint; as Sir Harold Macmillan pointed out: "To be alive at all involves some risk."

One of my personal challenges when I begin consultation with a pharmaceutical company is to learn the lexicon which is the in-house language but which may not be readily transparent to new visitors. We have tried to be consistent within and have decided arbitrarily to use such terms as FIH [rather than FTIM (first time in man)], NCE [rather than NME (new molecular entity) or NCD (new candidate drug)], and nonclinical (rather than preclinical, though both will be found).

I would like to thank Jonathan Rose at John Wiley & Sons for inviting me to put this book together and for his guidance during the process. I am very grateful to the authors of the various chapters for their dedication and patience, and for providing this project with their vast array of experience and expertise.

It is my joy to dedicate this book to my wife, Judy, who was instrumental in encouraging me to take on this project and whose love and support were absolutely invaluable during its course.

MITCHELL N. CAYEN

Bedminster, New Jersey
September 2009

PART I

INTRODUCTION

1

DRUG DISCOVERY AND EARLY DRUG DEVELOPMENT

MITCHELL N. CAYEN

1.1 THE DRUG DISCOVERY AND DEVELOPMENT SCENE

1.1.1 Pharmaceutical Research and Development Challenges

Although it is common practice to envisage the launching of a therapeutic as a linear paradigm comprising a drug discovery phase gradually bridging into a development phase, it should be noted that such a process is rarely so straightforward. There are many potential intersecting paths to a successful new therapy, often involving a mixture of successive or concurrent intellectual, scientific, practical, commercial, regulatory, and other considerations among academia, industry, and government. However, for the purposes of the focus of this book, the road to therapeutic success is being presented generally as a linear continuum starting with drug discovery, continuing to drug development, then submission to regulatory agencies and approval, and ending with what is hopefully a high-quality medication that exhibits optimal safety and efficacy in the target population.

Given the achievements in the past several decades in our understanding of the underlying mechanisms of disease, huge technological advances, and the goal of optimizing monetary, staff, and time resources, it would be expected that in the ideal world, in recent years we should have been witnessing an increase in the availability of new and improved medicinal products. However, anyone involved in health care delivery is well aware that this is not the case. The past five years have witnessed a dramatic decline in the number of new drugs approved by the U.S. Food and Drug Administration (FDA) compared to a decade ago. Compared

Early Drug Development: Strategies and Routes to First-in-Human Trials, Edited by Mitchell N. Cayen

to the highs of 53 in 1996 and 39 in 1997, the numbers of new drugs approved by the FDA was 21 in 2003, a decade high of 36 in 2004, 20 in 2005, 22 in 2006, 19 in 2007 (the fewest in 24 years), 25 in 2008, and 26 in 2009. Concurrently, the costs to discover, develop, and register an approvable new drug is compelling, and has been escalating from about $800 million in 2001 [1] to $900 million in 2004 [2] to about $1.3 billion today (comprising approximately $425 million for nonclinical and $850 for clinical development, although such estimates do vary, depending on the source material and analyses techniques), and the time from discovery to commercialization ranges from 10 to 15 years. The good news is that the average time for FDA approval has declined to an average of 1.1 years in 2005–2007 from around 2 years previously. With patent protection lasting for 20 years, at least in the United States, the time frame for profitability remains relatively narrow, although a patent-protected drug is generally highly profitable during this protected period. Following are some of the contemporary perspectives, challenges, and pressures inherent in the pharmaceutical industry that affect the timely availability of novel therapeutics.

Research and Development Challenges

- Research and development productivity has been declining.
- Late-stage pipelines have become relatively thin.
- Industry is tackling diseases of greater complexity [e.g., oncology and central nervous system (CNS) malfunctions such as Alzheimer's disease, Parkinson's disease, schizophrenia, and bipolar disease], necessitating complex clinical design protocols.
- No drug is perfectly safe or spectacularly efficacious at all doses.
- The concept of risk/benefit ratio is changing with the realization that the balance may not only be determined by dose, but that different patients may be more likely to gain the benefit, whereas others may be more prone to risk.
- Marketing pressures within pharmaceutical companies may be at odds with research and development goals, including risk/benefit analyses.
- Many companies are pulling potentially good drugs out of the pipeline because of regulatory agencies' diminished tolerance for side effects.

Business Perspectives

- Industry is struggling with greater scrutiny, patent expirations, major mergers, poor stock performance, thousands of layoffs, and thinning pipelines.
- Generic competition will eliminate $67 billion annual revenues for U.S. pharmaceutical sales between 2007 and 2012; more than three dozen drugs will lose patent protection during this interval.
- Accordingly, the first annual revenue decline in four decades will occur between 2011 and 2012.

- New blockbusters are lacking to replace old ones such as Lipitor and Plavix. There remains a mindset by many organizations that only blockbusters are worth developing.
- However, blockbuster mentality restricts research direction and diversification.
- To remain competitive, drug companies must adjust to shifting market conditions (including enhanced standard of care), which may become altered during the course of drug development.

1.1.2 Attrition During Discovery and Development

It is thus well known that the odds of a new chemical entity (NCE) finding its way to becoming a successful therapeutic agent are extremely low. Only one in 5000 to 10,000 NCEs are approved and, in both the United States and Europe, approximately one in nine compounds that enter clinical development end up as approved products. Emerging data seem to indicate that the approval rate is somewhat higher for biopharmaceuticals than for small-molecule drugs. In the early 1990s, one of the main causes of this high attrition was pharmacokinetics and bioavailability (including problematic clinical drug–drug interactions); however, with the recent focus on the very early assessment of such characteristics (Chapter 2), these properties can be identified to a great extent prior to the first-in-human (FIH) study, resulting in early elimination of compounds unlikely to elicit undesirable absorption, distribution, metabolism, and excretion characteristics in patients. In the past several years, the principal reasons for attrition are generally in the following order: clinical efficacy > nonclinical toxicology > commercial > clinical safety > pharmacokinetics/bioavailability > cost of goods > formulation [2]. Success rates can vary with the therapeutic area: For those NCEs entering an FIH trial, the percentages that end up as marketed drugs are approximately 20% for cardiovascular, 16% for arthritis/pain and infectious diseases, and 5 to 8% for oncology and CNS malfunctions.

The chapters in this book are designed to aid in the determination of the most efficient and effective path to the FIH trial with NCEs that have a high likelihood of morphing into successful therapeutics. It should be noted that the mindset of reducing attrition in clinical development should be in place from the earliest stages of discovery, given that research, development (nonclinical and clinical), and marketing personnel should be aligned as early as possible in the discovery process. In this manner, all relevant disciplines can help create the animal pharmacology models best predictive of clinical efficacy, and later to design a proof-of-concept endpoint in the FIH study to provide evidence that the molecular target is being hit and that hitting such a target will elicit the anticipated physiological response [the exploratory investigational new drug (IND) approach to rapid attainment of such information is discussed in Chapter 11]. Early coordination among disciplines can also help reduce attrition by the early elimination of compounds with poor pharmaceutical properties (e.g., solubility; permeability), insufficient chemical and metabolic stability, low bioavailability, potent enzyme inhibition or induction, mechanism-based toxicity, and other characteristics that would affect the clinical safety and efficacy of an NCE. Whether within a "big pharma" company, a smaller pharma/biotech organization, or a virtual company, strategic planning at all stages of discovery and development are critical, and can make or break a company (Chapter 13).

1.1.3 Corporate Strategy Perspectives

Given the extraordinary challenges and extensive commitment of time, financial, and human resources necessary to achieve marketing of a successful drug, the end result is usually a relatively profitable enterprise for the pharmaceutical company compared with many other industries. Such profitability is important, as it enables the industry to reinvest in research and development for those debilitating diseases that require improved therapies. The pharmaceutical industry has witnessed more major changes in the past century than, arguably, has any other major industry. This is probably because as we learn more about the causes and etiology of disease, which continue to remain elusive because of the complexities of normal and abnormal biological systems, adjustments must be made continuously based on our emerging understanding of the continuum between efficacy and safety. The basic principle of pharmacology (i.e., that no drug is perfectly safe and that safety is dose dependent), is sometimes overlooked by those intricately involved in the process. Despite all the knowledge we have accumulated, most contemporary therapies still alleviate disease symptoms rather than resulting in a cure of the target disease.

Although discrete pharmaceutical companies have been developing drugs for well more than a century, no optimal business model has emerged that would be predictive of success. With the numerous scientific, medical, marketing, financial, and regulatory pressures and challenges of recent years, some companies prescribe to the "bigger is better" philosophy, such as the recent megamergers of Pfizer and Wyeth, Merck and Schering-Plough, and Roche and Genentech; whether such consolidation results in industry stabilization remains to be determined. Other big pharma companies have been establishing relatively independent small research units that seem to mimic those in smaller biotech companies. Small to midsized pharmaceutical companies, virtual companies, and smaller biotech companies often try to develop new drug candidates through to successful proof of principle in humans, and then attempt to partner with a larger organization with more extensive clinical development and marketing muscle. The smaller the company, the more likely it is to exit product development early. Virtually all companies—small and large—utilize the services of contract research organizations (CROs) to supplement their programs, and this resource is discussed later in the chapter.

For companies of all sizes, it is critical to have a portfolio management strategy which is dependent on such considerations as the inherent size, research/

development/marketing staff skills, tolerance for risk, geography, corporate culture, and unfortunately, internal politics. Once a decision is made to embark on the development of an NCE, a plan is put in place that incorporates time lines through to the anticipated new drug application (NDA). There are numerous strategies that can comprise such a plan. One approach, which can be extremely useful, in particular for staff scientists within specific disciplines who may not be privy to the "big picture," is to write the outline of the drug label first. Although this may seem to be counterintuitive, focusing on and writing the target therapeutic qualities of a medicinal product can help in the design of specific studies that will determine whether the NCE meets those qualities.

The development plan should comprise several go/no go decision points (e.g., proof of principle), which will help determine whether a program should continue to progress through several gates. Often, however, other problematic data may emerge that are outside the formal decision points. One of the most difficult decisions is the timing regarding when a development program should be terminated, based on emerging problematic safety, efficacy, and/or pharmacokinetic data. A development program will typically have one or more "champions" and several stakeholders from numerous disciplines who may rationalize why the drug candidate should continue along the development path instead of intaking the difficult decision to terminate the program. The basic paradigm will continue to comprise intense planning, strategic decision making, extensive research, long-term nonclinical safety, and clinical safety and efficacy studies, comprehensive data collection and statistical analyses, and relevant support programs. Whatever the strategy, it is ultimately the drug that speaks, and it is incumbent upon all those within large or small organizations and all contributing disciplines to conduct the most appropriate studies that will enable all relevant aspects of efficacy and safety to be uncovered. Small and large studies in all disciplines must be conducted based on sound scientific disciplines, to avoid "garbage in–garbage out" results with equivocal interpretation. One cannot force a drug candidate to exhibit properties that it does not possess.

In light of the perspectives noted above, a primary goal of the chapters that follow is to help guide those involved in the exciting field of pharmaceutical discovery and development to plan and conduct those studies beginning with lead optimization (discovery support), to early development, through to the FIH trial. The goal is to evaluate NCEs that have the greatest likelihood of leading to valuable therapeutics, and to develop strategies that will optimize what are often limited monetary, time, and human resources. Moving forward, it will be important to adjust the focus of the various disciplines as new advances in biomedical and genomic technologies emerge, and to determine which of these technologies are really useful in predicting human safety and efficacy, thereby affecting the drug development process. It must always be kept in mind that the ultimate goal in drug development is not the NDA submission process but the attainment of an approved NDA.

1.2 DRUG DISCOVERY

1.2.1 Target Identification

Drug discovery is a process whereby potential therapeutics are designed and identified. Historically, most drugs have been discovered either by isolating the active ingredients from natural sources such as plants, animals, or minerals, or by empirical approaches that capitalized on enlightened serendipity (such as the discovery of penicillin in a dirty petri dish in Alexander Fleming's laboratory, or the invention of aspirin—still the most widely used drug worldwide). Indeed, in developed nations, herbal remedies have become more popular. With rapid advances beginning in the twentieth century in the understanding of the origins and pathology of human disease, modern drug discovery typically focuses on studying the metabolic pathways related to a disease state or pathogen, and manipulating these pathways using medicinal chemistry, biochemistry, physiology, microbiology, and/or molecular biology. Genetic and genomic information also offers great promise in drug discovery and therapeutic success [3].

The first step in the process is *target identification*, and it is this critical step that necessitates a true understanding of the pathogenesis of the disease. Target identification for numerous serious diseases is being pursued aggressively by laboratories in the pharmaceutical industry, universities, and government institutions worldwide. The ideal target is generally a clearly identified molecular entity (such as an enzyme or a receptor) known to be directly associated with the disease pathophysiology. Certain targets are considered to be more likely than others to be amenable to changes that the medicinal chemist can target with compounds that might ultimately lead to a successful medicine. The term *druggability* of a given target (*druggable target*) is being used to indicate the likelihood of being able to modulate a target with a small-molecule drug or antibody, and it is important to predict the potential druggability of a novel target. Parameters that influence druggability include cellular location, specificity, development of resistance, transport mechanisms, side effects, and toxicity. Some target classes, such as protein kinases or the large family of transmembrane receptors such as the G-protein-coupled receptors (GPCRs) have been targeted successfully, and a large number of approved drugs, such as many biogenic amines, eicosanoids, lipid-signaling molecules, and numerous peptide and protein ligands, exhibit their mechanism of action by interfacing with GPCR receptors. The many serious diseases that remain poorly treated may witness breakthroughs due to the exploitation of many unexplored targets.

However, many safe and effective drugs have been and continue to be discovered and developed without a true understanding of the actual target; that is, the mode of action may be known, but the mechanism of action may not be uncovered until later, or not at all. With their longer history, small-molecule drugs currently tend to be focused on the better established targets, while extensive research has been ongoing on new targets for biotherapeutics (i.e., biotechnology-derived drugs such as therapeutic proteins, peptides, oligosaccharides, and monoclonal antibodies). Also, the concept of "druglike" properties is used by medicinal chemists as a guide to the likelihood of an NCE becoming a successful drug [4]. Such characteristics include physicochemical properties such as lipophilicity, as well as optimal absorption, distribution, metabolism, and excretion (ADME) profiles (Chapter 2), which enable the compound to exhibit targeted efficacy for a sufficient length of time. Indeed, it appears that lipophilicity has emerged as the single best physicochemical characteristic that is predictive of the drug-like property of a chemical regarding potency, efficacy, ADME, and toxicity [4]. This is exemplified by the *Lipinski rule of five* [5,6], which is a rule of thumb describing the molecular properties of a drug that can predict the high absorption and permeability of small-molecule drugs, although the rule does not predict if a compound is pharmacologically active. The rule states that, in general, an orally active drug should not violate more than one of the following four criteria:

1. No more than five hydrogen bond donors (nitrogen or oxygen atoms with one or more hydrogen atoms)
2. No more than 10 hydrogen bond acceptors (nitrogen or oxygen atoms)
3. Molecular weight below 500 Da
4. Calculated octanol–water partition coefficient ($c\log P$) below 5

The Lipinski rule is only applicable for those compounds that are not substrates for active transporters (Chapter 2). An analysis of databases of the past decade of NCE hits and leads have shown that advanced lead compounds and early clinical candidates that have undergone attrition tend to differ in the desirable physicochemical properties described above, and that the undesirable phenomena were traced back to the nature of the high-throughput screening tests and hit-to-lead optimization practices [7]; this reinforces the value of studying druglike properties as early as feasible.

1.2.2 Hit-to-Lead Identification

Following target identification, and for small-molecule chemicals, the medicinal chemist is charged with the responsibility of compound synthesis (e.g., combinatorial chemistry, high-throughput chemistry, classical organic chemistry synthesis, compound libraries) based on numerous strategies and considerations [8]. This is followed by appropriate in vitro [usually by actual or virtual (using computer-generated models) high-throughput screening] and in vivo screens of the new compounds for potential potency and selectivity, and an evaluation of how NCEs with the appropriate characteristics are selected for specific targets of interest. Novel pharmacophores can also emerge by drug design, which involves the prediction of which NCEs might "fit" into an active site based on the biological and physical properties of the target. Thus, these initial evaluations focus on efficacy and potency rather than on potential safety. High-potency drugs are associated with low-efficacious doses, and in general, the lower the efficacious dose, the less the likelihood of toxicity and side effects.

It is rare that a perfect drug candidate will emerge from these early screens. Typically, several compounds will be uncovered with some degree of activity, and if these compounds share common chemical features, one or more pharmacophores can then be developed. Collaboration between biology and medicinal chemistry is critical such that medicinal chemists can attempt to use structure–activity relationships (SARs) to improve the characteristics of the lead compound(s) [e.g., increase activity against the target selected (potency)], decrease activity against unrelated targets (selectivity), and/or improve druglike properties (e.g., lipophilicity, as described above; metabolic stability). The goal is to improve the properties of the NCEs to allow the most favorable compounds to move forward to later-stage testing (e.g., disease models) in discovery and to enter the early stages of development. This process of drug discovery is discussed in detail in other treatises [e.g., 9,10] and is beyond the scope of this book. A variety of terms are used to define the major consecutive steps of the discovery and early development process following target identification: *hit identification, hit confirmation, hit to lead, lead identification, lead characterization, lead optimization*, and *bridging from discovery to development*. Realistically, these are not discrete stages of the discovery/early development process but should be viewed as a continuum as an NCE gradually morphs into a candidate drug. These terms are used only rarely in this book; instead, pre-FIH drug discovery implies those activities that occur, starting with lead optimization: that is, those studies that begin to define whether an NCE emerging from discovery is a realistic candidate to enter human trials.

As a general rule, pharmaceutical companies prefer to develop orally active small-molecule drugs, which can be administered conveniently to the patient, ideally once a day. However, many life-threatening diseases have not been attacked successfully by small molecules, and the evolution of biotherapeutics such as therapeutic proteins and peptides, monoclonal antibodies, oligosaccharides, and nucleic acids has revolutionized the industry. These macromolecular drugs pose specific challenges in terms of production, drug delivery, interpretation of animal toxicity studies, and administration to patients (Chapter 12).

1.2.3 Lead Optimization Strategies

To this point we have provided a brief overview of some of the early aspects of the discovery process. As stated, "discovery" and "development" can be considered a continuum; where one ends and the other begins—indeed, whether such a sharp distinction exists—varies among drug sponsors. For purposes of the discussions in subsequent chapters, the development phase is considered to begin when a decision is made to select an NCE for nonclinical development and the initial good laboratory practices (GLP) toxicity studies are planned. The chapters herein describe those discovery support activities, development programs, and support functions, starting when one or more NCEs emerge from in vitro and in vivo pharmacological testing as potentially efficacious new candidate drugs through to the recommended plan for the dosage regimen for the FIH trial.

The key challenge in drug development institutions, whether small or large organizations, is to establish a strategy whereby as many of the key properties of NCEs emerging from pharmacological testing as possible are evaluated in the most efficient and effective manner. There is, of course, no ideal drug, but some of the characteristics that can be considered important in the decision as to which of several compounds will be selected for pre-FIH development are listed in Table 1.1. This list should not be considered a boiler plate compendium, as the common thread throughout the pharmaceutical industry is that no two

TABLE 1.1 Some Optimal Characteristics Evaluated During the Discovery Phase for Orally Administered Drugs

Drug Property	Characteristic	Purpose
Potency	High target affinity	Lowest efficacious dose is desirable
Selectivity	Low affinity for related targets	Minimize side effects associated with other targets
Biology	Significant activity in a cellular assay	Demonstration of activity in a whole cell system
Chemical stability	Should be chemically stable	Pharmaceutical and bioavailability goals
Chirality	Should be a single stereoisomer if the NCE has a chiral center	Racemates should not be developed
Patent status	Free of intellectual property	Hit compound structures must be patentable
Physicochemistry	Appropriate lipophilicity	Desire druglike properties
Metabolism	High metabolic stability in vitro	Can predict relative clearance and dose frequency
Enzymology	Not a potent enzyme inhibitor or inducer	Can predict potential clinical drug–drug interactions
Bioavailability and pharmacokinetics	Oral bioavailability should be sufficiently high and dose related	Activity requires systemic exposure
Permeability	Exhibits cell membrane permeability	Drug must be absorbed and reach target
Drug transport	Not a potent inhibitor of P-glycoprotein	Transporters are barriers to drug uptake and distribution
Toxicity	Not cytotoxic (exception: some anticancer drugs) or mutagenic	Early signal of unwarranted toxicity
Safety pharmacology	Cardiac hERG channels	Major undesirable side effect for most drugs

companies would have identical strategies as to what should be included in, or excluded from, this list. For example, protein binding has not been included, as it is not considered by this author to be a key variable in the early decision-making process, although other investigators may view its importance as greater in the discovery paradigm. However, most drug sponsors would want to assure that most of these key properties have been studied prior to recommendation for pre-FIH development. In the chapters that follow, the assumption is made that the first seven properties—potency, selectivity, biology, chemical stability, chirality, patent status, and physicochemistry—have been studied appropriately such that the emerging NCEs can proceed through the gate for evaluation. Discussions are presented on the lead optimization and pre-FIH development programs principally for orally administered small-molecule drugs and systemically administered biotherapeutics, along with the regulatory expectations and various planning strategies for the critically important FIH trial.

1.3 PRE-FIH DRUG DEVELOPMENT

1.3.1 Introduction

Drug development refers to the activities undertaken after an NCE has been identified as a potential drug candidate to evaluate its suitability as a medication. In the context of this book, NCEs are considered to be compounds that emerge from the drug discovery process based on promising activity against a biological target(s) thought to be important in the target disease, and have been selected for GLP toxicity trials based on optimal lipophilicity, in vitro metabolism, nonclinical pharmacokinetics/bioavailability, and possibly preliminary safety pharmacology and/or in vitro toxicity tests. In the next few sections of this chapter we present some general perspectives of pre-FIH development and the FIH trial, most of which are covered in detail in subsequent chapters.

1.3.2 Pre-FIH Toxicology

Once an NCE has been selected as a feasible drug candidate, in vitro and in vivo studies are initiated to evaluate the drug's toxicity (Chapter 7). Acute toxicity involves harmful effects in an organism through a single or short-term administration, although its utility in the overall toxicology program may be waning. Chronic toxicity is the ability of a drug candidate to cause untoward effects after multiple administrations over an extended period of time. The goals are to identify organs targeted by the drug, effects on mammalian reproduction, and for drugs to be administered chronically, whether there are any long-term carcinogenic effects. These nonclinical safety evaluations are conducted according to strict regulatory procedures called *good laboratory practices* (GLPs) (Chapter 9). Toxicity evaluations are among the first development studies to be conducted on a candidate drug, and will continue concurrently through the course of the clinical development phases. The interpretation of toxicity findings is often different for small-molecule drugs than for biopharmaceutics; for some biologics, there are issues with "superpharmacology," wherein there is too much of a desired response being responsible for the adverse effects observed.

During the pre-FIH phase, the in vivo studies typically conducted are limited to a 2-week to 3-month duration (depending on the duration of use in humans) in a rodent and nonrodent species, whose choice is based on which is believed most closely correlated to humans. Species differences in gastrointestinal tract physiology, intrinsic enzyme activities, circulatory system, bioavailability, or metabolic profiles will render some species more appropriate than others. Also, certain classes of drugs may not be relevant in some species; for example, rodents are poor models for antibiotic drugs because the resulting alteration to their intestinal flora can cause significant adverse events that are not relevant for humans. Some species are used for similarity to specific human organ systems (e.g., swine for dermatological products, dogs for gastric studies). Species selection for pre-FIH toxicity studies should be made very carefully in light of the delays and additional expense that might occur (e.g., for new dose-ranging studies; see Chapter 7) should it be considered advisable to change the species at later stages of development.

The promising young field of toxicogenomics is emerging as a possible alternative to animal toxicology testing. These cell-based assays offer a compelling strategy for the evaluation of specific potential toxicity (e.g., the effect on gene expression in hepatocytes) with the hope that this discipline can be employed to reduce the use of whole animals. The dilemma is whether such in vitro models or toxicity biomarkers can be roughly equivalent to the classically used in vivo models and whether cell-based screens can ever replace animal testing. Perhaps toxicogenomics may best be employed at the early screening stages as a predictive toxicology tool to eliminate NCEs in the discovery phase. There is a critical need to develop and "validate" toxicogenomic high-throughput assays and other models which can at least partially replace current resource-intensive animal testing. Of course, all whole-animal models themselves have shortcomings in predicting human safety, although some modified animals, such as genetic knockouts, knock-ins, or transgenic models, can be used for specific purposes. In the meantime, it appears that the classical testing of a rodent and a nonrodent species for toxicity properties will remain the gold standard for the foreseeable future.

1.3.3 Formulation and Drug Delivery

The formulation and delivery of drugs into the human body forms an integral part of the drug discovery and development process (Chapter 5). Indeed, formulation issues can influence the design of the lead molecules and feed back into the iterative lead optimization cycle as well as nonclinical and clinical evaluations. The goals of formulating drug substances into drug products is to assure optimal stability and absorption for oral products (e.g., by enhancing absorption through their interaction with the cell membrane of the gastrointestinal tract) and solubility for systemically administered drugs. Indeed, a significant number of drug discovery and development programs center around new ways of formulating known or marketed drugs in order to improve on their pharmacokinetic profiles, thereby enhancing their safety and/or efficacy characteristics, or improving on the dose regimen (dose level or dose frequency). Components of formulation substances that are not generally regarded as safe (GRAS) become part of the nonclinical safety assessment program (i.e., they must be "qualified"). Sometimes side effects such as local irritation or allergic reactions are attributable to drug formulation rather than the active pharmaceutical ingredient (API).

One of the key logistical challenges in the initiation of pre-FIH toxicity studies is the timely availability of drug substance (or drug product, if formulation is required). It is not uncommon, upon deciding that a lead candidate is to become a candidate drug to undergo toxicity testing, for a drug sponsor to experience the frustration of delays in the synthesis and testing of sufficient amounts of drug required for the animal studies. In most instances, the synthetic route used to generate milligram (or low-gram) quantities of the drug in support of discovery and early development is not feasible for scale-up to the high-gram or possibly kilogram amounts needed for rodent and nonrodent toxicity evaluations. Accessibility of cost-effective starting material can become an issue. There is a "catch-22" element to such delays, in that resources should not be devoted to scale-up synthesis of compounds which may not become candidate drugs, yet once a decision is made to proceed to humans, it is desirable to schedule the toxicity studies as rapidly as possible with sufficient amounts of high-quality drug. It is thus important that representatives of the various disciplines that comprise the project team (Chapter 13) work closely together so as to minimize such inherent delays in the early development process.

1.3.4 Pre-FIH Drug Metabolism and Pharmacokinetics

As with the other major disciplines that comprise the nonclinical and clinical evaluations of candidate drugs [toxicity testing; CMC (chemistry, manufacturing, and controls)], evaluation of the ADME and pharmacokinetic properties of a drug candidate (Chapter 2) is a continuum beginning with support of discovery through to the NDA. This also applies to bioanalytical support of the discovery and development programs (Chapter 4) and the toxicokinetic evaluations (Chapter 8) required to demonstrate that there is a correlation between dose regimen in the toxicity studies with systemic exposure to relevant drug-derived material [parent drug and/or metabolite(s)].

As stated previously, the reason that pharmacokinetic (PK) and ADME characteristics are no longer the principal cause of attrition during drug development or of drug withdrawals postmarketing due to untoward drug–drug interactions (e.g., withdrawals of Posicor in 1998 or Hismanal in 1999) is that technologies are now being utilized during the discovery phase to weed out those NCEs that have poor such characteristics. Within the armamentarium of available rapid ADME, bioavailability, and bioanalytical testing procedures and laboratory equipment, the discovery unit must decide what to do when and with what; that is, medicinal chemists can rapidly generate numerous compounds which, with high-throughput techniques, can rapidly be evaluated for biological activity. Thus, discovery support ADME groups can become flooded with numerous NCEs and be asked to "tell us which compounds have good ADME/PK properties."

Strategic planning is critical in determining which studies should be done early and which can be deferred until later. Certainly, it is desirable to have an early assessment in vitro in human preparations of metabolic stability and cytochrome P450–mediated enzyme inhibition, as well as some indication of oral bioavailability in laboratory animals (pharmacology and/or putative toxicity species) (Table 1.1). Other possible discovery support tests are decided on a case-by-case basis; for example, although it is necessary to evaluate plasma protein binding of a drug undergoing clinical development, it is probably not necessary to have this information as part of the go/no go decision package during discovery or during pre-FIH development. Permeability and transporter assays are readily available to characterize drug uptake into, or efflux from, the target organ(s), and depending on the emerging properties of the NCEs being examined, the project team will decide if this assay is also relevant in compound selection. As most drugs undergo at least some biotransformation, a strategy is recommended regarding how much metabolism work should be conducted at this stage, as metabolites may also contribute to pharmacological activity, or with in vitro tests that do not involve metabolic activation [e.g., cardiac hERG (human ether-a-go-go related gene) channel assay; Table 1.1], a negative finding is valid for a parent drug but not for putative metabolite(s).

Once the decision is made to proceed to conduct pre-FIH toxicity studies, it is necessary to develop and fully validate the bioanalytical assay for the drug in plasma of the animal species selected (Chapter 4), to analyze the plasma samples, and to perform the toxicokinetic analyses to assess systemic exposure (Chapter 8). During this stage it is also advisable to time the validation of the bioanalytical assay for human plasma such that there will be no delay in such analyses once the FIH trial is initiated. The only regulatory ADME/PK requirements or expectations for ADME/PK in IND submissions are typically comparative in vitro data on metabolism across species (toxicity species and humans) and toxicokinetic support of the pre-FIH toxicity trials. Often, however, it is in the interest of the sponsor and for investigational review boards to have additional information that can help support predictions of safety and efficacy in initial human studies.

1.4 THE FIH TRIAL

The first administration of a drug candidate to human subjects is arguably the most exciting moment on the development path and the time that probably generates the highest anxiety, for this study represents the culmination of all the pre-FIH activities and results in the generation of initial data on the safety and possibly pharmacokinetics of the candidate drug in the target species. Up to this point, all of the information available has been based on in vitro and nonclinical pharmacology, toxicology, and ADME models, some of which may or may not be reliable indicators of human response. Also, this stage often involves change from a nonclinical champion of the NCE to a clinical champion on the development team.

It is critical that the FIH trial be designed appropriately so as to address its primary purpose: that is, to characterize the safety, tolerability, and pharmacokinetics of the NCE, including an evaluation of its maximum tolerated dose. Efficacy is rarely a primary goal of the FIH trial, as they are generally insufficiently powered to assess a relevant pharmacodynamic endpoint and the studies are typically conducted in healthy volunteers rather than in patients. However, it could be extremely useful if some biomarker of pharmacodynamic activity were available to be included in the FIH trial.

There are several challenges in the design and implementation of an FIH trial. The primary challenge is selection of the starting dose, the dose escalation strategy, and the stopping dose (Chapter 10), based generally on the totality of safety and plasma exposure data emerging from the pre-FIH toxicity studies (Chapter 7) as well as the results from the safety pharmacology studies (Chapter 6). The second challenge is to assure that all resources are available in a timely manner (e.g., sufficient appropriately tested drug product and fully validated bioanalytical assay). Thus, it is important that representatives from all the various disciplines involved in generating the relevant data—nonclinical pharmacology, toxicology, safety pharmacology, drug metabolism and pharmacokinetics, formulation development—contribute to the important decision regarding the starting dose and study design of the FIH trial.

1.5 THE REGULATORY LANDSCAPE

Drug development is different from other high-tech ventures in that it is highly regulated, although some outside the industry would argue that it is not regulated enough. There is no doubt that the tough new regulatory landscape is altering drug development strategies. It is important that the pharmaceutical industry appreciate that regulatory authorities in the United States [11], Europe [12], and elsewhere have become more demanding regarding the adequacy of benefit/risk assessments, particularly in the wake of high-profile withdrawals by the FDA of drugs such as Vioxx. Industry commentators have suggested that the increased risk aversion by regulatory agencies, resulting in larger clinical trials, is a contributor to the recent decreases in new drug approvals. On the other hand, regulatory authorities tend to argue that fewer drugs are being approved because pharma has filed fewer NDAs, due to faltering research efforts. More clarity is being sought by drug sponsors as to the regulatory tolerance for risk, which hopefully will not be a moving target given the myriad medical, scientific, political, and business interests that are interacting with government officials. Also, uncertainty exists as to how the some 200 new provisions in the FDA Amendments Act of 2007 will affect agency requirements. Although some drugs still reach the market without adequate assessment of efficacy, it is important to note that marketed drugs are rarely withdrawn due to poor quality or efficacy, and that the percentage of marketed actually drugs withdrawn due to patient risk is quite low. The latter include:

- *2007:* aprotinin (Trasylol)—increased complications or death
- *2007:* tegaserod (Xelnorm)—heart attack and stroke
- *2007:* pergolide (Permax)—risk of heart valve damage; still available outside the United States.
- *2006:* ximelagatran (Exantia)—increased hepatotoxicity
- *2005:* pemoline (Cylert)—increased hepatotoxicity
- *2004:* rofecoxib (Vioxx)—risk of myocardial infarction (the most publicized withdrawal in recent years)

Although marketing of approved therapeutics is generally targeted worldwide, our heterogeneous world results in regional differences, such as varying standards of care, population dynamics such as ethnic and metabolic features, and emerging markets (Asia-Pacific; Latin America; Eastern Europe; Middle East/Africa) with different regulatory challenges and opportunities (Chapters 14 and 15). Historically, three main regulatory bodies have dominated the global oversight of drug approvals:

1. The U.S. Food and Drug Administration (FDA)
2. The European Medicines Agency (EMEA)
3. The Japanese Ministry of Health, Labor, and Welfare (MHLW)

A gigantic step in attempts to globalize and harmonize regulatory guidelines was the establishment in 1992 of the International Conference of Harmonization of Technical Requirements for the Registration of Pharmaceuticals for Human Use (ICH), which brought together representatives from the FDA, EMEA, and MHLW, together with their industry counterparts from the U.S. Pharmaceutical Research and Manufacturers Association (PhRMA), the European Committee for Proprietary Medicinal Products (EC-CPMP/EFPIA), and the Japanese Pharmaceutical Manufacturers Association. Representatives from other countries, including Canada (Health Canada) and Australia (Therapeutic Goods Administration), also participated. The goal was to attempt to develop an international consensus on the scientific, technical, and regulatory aspects of drug development and product registration, and to make the regulatory processes more transparent with the generation of "harmonized" guidelines that would be applicable worldwide (www.fda.gov/cber/ich/ichguid.htm). These common requirements agreed upon by the major regulatory bodies have simplified at least some of the drug development processes, have reduced duplication due to regional regulatory differences, although regional guideline documents that remain still take precedent within the respective geographical areas. Regarding IND submissions, one of the major benefits that emerged from ICH is the ability to submit INDs electronically worldwide using the common technical document format (eCTD). The ICH process is a growing initiative which continues today, and the FDA, EMEA, and MHLW continue to harmonize their policies on a broad range of regulatory issues, much of which is discussed in later chapters.

In addition to the sections that describe the common technical document (CTD) (with prefix letter "M") format for submission of marketing applications to regulatory agencies (Chapter 15), the ICH guidance documents, some of which are relevant to pre-FIH development studies, are divided into three general categories:

1. *Safety*. These guidances, designated with the prefix letter "S," refer to nonclinical safety, but not clinical safety, and describe the short- and long-term toxicity studies for small-molecule drugs and biopharmaceutics. Included are genotoxicity tests, reproductive toxicology, immuntoxicity evaluations, and carcinogenicity studies. Also included in this category are support functions such as toxicokinetics, safety pharmacology (including QT-interval prolongation), and tissue distribution studies.

2. *Quality*. These documents, designated with the prefix letter "Q," fall under the general category of chemistry, manufacturing, and controls (CMC) for small-molecule drugs and biopharmaceutics. Included are stability testing procedures, validation of analytical methodologies for drug substance and impurities, dissolution testing, good manufacturing practices (GMPs), and other relevant guidances.

3. *Efficacy*. These documents, designated with the prefix letter "E," describe various aspects of efficacy as well as safety evaluations conducted in human subjects. Included are good clinical practices (GCPs), dose–response approaches, special populations (e.g., pediatrics and geriatrics), statistical principles, data management, structure and content of clinical study reports, acceptability of foreign clinical data, and other clinical support documents.

Regulatory authorities continue to issue guidances or guidelines independent of ICH. It should be noted that although a *regulation* is legally binding (such as GLP regulations, Chapter 9; GMPs; GCPs), *guidances* are technically just a recommendation and are nonbinding. As stated in the preamble to the FDA guidance Web page (www.fda.gov/CDER/GUIDANCE), "Guidance documents represent the agency's current thinking on a particular subject." However, it is wise for sponsors to consider the contents of regulatory guidances as expectations, and any planned deviations should be subject for discussions with the FDA or other relevant agencies (Chapter 14).

1.6 CONTRACT RESEARCH ORGANIZATIONS

One of the most valuable resources available for sponsors to support discovery and development programs is the wide variety of institutions known as contract research organizations (CROs). The use of such organizations is mentioned in passing in several chapters of this book. The term *CRO* originally referred to "clinical research organization," as initially, in the early 1980s, such discrete institutions were involved solely in phase III clinical trials. At that time, various government entities were outsourcing clinical testing under grants and contracts. Throughout the past three decades, CRO functions have expanded to encompass a wide array of discovery and development functions (Table 1.2), to include both nonclinical and clinical activities, and to support functions such as CMC (for contract formulation and testing) and analytical/bioanalytical assay

TABLE 1.2 Some Contract Research Organization Functions and Activities

Stage of R&D	Function	Activity
Drug discovery	Basic research	Target identification and validation
		Hit-to-lead optimization
		Lead optimization
	Chemistry	Medicinal chemistry
		Custom synthesis
	In vitro studies	Target enzyme kinetics
		Receptor binding
		ADME screens (e.g., metabolic stability, enzyme inhibition)
		Toxicity screens (e.g., Ames test)
	Bioanalytical	Partially validated assay (non-GLP)
	In vivo studies	Efficacy evaluation
		Preliminary bioavailability
Nonclinical development	CMC	Drug substance synthesis
		Preformulation design
		Formulation development
		Specification analyses (e.g., stability, impurities)
		Analytical services
	Toxicology	Pre-FIH safety in rodent and nonrodent (GLP)
	Bioanalytical	Validated assays for toxicology species (GLP)
	ADME/PK	Toxicokinetics and additional ADME
	Safety pharmacology	
Clinical development	CMC	Manufacture of GMP drug product
		Other activities similar to nonclinical
	Clinical trials	Trial design and protocol preparation
		Trial conduct and management
		Central laboratory services
		Medical writing
	Bioanalytical	Validated assay(s) for human matrices
Support services	Quality assurance	Both nonclinical and clinical development
	Regulatory	Data management (nonclinical and clinical)
		IND preparation and filing
		NDA preparation and filing

development, validation, and sample analyses. The advent of liquid chromatography-mass spectrometry (LC-MS/MS) as a sensitive and specific bioanalytical tool led to an explosion of new specialty CROs in the early 1990s. Today it is possible to outsource virtually all components of drug discovery and development. The role of the CRO is to provide complementary capabilities for a sponsor company's in-house operations. At the other end of the scale, the range of expertise of CROs can enable "virtual" companies to develop and register drug candidates with no internal resources with the exception of management personnel in collaboration with outside scientific, clinical, and regulatory consultants.

The availability of CROs enables drug research and development institutions to develop strategies that combine internal and external resources in the most efficient possible manner. This is certainly the case when considering the use of nonclinical CROs that specialize in discovery support and nonclinical development. In the ideal world, drug sponsors would conduct all studies in-house; in this manner, resources (time/staff/cost) and flexibility are under the direct control of the sponsor company. However, even big pharma companies find the need to utilize the services of CROs for those studies for which expertise is not available internally, or it is deemed more efficient to outsource. Indeed, given the growing number of available services and the attraction for high-quality scientists to become part of the CRO industry, it is often advisable to outsource to CROs even though studies could be set up and performed in-house. Such considerations are company specific.

CROs come in all shapes and sizes: from the multinational "one-stop shopping" (or so they say) organizations to smaller specialty laboratories, some of which are associated with academic institutions; there are currently some 500 CROs worldwide competing for business [13]. When a sponsor firm decides to outsource to a nonclinical CRO or contract formulator for their pre-FIH programs, many considerations must be taken into account. Although too numerous to include, some of those considerations, many of which also apply to clinical CROs, include the following:

1. *Choose the CRO carefully.* There is nothing more wasteful in the drug discovery and development business than to conduct poor quality studies which generate equivocal answers (i.e., garbage in–garbage out). This will often occur if a sponsor uses cost as the primary variable in CRO selection. Although it is important to generate competitive bids for study conduct from two or more CROs, those companies selected to submit bids should be high-quality organizations with an established positive reputation. CRO providers can be located by attending relevant scientific meetings. Sponsors should make independent inquiries about the CRO and/or to arrange for qualified personnel to visit the CRO site for a due-diligence evaluation. Some key criteria for CRO selection include, but are not limited to, the following:

- Quality of the scientific staff (especially the study director) and equipment
- Problem-solving abilities and data interpretation capabilities

- Company and staff stability (e.g., whether economics has resulted in recent staff reductions or changes that may affect their operations)
- Experience in specific study and/or therapeutic area
- Operational efficiency and flexibility
- Relations with regulatory agencies (including results of recent FDA inspections and severity of FD-483 citations, which should be requested for review)
- Record keeping (including sample-handling procedures) and documentation [including standard operating procedures (SOPs)]
- Management oversight of operations
- Quality and efficiency of quality assurance oversight of operations and review of data (if applicable)
- Quality of written documentation

If overall quality, experience, and level of service are deemed to be similar, cost and other variables, such as turnaround time, should affect the selection. When bids are received, the sponsor should assure that they understand the rationale for the cost of each line item and should request more detailed breakdown should such clarity not be readily apparent. Although this may appear to be obvious, it is important to assure that bid comparisons are made based on identical study designs and deliverables and that no hidden costs will emerge after study initiation. It should also be noted that with the globalization of larger CROs, the due-diligence results from one site may not apply to newer sites of the same company, such as in Eastern Europe, India, China, or Latin American; if outsourcing to such sites is considered because of potential cost savings, they should be treated as discrete companies which should be subject to a separate due-diligence evaluation.

2. *Review the sponsor/CRO culture.* It is important that the drug sponsor view the putative CRO as an extension of their own institution. The relationship between the two organizations must develop into a business partnership, and thus it is critical that smooth communication be established between the sponsor and the CRO. A sponsor project manager or management team (see also consideration 4 below) should be responsible for the supervision of the CRO and would interface with one or more point persons from the CRO. Such interactions should occur on several relevant occasions during performance of the study. Once a relationship has been established with initial studies, subsequent studies should run more smoothly. It should be noted that the CRO should not be asked to provide overall program leadership; this must remain the responsibility of the sponsor. Project management within the sponsor company will act in its best interests: for example, to determine whether multiple providers with specific specialists are advisable, or whether a single large CRO with multifaceted capabilities works to the sponsor's advantage.

3. *Prepare with great care.* The sponsor must recognize that CROs are for-profit businesses and that there is nothing more wasteful, stressful, or frustrating

for a CRO than dealing with an unprepared client. "High-maintenance" sponsors may be charged more for the same study than a client known to be well prepared [14]. Preparation involves proper planning by the client company regarding study goals and anticipated deliverables, including agreement on report format. Small pharma/biotech or virtual companies with minimal internal scientific expertise should not only rely on advice from CROs but should utilize an independent consultant working on behalf of the client. Proper preparation also involves assurance that the drug substance or drug product is available to the CRO on time; lack of drug availability is the principal cause for study delay and may result in increased cost due to disruption of the CRO schedule. The sponsor should also provide other appropriate information to the CRO, such as any documentation or reports (e.g., certificate of analysis, bioanalytical report for toxicokinetics) for inclusion in the final report.

4. *Monitor the studies.* With the possible exception of small or specialty studies for which the CRO has a reputation for excellence (e.g., receptor binding, in vitro metabolism; enzyme inhibition, Ames test), it is in the sponsor's interest to monitor critical aspects of the study with a well-trained sponsor representative who will be charged with auditing the conduct of the study for, where relevant, protocol, SOP, and GLP compliance as well as critical components such as the first day of animal dosing for toxicity or ADME/bioavailability studies and necropsy for toxicity studies. Reputable CROs are usually very comfortable with such a monitor, as they welcome the independent eyes of the external representative. Study monitoring also helps to solidify the partnership that should develop between the CRO and the drug sponsor.

5. *Review all documentation carefully.* It is important to critically review the contract with the CRO, and for the sponsor to understand the fee structure and the CRO's policies on study changes, delays, cancellation fees, and so on. The second document that requires very close scrutiny is the study protocol, and it is important that the sponsor spend sufficient time with the CRO regarding protocol preparation and careful review to assure that it satisfies the study goal(s) (which should be clearly stated). As all studies are protocol driven, this document determines the subsequent path moving forward. Finally, draft and final reports require careful review by experts of the various disciplines that comprise the study conduct.

1.7 CONCLUDING REMARKS ON INTRODUCTORY PERSPECTIVES

The interval from lead optimization through to initiation of the FIH trial represents the first opportunity to evaluate the potential of the NCE, selected on the basis of its initial positive pharmacological properties, to become a successful therapeutic. Those involved at this pre-FIH stage, as well as the clinical phases of drug development, are subject to numerous forces, not the least of which is the pressure for corporate profit and therefore the tendency to try to force the NCE to possess optimal safety and efficacy. This becomes a balancing act, because independent of such factors as resources (time/cost/staff), internal champions, corporate strategies, and portfolio management goals, the NCE must be viewed as the boss of the exercise. This is very tricky, since there is no such thing as a perfectly efficacious and safe drug. Also, an NDA that has been submitted may be approvable, but will the resulting marketed drug really be a valuable addition to the therapeutic armamentarium and thereby generate sufficient profits for the drug sponsor? All studies must be designed carefully and the results interpreted dispassionately such that appropriate decisions can be made as to whether development should continue. One of the most difficult tasks within any size of a drug development organization is to make the difficult decision to terminate development of what had seemed to that stage to be a promising candidate drug. However, there is nothing more wasteful than to continue to push for a drug candidate to elicit therapeutic properties that it does not possess. It is thus incumbent upon all disciplines, certainly at the pre-FIH stage when several go/no-go decisions should be in place, to work together and determine unemotionally the true risk/benefit potential for the specific target disease and patient population.

REFERENCES

1. DiMasi JA, Hansen RW, Grabowski HG. The price of innovation: new estimates of drug development costs. *J Health Econ*. 2003;151–185.
2. Kola I, Landis J. Can the pharmaceutical industry reduce attrition rates? *Nat Rev Drug Discov*. 2004;3:711–715.
3. Vallance P, Levick M. Drug discovery and development in the age of molecular medicine. *Clin Pharmacol Ther*. 2007;82:363–366.
4. Leeson PD, Springhorpe B. The influence of drug-like concepts on decision-making in medicinal chemistry. *Nat Rev, Drug Discov*. 2007;6:881–890.
5. Lipinski CA, Lombardo F, Dominy BW, Feeney PJ. Experimental and computational approaches to estimate solubility and permeability in drug discovery and development settings. *Adv Drug Deliv Rev*. 1997;23:3–25.
6. Lipinski CA. Lead- and drug-like compounds: the rule-of-five revolution. *Drug Disc Today Technol*. 2004;1:337–341.
7. Keseru GM, Makara GM. The influence of lead discovery strategies on the properties of drug candidates. *Nat Rev Drug Discov*. 2009;8:203–212.
8. Thomas G. *Medicinal Chemistry: An Introduction*. Hoboken, NJ: Wiley; 2008.
9. Chorghade MS. *Drug Discovery and Development*, Vol. 1, *Drug Discovery*. Hoboken, NJ: Wiley; 2006.
10. Gad SC. *Drug Discovery Handbook*. Hoboken, NJ: Wiley; 2005.
11. Guidance for Industry: Development and Use of Risk Minimization Action Plans. U.S. Department of Health and Human Services, Food and Drug Administration; 2005.

12. Guideline on Risk Management Systems for Medicinal Products for Human Use. European Medicines Agency, Committee for Medicinal Products for Human Use; Nov. 2005.
13. Snyder S. Business smarts. *Contract Pharma*. Mar. 2009;36–38. Available at: www.contractpharma.com.
14. Hoang T. *Contract Research Helps Keep Drug Pipelines Flowing*. Sector Focus Report. Berwyn, PA: Turner Capital Investment; July 2008. Available at: www.turnerinvestments.com/index.cfm/fuseaction/commentary.detail/ID/2661/CSID/387/.

PART II

LEAD OPTIMIZATION STRATEGIES

2

ADME STRATEGIES IN LEAD OPTIMIZATION

Amin A. Nomeir

2.1 INTRODUCTION

Drug discovery is a highly complex, dynamic, and evolving process; it requires highly skilled and trained people of many scientific disciplines who not only must master the relevant science but must also be able to work together as a team. A successful drug discovery program requires continuous, effective, and timely communication, participation, and interactions among team members.

In the simplistic approach, drug discovery involves all research activities that are carried out to identify and characterize a new chemical entity (NCE) that is deemed suitable for development as a therapeutic agent. This includes creation of a working hypothesis for a target receptor or enzyme for the target disease, then developing and setting up in vitro and in vivo models to screen the new NCEs for biological activity [1]. For small molecules, this involves evaluation of a large number of compounds in various in vitro and in vivo assays to recommend a candidate for development. Drug development includes research and other activities that are carried out to evaluate the safety of the recommended NCE in laboratory animals, and its safety and efficacy in humans. The results of these studies are submitted to regulatory agencies as the basis for approval and marketing of the new drug candidate. The stages of modern drug discovery that most pharmaceutical companies follow include target identification and characterization, hit finding, lead identification, lead optimization, and lead characterization [2]. However, many successful drugs have been discovered outside this traditional path.

Early Drug Development: Strategies and Routes to First-in-Human Trials, Edited by Mitchell N. Cayen

With the pressure on pharmaceutical companies to develop safe and effective drugs with optimal resources (cost; staff; time), it becomes critical to reduce the attrition rate, since the cost of failure becomes astronomical as the compound advances through the sequential stages of drug development (Chapter 1). The cost estimate for discovering and developing a new drug was $900 million in 2004 [3] and is increasing; and any efforts that could lead to a candidate with a better chance of success in development are welcome. Therefore, it is advisable to evaluate the NCE thoroughly in the discovery stage to select those with the best chance of success. It would be ideal to eliminate undesirable compounds as early as possible in the discovery process; however, compound discontinuation, even in the last stage of discovery, should not be considered a failure, as it saves downstream resources and would probably lead to a better candidate. Furthermore, it is faster and more cost-effective to resolve putative problems with the NCEs during the discovery stage than during development.

NCEs are evaluated for potency, efficacy, safety, pharmaceutical properties, drug metabolism [absorption, distribution, metabolism, and excretion (ADME)] and pharmacokinetic attributes. It is highly unlikely for a compound to possess ideal profiles in all properties; therefore, compounds with the best overall characteristics, without major deficiencies, are selected for development [4]. ADME properties are usually evaluated in lead optimization; however, during the hit-to-lead stage, ADME attributes could be helpful in the selection of a chemical class over another or in prioritizing several chemical scaffolds. ADME characteristics considered for evaluation by drug sponsors generally include potential for oral absorption (for orally intended NCEs), metabolism, pharmacokinetics, potential drug–drug interactions, brain penetration, protein binding, and isozyme profiling. Many small or virtual companies do not possess the capabilities to perform such screens, as resources devoted for ADME evaluation are limited and vary depending on the size of the company. These small companies are more concerned with the evaluation and validation of their novel discovery targets and developing the necessary assays for screening and counter screening. Depending on the corporate goals, ADME evaluation in these companies may be outsourced to contract research organizations (CROs) (Chapter 1), and may be performed at a later development stage or after landing a joint venture agreement with a big pharma company [5]. However, it is important to appreciate that, independent of the size of a sponsor company, the discovery and development paradigm must be planned in the most efficient manner, and this includes an assessment of the relevant ADME properties that enable appropriate go/no go decisions to be made.

The desirable ADME attributes vary considerably based on the disease target, the route and frequency of administration, pharmacokinetic–pharmacodynamic (PK-PD) relationships, and the competitive landscape. These variables make it impossible to devise one general strategy for ADME screening for all drug discovery programs (i.e., there is no "one size fits all"). In general, the NCE must be able to reach the pharmacological target and maintain sufficient concentrations at the target site for the duration required to solicit the desired response. Desirable ADME and pharmacokinetic properties include those that fulfill the goal noted above in addition to minimal or no potential for undesirable drug–drug interactions in humans, elimination by several metabolic and/or excretion pathways, minimal biotransformation by a polymorphic enzyme, low intersubject variability, and linear pharmacokinetics.

In the 1990s, approximately 40 to 50% of drug candidates' failure in development was attributed to unacceptable ADME and pharmacokinetic properties [6]. This high failure rate has been reduced dramatically in recent years, accounting for only 10% of failures in the year 2000. This considerable improvement was driven primarily by the allocation of appropriate resources, particularly in big pharma, for early evaluation of critical ADME and pharmacokinetic properties of NCEs. Concurrent with the emergence of numerous technological advances, innovative ADME testing has been incorporated into early NCE evaluation. The overriding principle of these assays is to screen out compounds with undesirable ADME and pharmacokinetic characteristics early, quickly, and cheaply, focusing resources on promising NCEs that pass the initial screening assays.

With the recent advances in synthetic chemistry, genomics, molecular biology, structural chemistry, and robotics, the number of new therapeutic targets and therefore NCEs has been increasing dramatically in big pharma, consequently increasing the number of NCEs requiring ADME evaluation. Major pharmaceutical companies have been challenged to develop focused strategies and resources designed to test numerous available NCEs in the most efficient manner possible. In vitro higher-throughput screens and counter screens designed to evaluate ADME attributes have been incorporated into drug discovery in addition to devising new approaches to increase the efficiency, speed, and capacity of traditional pharmacokinetic evaluations. Because of its speed, sensitivity, versatility, and specificity, liquid chromatography coupled with tandem mass spectrometry (LC-MS/MS) has become the bioanalytical tool of choice (Chapter 4), not only for in vitro screening assays but also for the analysis of biological samples from in vivo pharmacokinetic studies. The in vitro models are easier to use, faster, and require small amounts of compound, resulting in dramatically accelerating the lead identification and characterization processes, allowing the timely assessment of ADME properties of NCEs.

As mentioned above, smaller pharma or startup biotech and virtual pharmaceutical companies do not possess the resources for full ADME and pharmacokinetic evaluation of their candidates. Again depending on the target disease, limited ADME and PK evaluation could be carried out in small pharma. For example, for a novel target first in class of a previously untreatable life-threatening disease (often how small and virtual pharma starts), with the drug candidate aimed at monotherapy, potential clinical drug–drug interactions may not be a major concern, and thus the company should focus on performing those ADME and pharmacokinetic studies that would facilitate the initiation of safety studies in animals to help move quickly into phase 1 studies in humans. This would include primarily pharmacokinetic studies in animals designed to show sufficient bioavailability and dose-related plasma drug concentrations. However, with a shortcut strategy there is always some level of risk. Alternatively, small pharmaceutical companies usually have a limited number of NCEs that can be fully evaluated for ADME and pharmacokinetic properties at CROs in a relatively more cost-effective (compared to setting up and validating ADME screens) and timely manner, allowing them to choose the candidate with the best overall profile.

When implementing these higher-throughput assays into a decision tree in big pharma's screening strategy, it is important to understand the relevance, precision, accuracy, and shortcomings of each assay. Also, setting up a sequence of ADME screens in a decision tree must be done on an evolving principle, allowing changes whenever warranted to maximize the benefits and shorten the lead optimization time. It is also crucial to understand how the results of higher-throughput data should be incorporated into the program-specific acceptance or rejection criteria. To optimize limited resources, strategies should be prepared prior to generating such data as to how the results will be used in the decision-making process.

In this chapter we present several higher-throughput ADME and pharmacokinetic screening assays that are performed primarily in lead optimization of small-molecule NCEs (nonbiologics). ADME and pharmacokinetic evaluations of biologics (e.g., proteins, monoclonal antibodies), although limited compared to small molecules, are discussed whenever warranted. The role of in silico ADME screening and the promise of metabolomics in drug discovery are discussed briefly. The methodologies in these assays are also presented.

It should be emphasized that various ADME screens described herein are carried out during lead optimization and are designed as high-throughput assays to screen a large number of NCEs as quickly as possible in order to select the best compound for development. The accuracy of these assays is sufficient for making go/no go decisions regarding the selection of NCE, but is not designed for regulatory submission. Therefore, the results of these screening assays are not intended to be investigational new drug (IND)-enabling studies and are not carried out under the guidelines of good laboratory practices (GLPs). Also, the majority of the data obtained from these assays are not required before phase I first-in-human (FIH) studies. However, the screening data could be submitted to regulatory agencies as part of the preliminary characterization of the potential drug, along with subsequent results obtained once the compound has been selected for development.

2.2 ABSORPTION

As oral drug delivery is the most common route of drug administration for systemically active drugs, the objective of most discovery programs is to select NCEs with a good potential for oral absorption in humans. It is obvious that for NCEs targeted for parenteral administration, evaluation for potential oral absorption is not warranted, but other ADME screens would be more relevant. The two important factors that are crucial for drug absorption from the gastrointestinal tract are solubility (and dissolution rate) and permeability across the enterocytes, as an NCE must be in solution in order to be absorbed. Therefore, determination of the aqueous solubility of the NCE is important in order to assess the potential for oral absorption. Several high-throughput methods of determining the aqueous solubility of NCEs which are usually carried out by chemistry or pharmaceutical sciences departments have been reported [7].

In the past two decades considerable attention has been focused on oral absorption from a mechanistic standpoint [8–11]. This has led to the development of various models for the prediction of oral absorption. In vivo animal models are the most reliable methods of evaluating oral pharmacokinetics that include absorption; this approach is preferred if a limited number of NCEs is being studied, as the case would be with small pharma, biotech, or virtual companies. However, in vivo pharmacokinetic evaluation of a large number of NCEs (as would be with big pharma) is costly, time consuming, and requires relatively large amounts of compounds and large number of animals. Also, animal models provide the net pharmacokinetic outcome of all processes that encompass absorption, distribution, metabolism, and excretion. As a result, it would be difficult to ascertain if the problem with the pharmacokinetics of an NCE is due to oral absorption and/or other factors. Utilizing physicochemical properties such as log P, pK_a, and molecular weight could provide a general idea regarding the transcellular passive diffusion mode of absorption and is useful as an initial screen in the design of chemical libraries [12], as discussed later. However, other modes of absorption, including transporter-mediated absorption, would be difficult to determine based on physicochemical properties alone [13]. Thus, in vitro models that can assess the potential for oral absorption of NCEs have become a major component of lead optimization in major pharmaceutical companies [14,15]. Several in vitro models, such as parallel artificial membrane permeation assay, and the Madin–Darby canine kidney and human colon adenocarcinoma (Caco-2) cell lines, have been in use to assess the potential for oral absorption, of which the Caco-2 monolayer has been the most utilized model [16]. When grown in culture as monolayers, Caco-2 exhibits properties resembling those of the intestinal enterocytes, such as the formation of microvilli, tight junctions, and P-glycoprotein (P-gp) and other transporter expression [17,18]. Several studies have shown a good correlation between oral drug absorption in humans and Caco-2 permeability [19,20]; therefore, it has generally been accepted that compounds with good permeability across the Caco-2 monolayer would have good potential for intestinal absorption in humans unless solubility and/or dissolution rate are limiting factors.

Drugs and other xenobiotics are absorbed from the gastrointestinal tract via four major pathways [15,18]. The majority of drugs are absorbed via transcellular passive diffusion across a single cell layer, the enterocytes, and the absorption is driven by the concentration gradient. Lipophilic compounds partition into the cell membrane and thereby cross the enterocytes. The compound must possess some degree of solubility in the intestinal lumen and lipophilicity in order to partition into the lipid membrane, as well as some degree of aqueous solubility to cross the enterocytes into the bloodstream. Small-molecular-weight hydrophilic compounds may be absorbed via the paracellular route by passing through cell–cell tight junctions. Since the junctions represent a small surface area compared to the enterocytes, this mode of transport is usually slow and is primarily for water-soluble compounds with molecular weights of 200 Da or less [21]. Molecular shape may be a factor in the molecular weight cutoff for the paracellular mode of absorption. Compounds could also be absorbed by facilitated diffusion via a transmembrane transporter without requiring energy (driven by concentration gradient) or by active transport with the expenditure of energy, which could proceed against the concentration gradient. Because a reversible drug–carrier complex is formed with the latter two modes of transport, these processes could be fairly selective. Also, since the number of a specific transporter is limited, the transport process is saturable either by the compound itself at higher concentrations or by other compounds that are substrates to the same transporter. It is worth mentioning that a compound is probably absorbed by means of one or more modes of transport at varying degrees.

It must be recognized that oral absorption is a highly complex process and that any factor that affects solubility and/or permeability of the compound will probably alter the extent of oral absorption. For example, a compound could be highly permeable, but because of low solubility and/or a low dissolution rate in the intestinal lumen, the extent of absorption would be low. A good example that is often encountered in late-stage drug discovery/early development is that an NCE is well absorbed when administered as an amorphous suspension (in early discovery), whereas it shows poor absorption when administered as a suspension of the crystalline form (late discovery/early development). The primary reason for this discrepancy is the limited dissolution rate of the crystalline form. Consequently, it may be important to assess as early as possible whether a potential drug candidate, which is well absorbed in its amorphous form, also exhibits good absorption in an acceptable pharmaceutical form (crystalline), and to base decisions on further development accordingly.

Another important aspect of oral absorption is the fact that the compound encounters different environments when moving down the gastrointestinal tract: a highly acidic pH in the stomach, a slightly acidic to neutral pH in the small intestine, and a neutral to slightly basic pH in the large intestine. Such dramatic changes in pH would affect solubility, ionization, and permeability of acidic and basic compounds. For example, a basic compound may be dissolved in the highly acidic environment of the stomach, and as it moves down through the less acidic environment of the small intestine, the compound could precipitate out, which may limit the extent of its absorption. On the other hand, a crystalline basic compound could be dissolved in the stomach acid and precipitate out in the small intestine as amorphous, which has a relatively higher dissolution rate, resulting in the enhancement of oral absorption.

2.2.1 Permeability

As indicated earlier, the Caco-2 monolayer is the most utilized in vitro model to screen NCEs for potential oral absorption, and its predictability to human absorption is discussed in Chapter 3. Robotic systems for growth and maintenance of Caco-2 monolayer, available from several vendors, eliminate the tedious manual labor involved in cell growth and maintenance and allow for an uninterrupted supply of monolayers. The monolayers are generally used after three weeks (or shorter under specific conditions) of growth in transwells, which are sufficient to form a differentiated polarized monolayer. A typical study design for the evaluation of permeability of NCEs in Caco-2 cells is shown in Table 2.1.

It must be recognized that the P_{app} can vary considerably depending on the experimental conditions. Therefore, when the Caco-2 assay is set up initially, it is highly advisable to evaluate the permeability of 20 to 30 known drugs with a wide range of the extent of absorption in order to develop a relationship between permeability and the extent of absorption under the specific laboratory conditions. This relationship should be used to classify the NCE in terms of permeability (low, moderate, or high). Also, it is always advisable to run control drugs with a known extent of human absorption, with each experiment as a quality control for each run.

Several limitations need be recognized when interpreting the Caco-2 data. The first is that the NCE concentrations in the gastrointestinal tract are not known nonclinically; therefore, the permeability determination at the preset screening conditions may be different than those encountered in humans, particularly in the presence of various solubilizing factors in the intestine, such as bile and other gastrointestinal fluids. Second, if a transporter is involved in absorption, Caco-2 may not be a good model for absorption, as the transporter may not be expressed in Caco-2. Third, for low-molecular-weight hydrophilic compounds, Caco-2 may underestimate the permeability, as it has been well documented that Caco-2 (21 to 25 days) has tighter junctions than those of the human intestine. Fourth, if the solubility and/or dissolution rate of the compound in the gastrointestinal fluid is low, the extent of absorption could be low even if it showed high permeability in Caco-2, as the compound must be in solution in order to partition into the membrane of the enterocytes. Nevertheless, Caco-2 is considered a good model for screening NCEs for potential oral absorption in lead optimization.

In the Caco-2 assay the NCE is best analyzed by liquid chromatography (LC)–mass spectrometry (MS)/MS; therefore, the assay is compound specific. Recent advances in mass spectrometry and robotics have largely enabled the automation of method development and sample analysis (Chapter 4). Paradoxically, with the automation of Caco-2 cell culture maintenance and experimental systems, the challenge to increasing throughput has become the analytical support. Several approaches have been successful in increasing the analytical capacity, such as using LC-MS/MS with the multiplexed inlet system (MUX), which allows for four data acquisitions simultaneously, where both method development and sample analysis time/NCE have been greatly reduced [23]. With this system, generic LC-MS/MS systems suitable for the analysis of the majority of NCEs received from various discovery programs have been developed [23].

To cite an example of the process, the Caco-2 permeability screening assay has been set up in our laboratory to be a one-week cycle [25]. The cycle starts on Tuesday, when methanolic or dimethyl sulfoxide (DMSO) solutions of NCEs

TABLE 2.1 Drug Absorption In Vitro: A Typical Study Design for Caco-2 Monolayer Permeability in Lead Optimization

Study Parameter	Specifications
Culture system	Caco-2 monolayers grown in culture for 21–25 days are used. The monolayers are preincubated at 37°C for 30 min in a CO_2 incubator with transport media (TM) prior to the initiation of the transport experiment.
TM for donor (apical) compartment	HBSS buffer with 4-morpholineethanesulfonic acid and D-glucose at pH 6.5.
TM for receiver (basolateral) compartment	HBSS buffer with HEPES, D-glucose at pH 7.4 with 4% bovine serum albumin (BSA) added to the TM to reduce nonspecific binding for lipophilic compounds, and to create "sinklike" conditions [22].
Monolayer integrity assessment	Transepithelial electrical resistance is measured before and after the transport experiment.
NCE concentrations	Usually, one concentration of 10 μM because of the limited solubility of the majority of discovery compounds. Higher concentrations are preferred if solubility allows.
Experimental procedure	A high (metoprolol or propranolol) and a low (mannitol) permeability marker are included with each run, in addition to the NCEs. The compounds are added to the apical side at 0 h in DMSO or methanol (not to exceed 1% by volume) and then incubated at 37°C in a CO_2 incubator for 2 h. Each compound is run in duplicate.
Sample analysis	Compound concentrations are determined in the apical (donor) side at 0 h (immediately after compound addition) and in both the apical and basolateral (receiver) sides at 120 min by LC-MS/MS after the addition of an internal standard in acetonitrile (3:1 dilution) followed by centrifugation using a 96-well plate format. The relative concentrations between the basolateral and apical samples (C_{R120}/C_{D0}; see below) could be calculated based on the peak area ratio between the analyte and the internal standard, possibly resulting in the elimination of calibration standard samples that use one-third of the total analysis time. This approach has been validated [23]. The linearity of response between the basolateral and apical samples is ensured by diluting the donor samples (D_0 and D_{120}, see below) with transport medium to concentrations that fall within approximately one order of magnitude of the C_{R120} samples.

TABLE 2.1 (*Continued*)

Study Parameter	Specifications
Calculations and results	The results of the transport experiment are expressed as the apparent permeability coefficient (P_{app}) in nm/s, which is calculated for each compound as follows: $P_{app} = (C_{R120}/C_{D0})V_R/(120SA)$ The total recovery is calculated as follows: $R = (C_{R120}V_R + C_{D120}V_D)/(C_{D0}V_D)$ where C_{R120} is the concentration of the NCE in the receiver side at the end of the study (120 min), C_{D0} is the concentration of the NCE in the donor side at the beginning of the study (0 time), V_R is the volume of the receiver side of the transwell, SA is the Caco-2 membrane surface area [24], and V_D is the volume of the donor side.
Statistics	If the difference in permeability between duplicates is $\geq$ twofold, the compound is flagged to be repeated.
Data interpretation	If the total recovery is $\geq$50%, the NCE is classified as having low, moderate, or high permeability, depending on the relationship between absorption and permeability developed under laboratory conditions (Table 2.2). If the recovery is <50%, the NCE is still classified based on permeability, although it may be underestimated.

are provided in 96-well plates. Automated method development efforts are initiated overnight on the day of compound receipt using a generic LC-MS/MS with the MUX system. On Wednesday morning, compounds that could not be analyzed with the generic analytical system (usually, 5 to 15%) are transferred to a second LC-MS/MS system for additional method development efforts. On the same day, sample lists are generated for both instruments. On Wednesday, the Caco-2 transport experiment is carried out and the samples are delivered in 96-well plates. Sample analysis is complete by Friday and the data are evaluated for errors and submitted electronically. On Monday the data are processed and the Caco-2 permeability reports are issued to individual discovery teams or deposited into a central database. Also, the instruments are subjected to preventive maintenance to be ready for the next cycle. With this arrangement, approximately 60 compounds could be evaluated weekly with a one-week turnaround time [25].

2.2.2 Efflux Transport

During the process of drug absorption from the intestinal lumen, efflux transporters such as P-gp, which is located in the apical membrane of the enterocytes, could expel certain drugs back into the intestinal lumen after they partition into the cell membrane [26]. These efflux transporters could hinder absorption and may influence the overall disposition of an NCE. It is noteworthy that P-gp and other transporters are also expressed in many other tissues, including brain, liver, and kidneys, and therefore could have a major impact on tissue uptake such as brain penetration. However, if a transporter is involved, the transport process is saturable. Therefore, for drugs that are highly soluble in the intestinal lumen and are administered at a relatively high oral dose, their oral absorption would be unlikely to be hindered by P-gp and other efflux transporters, as the concentrations in the intestinal lumen would be high and therefore saturate the efflux transporter. On the other hand, P-gp efflux could hinder the absorption of drugs that are highly insoluble and/or administered at a relatively low oral dose if they are substrates to efflux transporters [27,28]. For uptake to brain and other tissues, saturation is unlikely, as the concentrations in plasma are usually much lower than those in the intestinal lumen [29,30].

Evaluation of NCEs as efflux substrates is not a typical screen in drug discovery. This is a relatively more resource-intensive assay with a lower throughput compared to the permeability screen and is usually carried out only on "as needed" basis. For example, if a chemical series showed poor oral absorption and/or low brain uptake (for central nervous system drugs), and the reason is delineated to be efflux transporter-related, the assay could be used as one of the screens to select compounds prior to evaluation in animal models.

It has been well documented that Caco-2 monolayers express P-gp as well as other transporters in the apical side [28]. A bidirectional transport experiment using Caco-2 monolayers is usually carried out to determine if an NCE is a substrate for an efflux transporter (primarily, P-gp) in lead optimization. An example of a study design to evaluate an NCE as an efflux substrate (primarily, P-gp) in Caco-2 cells is outlined in Table 2.2.

The role of efflux transporters in limiting the permeability of a drug candidate could be further delineated by using specific inhibitors. If a compound is a substrate for the efflux system, the apparent A-to-B (apical-to-basolateral) permeability would be enhanced by an inhibitor of the transporter. It is obvious that if a discovery program determined that P-gp interaction screening is needed for a chemical series, Caco-2 permeability screening would not be necessary, as the bidirectional experiment will generate the permeability from the apical to basolateral side, which is the product of the permeability screen.

2.3 DISTRIBUTION

2.3.1 Plasma Protein Binding

Although it has generally been believed that the free (unbound) fraction of a drug is responsible for pharmacological activity, toxicity, and tissue distribution [31–33], plasma protein binding per se is rarely used for a go/no

TABLE 2.2 Drug Absorption: Assessment of the Efflux Substrate Potential (Probably P-Glycoprotein) in Lead Optimization

Study Parameter	Specifications
Bidirectional permeability assessment	Two transport experiments are conducted; one for the apical-to-basolateral (A to B) direction and the other for the basolateral-to-apical (B to A) direction. Caco-2 monolayers grown in culture for 21–25 days are used.
Preincubation	Prior to the transport experiment, Caco-2 monolayers are incubated at 37°C for 30 min in a CO_2 incubator with transport media (TM).
TM for donor compartment	HBSS buffer with HEPES and D-glucose at pH 7.4.
TM for receiver compartment	HBSS buffer with HEPES and D-glucose at pH 7.4, with 4% BSA to reduce nonspecific binding for lipophilic compounds and to create "sinklike" conditions [22].
Monolayer integrity assessment	Transepithelial electrical resistance is determined before and after the transport experiment.
NCE concentrations	One concentration of 5 μM is used because it is more in line with expected NCE plasma concentrations.
Experimental procedure	A positive-control P-gp substrate (digoxin) and a negative-control non-P-gp substrate (metoprolol or probenecid) are included with each run in addition to NCEs. The compounds are added to the donor side at 0 h in DMSO or methanol (not to exceed 1 vol%) and then incubated at 37°C in a CO_2 incubator for 2 h. Each compound is run in duplicate.
Sample analysis	The NCE concentrations are determined in the donor side at 0 h (immediately after compound addition) and in both the donor and receiver sides at 120 min by LC-MS/MS after the addition of internal standard in acetonitrile (3 : 1 dilution) followed by centrifugation using 96-well plates.
Calculations	Results of the transport experiments are expressed as an apparent permeability coefficient (P_{app}), calculated for both the A-to-B and B-to-A directions as indicated in Table 2.1. The total recovery of each compound is also calculated for each direction.
Statistics	If the difference in permeability between duplicates is ≥ twofold for either direction, the compound is flagged to be repeated.
Data interpretation	If the total recovery for both directions is similar and ≥50%, the permeability ratio (B to A/A to B) is calculated for each NCE and standard compound. The ratio for metoprolol or probenecid should be <2, while for digoxin it should be ≫2 (usually 10–25). If the ratio for the NCE is ≥2, the compound is considered to be an efflux substrate (usually, P-gp). If the ratio is <2, the compound is considered not to be a substrate for an efflux transporter. If the positive and negative controls did not show the expected ratios or if the recovery is low and/or highly different in both directions, no conclusion is made as to whether the compound is a P-gp substrate.

go decision with regard to advancing an NCE. Furthermore, the notion that clinically relevant drug–drug interactions could result from protein-binding displacement by coadministered drugs appears to be exaggerated [34,35]. Nevertheless, it has been well recognized that plasma protein binding is relevant in pharmacokinetic (PK) modeling, such as extrapolation from laboratory animals to humans and in developing in vitro–in vivo correlations. Consequently, determination of plasma protein binding could be important in understanding the pharmacokinetics as well as the PK-pharmacodynamic (PD) relationship of NCEs. Also, species differences in plasma protein binding could affect animal and human exposure multiple calculations in nonclinical safety evaluation studies [36]. In lead optimization, protein binding is not used for screening NCEs; rather, it is used to address certain issues in discovery, such as weak or lack of in vivo pharmacological activity despite high in vitro potency against the target. Also, determination of human plasma protein binding is important in the risk assessment of a hERG (human ether-a-go-go related gene) signal, by determination of the ratio of the IC_{50} of the hERG signal relative to free concentration at the projected human plasma concentration [37,38].

Two major procedures have generally been used for the determination of plasma protein binding (i.e., ultrafiltration and equilibrium dialysis), although other methods, such as ultracentrifugation, have been reported [39]. These two assays produce comparable data for most compounds; however, each has advantages and limitations. One of the major advantages of equilibrium dialysis is that it is not greatly affected by nonspecific binding; therefore, it is more suitable for use with NCEs in the discovery stage, where nonspecific binding potential is unknown. Equilibrium dialysis is not suitable for NCEs that are unstable in plasma because of the long equilibrium time of the current systems (ca. 20 hours), although newer systems with shorter equilibrium times have recently been reported, but still under evaluation in many laboratories. In these cases, ultrafiltration would be a better substitute, but nonspecific binding could greatly distort the outcome; therefore, mass balance must be determined at the end of the experiment. In the drug discovery setting, the great majority of protein-binding studies are carried out by equilibrium dialysis. An example of a study design for the determination of protein binding of NCEs using equilibrium dialysis is outlined in Table 2.3.

The designation of a drug as being “highly,” “moderately,” or “poorly” protein bound is very often a matter of compound-specific interpretation. In addition to utilizing the data for potential extrapolation from animal species to humans, as described above, the ultimate goal is to evaluate the potential for protein binding–mediated clinical drug–drug interactions. Unless the drug has a narrow therapeutic index and is very highly protein bound (e.g., warfarin), it is rare that the pharmacokinetic changes of protein-binding interactions have clinical relevance [35]. Because of the high competition and regulatory expectations, most drugs approved today have high therapeutic indices, at least for non-life-threatening indications. Indeed, a drug that is, for example, 95% protein bound may seem to be designated as “high,” but from a clinical perspective, such binding

TABLE 2.3 Plasma Protein Binding: Typical Study Design Using Equilibrium Dialysis in Lead Optimization

Study Parameter	Description
Species	Usually the pharmacology species, toxicity species and human.
NCE concentrations	One concentration of 10 μM run in duplicate.
Experimental procedure	A 96-well [40,41] equilibrium dialysis device (Harvard Apparatus, Holliston, MA) is used. Each well consists of top and bottom chambers separated by a semipermeable membrane with a molecular weight cutoff of 5000 Da. A volume of 200 μL of plasma containing the NCE is placed into the top chamber (plasma side) followed by the addition of an equal volume of phosphate buffer saline (PBS), pH 7.5, into the bottom chamber (buffer side or dialysate side). The dialysis device is kept for about 20 h at 37°C in a revolving CO_2 incubator.
Sample analysis	A volume of 20 μL from the plasma side and 100 μL from the buffer side is placed into an analytical sampling plate; 100 μL of PBS and 20 μL of blank plasma are added to plasma and buffer samples, respectively, to make the analytical matrix uniform. Samples are then mixed with 2 volumes of acetonitrile containing an analytical internal standard, vortexed, centrifuged, and analyzed by LC-MS/MS.
Calculations	The percentage of plasma protein binding is calculated as $= 100(C_{pl} - C_{bu})/C_{pl}$, where C_{pl} and C_{bu} are the NCE concentrations in plasma and buffer chambers, respectively.

typically may not result in any pharmacokinetic interaction. As more clinical data emerge on the true role (or lack thereof) of protein binding in a clinical setting, many investigators would not call a drug "highly" protein bound unless the extent exceeds 98%.

Although protein-binding assessment per se is not an expectation nor a pre-FIH regulatory requirement, a sponsor may decide on a case-by-case basis that such data are prudent to generate prior to FIH. A good example is that non-clinical cardiovascular safety studies in animals are usually submitted with the IND and extrapolation of the findings (if any) from animals to humans requires consideration of the free fraction in plasma of both species. For compounds that have progressed beyond FIH (usually, during phase II), protein-binding studies are conducted by a more rigorous procedure. At this stage it is carried out in humans and the pharmacology and toxicology species using both genders (can be combined) of the same strains. The experiments are performed at several concentrations encompassing those observed in the safety evaluation studies and those determined in humans. The studies are usually performed with more replicates than done in discovery [3,4].

2.3.2 Brain Uptake

NCEs targeted for the central nervous system (CNS) must be able to reach the target organ in order to exert their pharmacological effect. On the other hand, extensive CNS uptake of non-CNS-targeted NCEs could result in adverse drug reactions. The uptake of endobiotics and xenobiotics into the CNS is controlled by the blood–brain barrier (BBB), a highly regulated membranous barrier of brain capillaries resulting from complex tight junctions formed by the microvessel endothelial cells. Although the endothelial cells of brain capillaries are clearly the principal cellular element of the BBB, the formation and regulation of intact BBB structure appear to require interactions of the endothelial cells with other cellular components, such as astrocytes and pericytes [42]. These endothelial cells also contain an array of metabolic enzymes and express efflux and uptake transporters, such as P-gp in the lumen side, constituting a biochemical barrier to a significant proportion of xenobiotics [43,44]. The combination of physical and biochemical barriers segregates the CNS from systemic blood circulation, resulting in tight control of the exchange of substances between blood and CNS to maintain a delicate homeostasis of the CNS environment [42]. It has been estimated that the BBB limits the brain uptake of more than 98% of potential neurotherapeutic agents [45].

Physicochemical parameters, which may include the lipophilicity (log D), van der Waals surface area of basic atoms, polar surface area, and others, have been shown to affect drug delivery across the BBB [46,47]. These in silico screens (discussed in Section 2.8) could be used as an initial evaluation of virtual compounds if a sufficient database exists. However, due to the presence of various uptake and efflux transporters, permeability of NCEs across the BBB may not be predicted accurately from physicochemical calculations alone.

Traditional methods for the evaluation of brain uptake of an NCE or a small number of NCEs have been carried out by determination of the compound concentrations in brain and plasma of laboratory animals, typically rats and mice. This is well suited for smaller pharmaceutical companies, as pharmacokinetics in rodents are usually the first in vivo ADME assays to be acquired. Also, mice and rats are often used as the animal models of efficacy, so no additional animal resources are needed. However, for screening a large number of compounds, in vitro models provide an initial evaluation in a resource-efficient manner. These models include primary cultures of microvessel endothelial cells from various animal species, including bovine, porcine, and rodent, and also from humans, which are cultured alone or co-cultured with astrocytes to form confluent monolayers [48–50]. Because of the availability of bovine brains in large quantities from slaughterhouses, cultured bovine brain microvessel endothelial cells (BBMECs) have been used more extensively [51]. The in vitro BBB screening assay is easier to perform, requires small amounts of test compounds (1 to 2 mg), and when coupled with LC-MS/MS analysis has a shorter turnaround time. This assay (Table 2.4) allows the categorization of compounds in terms of potential brain penetration, which is suitable for the early stage of drug discovery. It provides

TABLE 2.4 Drug Penetration Through the Blood–Brain Barrier: In Vitro Assay Using Bovine Brain Microvessel Endothelial Cells (BBMECs) in Lead Optimization

Study Parameter	Description
Isolation of BBMECs	The BBMECs are isolated from the gray matter of freshly obtained bovine cerebrum [43,51]. The gray matter is incubated with protease to separate the microvessels from fat, myelin, and other tissues, followed by digestion with collagenase/dispase to separate the endothelial cells from the basement membrane. Percoll gradient is then used to separate the BBMECs. The BBMECs are aliquotted and frozen in liquid nitrogen with 20% horse serum and 10% DMSO until use. The isolation process takes approximately 12 h. The cells could be used for about three months after isolation and freezing.
Culturing BBMECs into monolayers	For potential brain uptake in vitro study, the BBMEC are cultured in 12-well transwell plates with a culture medium made of 1 : 1 ratio of MEM and F-12 Ham containing 10% horse serum in an incubator at 37°C with 5% CO_2 [51]. Confluent monolayers ready for transport experiments are formed within 11–13 days.
Transport experiment	The transport experiment is carried out essentially as described for the Caco-2 study (Table 2.1), where the NCE or the high-permeability control propranolol [51] is added to the donor (apical) side of the transwell as a solution in DMSO (final concentration of DMSO <1%). Samples are taken at 0 and 60 min from both the donor and receiver sides.
Sample analysis and calculations	The samples are mixed with an internal standard in acetonitrile, centrifuged, and the supernatant is subjected to LC-MS/MS analysis. The BBB permeability is calculated as described for Caco-2 permeability. Compounds are rank-ordered according to permeability.

a system for screening compounds prior to the performance of the in vivo brain uptake studies.

The reliability of this in vitro BBB model was evaluated in our laboratory by comparing the in vitro BBB permeability to brain/plasma AUC (area under the plasma–serum concentration–time curve) ratios of 28 NCEs administered orally to rats. A good concordance with a correlation coefficient (r) of 0.87 [51] was established, which is comparable to data reported by other investigators [43,52].

2.3.3 Tissue Distribution

Tissue distribution studies of radioactivity and/or parent compound are not generally conducted in lead optimization or required prior to an FIH trial, and therefore are not discussed in this chapter. However, for compounds targeted for specific tissues, such as CNS (discussed above) or liver (e.g., hepatitis C virus), it is highly desirable to determine the concentration of the compound in target tissues following compound administration to laboratory animals (usually, rats and mice). To measure parent compound in tissues, limited assay validation will be required, the process of which can be more difficult than validation in a matrix such as plasma or urine, due to possible drug binding to tissues. Thus, such distribution studies are often conducted based on radioactivity content in the target tissue from administered ^{14}C- or ^{3}H-labeled drug, with the caveat that these results will encompass total drug-derived material [i.e., parent drug + metabolite(s)] rather than a single analyte. If deemed necessary pre-FIH, these studies can be carried out as part of pharmacokinetic studies in rodents, with either radiolabeled or unlabeled drug, as the tissues could be excised at the termination of the experiment and analyzed for compound or radioactivity concentrations (Section 2.6).

2.4 METABOLISM

Metabolism (biotransformation) is considered the most important of the ADME variables affecting the totality of the oral bioavailability, systemic exposure, intersubject variability, and drug–drug interactions. It is also the most complex of the ADME parameters to be evaluated. Accordingly, decisions are required at each stage of drug discovery and development as to which metabolism studies best support ongoing evaluation of the safety and efficacy of the NCE. The U.S. Food and Drug Administration (FDA) 1997 guidance "Drug Metabolism/Drug Interaction Studies in the Drug Development Process: Studies In Vitro" [53] states the following regarding timing of metabolism studies: "An early understanding of how a compound is metabolized could influence selection among several pharmacologically similar agents and could lead to dose regimens that would be more likely to detect a positive clinical effect." The following discussion relates to approaches that sponsors should consider in using metabolism assays in the most efficient manner to help both in the selection of an NCE for development and in characterization of relevant metabolic properties prior to the decision to conduct a FIH trial.

2.4.1 In Vitro Metabolism Studies

Metabolic Stability in Liver Microsomes and Hepatocytes For orally administered drugs, bioavailability is a product of absorption and first-pass (presystemic) elimination, which includes intestinal and hepatic metabolism as well as biliary excretion of unchanged drug. It is thus important to note that a drug can be very well absorbed but because of high presystemic metabolism exhibit low bioavailability. Also, metabolism is a major determinant of systemic clearance, which is one of the two parameters (volume of distribution is the second parameter) that determine the elimination half-life ($t_{1/2}$). Therefore, metabolic stability evaluation is not only relevant for NCEs intended for enteral routes but also for those targeted for parenteral administration. Hence, the most prudent first in vitro ADME test for an NCE in lead optimization is the assessment of metabolic stability. This assay determines the inherent metabolic potential of the NCE and is usually conducted along with other compounds (standard drugs with known pharmacokinetics in humans as well as best drugs within the same chemical series) such that the comparative extent of metabolism can be determined. With the powerful tools of robotics, automated liquid handlers, LC-MS assays, and the multiwell plate format (96-well and higher), coupled with bioinformatics software to capture, manipulate, and distribute the data, these screens are largely automated and can provide rapid throughput. Hence, timely feedback as to structure–metabolic stability relationship development can be provided to chemists. Although metabolism can proceed via both phase 1 (oxidation, reduction, and hydrolysis) and phase 2 (conjugation) pathways, the majority of metabolic stability screening is carried out using liver microsomes, cDNA-expressed recombinant cytochrome P450 (rCYP) enzymes, or a cocktail of rCYPs, all of which essentially evaluate phase 1 metabolism. This is well justified for several reasons. First, from a practicality standpoint, it is much easier, faster, and cheaper to work with liver microsomes (or expressed enzymes) than with hepatocytes or liver slices, which contain both phase 1 and phase 2 drug-metabolizing enzymes. Second, the majority of NCEs encountered in drug discovery do not contain a functional group amendable for phase 2 metabolism, and they must be metabolized first by phase 1 enzymes before being subjected to phase 2 metabolism; therefore, phase 1 reactions are probably the rate-limiting steps in the biotransformation of the NCEs. Third, the majority of drugs are eliminated by hepatic metabolism via CYP-dependent oxidation [54]. Fourth, CYP-mediated metabolism is the major ADME factor for drug failure in the market [55]. Fifth, even if an NCE is metabolized primarily by phase 2 enzymes, it would be a false positive (acceptable) and would probably be eliminated by subsequent screens.

Liver microsomes from various animal species, including humans, are available from many vendors. It is usually advisable to conduct initial screens for metabolic stability using human liver microsomes, so that an early evaluation in the target species is obtained. Other species (generally, rats) are sometimes used, but the results may not be predictive of the human setting. A sample protocol for such a study in human liver microsomes is outlined in Table 2.5.

The microsomal stability assay is usually set up in a sponsor company with sufficient resources or in a specialty CRO in a high-throughput automated assay format, wherein a large number of compounds are evaluated with a rapid turnaround time. The screen could also be developed in a nonautomated low-throughput format, as the case would be in small pharma, as soon as the company acquires the analytical resources needed [usually LC-MS (preferred) or even LC-ultraviolet] and can be used to evaluate a limited number of compounds. This screen is probably one of the earliest ADME screens that

TABLE 2.5 Study Design for the Evaluation of High-Throughput Metabolic Stability Using Human Liver Microsomes in Lead Optimization

Study Parameter	Description
Species, strain, gender	A pool of human liver microsomes from 20–30 subjects (both males and females) is used. Other species, such as rats and the pharmacology species, may be used, depending on the objective.
Assay setup	Differentiate between low, medium, and high metabolic stability by different combinations of experimental variables (protein concentration, incubation time, and compound concentration).
Assay validation	The assay is validated in advance of screening NCEs. The validation is carried out using drugs or chemicals of known and variable metabolic stability (20–30 compounds), which should be consistent with human or animal pharmacokinetic data.
Incubation conditions	Microsomes are suspended in phosphate buffer, pH 7.4, at a protein concentration of usually 1 mg/mL or lower, and incubated at 37°C with individual NCE (usually 1–5 μM). A reduced NADPH or NADPH-generating system, a cofactor of CYP-mediated metabolism, is added at approximately 1 mM to initiate the reaction. The reaction is allowed to proceed for 10–60 min. The reaction may be set up for one or several time points, depending on the objective.
Sample analysis	Following incubation, the reaction is quenched by the addition of an organic solvent (methanol or acetonitrile), centrifuged, and the supernatant is analyzed by LC-MS or LC-MS/MS after the addition of an appropriate internal standard. Incubations and assays are carried out in the same 96-well plate, to minimize sample handling.
Quality control	Several standards with known metabolic stability (low, medium, and high for each species) are usually included with each plate as a quality control for both the incubation and the LC-MS/MS analysis [56]. It is sufficient to use this initial screen to rank-order compounds; however, the data could be subjected to more rigorous analysis to project intrinsic clearance.
Acceptance criteria	The acceptance criteria vary depending on the discovery program and the stage of the program. It is preferable for the early stage that the acceptance criteria should be wide enough to allow moving compounds with borderline stability farther down the decision tree to allow for SAR development. When the program is more mature, a combination of SAR understanding and metabolic stability could tighten the acceptance criteria.

could be set up in-house in smaller companies, as it does not require cell culture growing and experimentation capabilities.

Depending on the goal of discovery program and/or corporate strategies, a sponsor may decide to perform metabolic stability in hepatocytes as the first in vitro ADME assay or subsequent to the microsomal stability assay. The hepatocyte assay (Table 2.6) is more elaborate, where cryopreserved hepatocytes are used because of practicality [57]. The major advantage of hepatocytes is that they contain both phase 1 and phase 2 drug-metabolizing enzymes, with their cofactors present in natural proportions within the intact cell architecture; therefore, they are one step closer to the in vivo situation. This is important particularly if the NCE contains a functional group amenable to conjugation. Also scaling from

TABLE 2.6 Study Design for the Evaluation of Intrinsic Clearance in Hepatocytes in Lead Optimization

Study Parameter	Description
Species, strain, gender	Human (pooled male + female) hepatocytes are best; however, other species may be used if needed.
Cryopreserved hepatocytes handling	Cryopreserved hepatocytes are usually thawed in a water bath at 37°C. The cell suspension is centrifuged and the hepatocyte pellets are gently resuspended in medium to a final density of approximately 1 million cells/mL.
Cell viability evaluation	Before using the hepatocytes, their viability is determined using trypan blue staining.
Incubation conditions	NCEs are dissolved in an organic solvent (methanol or DMSO) if insoluble in water and added to the hepatocyte suspension in a Waymouth medium at a final concentration of 1 to 10 μM (1 μM is generally used for screening). Incubations are carried out in multiwell plates with a shaker at 37°C in a CO_2 incubator for 2 h.
Sample analysis	A volume of the incubation mixture is taken at several time points and the reaction is quenched with methanol or acetonitrile in a 96-well plate. The plates are subjected to sonication, vortexed, and centrifuged prior to LC-MS/MS analysis.
Calculation of intrinsic clearance	The intrinsic hepatocyte clearance is calculated as follows [56]: $CL_{intrinsic}$ (in μL/min per million cells) $= [(C_0 - C_{2h})/AUC_{(0-2h)}](V/N)$, where C_0 and C_{2h} are the concentrations of the compound in μM at 0 and 2 h, respectively. $AUC_{(0-2h)}$ is the area under the concentration versus time curve (from 0 to 2 h) in μM · min, V is the volume of incubation mixture in μL, and N is the number of hepatocytes in millions.

hepatocyte clearance to systemic clearance in animals could be a way to add some certainty (or uncertainty) to scaled human clearance (from animal pharmacokinetic studies), as systemic clearance in animals is obtained from intravenous pharmacokinetic studies.

The predictability of this in vitro model should be evaluated with each new class of compounds, and this could be carried out in animals by determination of the intrinsic clearance, which could be scaled to in vivo clearance and comparing the values to the actual in vivo clearance. Some fundamental assumptions need to be kept in mind when using this model: (1) in vitro enzyme kinetics are applicable to the in vivo kinetic properties; (2) intrinsic clearance follows first-order kinetics; and (3) liver metabolism is the major pathway for the clearance of the NCEs evaluated.

Metabolite Characterization In addition to metabolic stability and intrinsic clearance, characterization and/or identification of the metabolites formed by the in vitro metabolic system are carried out in lead optimization, but less frequently. However, if a highly desirable chemical scaffold (based on potency, safety, and/or physicochemical properties) is metabolically unstable, it is worthwhile to understand the reason behind this instability and try to remedy the problem. This is usually carried out by the characterization of the metabolites formed by the in vitro system and thereby identifying the metabolic "hot spot(s)" in the molecules. This is followed by devising a strategy to block or slow down the metabolism in the newly synthesized compounds without the loss of the desired pharmacological attributes, based on an understanding the structure–activity relationship (SAR). Those newly synthesized NCEs are then subjected to in vitro metabolic stability evaluation to test and refine the strategy. Several iterations may be required to achieve the outcome desired.

In lead characterization where one or several compounds are identified as leads, the synthesis and targeted evaluation of ^{3}H-labeled compounds (in some cases, ^{14}C-labeled) can provide an efficient mechanism for rapid identification of metabolic issues. In vitro metabolism studies with the radiolabeled compounds directed toward characterization and/or identification of the major metabolites in animal and human liver microsomes and/or cryopreserved hepatocytes (as well as in animals in vivo) can be carried out. These studies are usually conducted by big pharma, where radiochemistry resources for the synthesis of radiolabeled compounds as well as various mass spectrometry instrumentations for metabolite characterization are available. Metabolite characterization is important in several respects:

1. The presence of significant amounts of reactive intermediates, such as unstable acyl glucuronides (and glutathione conjugates as indicative of possible reactive intermediates) and potentially toxic metabolites, could result in reassessment of the viability of the candidate.

2. Sponsors should avoid NCEs that generate human-specific metabolites [i.e., compounds that form certain metabolite(s) by the human systems only], as the development of such candidates will be extremely costly.

3. If a pharmacologically active metabolite is formed, this could lead to a better understanding of PK-PD relationships or can even result in the development of a candidate that has a better profile than the parent compound [58].

4. The presence of an active or major metabolite may trigger its synthesis and characterization to ensure minimum liabilities and the development and validation of an analytical method to monitor the metabolite in the safety and FIH studies.

5. By comparing the metabolite profiles across species, the selection of toxicology species that cover all human metabolites formed in vitro would be facilitated. This is usually important in selection of the nonrodent species for the pre-FIH toxicity studies (Chapter 7). This point was cited in the FDA 1997 guidance on in vitro metabolism studies [53], which states: "Early identification of human metabolic routes of elimination and metabolites by studies in vitro can provide clear direction for nonclinical studies in animals."

Metabolic Drug–Drug Interactions Drug–drug interactions occur when one drug changes the pharmacodynamics, safety, and/or the pharmacokinetics of a coadministered drug. Pharmacodynamic drug–drug interactions could be independent of, or a consequence of, pharmacokinetics. Also, pharmacokinetic drug–drug interaction does not necessarily result in a pharmacodynamic interaction. Pharmacokinetic drug–drug interactions result when one drug changes the absorption rate, distribution, metabolism, and/or the excretion rate of a coadministered drug. The net effect is an increase or decrease of plasma concentrations and/or the duration of action of a coadministered drug (i.e., its pharmacokinetics). Despite the fact that drugs are metabolized by both phase 1 and phase 2 enzymes, oxidation reactions via CYP enzymes are the most prevalent biotransformation pathways of administered drugs and other xenobiotics [54]. Metabolic drug–drug interactions could result from inhibition, induction, and to a much lesser extent, activation of various CYP isozymes.

In recent years, regulatory authorities worldwide have been focused increasingly on the utility of in vitro drug–drug interaction models as predictors of potential drug–drug interactions in humans and on the advisability of performing such studies early in development. The 2006 draft FDA guidance entitled "Drug Interaction Studies: Study Design, Data Analysis, and Implications for Dosing and Labeling" [59] states: "Using suitable in vitro probes . . ., the potential for drug–drug interactions can be studied early in the development process." Also, the European Agency for the Evaluation of Medicinal Products (EMEA) guidance entitled "Note for Guidance on the Investigation of Drug Interactions" [60] states: "The potential for the new drug to inhibit specific drug metabolizing enzymes including important enzymes for which the drug is not a substrate should be defined."

Cytochrome P450 Inhibition The majority of drugs are oxidatively metabolized, primarily in the liver, by the superfamily of heme-containing CYPs [61]. With completion of the sequencing of the human genome, the number of active human CYP genes is 57 [62]; however, only six enzymes, with different prevalence in human liver (Figure 2.1), are known to play a major role in drug metabolism. In particular, CYPs 1A2, 2C8, 2C9, 2C19, 2D6, and 3A4 are the major isoforms that catalyze drug metabolic transformation reactions (Figure 2.1), of which CYPs 3A4 and 2D6 participate in the metabolism of nearly 80% of commercially available drugs [63]. Inhibition of one or more of these enzymes by a coadministered drug is the major source of pharmacokinetic drug–drug interactions encountered. The net result of CYP inhibition is a decrease in the metabolic clearance of a coadministered drug that is a substrate of the inhibited enzyme, resulting in increased plasma concentrations, which may cause adverse drug reactions and/or enhanced therapeutic effects. Also, the inhibited metabolic pathway could lead to decreased formation of an active metabolite, or a drug from a prodrug, resulting in decreased efficacy. The increased plasma concentrations could be substantial, as

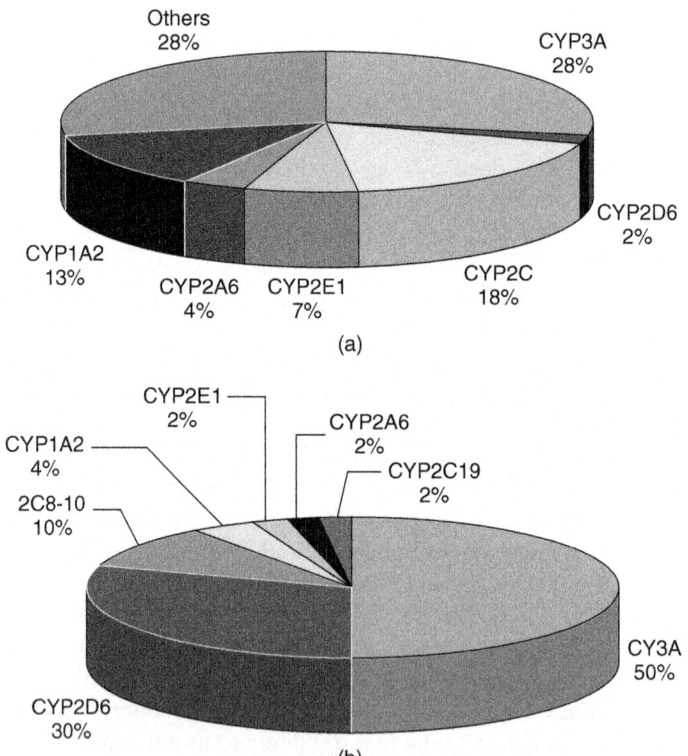

FIGURE 2.1 (a) Prevalence of CYP isoforms in a typical human liver; (b) their contribution to the metabolism of known drugs.

reported for the interaction between fluvoxamine (a potent CYP1A2 inhibitor) and remelteon (Rozerem, metabolized primarily by CYP1A2), where the area under the plasma concentration versus time curve extrapolated to infinity [AUC_{inf}] and peak plasma concentration (C_{max}) of remelteon increased by 190- and 70-fold, respectively [64]. The increase in plasma concentration could in some cases lead to adverse drug reactions, including fatalities, especially for drugs with a narrow therapeutic index [65]. Inhibitory drug–drug interactions are particularly important for patients on multiple medications and those on long-term drug therapy, such as the elderly population. Consequently, in vitro CYP inhibition evaluation of NCEs has become an important early screen in lead optimization [66]. These inhibition assays have become of higher throughput, are easier to perform, and provide an unambiguous outcome: for the most part allowing a go/no go decision with regard to advancing an NCE.

Inhibition of CYPs could be classified into direct and time-dependent, also called metabolism/mechanism-based [4]. Direct inhibition is reversible, where the drug itself reversibly (noncovalently) binds to the enzyme, resulting in alteration of the Michaelis–Menten kinetic parameters (K_m and/or V_{max}). This interaction could be competitive, noncompetitive, uncompetitive, or mixed inhibition [67]. Metabolism/mechanism-based inhibition results from the binding of a metabolic product to the enzyme. Metabolism- and mechanism-based inhibitions could be differentiated further; the first results from the direct inhibition of a CYP isoform by a metabolite of the compound. Mechanism-based inhibition (the earlier term was "suicide substrate") results from irreversible covalent or noncovalent tight binding (quasi-irreversible) of a metabolic product to the enzyme that catalyzes its formation, resulting in inactivation of the enzyme [68].

Earlier studies to evaluate CYP inhibition in human liver microsomes were carried out using a prototype substrate (with a specific metabolic reaction) for each CYP individually to determine the effect of an NCE on CYP activity at several concentrations [66,69,70]. Some laboratories have used recombinant CYPs for CYP inhibition screening; this is not recommended, for reasons beyond the scope of this chapter to describe. More recent screening assays are carried out by combining several CYP inhibition assays in a single incubation using human liver microsomes coupled with LC-MS/MS analysis. This has resulted in an increase in throughput without compromising the quality of the data. The combined approach has been developed and validated in several laboratories, including ours, over the past several years [40,71–74]. As the majority of drugs (90%) are metabolized by CYPs 3A4, 2D6, and 2C9 [63], evaluation of the inhibition of these three enzymes in one assay has been carried out in our laboratory as the first CYP inhibition screen in lead optimization [40]. Although this high-throughput assay has been largely automated using liquid handlers, it can also be performed manually on a small number of compounds, as the case would be with smaller pharma companies. An example of a study design to evaluate direct and metabolism/mechanism-based inhibition using the combined three substrates in one assay is outlined in Table 2.7.

TABLE 2.7 Enzyme Inhibition In Vitro: Study Design for the Evaluation of Direct and Metabolism/Mechanism-Based Inhibition in Human Liver Microsomes Using the 3-in-1 Screening Assay in Lead Optimization

Study Parameter	Description
Species	A pool of human liver microsomes from 20–30 subjects (pooled male + female).
Assay setup	To evaluate both direct and time-dependent inhibition, coincubation and preincubation experiments are performed [75,76]. For coincubation, the NCE is incubated at several concentrations with human liver microsomes, NADPH (or NADPH-generating system), and probe substrates. For preincubation, the NCE is first incubated with liver microsomes and NADPH for 30 min in the absence of substrate, then the substrate is added and the reaction with the substrate is initiated as with the coincubation experiment.
Coincubation conditions	The CYP inhibition screening assay (both incubation and analyses) is performed in 96-well plates [40]. NCE is incubated at several concentrations (usually 0.3, 3, and 30 μM) in wells containing microsomal protein (final concentration 0.4 mg/mL). The probe substrates are added at concentrations equal to or slightly below the K_m value of each reaction; therefore, a good estimate of K_i is obtained from the IC_{50} value ($K_i = IC_{50}$ or one-half the IC_{50}, depending on the type of inhibition). Substrate concentrations for the combined assay are 200 μM of tolbutamide (for CYP2C9), 4 μM of dextromethorphan (CYP2D6), and 100 μM of testosterone (CYP3A4). Reactions are conducted in 100 mM phosphate buffer, pH 7.4, containing 150 mM KCl. Plates are prewarmed at 37°C for 5 min. The reactions are initiated by adding 20 μL of 10 mM NADPH prepared in buffer (final NADPH concentration is 1 mM) followed by brief shaking. The total reaction mixture volume is 200 μL. The samples are incubated at 37°C for 10 min.
Preincubation conditions	The NCE is first incubated with liver microsomes and NADPH for 30 min at the same concentrations as with the coincubation, probe substrates are added, and the reactions proceed for 10 min at 37°C as with the coincubation experiment.
Sample analysis	Following both the coincubation and preincubation experiments, the reactions are terminated by adding 20 μL of 35% perchloric (or organic solvents) acid followed by shaking and centrifugation to precipitate microsomal proteins [40]. The supernatant is analyzed by LC-MS/MS after the addition of an internal standard (better isotopically stable labeled metabolites) to quantify the metabolites of the CYPs 2C9, 2D6, and 3A4 reactions. The LC-MS/MS assay is carried out in the positive-ion multiple reaction monitoring mode.

TABLE 2.7 (*Continued*)

Study Parameter	Description
Calculations	The IC_{50} values are determined by semilog plotting of NCE concentration vs. % remaining activity. The concentration of NCE that inhibits 50% of the enzyme activity (IC_{50}) relative to solvent control (with the same solvent used to solubilize the NCE at the same concentration, which should be $\leq$1 vol%) is calculated for each CYP. This step is carried out using software programs.
Quality control	For both co- and preincubation experiments, blank solvent and positive-control incubations are included (prototype direct and mechanism-based inhibitors for each CYP at one concentration each). These serve as quality control for the CYP inhibition assay.
Data interpretation	Based on data from co- and preincubation experiments, the NCE is classified as a direct inhibitor if the IC_{50} values under both conditions are similar (within twofold) or higher under preincubation conditions. If the IC_{50} under preincubation conditions is lower than for coincubation ($\geq$ twofold), the NCE is likely to be a time-dependent inhibitor. For direct inhibition, NCEs with IC_{50} values of >10 μM are considered to be less likely to cause inhibitory drug–drug interactions. NCEs with IC_{50} values of <1 μM are considered potent inhibitors and are likely to cause drug–drug interactions. The fate of NCEs with IC_{50} values between 1 and 10 μM is determined by additional factors such as potency, which CYP isoform is inhibited, therapy area, the stage of the discovery program, and projected efficacious plasma concentrations.
Subsequent studies	If an NCE advances to become a potential recommendation candidate, more rigorous inhibition assays are carried out in which the three isoforms discussed above as well as the CYPs 1A2, 2A6, 2B6, 2C8, 2C19, and 2E1 are evaluated in individual assays. Table 2.8 lists the substrates recommended in an FDA Guidance document [59]. Because of the well-documented substrate-dependent inhibition of CYP3A4 [77], a second substrate (midazolam) is used to evaluate the inhibition of CYP3A4. These individual CYP assays are of low throughput and are usually carried out on a few compounds in the lead characterization stage. In these more robust assays, extended concentration ranges of NCEs are used. These individual assays were reported previously [78].

To distinguish between metabolism- and mechanism-based inhibition, additional experiments beyond the scope of this chapter are required [76]. Both direct and mechanism-based inhibitors could result in drug–drug interactions. In addition, mechanism-based inhibitors are thought to carry an additional risk of potential idiosyncratic drug effects. It should be recognized that a compound could be a weak direct inhibitor but a potent metabolism/mechanism-based inhibitor; therefore, it is highly advisable to evaluate both types of inhibition. Usually, potent mechanism-based inhibitors of a major CYP isoform are excluded from development except under special circumstances, such as a first in class for an unmet medical need of a life-threatening disease.

It must be emphasized that CYP inhibition is not the only factor that determines the potential for metabolically based clinical drug–drug interactions. Other factors include the relative contribution of inhibited enzyme to the overall clearance of a drug (i.e., if the drug is excreted unchanged in urine and/or bile and/or metabolized by multiple CYPs or other enzymes), the concentration of the inhibitor at the enzyme active site, and the rate of depletion of the inhibitor concentration. It is worth mentioning that it is not advisable to follow-up a positive in vitro finding in human liver microsomes with a drug–drug interaction study in laboratory animals, as the substrate specificity and interactions of animal CYPs with various inhibitors are probably different from those in humans, and thus the predictability to humans of such an in vivo study in animals is questionable.

A decision regarding advancing a CYP inhibitor toward recommendation should be dependent on many factors, such as the potency of the inhibition, which CYP is inhibited, the intended therapy, the projected dose level, the frequency and duration of administration, other medications that are likely to be coadministered with the intended drug, and the competitive landscape. For example, since CYP3A4 is involved in the metabolism of approximately 50% of commercially available drugs (Figure 2.1), advancing a potent CYP3A4 inhibitor could result in drug–drug interactions with many coadministered drugs; hence, it is a major concern. However, if an NCE inhibits a CYP with much less contribution to drug metabolism (e.g., 1A2, Figure 2.1) this would be of less concern. Also, many CNS drugs are CYP2D6 substrates; therefore, a compound intended to be coadministered with these drugs should be devoid of (or minimally inhibit) CYP2D6 inhibition. Furthermore, from a competitive advantage standpoint, if marketed drugs that treat the same disease have a clean CYP profile, it would be commercially disadvantageous to recommend and advance a compound with such a liability.

The substrates recommended in the FDA guidance [59] for the conduct of in vitro drug–drug interaction studies (preferred and acceptable) are listed in Table 2.8. Also, the guidance recommends that no more than 10 to 30% of the substrate or inhibitor depletion occurs during the incubation. Furthermore, the guidance suggests that reactions should be carried out within the linear range of the relationship between time and amount of product formed.

In lead optimization, the goal is to avoid advancing NCEs that are potent inhibitors of major CYPs toward recommendation. In lead characterization, data

TABLE 2.8 CYP Inhibition In Vitro: Probe Substrates and Metabolic Reactions Recommended in the FDA Drug Interaction Guidance

CYP	Preferred	Acceptable
1A2	Phenacetin-O-deethylation	7-Ethoxyresorufin-O-deethylation Theophylline-N-demethylation Caffeine-3-N-demethylation Tacrine 1-hydroxylation
2A6	Coumarin-7-hydroxylation Nicotine C-oxidation	
2B6	Efavirenz hydroxylase Bupropion hydroxylation	Propofol hydroxylation *S*-Mephenytoin N-demethylation
2C8	Taxol 6-hydroxylation	Amodiaquine N-deethylation Rosiglitazone-*p*-hydroxylation
2C9	Tolbutamide methyl-hydroxylation *S*-Warfarin 7-hydroxylation Diclofenac 4′-hydroxylation	Flurbiprofen 4′-hydroxylation Phenytoin-4-hydroxylation
2C19	*S*-Mephenytoin 4′-hydroxylation	Omeprazole 5-hydroxylation Fluoxetine O-dealkylation
2D6	(±)-Bufuralol 1′-hydroxylation Dextromethorphan O-demethylation	Debrisoquine 4-hydroxylation
2E1	Chlorzoxazone 6-hydroxylation	*p*-Nitrophenol 3-hydroxylation Lauric acid 11-hydroxylation Aniline 4-hydroxylation
3A4/5	Midazolam 1-hydroxylation Testosterone 6β-hydroxylation	Erythromycin N-demethylation Dextromethorphan N-demethylation Riazolam 4-hydroxylation Terfenadine C-hydroxylation Nifedipine oxidation

Source: From [59].

on the approximate plasma concentrations required for efficacy are generally available. Therefore, a more rigorous projection of potential drug–drug interaction could be made. The likelihood of in vivo interaction for direct CYP inhibitors is projected based on the $[I]/K_i$ ratio, where [I] represents the projected mean steady-state C_{max} for total drug concentration (bound plus unbound) following administration of the highest proposed clinical dose, and K_i is the inhibition rate constant [59], which could be obtained experimentally or estimated as one-half of the IC_{50} if the CYP inhibition evaluation studies are conducted near the K_m values for the reaction. This is a conservative estimate, as it is true for competitive inhibition, while for noncompetitive inhibition the K_i would approximate the IC_{50}. As the $[I]/K_i$ ratio increases, the likelihood of drug–drug interaction increases. Table 2.9 shows the likelihood of in vivo drug–drug interaction based on the estimated $[I]/K_i$ ratios as reported in the FDA guidance. An estimated $[I]/K_i$ ratio greater than 0.1 is considered positive and a follow-up in vivo evaluation is

TABLE 2.9 Prediction of Clinical Drug–Drug Interaction Based on In Vitro Data for Direct CYP Inhibitors)

$[I]/K_i$[a]	Drug–Drug Interaction Prediction
>1	Likely
>0.1 and <1	Possible
<0.1	Remote

Source: From [59].
[a] $[I] = C_{max}$ in humans at steady state at the highest therapeutic dose.

recommended. When $[I]/K_i$ ratios are obtained for the major CYPs, an in vivo drug–drug interaction study starting with the CYP with the largest $[I]/K_i$ may be appropriate. If the CYP with the largest $[I]/K_i$ shows no drug–drug interaction in vivo, evaluation of the other CYPs with smaller $[I]/K_i$ values may not be needed [59]. As indicated earlier, for CYP3A4 inhibition, two structurally unrelated substrates are evaluated. If one of the two suggests a potential interaction (i.e., $[I]/K_i > 0.1$), an in vivo evaluation study should be conducted [59].

Projection of the extent of a potential drug–drug interaction for mechanism-based inhibitors is more complex and requires additional experiments. These studies are carried out to determine the inactivation kinetic parameters: K_{inact}, which is the maximum inactivation rate constant, and K_i, which is the inactivator concentration that produces half the maximal rate of inactivation. The science of using these parameters to estimate the extent of in vivo drug–drug interactions by mechanism-based inhibitors is evolving rapidly. More detailed discussions are available in recent publications [79–82].

Cytochrome P450 Induction Induction of drug-metabolizing enzymes could also result in adverse clinical drug–drug interactions. In most cases, CYP induction results from increased gene transcription and consequently an increased rate of synthesis of drug-metabolizing enzymes. Other mechanisms such as reduction of the rate of degradation of the enzyme itself (stabilizing the enzyme) or its mRNA (stabilizing the mRNA) have been reported [83]. The drug-induced enzyme could metabolize the drug itself (autoinduction) or a coadministered drug, resulting in increased metabolic clearance and subsequent decrease in drug concentrations to subtherapeutic levels. The consequences could be serious, such as reduction of therapeutic efficacy of a lifesaving drug, enhanced toxicity by increasing the rate of synthesis of a reactive or toxic metabolite, or increased activation of prodrugs, causing alteration of their pharmacokinetics and thus possibly their efficacy and/or toxicity [84,85]. Enzyme induction becomes more critical when multiple medications are coadministered, as the addition or elimination of a drug that is an inducer could affect the pharmacokinetics and therefore the efficacy and/or safety of the other medications. Unlike CYP inhibition, induction is not spontaneous but is a rather slow process, taking days to weeks for the attainment of a new enzymatic steady-state level [75].

It has been well established that the nuclear receptors (also called *xenosensors*) pregnane X receptor (PXR), constitutive androstane receptor (CAR), and aryl hydrocarbon receptor (AhR) are involved in gene regulation and induction of the major drug-metabolizing enzymes, including phase 1 and phase 2 as well as transporters [83,86–88]. It is generally believed that CYP induction regulations are similar across animal species; however, qualitative and quantitative differences in response to various inducers are considerable among animal species [83], with major individual variability at least in humans [89]. Therefore, the potential of CYP induction in humans could only be assessed reliably in human-derived in vitro systems.

Because of the induction liabilities, it is highly desirable that potent human CYP inducers not be recommended for development. Many pharmaceutical companies have recognized the impact of CYP induction and have included this evaluation as part of their ADME screens in the discovery stage. The discovery of PXR as the xenosensor for CYP3A4 induction has led to the development of PXR reporter gene assays for higher-throughput induction screening [90,91]. Several other in vitro models, including liver slices, immortalized cell lines, and primary hepatocytes, have been established [92–96]. Among these systems, the primary culture of human hepatocytes is the most reliable and is considered the gold standard [54,83,85,97]. However, the problem with primary culture of human hepatocytes is the sporadic and unpredictable supply as well as interindividual variability in the activity and response to various inducers. Recent advances in cryopreservation technology have made available cryopreserved human hepatocytes that could be used for the assessment of CYP induction potential.

The FDA guidance on drug–drug interactions states that the most reliable method to assess CYP induction potential in vitro is to determine the activity of the induced CYP in the primary culture of human hepatocytes following treatment with the NCE [59]. Both positive (listed in Table 2.8), and negative (vehicle-treated hepatocytes) controls should be included in the experiment. The positive controls should be potent inducers, producing a better than twofold increase in enzyme activity at inducer concentrations below 500 μM. A study design to conduct CYP induction in human hepatocytes consistent with the FDA guidance is outlined in Table 2.10, and chemical inducers for human hepatocytes are listed in Table 2.11. It has been suggested that CYP3A4, CYP2C8, CYP2C9, and CYP2C19 are coregulated and induced primarily via interaction with the nuclear receptor PXR [88,96,98]. Therefore, if an NCE it is not an inducer of CYP3A4, it could be concluded that it is not an inducer of CYP2C8, CYP2C9, or CYP2C19.

Cytochrome P450 Activation Drug–drug interactions could also occur as a result of CYP activation, although they are much less frequently reported than CYP induction and inhibition. Unlike CYP induction, activation does not involve an increase in the amount of drug-metabolizing enzymes and occurs spontaneously between coadministered drugs, as is the case with CYP inhibition. The net

TABLE 2.10 Enzyme Induction in Human Hepatocytes In Vitro: Study Design Consistent with the FDA Guidance on Drug Interactions [59] During Lead Characterization

Study Parameter	Description
Test system	Cryopreserved human hepatocytes are used from at least three donor livers (separate incubations) because of the interindividual variability in the induction potential.
Assay setup	Hepatocytes are thawed, cultured on a collagen substratum, and allowed to adapt to the culture conditions for 2–3 days before study initiation. Cultures are examined under light microscopy, and those dedifferentiated into fibroblast-like cells or having undergone extensive apoptosis are discarded [96].
Compound treatment	The hepatocyte cultures are treated daily for 3 days with the NCE, and with positive and negative controls (negative control is the vehicle, usually DMSO at a final concentration not to exceed 0.1% v/v). Treatments are carried out by changing the media containing test compounds and vehicle daily. The NCE concentrations are selected based on the expected human plasma drug concentrations. At least three concentrations spanning the therapeutic range, including at least one concentration that is an order of magnitude greater than the average plasma drug concentration expected, are used.
Sample analysis	Either intact cells or isolated microsomes are used to monitor compound-induced changes in enzyme activity [59]. At 24 h after the final treatment, the activity of various enzymes is determined using probe substrates. Alternatively, the hepatocytes are scraped and the microsomes prepared by differential centrifugation are used to determine enzyme activity using probe substrates, or are frozen at −80°C until use. The substrates recommended are phenacetin for CYP1A2, coumarin (CYP2A6), tolbutamide (CYP2C9), *S*-mephenytoin (CYP2C19), and testosterone (CYP3A4). The assays are conducted by LC-MS/MS. Also, microsomes could be used for Western immunoblotting to determine the amount of a specific CYP.
Quality control	A positive control for each CYP is included. Positive controls (both preferred and acceptable) and their properties, as recommended in the FDA Guidance, are listed in Table 2.11.

TABLE 2.10 ***(Continued)***

Study Parameter	Description
Calculations	The % induction relative to positive control is calculated as follows: % of positive control $$= \frac{\text{activity of NCE- treated cells} - \text{activity of negative control}}{\text{activity of positive control} - \text{activity of negative control}} \times 100$$
Data interpretation	An NCE that produces a change that is equal to or greater than 40% of the positive control in at least one subject is considered an in vitro inducer. Induction implication would depend on therapeutic area, dose regimen, the projected human plasma concentration, and whether the compound is going to be dosed as monotherapy or in combination with other drugs.

effect is similar to induction, resulting in an increase in clearance of a coadministered drug, thereby reducing its plasma concentration. CYP activation has been proposed as the mechanism of drug–drug interactions between the antiepileptic drugs felbamate and carbamazepine [99], where the addition of felbamate to carbamazepine monotherapy resulted in a decrease in carbamezapine concentrations and an increase in the plasma concentration of the CYP-mediated metabolite carbamazepine-10,11-epoxide [100]. Usually, CYP activation is not evaluated separately in lead optimization or characterization as it could be observed in CYP inhibition studies, but it is prudent to be aware of such a potential.

CYP Isozyme Profiling Determination of the major CYPs responsible for the metabolism of an NCE is necessary to assess the risk of potential drug–drug interactions with coadministered drugs that are inhibitors or inducers of drug-metabolizing enzymes, as well as assessment of the risk of genetic polymorphism. The FDA guidance [59] states: "If human in vivo data indicate CYP enzymes contribute >25% of a drug's clearance, studies to identify drug metabolizing CYP enzymes in vitro should be conducted." However, in lead optimization/characterization, the contribution of CYP enzymes to the metabolism of the NCE is not yet known; therefore, only limited studies are warranted, to minimize the risk of recommending an NCE that is primarily metabolized and cleared by a polymorphic enzyme (CYPs 2D6, 2C9, and 2C19).

Isozyme profiling (also called *reaction phenotyping*) is usually carried out in lead characterization, although preliminary information could be obtained in lead optimization as a screen, if the chemical scaffold is known to be metabolized primarily by a polymorphic CYP. This is particularly important for drugs with a narrow therapeutic index, even though the NCE itself may not be an inhibitor of a major CYP. The case of terfenadine, which is metabolized primarily by CYP3A4, is a good example. When coadministered with the potent CYP3A4 inhibitor

TABLE 2.11 Chemical Inducers (Preferred and Acceptable), Their Concentrations, and Expected Fold of Induction for In Vitro Induction Experiments in Human Hepatocytes

CYP	Preferred Inducer	Inducer Concentrations (μM)	Fold Induction	Acceptable Inducer	Inducer Concentrations (μM)	Fold Induction
1A2	Omeprazole	25–100	14–24	Lansoprazole	10	10
	β-Naphthoflavone	33–50	4–23			
	3-Methylcholanthrene	1–2	6–26			
2A6	Dexamethasone	50	9.4	Pyrazole	1000	7.7
2B6	Phenobarbital	500–1000	5–10	Phenytoin	50	5–10
2C8	Rifampin	10	2–4	Phenobarbital	500	2–3
2C9	Rifampin	10	3.7	Phenobarbital	100	2.6
2C19	Rifampin	10	20			
3A4	Rifampin	10–50	4–31	Phenobarbital	100–2000	3–31
				Phenytoin	50	12.5
				Rifapentine	50	9.3
				Troglitazone	10–75	7
				Txol	4	5.2
				Dexamethasone	33–250	2.9–6.9

Source: Adapted from [59].

ketoconazole, the concentrations of terfenadine in plasma increased dramatically, causing significant QT prolongation, leading to cardiotoxicity and fatalities [65]. Hence, terfenadine was given a black box warning and was voluntarily withdrawn from the market. It is highly preferable that an NCE be metabolized by more than one enzyme or eliminated by multiple mechanisms so that if one is inhibited, the compound will still be eliminated by the alternative pathways, minimizing the potential for drug–drug interactions and toxicity. Also, it is undesirable that NCEs with a narrow therapeutic index be metabolized solely by a polymorphic CYP, as this could lead to major interindividual variability.

Isozyme profiling is carried out using three well-characterized methods [59]: (1) chemical inhibitors or antibodies as specific CYP inhibitors in human liver microsomes; (2) individually expressed human rCYP enzymes; or (3) a bank of human liver microsomes characterized for CYP activity prepared from individual donor livers (used less frequently and not discussed here). The FDA guidance recommends that at least two of the three methods be performed to identify the specific enzyme(s) responsible for the metabolism of a new drug. Examples of study designs to evaluate reaction phenotyping of an NCE in lead optimization/characterization using human liver microsomes with specific chemical inhibitors as well as individually expressed human rCYPs are shown in Table 2.12. The FDA-recommended CYP inhibitors used in these studies are shown in Table 2.13.

TABLE 2.12 Study Design for the Evaluation of Initial Isozyme Profiling in Human Liver Microsomes and in Individually Expressed Recombinant Human CYPs in Lead Characterization

Study Parameter	Description
Species, strain, gender	A pool of human liver microsomes from 20–30 subjects (males + females) and/or recombinant individually expressed human CYPs are used.
Evaluation using human liver microsomes	A preliminary experiment to select the appropriate incubation time and protein concentration is carried out in which human liver microsomes (0.2–1.0 mg protein/mL) are incubated with the NCE (1–5 μM) in the presence and absence of NADPH (1 mM) for several intervals (15 min to 2 h). The reaction is terminated by an organic solvent (acetonitrile or methanol) followed by centrifugation to precipitate microsomal proteins. The supernatant is analyzed for the parent compound and metabolite(s) (if possible) by LC-MS or LC-MS/MS. Incubation time and protein concentration are selected for subsequent studies of linear metabolite production. Microsomes are then incubated with the NCE and NADPH in the presence and absence of individual CYP inhibitors at the proper concentration that primarily inhibits the intended enzyme (Table 2.13). For mechanism-based inhibition, microsomes are first incubated with the inhibitor and NADPH in the absence of the NCE for 15–30 min prior to NCE addition. Samples are then treated as above and the supernatant is analyzed for metabolite(s). Significantly, inhibition of metabolite formation would suggest that the NCE is metabolized by the CYP(s) inhibited. An NCE with a potentially narrow therapeutic index that is metabolized primarily by a polymorphic CYP (2D6, 2C9, or 2C19) and is not cleared by other mechanisms should be discontinued unless it is a first-in-class for a previously untreated life-threatening disease (unmet medical need). Experiments designed to quantify the relative importance of individual CYPs in the metabolism of an NCE should be carried out at an NCE's concentration of $\leq K_m$. Therefore, the K_m must be determined in advance.
Evaluation using recombinant individual human CYPs	Individually expressed recombinant human CYPs (0.25 nmol CYP/mL) are incubated with the NCE (1–5 μM) in the presence of 1 mM NADPH for approximately 1 h. Control microsomes devoid of CYPs are also used to ensure that the reaction is CYP mediated. Following incubation, the reactions are terminated and protein precipitated as above. The supernatant is analyzed for the metabolite(s) and parent compound by LC-MS or LC-MS/MS. CYP incubations resulting in a significant formation of metabolite(s) and/or disappearance of the parent drug are probably involved in the metabolism of the NCE.
Assay validation	It is highly advisable to validate the assays when they are first set up. The validation is carried out using several drugs with known and varied reaction phenotypes (i.e., each with different CYPs).

TABLE 2.13 FDA Preferred and Acceptable CYP Inhibitors and Their K_i Values for Reaction Phenotyping Using Human Liver Microsomes

CYP	Preferred Inhibitor	K_i (μM)	Acceptable Inhibitor	K_i (μM)
1A2	Furafylline[a]	0.6–0.73	α-Naphthoflavone	0.01
2A6	Tranylcypromine	0.02–0.2	Pilocarpine	4
	Methoxsalen[a]	0.01–0.2	Tryptamine	1.7
2B6			3-Isopropenyl-3-methyl diamantin	2.2
			2-Isopropenyl-2-methyl adamantine	5.3
			Sertraline	3.2[b]
			Phencyclidine	10
			Triethylenethiophosphoramide (thiotepa)	4.8
			Clopidogrel	0.5
			Ticlopidine	0.2
2C8	Montelukast		Trimethoprim	32
	Quercetin	1.1	Gemfibrozil	69–75
			Rosiglitazone	5.6
			Pioglitazone	1.7
2C9	Sulfaphenazole	0.3	Fluconazole	7
			Fluvoxamine	6.4–19
			Fluoxetine	18–41
2C19			Ticlopidine	1.2
			Nootkatone	0.5
2D6	Quinidine	0.027–0.4		
2E1			Diethyldithiocarbamate	9.8–34
			Clomethiazole	12
			Diallyldisulfide	150
3A4/5	Ketoconazole	0.0037–0.18	Azamulin	[c]
	Itraconazole	0.27, 2.3	Troleandomycin	17
			Verapamil	10, 24

Source: Adapted from [59].

[a]Furafylline and methoxsalen are mechanism-based inhibitors and should be preincubated with the microsomes and NADPH before the addition of substrate.

[b]IC_{50} values.

[c]Specific time-dependent inhibitor.

Prior to the FIH trial, human metabolites (and their contribution) of an NCE are largely unknown, as only preliminary data are available from in vitro systems. Therefore, it may be sufficient to use one of the systems described in Table 2.12 to obtain preliminary information on the CYP isoforms that metabolize the NCE, to avoid advancing compounds that are metabolized primarily by a polymorphic

CYP. Comprehensive studies with more than one system should be deferred after the FIH when the major human metabolites are identified.

2.5 EXCRETION

In vivo excretion studies are not usually performed in lead optimization and are not required prior to the initiation of FIH studies. However, with the availability of radiolabeled compounds in lead characterization, some big pharma companies perform excretion studies as part of metabolite identification (identification of urinary and biliary metabolites) or as a limited mass balance study to avoid NCEs that are retained persistently in the body. These studies are usually carried out in rats and occasionally in large animals.

Renal and biliary excretion of unchanged drug in the urine and/or bile is the primary nonmetabolic route of drug elimination. In vitro models to investigate renal excretion are very limited. The primary in vitro renal excretion model is the isolated perfused rat kidney [101], which is of low throughput and rarely used in drug discovery. Biliary excretion is one of the major components of the overall first-pass effect that could affect the bioavailability of orally administered drugs. Biliary excretion is a complex process involving a network of biliary canaliculi with uptake and efflux transporters, each specifically located on the sinusoidal (basolateral) or the canalicular (apical) membrane of the hepatocytes [102,103]. This polarized architecture is critical to hepatic function, including biliary excretion of endogenous and exogenous compounds. Potential biliary excretion of NCEs has been investigated using several in vitro systems, including hepatocytes and membrane vesicles prepared from cell lines transfected with specific transporter proteins [102]. However, in the process of hepatocyte isolation, the liver is subjected to collagenase digestion, which results in the loss of polarization, which causes a loss of their ability to excrete compounds in a vectorial manner [104,105]. As a result, in vitro models to evaluate potential biliary excretion in animals, and most important in humans, have been slow and difficult to emerge. More recently, it has been recognized that primary rat hepatocytes cultured between two layers of gelled collagen in a sandwich configuration reestablish polarization in culture, form intact sealed bile canalicular networks, express liver-specific proteins and transporters, and excrete a variety of endogenous and exogenous compounds into the newly formed biliary canalicular networks [106–108]. This in vitro sandwich-cultured hepatocyte system has been used successfully to investigate the hepatobiliary disposition of drugs and to estimate biliary excretion [109,110]. An example of a study design to evaluate hepatobiliary excretion using sandwich-cultured rat hepatocytes is outlined in Table 2.14.

Validation of the sandwich-cultured rat hepatocytes was accomplished by comparing the in vitro biliary excretion index and biliary clearance to the in vivo biliary excretion of seven compounds in rats following intravenous administration to bile duct–cannulated animals [109,110]. The in vitro biliary excretion

TABLE 2.14 In Vitro Assay for Biliary Excretion: Evaluation of Hepatobiliary Excretion Using the Sandwich-Cultured Rat Hepatocyte System

Study Parameter	Description
Isolation of hepatocytes	The experiment is conducted by the isolation of hepatocytes in a two-step collagenase perfusion method under sterile conditions [111,112]. Rats are anesthetized with ketamine and xylazine (60 and 12 mg/kg i.p., respectively) before portal vein cannulation. The liver is perfused in situ with oxygenated Ca^{2+}-free Krebs–Henseleit bicarbonate buffer containing 5.5 mM glucose for 10 min at 37°C followed by perfusion with Krebs–Henseleit bicarbonate buffer containing collagenase type I (0.5 mg/mL) for 10 min. The hepatic capsule is removed and the hepatocytes are released by shaking the liver gently in 100 mL of Dulbecco's modified Eagle's medium (DMEM). The cells released are filtered through a sterile nylon mesh (70 μm) and centrifuged at 50 g for 3 min. The cell pellet is suspended in 25 mL of DMEM and an equal volume of 90% isotonic Percoll (pH 7.4), and then centrifuged at 150*g* for 5 min. The hepatocytes are resuspended in 50 mL of DMEM and the suspensions are combined into one tube followed by centrifugation at 50 *g* for 3 min. Hepatocyte viability is determined by trypan blue exclusion. Only those hepatocyte preparations with viability >90% are used.
Preparation of the sandwich culture of rat hepatocytes	Sandwich-cultured rat hepatocytes are prepared in 60-mm plastic culture dishes coated with neutralized rat tail collagen. Hepatocyte suspensions are added to the precoated culture dishes at a density of 2×10^6 cells/dish. At approximately 1 h after plating the cells, the medium is removed and fresh medium is added. The sandwich culture is prepared by the addition of neutralized collagen solution to the hepatocyte monolayers at 24 h after the cells have been seeded. Cultures with collagen overlay are incubated for 45 min at 37°C in a humidified incubator to allow the collagen to gel before addition of the medium. The medium is changed daily until the fourth day after seeding. These 4-day sandwich-cultured hepatocytes are used for the estimation of in vitro biliary excretion.
Compound treatment	Two dishes of sandwich-cultured hepatocytes are first incubated, one in a standard complete buffer and the other in a Ca^{2+}-free buffer (to disrupt the sealed-tight junctions of the biliary canaliculi) at 37°C for 10 min, and then the buffer is removed [112]. The uptake study is initiated by adding the NCE in standard buffer to each of the two dishes. Following 10–30 min of incubation, cumulative uptake is terminated by aspirating the incubation medium and rinsing the cultured hepatocytes with compound-free buffer to remove extracellular compound. Cells of both preparations of hepatocytes (complete and Ca^{2+}-free media) are lysed.
Sample analysis	Aliquots of cell lysates are analyzed for the compound by LC-MS/MS.

TABLE 2.14 *(Continued)*

Study Parameter	Description
Calculations	The difference in the uptake between the hepatocytes treated with complete buffer and those treated with Ca^{2+}-free buffer reflects the compound taken up by the hepatocytes and excreted into the biliary canaliculi. The biliary excretion index (BEI) and biliary clearance [$CL_{B(culture)}$] are calculated as follows [109,110]: $$BEI = \frac{\text{uptake}_{\text{standard buffer}} - \text{uptake}_{Ca^{2+}-\text{free buffer}}}{\text{uptake}_{\text{standard buffer}}} \times 100$$ $$CL_{B(culture)} = \frac{\text{uptake}_{\text{standard buffer}} - \text{uptake}_{Ca^{2+}-\text{free buffer}}}{\text{time}_{\text{incubation}}\ \text{concentration}_{\text{medium}}}$$ where $\text{uptake}_{\text{standard buffer}}$ and $\text{uptake}_{Ca^{2+}-\text{free buffer}}$ represent the cumulative uptake of compound over the time interval in the hepatocytes preincubated in standard and Ca^{2+}-free buffers, respectively. $\text{Time}_{\text{incubation}}$ and $\text{concentration}_{\text{medium}}$ are the incubation time of the compound with the hepatocytes and its initial concentration in the incubation medium, respectively.

index was consistent with the percentage of dose excreted in bile from in vivo studies. Also, the in vitro biliary clearance or five compounds (inulin, salicylate methotrexate, [D-peb^{2,5}]enkephalin, and taurocholate) well correlated with their intrinsic in vivo biliary clearance with a correlation (r^2) of 0.99.

It has been also demonstrated that primary human hepatocytes grown in a sandwich culture repolarize, establish canalicular networks, and express MRP-2 as well as P-gp in the canalicular side, similar to rat hepatocytes [104]. However, the validity of the sandwich-cultured human hepatocyte system to estimate biliary excretion has been subjected to limited evaluation because of the complexities of the procedures required to measure hepatobiliary clearance in humans. One study reported on the excretion of [^{3}H]taurocholate in sandwich-cultured human hepatocytes and the effect of the anti-HIV drugs ritonavir, sequinavir, efavirenz, and nevirapine on the biliary excretion index of [^{3}H]taurocholate [113]. The biliary excretion index of [^{3}H]taurocholate was reduced by 59, 39, and 20% by ritonavir, sequinavir, and efavirenz, respectively, whereas nevirapine had no effect. Similar results were observed in sandwich-cultured rat hepatocytes. More recently, biliary clearance of the compounds ^{99m}Tc sestamibi, ^{99m}Tc mebrofenin, and piperacillin was determined using sandwich-cultured human hepatocytes from four donors, and the results were compared to the biliary clearance measured in vivo. The rank order of biliary clearance predicted from the sandwich-cultured hepatocytes corresponded well with the in vivo biliary clearance values [114].

The sandwich-cultured hepatocyte system is not a high-throughput assay. It could be used in lead characterization to understand the hepatobiliary disposition of an NCE recommended for development using both human and rat systems. The rat system is recommended in order to generate in vivo and in vitro data on the NCE as a limited validation with the specific NCE. Also, in certain cases where biliary excretion is the major determinant of low oral bioavailability, this assay could be used to screen a limited number of compounds to select an NCE with the desired hepatobiliary disposition characteristics.

The sandwich-cultured hepatocytes is a patented technology (B-Clear) available from Qualyst, Inc, Research Triangle Park, North Carolina.

2.6 PHARMACOKINETICS

After the NCE passes the initial ADME in vitro screens, evaluation of its pharmacokinetics in animals is often considered the next step in the lead optimization/characterization process typically conducted in big pharma. Small pharma may opt to bypass initial in vitro screens and to evaluate their candidates directly in in vivo animal pharmacokinetic studies, either in-house or most likely at CROs. The appropriate strategy is obviously dependent on the program goals and corporate resources.

Understanding the behavior of an NCE in an integrated system of absorption, distribution, metabolism, and excretion (i.e., its pharmacokinetic profile in animal models) is crucial for drugs designed to be systemically active. This is important in several respects. First, it is a validation of the in vitro ADME screens which are performed primarily to select a compound with an acceptable pharmacokinetic profile. Second, pharmacokinetics in animals are used to approximately project the human pharmacokinetic profile of an NCE, and along with in vitro and in vivo pharmacodynamic data, the human dose and pharmacokinetic profile needed to elicit the intended pharmacological response are projected (Chapter 3). Third, the pharmacokinetic profile in laboratory animals can aid in the design of the pre-FIH nonclinical safety studies. It is not uncommon that an NCE emerges successfully from the in vitro ADME screens, but is subsequently discontinued because of an unacceptable pharmacokinetic profile in animals. For compounds intended to be administered by the intravenous route in humans, only pharmacokinetic studies in animals after intravenous administration (either as bolus and/or infusion) should be considered, whereas for those intended for oral administration, pharmacokinetic evaluation after both oral and intravenous administration in animals is warranted.

An acceptable pharmacokinetic profile of an NCE would be dependent on many factors, such as the target disease, the intended route of administration, the stage of the discovery program, the competitive landscape, and the PK-PD relationship. In general, the aim to attain sufficiently high bioavailability and slow clearance such that the NCE attains the desired therapeutic efficacy under conditions of a convenient dose regimen. Thus, a compound that would produce a pharmacokinetic profile in animals that is probably consistent with once (qd) or twice (bid) daily administration in humans (based on projection of human pharmacokinetics) would be acceptable, with qd usually preferable. Also, the compound should achieve sufficient plasma exposure (C_{max} and/or AUC) in animal species at higher doses (rodent and nonrodent species) to conduct successful nonclinical safety evaluation studies prior to the FIH trial. For orally intended drugs, for example, an oral bioavailability of $\geq$20% is considered acceptable [115], along with a projected half-life sufficient for qd or bid dose regimen. Compounds with high oral bioavailability are also likely to show lower interindividual variability, a highly desirable attribute for a drug candidate. The minimum desired pharmacokinetic profile in animals would be species dependent, as the scaling factors from animal to human vary among species. A cutoff AUC value following oral administration could be set up in the beginning of the discovery program and refined as the program progresses.

Some major drawbacks of in vivo pharmacokinetic studies are that they are complex (requiring animal dosing, sample collection, and plasma and pharmacokinetic analyses), time consuming, require relatively large amount of compounds, and are of low throughput. These studies are usually considered the "bottleneck" in lead optimization. As a result, for the majority of pharmaceutical companies, in vivo pharmacokinetic studies are usually carried out during late-stage drug discovery. However, several ingenious approaches have been employed in recent years with the use of LC-MS/MS technology to increase throughput, resulting in moving these studies earlier in the screening paradigm. One such approach is cassette dosing or "*n*-in-1," where several compounds (usually, 10 NCEs or less) are administered simultaneously to one animal and the pharmacokinetics are determined. This would result in a higher throughput and faster turnaround time (per compound) and would reduce the number of animals and the amounts of NCEs used, as the dose of each compound in the cassette would be reduced. Several precautions must be considered when selecting compounds for each cassette [4]. Also, coadministration of multiple compounds may result in pharmacokinetic drug–drug interactions, which presumably could lead to misleading results, an issue that has been subject to much debate [116–118]. Cassette dosing has been reported to be used in drug discovery by several sponsors [119–124], while others have suggested that it is probably unsuitable, due to nonlinear pharmacokinetics and/or drug–drug interactions [116,125]. It is therefore recommended that cassette dosing be considered with caution and that, if used, the results be interpreted with full awareness of the inherent caveats of this animal model.

Alternative approaches to cassette dosing that avoid the potential for drug–drug interactions are recommended. The first of such approaches is pooling plasma samples from several animals dosed with different compounds (one compound per animal), followed by LC-MS/MS analysis and pharmacokinetic calculation on the pooled samples. This results in a reduction in the number of samples subjected to LC-MS/MS analysis [126]. A second approach is pooling the samples from one animal dosed with one compound across six time points (usually, 1 to 6 hours equally spaced), generating one sample per animal per compound for LC-MS/MS analysis [127]. When the concentration from the pooled sample is multiplied by the time interval (6 hours), an approximate area under the curve [$AUC_{(0-6h)}$] sufficient for ranking-order compounds is obtained [127]. A third approach that also has no potential for drug–drug interactions has more recently been reported from our laboratory and termed *cassette-accelerated rapid rat screen* (CARRS) [128]. An example of a study design to evaluate the oral pharmacokinetic profile of NCEs using the CARRS approach is outlined in Table 2.15. The CARRs system, even though well structured for higher-throughput and quick turnaround time (two weeks from sample submission), has enough flexibility to analyze tissues and targeted metabolites when required.

In addition to the evaluation of pharmacokinetics in animals, understanding the PK-PD relationship of the disease target in animal models of efficacy is crucial in the projection of the human pharmacokinetic profile and dose regimen needed for efficacy, as well as in devising the appropriate strategy for disease treatment. Such studies (the details and design of which would depend primarily on the disease) are usually carried out by dosing the animal model of efficacy at several dose levels (including a no-effect dose) and the measurement of the pharmacological response (directly and/or biomarkers of efficacy) as well as compound (and active metabolites, if any) concentrations in plasma and target tissue (if possible). The time dependency of the response and pharmacokinetics are also important. These valuable data are then used to develop the PK-PD model, which is then used for projections of the human pharmacokinetics and dose regimen.

After the compound survives the initial ADME and pharmacokinetic screens, it is usually subjected to more rigorous pharmacokinetic evaluation, the details of which are beyond the scope of this chapter. Briefly, these studies are designed for two purposes. The first is to project the human pharmacokinetics and dose regimen (by the performance of oral or intravenous pharmacokinetics in rats, dogs, and/or monkeys for orally targeted NCEs), and the second is to ensure that sufficient exposure would be achieved in the pre-FIH safety evaluation species. This is carried out by the performance of single-rising-dose studies in the proposed toxicology species (usually, rodent and nonrodent). These studies are initially conducted using the amorphous material and are repeated after a developable crystalline form becomes available (in most cases) (Chapter 5), usually during the bridging-to-development phase (after the compound is recommended and before the initiation of GLP safety studies). Also, additional pharmacokinetic studies may be carried out, such as dose formulation selection for humans and for animal GLP safety studies. The majority of these are single-dose studies, although on occasion multiple-dose pharmacokinetic studies have been performed to address a specific issue.

It is important to emphasize that the relevant ADME and PK studies for biotherapeutics would be limited primarily to pharmacokinetic evaluation, typically in rats and monkeys. In rats, it would be more prudent to use the rat homolog of the protein, if available. These studies are carried via the intended route of

TABLE 2.15 Study Design for the Evaluation of Oral Pharmacokinetics in Rats Using the CARRs Approach in Lead Optimization

Study Parameter	Specifications
Species, strain, gender	The femoral artery of male Sprague–Dawley rats is precannulated to facilitate rapid and precise timing of blood collection.
Compound administration	NCEs are orally dosed individually at 10 mg/kg to 2 rats/compound in batches of 6 compounds/set. Dose formulation is prepared in 0.4% hydroxypropyl methylcellulose as a solution or suspension. Other vehicles, such as 20% hydroxyypropyl-β-cyclodextrin, can be used, depending on the chemical series.
Sample collection	Blood samples (ca. 200 μL) are collected at 0.5, 1, 2, 3, 4, and 6 h after dosing. In some cases, brain or liver is harvested at 6 h. Separated plasma samples (50-μL pool from two animals/time point per compound) are transferred to 96-well plates and frozen at −20°C until analysis. Liver and brain tissues are homogenized in distilled water (1 g of tissue + 3 mL of distilled water), stored frozen, and treated like plasma samples.
Sample preparation	A semiautomated protein precipitation procedure is used. Acetonitrile containing an analytical internal standard is added at a 3 : 1 ratio to plasma or tissue samples in a 96-well plate format. The samples are mixed and centrifuged to precipitate plasma or tissue proteins. An aliquot of the supernatant is transferred from each well to a fresh 96-well plate for LC-MS/MS analysis.
Sample analysis	A minicalibration curve with three concentrations (usually 25, 250, and 2500 ng/mL) and a blank (zero) in rat plasma is prepared in duplicate. Thus, for each compound a total of 14 plasma and standard samples are analyzed. Liquid chromatography/atmospheric pressure ionization tandem mass spectrometry assay is streamlined by analyzing the samples as cassettes of six [128].
Data reporting	Plasma concentrations at each time point are expressed as ng/mL and nM. The AUC (0–6 h) for each compound is also calculated as ng · h/mL and nM · h. Tissue concentrations are reported as ng/g wet weight and as tissue/plasma ratio at 6 h.
Data interpretation	An AUC value of ≥500 ng · h/mL for a 10-mg/kg oral dose is considered acceptable to keep the NCE moving forward [115].

Source: Adapted from [128].

administration in humans, and it is preferable to perform a single-rising-dose pharmacokinetic study to understand the pharmacokinetics over a wide range of doses in animals prior to FIH. These studies should be initiated as early as possible because of the usually long half-life of biotherapeutics. Also, the performance of PK-PD studies in the animal model of efficacy would be important in order to select the starting clinical dose and to demonstrate target engagement. Other studies, such as neutralizing antidrug antibodies and tissue distribution, would probably be deferred to after the FIH studies.

2.7 PRIORITIZING ADME SCREENS

Lead optimization involves the use of several screens to select an NCE with the best overall efficacy, safety, and ADME/pharmacokinetic profile. The ADME/pharmacokinetic screens could be performed in parallel or in sequence, depending on staff, cost, and time resources, the company's overall strategy, and the therapeutic area as well as the stage of the discovery program (early or late stage). Parallel screening has the advantage of allowing earlier decisions regarding the fate of an NCE and provides a large amount of data for a chemical space, allowing a quick SAR development for each screen; however, it is resource intensive. Sequential screening is streamlined and less resource intensive, but more time consuming. Many pharmaceutical companies use a mixture of both, depending on the project and its priority and the corporate portfolio management strategy. A drug discovery screening paradigm should be flexible, discriminatory, and under continuous examination to take advantage of emerging changes in the state of the art. Screens that do not add value should be eliminated. For example, if the majority of NCEs passes a specific screen, this assay should not be employed. Also, if the data could be obtained by other means (faster and/or cheaper, or could be part of another screen), the screen should also be eliminated. A good example is that in the CARRS study for CNS-targeted NCEs, brain concentrations are obtained 6 hours after dosing from rats dosed with an NCE; therefore, an in vitro BBB model became unnecessary [128]. In the sequential approach it is important that the screens be prioritized to maximize the outcome (i.e., screening out as many undesirable compounds as early and as cheaply as possible). To this end, assays with the best combination of relevance and speed should be first in a sequence of screens [4]. The data from these early screens should be unambiguous, allowing for a go/no go decision. Usually, the first screen is a high-throughput in vitro assay for target interaction. The second set of screens may be receptor-subtype counterscreens to evaluate the selectivity (safety) toward the target or a cell-based assay related to the pharmacology target. Many big pharma companies employ ADME screens and counterscreens (such as metabolic stability, permeability in a monolayer, and CYP inhibition) as the second set of screens, as they have become of much higher throughput. Pharmacokinetic studies in animals are usually carried out subsequent to in vitro screens by most sponsors; however, some companies have streamlined and increased their throughput to the extent that they are used subsequent to pharmacology evaluation [128]. The in vivo pharmacokinetic studies usually provide an unambiguous outcome, allowing for a go/no go decision. An example of the sequence of ADME and pharmacokinetic studies that may be advisable to employ prior to the FIH trial (excluding toxicokinetics and other tests that support toxicology assessment directly) is shown in Table 2.16.

2.8 IN SILICO ADME SCREENING

Computational ADME has been receiving considerable and increasing attention in the past several years. It has been estimated that in silico modeling represented 10% of pharmaceutical R&D expenditure in 2006, and it is expected to rise to 20% by 2016 [129]. In silico modeling is a complex subject that involves practically all ADME properties; and extensive discussions are beyond the scope of this chapter. Hence, a brief overview of in silico ADME and its potential for accelerating drug discovery will be given. For more detailed discussions, comprehensive reviews are available [129–133].

The availability of massive ADME and pharmacokinetic data in the literature and within the pharmaceutical company databases has led to the initiation of data-mining efforts in order to understand the SAR for ADME properties. In silico *prediction* is the process of learning from available experimental data with known compounds to predict ADME properties of new compounds. The main hypothesis behind in silico approaches is that similar molecules and/or molecules with similar molecular descriptors are likely to have similar ADME attributes. Although considerable progress has been made in in silico screening, some skepticism still surrounds these efforts [134]. The major advantage of in silico modeling is that it is the only option available for "screening" NCEs before they are synthesized (virtual screening), allowing the synthesis of only those compounds that are predicted to have superior ADME characteristics. Accordingly, its utility rests in the initial elimination of compounds among a large number of potentially available NCEs but is not useful for sponsors evaluating relatively few compounds.

One of the earliest approaches in this regard is Lipiniski's analysis of the World Drug Index, which led to his well-known *rule of five*, which predicts that poor absorption or permeability of a compound is more likely to occur when there are more than five hydrogen bond donors (OH and NH), 10 hydrogen bond acceptors (N and O atoms), the molecular weight is greater than 500 Da, and the calculated log octanol : water partition coefficient [log P(C log P)] is greater than 5 (or M log $P > 4.15$) [135,136]. Following Lipinski's pioneering work, other investigators proposed similar druglike rules, which included parameters such as the number of rotatable and rigid bonds [131].

TABLE 2.16 ADME and Pharmacokinetic Screens and Studies for Consideration Prior to the FIH Trial

Screen/Study	Information Provided	Factors Affecting the Conduct of Pre- or Post-FIH Program	Timing
In silico ADME screening	Prediction of ADME properties based on chemical structure and molecular descriptors (Section 2.8).	Allows the synthesis of NCEs with best predicted ADME properties.	Lead identification/early lead optimization
Metabolic stability in human liver microsomes	Relative extent of phase 1 metabolism as compared to other NCEs and known drugs.	Aids in selection of NCE for further evaluation; recommended as the first ADME screen.	Lead identification and/or lead optimization
Metabolic stability in human hepatocytes	Relative extent of phase 1 and phase 2 metabolism as compared to other NCEs and known drugs.	Allows for human PK and dose projection and confirms allometric scaling.	Lead optimization and lead characterization
Aqueous solubility	Along with permeability, projects the potential for oral absorption. Also helps assess the validity of in vitro ADME data.	Affects the strategy and timing for the development of human and animal dose formulations.	Lead optimization
Caco-2 permeability	Potential for oral absorption in humans and initial Biopharmaceutical Classification System (Chapter 3) assessment for oral NCEs.	Affects the strategy and timing for the development of human dose formulation.	Lead optimization

CYP inhibition in human liver microsomes	Evaluation of the potential for inhibitory drug–drug interactions with coadministered drugs.	Could affect the decision to select an NCE. If a CYP inhibitor is selected, could affect the design, timing, and the number of in vivo clinical drug–drug interaction studies.	Lead optimization
CYP induction in human PXR	Evaluates the potential for drug–drug interactions with coadministered drugs as a result of CYP induction.	Affects the timing of CYP induction studies in human hepatocytes.	Lead optimization
CYP induction in human hepatocytes	Confirms the PXR findings. Considered the definitive in vitro CYP induction experiment.	Could affect the decision to select an NCE. If a CYP inducer is selected for development, the design, timing, and number of in vivo clinical drug–drug interaction studies could be affected.	Lead characterization
Plasma protein binding in animals and human	Provides a safety margin for hERG signal (if any) and helps in the estimation of animal-to-human exposure multiples from nonclinical cardiovascular and safety studies.	If the hERG multiples are low, a cardiovascular (CV) safety study in animals is performed, which could result in NCE discontinuation. If an NCE with CV liabilities is selected for development, this could affect the speed and progression of the clinical program. Also, the animal/human exposure multiples from safety studies could affect the progression of the clinical program.	Lead characterization

(*Continued overleaf*)

TABLE 2.16 ***(Continued)***

Screen/Study	Information Provided	Factors Affecting the Conduct of Pre- or Post-FIH Program	Timing
Metabolite profiling in hepatocytes of animals and humans	Aids in the selection of the toxicology species. Evaluates the presence of human-specific metabolite(s) and/or reactive or toxic metabolite(s).	NCEs that show human-specific metabolites or a large amount of reactive or toxic metabolite(s) are usually discontinued. Affects the selection of nonclinical toxicology species.	Lead characterization
CYP reaction phenotying	Evaluates the potential for drug–drug interactions, genetic polymorphism, and intersubject variability.	Could affect the timing for drug–drug interaction studies and genotyping screening for slow and fast metabolizers.	Lead characterization
I.v./p.o. PK in rats, dogs, and monkeys	Projection of human pharmacokinetics and the potential for a successful toxicology program.	Will affect the selection of the NCE for development, as compounds with poor PK in animals will be discontinued.	Lead characterization
Projection of human PK and dose regimen	Estimates the human pharmacokinetics and the dose regimen needed for the pharmacological response intended.	Projects the potential for a successful drug.	Lead characterization
PK/PD studies in animal models of efficacy	Provides plasma and target tissue concentrations of NCE (and active metabolite, if any) required for in vivo efficacy. Also provides the duration of exposure required to elicit the pharmacological response.	Important for the projection of the initial human pharmacokinetics and dose regimen required for efficacy. Also, helps in devising a strategy for disease treatment.	Lead characterization

Single-rising-dose PK in rats and large animals (dogs and/or monkeys)	Projects the potential for achieving acceptable exposure multiples in rodent and nonrodent toxicology species during nonclinical safety evaluation.	The selection of the candidate is affected, as a candidate with low multiples will probably be difficult to develop. Affects the amount of compound to be synthesized for safety studies.	Lead characterization
Metabolite profiling in rats and nonrodents (projected toxicology species)	Evaluates the presence of a potentially toxic metabolite and/or reactive intermediate. Confirms the hepatocyte metabolite identification findings and provides an initial look at potential human metabolites.	Could affect the selection of an NCE, as if a reactive or toxic metabolite is present in a significant amount, the NCE may not be recommended. If recommended, the metabolites should be monitored in humans.	Lead characterization
Oral PK in animals with a developable crystalline form and food-effect study	A developable stable crystalline form with an acceptable PK profile in animals would probably ensure a successful safety evaluation program and the timely development of an acceptable human dosage form for clinical studies. The food effect will aid in the selection of a dosing schedule in animals and could provide an indication of the potential food effect in humans.	This could speed up the development program, as it will allow the initiation of safety studies as soon as the compound is available, with minimal formulation support to develop animal and human dosage forms. Affects the timing of a food-effect study in humans.	Lead characterization/ bridging to development

Current in silico ADME approaches involve the use of two main modeling methods: molecular-based and data-based. In molecular-based modeling, molecular mechanics, pharmacophore, molecular docking, and quantum mechanics are used to explore the potential interaction between the compound of interest and proteins known to be involved in the ADME manifestation, such as CYPs and transporters. This requires the three-dimensional structural information of the protein (available for several CYPs), which could be built by homology modeling of related structures if the human protein structure is not available. An alternative method is to use pharmacophore models which are built from superposition of the known ligand of the protein. For the data-based modeling approach, a quantitative structure–property relationship is typically used. This approach uses statistical tools to derive correlations between an ADME property and a set of molecular descriptors. These molecular descriptors could be based on one-, two-, and/or three-dimensional chemical structures of the compounds [129,130].

Several statistical algorithms with varying degrees of complexities to relate an ADME property with molecular descriptors have been reported. These include (but are not limited to) multiple linear regression, the partial least-squares method, linear discriminating analysis, artificial neural networks, and genetic algorithms. Also, several physicochemical descriptors have been used to develop in silico models, including lipophilicity parameters such as log P, log D (log P using buffer at pH 7.4), and Δ log P (the difference between the log octanol:water partition coefficient and the log cyclohexane:water partition coefficient); properties associated with hydrogen bonding (or lack thereof), such as polar surface area, nonpolar surface area, and dynamic polar van der Waals surface area, in addition to other descriptors, such as calculated molar volume and Abraham descriptors [130,133].

The basic requirements for successful in silico modeling include a high-quality in vitro data set for diverse molecular structures, with a wide range of activity for each property, multiple integrated molecular descriptor generating tools, statistical algorithms for structure–property relationship derivations, statistical methods to test and validate the models, and the ability to integrate the models with other available tools. Furthermore, the models should be flexible and updated and refined continuously with the availability of new in vitro data [137].

The process of data modeling starts by choosing the ADME property to be modeled and dividing the available data into those to be used for model generation (training or learning set) and those for model evaluation (validation or test set). There are several considerations in selecting the two data sets to maximize the validity of the model [133]. The model is developed by generating various molecular descriptors (could be as simple as the number of N and O atoms or more complex, such as quantum mechanics–related parameters) and statistically correlating the descriptors to the ADME property. Several statistical approaches could be used for the same data set to select the best model or to develop several models. The model is subjected to several iterations to select the most relevant descriptors for the particular ADME property, by eliminating one descriptor at a time, followed by reevaluation of the model's statistics. The accuracy of the models is evaluated by predicting the ADME attribute of the test set and comparing the computed data to the experimental data. Statistical approaches are used to test the accuracy of the model quantitatively [138]. These models could be local, which are generated for compounds of a limited chemical space (closely related compounds, i.e., within one discovery target program) which are used for prediction within the same chemical space, or global which would require a much larger data set for model development and validation.

Several physicochemical and ADME properties have recently been modeled with a great deal of success. The most modeled properties include log *P*, solubility, intestinal or Caco-2 permeability, plasma protein binding, and blood–brain barrier permeability [130,133]. For example, a computational linear model for passive brain permeability has been developed using three descriptors: log *D*, van der Waals surface area of basic atoms, and polar surface area [139]. The model showed a good correlation between calculated and experimentally obtained data using in situ rat perfusion technique with a correlation (r^2) of 0.77 to 0.94 and a standard deviation (SD) of 0.38 to 0.51.

Two in silico models to predict CYP2D6 and CYP3A4 inhibition have recently been reported [140]. Data used for modeling consisted of diverse sets of 1153 and 1382 NCEs for CYP2D6 and CYP3A4 inhibition in human liver microsomes, respectively. For CYP2D6, 82% of the test set was predicted correctly. For CYP3A4, 88% of compounds were classified correctly as inhibitors and noninhibitors. More important, fragment analysis was performed, and structural fragments frequent in CYP2D6 and CYP3A4 inhibitors and noninhibitors have been elucidated.

A combined in silico neural network and Bayesian models to predict hERG (human ether-a-go-go related gene) channel blocking (about 46,000 compounds for the training set and 12,000 compounds for the validation set) and CYP2D6 inhibition (about 2400 compounds for the training set and 600 compounds for the validation set) have been reported [141]. Both modeling methods were developed for each of the two properties. The combination of the two models (consensus model) resulted in the correct prediction of >90% of the compounds from the validation sets.

More recently, metabolic stability in human liver microsomes has been modeled using several in silico modeling systems [142]. For model building, 1952 proprietary compounds comprising two classes (stable/unstable) were used with 193 descriptors calculated using the Molecular Operating Environment [142]. The results of the test compounds have demonstrated that all classifiers yielded satisfactory results (accuracy >0.8, sensitivity >0.9, specificity >0.6, and precision >0.8).

Commercial in silico ADME and toxicity software programs have been available for the past several years [129,130]. Current commercial models are limited to specific ADME properties. Examples include VolSurf (accelrys, tripos; www.tripos.com), which predicts solubility, Caco-2, and blood–brain barrier permeabilities and distribution. Another example is Ceius^2.ADME (accelrys; www.accelrys.com), a package of six predictive ADME/toxicity models, including human intestinal absorption, aqueous solubility, CYP2D6 inhibition, blood–brain barrier penetration, protein binding, and hepatotoxicity. These models have been developed from published experimental in vitro data.

It must be recognized that there is no single established model that can predict pharmacokinetics, as this process represents the totality of several variables. Nevertheless, in silico approaches are evolving rapidly [132]. Several prediction models for the same property are available, and any one in silico prediction model may not be sufficient. The emerging consensus models, a combination of two or more models for the same property based on different principles, would probably improve the quality and reliability of ADME predictions [130]. In silico ADME screening certainly has a role in drug discovery, a role that is likely to grow in the future, with the potential to become more dominant as the models become simpler and more reliable.

2.9 THE PROMISE OF METABOLOMICS

Metabolomics is defined as the comprehensive and simultaneous systematic determination of endogenous metabolites in whole organisms and their change over time as a consequence of stimuli such as diet, lifestyle, environment, genetic effects, disease state, and pharmaceutical and toxicological interventions [143,144]. Metabolomics, the most recent "omic" science, provides a dynamic portrait of the metabolic status of a living system [145]. The field of metabolomics holds the potential of filling the gap between genotype and phenotype, as it more directly reflects the phenotype features of an organism (Figure 2.2). Like the preceding "omic" sciences (i.e., genomics, transcriptomics, and proteomics), metabolomics deals with a large amount of information extracted from the living system. Metabolite profiling (metabolomics) could be performed in tissues or isolated cells; however, from the drug discovery and development standpoints, urine, plasma, and saliva are the most relevant.

In general, the field of metabolomics involves the analysis of low-molecular-weight compounds that serve as substrates and products of various metabolic enzymes [145], which include sugars, lipids, amino acids, intermediary metabolites, and disease-associated metabolites as well as bioactive products acting at very low concentrations in signaling pathways [146]. Although the number of

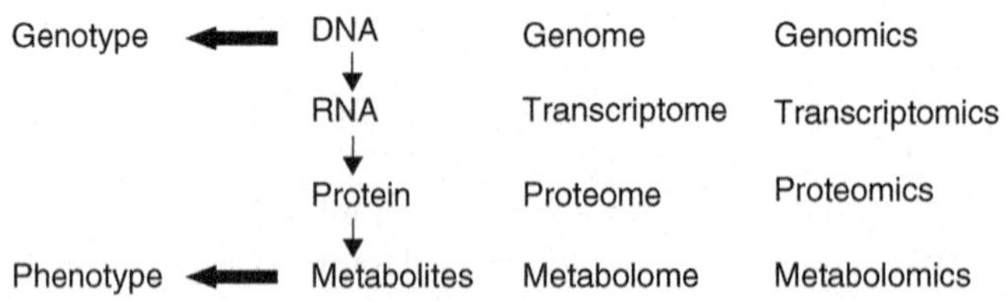

FIGURE 2.2 Terminolomy used in "omic" sciences and their interrelationships.

different metabolites in humans is unknown, it is estimated to be in the range of 2000 minimum and 20,000 maximum, compared to an estimated 23,000 genes and 60,000 proteins [145,147].

Metabolomics holds great promise for drug discovery, development, and drug treatment [148]; below are a few examples:

1. Biomarkers or fingerprints of various diseases, disease stage, and prognosis could be identified.
2. Biomarkers responding to drug treatment could be discovered and used to monitor a patient's progress, allowing for quickly changing treatment, dose adjustment, and comedication.
3. Metabolomics could be applied to the discovery of a metabolic pathway altered in a specific disease (such as cancer using cancer cells), allowing an understanding of the mechanism of response to certain treatment and the identification of biomarkers.
4. Metabolomics may lead to the discovery of new drug targets by understanding the cascade that leads to a certain phenotype, allowing intervention at several points in the cascade.
5. In the safety evaluation of an NCE, metabolomics could provide a relatively noninvasive approach by an analysis of plasma or urine to determine a no-effect dose, target organ toxicity, mechanisms of a toxic response, and the time course of its onset [149].

The choice for analysis of the metabolome (the totality of the metabolites) depends on the objective. Proton nuclear magnetic resonance spectroscopy (^{1}H-NMR) and mass spectrometry (MS) coupled with a separation stage(s) (such as liquid or gas chromatography) are the major analytical platforms used in metabolomics [144,148,150,151]. Each of these techniques has its advantages and limitations in quantification, scope, and throughput. ^{1}H-NMR has the advantage of not requiring a separation step or sample preparation (which could result in the loss of some metabolites), it is nondestructive, cost-effective, more reproducible, and fast, but of lower sensitivity. Mass spectrometry has the advantage of higher sensitivity and a better chance of metabolite resolution and identification. None of these techniques alone can identify and quantify the diverse range of metabolites, and an integrated set of both techniques is needed to address the entire spectrum of metabolomics [152]. More comprehensive discussions of both technologies have been published in several recent excellent reviews [144,145,150].

The role of metabolomics in drug discovery and development is increasingly gaining ground. The majority of big pharma companies have incorporated metabolomics in their research and development programs, particularly in biomarker discovery. Many recent examples of metabolomics application in drug discovery and development have been reported [148,149,153–155]. In one recent study ^{1}H-NMR–based metabolomics approach has been used to establish a metabolic biomarker pattern in a transgenic murine model of rheumatoid arthritis [151]. Serum ultrafiltrates from arthritic and control mice with the same genetic background (but lacking the arthritogenic T-cell receptor) were compared by ^{1}H-NMR spectroscopy. A highly significant subset of 18 spectral features was identified as biomarkers, which were termed a *metabolic bioprofile*. Metabolites related to nucleic acid, amino acid, and fatty acid metabolism as well as lipolysis, reactive oxygen species generation, and methylation were identified. Pathway analysis suggested a shift from metabolites involved in numerous reactions toward intermediates and metabolic endpoints associated with arthritis. This is a good demonstration of the power of metabolomics for identifying a wide variety of disease-associated markers [151].

Although metabolomics is a more recent science, its utilization in drug discovery and development is increasing rapidly. This has been made possible by major advances in analytical techniques (i.e., NMR and MS coupled with separation technologies) which allow the qualitative and quantitative analysis of a large number of components in complex mixtures. Together with other, more mature "omic" sciences, advances in our understanding of major disease, disease progression, disease treatment, and target identification will continue to be forthcoming.

2.10 CONCLUSIONS

Modern drug discovery has been evolving in the past two decades as a result of advances in science and technology. The sequencing of the human genome, coupled with advances in molecular biology and genetics, major breakthroughs in structural chemistry and x-ray crystallography, advances in organic chemistry (including parallel and combinatorial synthesis), the availability of highly dependable programmable robotics with miniaturization technology, and the availability of highly sensitive, selective, and user-friendly analytical instrumentation have shaped modern drug discovery. As a result, the number of NCEs that requires ADME and pharmacokinetic screening has been increasing substantially, creating a need for higher-throughput assays. Cost-effective and less labor intensive in vitro models have been incorporated into drug discovery to weed out compounds with undesirable ADME and pharmacokinetic attributes, thereby fine-tuning the ADME profile of those NCEs moving forward into development. Several in vitro screening assays, including microsomal stability, CYP inhibition, Caco-2 permeability, efflux transport evaluation, hepatocyte clearance, protein binding, and isozyme profiling, have been incorporated into drug discovery. It must be recognized that there is no single strategy that should be used for all discovery programs, as it is dependent on the company's resources (staff, time, and cost), portfolio management philosophy, the discovery program, the target therapeutic area, and priorities. It is crucial to understand the relevance, precision, and limitations of each higher-throughput assay, particularly if it is positioned for a go/no go decision. Such decisions should be program dependent and are likely to change as the program advances. Continual interpretation and "value added" assessments should be part of all discovery paradigms. Another important consideration is that when setting up a sequence of screens, the decision tree should be designed to eliminate compounds with undesirable attributes as early in the discovery process as possible. In this way, resources are focused on those candidates with optimal chances for success in the clinic.

More recent technologies, such as in silico ADME screening and metabolomics, are quickly gaining ground in the drug discovery landscape. The potential of these technologies to improve the quality of NCEs and speed up the discovery and development processes is high. These approaches are evolving quickly and would probably help in the design of targeted chemical libraries with druglike properties, therefore reducing the attrition rate in lead optimization. Although metabolomics is a more recent science, its utilization in drug discovery and development is increasing rapidly. Together with the other more mature "omic" sciences (i.e., genomics, transcriptomics, and proteomics), the potential advances in our understanding of major disease, disease progression, disease treatment, and target identification are limitless.

REFERENCES

1. Lin JH, Lu AYH. Role of pharmacokinetics and metabolism in drug discovery and development. *Pharmacol Rev*. 1997;49:403–449.
2. Wienkers LC, Heath TG. Predicting in vivo drug interactions from in vitro drug discovery data. *Nat Rev Drug Discov*. 2005;4:825–833.
3. Kola I, Landis J. Can the pharmaceutical industry reduce attrition rates? *Nat Rev Drug Discov*. 2004;3:711–715.
4. White RE. High-throughput screening in drug metabolism and pharmacokinetic support of drug discovery. *Annu Rev Pharmacol Toxicol*. 2002;40:133–157.
5. Wiederrecht GT, Hill RG, Beer MS. Partnership between small biotech and big pharma. *Drugs*. 2006;9:560–564.
6. Frank R, Hargreaves R. Clinical biomarkers in drug discovery and development. *Nat Rev Drug Discov*. 2003;2:566–580.
7. Kerns EH, Di L, Carter GT. In vitro solubility assays in drug discovery. *Curr Drug Metab*. 2008;9:879–985.
8. Stenberg P, Luthman K, Artursson P. Virtual screening of intestinal drug. *J Control Release*. 2000;65:231–243.
9. Amidon GL, Lennernäs H, Shah VP, Crison JR. A theoretical basis for a biopharmaceutic drug classification: the correlation of in vitro drug product dissolution and in vivo bioavailability. *Pharm Res*. 1995;12:413–420.
10. Johnson KC, Swindell AC. Guidance in the setting of drug particle size specifications to minimize variability in absorption. *Pharm Res*. 1996;13:1795–1798.
11. Norris DA, Puri N, Sinko PJ. The effect of physical barriers and properties on the oral absorption of particulates. *Adv Drug Deliv Rev*. 1998;3:135–154.

12. Camenisch G, Alsenz J, van de Waterbeemd H, Folkers G. Estimation of permeability by passive diffusion through Caco-2 cell monolayers using the drugs' lipophilicity and molecular weight. *Eur J Pharm Sci*. 1998;6:317–324.
13. Brayden DJ. Human intestinal epithelial cell monolayers as prescreens for oral drug delivery. *Pharm News*. 1997;4:1–15.
14. Wilson G, Hassan IF, Dix CJ, et al. Transport and permeability properties of human Caco-2 cells: an in vitro model of the intestinal epithelial cell barrier. *J Control Release*. 1990;11:25–40.
15. Stevenson CL, Augustijns PF, Hendren RW. Use of Caco-2 cells and LC/MS/MS to screen a peptide combinatorial library for permeable structures. *Int J Pharm*. 1999;177:103–115.
16. Yamashita S, Furubayashi T, Kataoka M, Sakane T, Sezaki H, Tokuda H. Optimized conditions for prediction of intestinal drug permeability using Caco-2 cells. *Eur J Pharm Sci*. 2000;10:195–204.
17. Hidalgo IJ, Raub TJ, Borchardt RT. Characterization of human colon carcinoma cell line (Caco-2) as a model system for intestinal epithelial permeability. *Gastroenterology*. 1989;96:736–749.
18. Wilson G. Cell culture techniques for the study of drug transport. *Eur J Drug Metab Pharmacokinet*. 1990;15:159–163.
19. Polli JE, Ginski MJ. Human drug absorption kinetics and comparison to Caco-2 monolayer permeabilities. *Pharm Res*. 1998;15:47–52.
20. Gres MC, Julian B, Bourrie M, et al. Correlation between oral drug absorption in human, and apparent drug permeability in TC-7 cells. A human epithelial intestinal cell line: comparison with the parental Caco-2 cell line. *Pharm Res*. 1998;15:726–733.
21. Lennernäs H. Intestinal permeability and its relevance for absorption and elimination. *Xenobiotica*. 2007;37:1015–1051.
22. Krishna G, Chen KJ, Lin CC, Nomeir AA. Permeability of lipophilic compounds in drug discovery using in-vitro human absorption model, Caco-2. *Int J Pharm*. 2001;222:77–89.
23. Fung EN, Chu I, Li CC, et al. Higher-throughput screening for Caco-2 permeability utilizing a multiple sprayer LC-MS/MS system. *Rapid Commun Mass Spectrom*. 2003;17:2147–2152.
24. Eddy EP, Maleef BE, Hart TK, Smith PL. In vitro models to predict blood–brain barrier permeability. *Adv Drug Deliv Rev*. 1977;23:185–194.
25. Chu I, Nomeir AA. In vitro DMPK screening in drug discovery. In: Chowdhury SK, ed. *Identification and Quantification of Drugs, Metabolites and Metabolizing Enzymes*. New York: Elsevier; 2005: 105–122.
26. Hunter J, Hirst BH, Simmons NL. Drug absorption limited by P-glycoprotein–mediated secretory drug transport in human intestinal epithelial Caco-2 cell layers. *Pharm Res*. 1993;10:743–749.
27. Lin JH. How significant is the role of P-glycoprotein in drug absorption and brain uptake? *Drugs Today*. 2004;40:5–22.
28. Hunter J, Hirst B. Intestinal secretion of drugs: the role of P-glycoprotein and related drug efflux systems in intestinal oral drug absorption. *Adv Drug Deliv Rev*. 1997;25:129–157.

29. Lin JH. Transporter-mediated drug interactions: clinical implications and in vitro assessment. *Expert Opin Drug Metab toxicol*. 2007;3:81–92.
30. Lin JH, Yamazaki M. Clinical relevance of P-glycoprotein in drug therapy. *Drug Metab Rev*. 2003;35:417–454.
31. Fichtl B, Nieciecki AV, Walter K. Tissue binding versus plasma binding of drugs: general principles and pharmacokinetic consequences. *Adv Drug Res*. 1991;20:117–166.
32. Kalvass JC, Maurer TS. Influence of nonspecific brain and plasma binding on CNS exposure: implications for rational drug discovery. *Biopharm Drug Dispos*. 2002;23:327–338.
33. Devane CL. Clinical significance of drug binding, protein binding, and binding displacement drug interactions. *Psychopharmacol Bull*. 2002;36:5–21.
34. Rolan PE. Plasma protein binding displacement interactions: Why are they still regarded as clinically important? *Br J Clin Pharmacol*. 1994;37:125–128.
35. Benet LZ, Hoener BA. Changes in plasma protein binding have little clinical relevance. *Clin Pharmacol Ther*. 2002;71:115–121.
36. Kosa T, Maruyama T, Otagiri M. Species differences of serum albumins: I. Drug binding sites. *Pharm Res*. 1997;14:1607–1612.
37. Nolan ER, Feng MR, Koup JR, et al. A novel predictive pharmacokinetic/pharmacodynamic model of repolarization prolongation derived from the effects of terfenadine, cisapride and E-4031 in the conscious chronic AV node—ablated, His bundle-paced dog. *J Pharmacol Toxicol Methods*. 2006;53:1–10.
38. Gintant GA, Su Z, Martin RL, Cox BF. Utility of hERG assays as surrogate markers of delayed cardiac repolarization and QT safety. *Toxicol Pathol*. 2006;34:81–90.
39. Nakai D, Kumamoto K, Sakikawa C, Kosaka T, Tokui T. Evaluation of the protein binding ratio of drugs by a micro-scale ultracentrifugation method. *J Pharm Sci*. 2004;93:847–854.
40. Chu I, Nomeir AA. Utility of mass spectrometry for in-vitro ADME assays. *Curr Drug Metab*. 2006;7:467–477.
41. Banker MJ, Clark TH, Williams JA. Development and validation of a 96-well equilibrium dialysis apparatus for measuring plasma protein binding. *J Pharm Sci*. 2003;92:967–974.
42. Lai CH, Kuo KH. The critical component to establish in vitro BBB model: Pericyte. *Brain Res Brain Res Rev*. 2005;50:258–265.
43. Eddy EP, Maleef BE, Hart TK, Smith PL. In vitro models to predict blood–brain barrier permeability. *Adv Drug Deliv Rev*. 1977;23:185–194.
44. Rubin LL, Staddon JM. The cell biology of the blood–brain barrier. *Annu Rev Neurosci*. 1999;22:11–28.
45. Pordridge WM. Log(BB), PS products and *in silico* models of drug brain penetration. *Drug Discov Today*. 2004;9:392–393.
46. Liu X, Tu M, Kelly RS, Chen C, Smith BJ. Development of a computational approach to predict blood–brain barrier permeability. *Drug Metab Dispos*. 2004;32:132–139.

47. Goodwin JT, Clark DE. *In silico* predictions of blood–brain barrier penetration: considerations to "keep in mind." *J Pharmacol Exp Ther*. 2005;315:477–483.

48. Garberg P, Ball M, Borg N, et al. In vitro models for the blood–brain barrier. *Toxicol In vitro*. 2005;19:299–334.

49. Smith M, Omidi Y, Gumbleton M. Primary porcine brain microvascular endothelial cells: biochemical and functional characterisation as a model for drug transport and targeting. *J Drug Target*. 2007;15:253–268.

50. Perrière N, Yousif S, Cazaubon S, et al. A functional in vitro model of rat blood–brain barrier for molecular analysis of efflux transporters. *Brain Res*. 2007;1150:1–13.

51. Chu I, Liu F, Soares T, Kumari P, Nomeir AA. Generic fast gradient liquid chromatography/tandem mass spectrometry techniques for the assessment of the in vitro permeability across the blood–brain barrier in drug discovery. *Rapid Commun Mass Spectrom*. 2002;16:1501–1505.

52. Lundquist S, Renftel M, Brillault J, Fenart L, Cecchelli R, Dehouck MP. Prediction of drug transport through the blood–brain barrier in vivo: a comparison between two in vitro cell models. *Pharm Res*. 2002;19:976–981.

53. Guidance for Industry: Drug Metabolism/Drug Interaction Studies in the Drug Development Process: Studies In vitro. U.S. Department of Health and Human Services, Food and Drug Administration; 1997.

54. Soars MG, McGinnity DF, Grime K, Riley RJ. The pivotal role of hepatocytes in drug discovery. *Chem Biol Interact*. 2007;168:2–15.

55. Roberts SA. High-throughput screening approaches for investigating drug metabolism and pharmacokinetics. *Xenobiotica*. 2001;31:557–589.

56. Drexler DM, Belcastro JV, Dickinson KE, et al. An automated high throughput liquid chromatography–mass spectrometry process to assess the metabolic stability of drug candidates. *Assay Drug Dev Technol*. 2007;5:247–264.

57. Lau YY, Sapidou E, Cui X, White RE, Cheng KC. Development of a novel in vitro model to predict hepatic clearance using fresh, cryopreserved and sandwich-cultured hepatocytes. *Drug Metab Dispos*. 2002;30:1446–1454.

58. Nomeir AA, Pramanik BN, Heimark L, et al. Posaconazole (Noxafil, SCH 56592), a new azole antifungal drug, was a discovery based on the isolation and mass spectral characterization of a circulating metabolite of an earlier lead (SCH 51048). *J Mass Spectrom*. 2008;43:509–517.

59. Guidance for Industry: Drug Interaction Studies: Study Design, Data Analysis, and Implications for Dosing and Labeling, Draft Guidance. U.S. Department of Health and Human Services, Food and Drug Administration; 2006.

60. Note for Guidance on the Investigation of Drug Interactions. Committee for Proprietary Medicinal Products, European Agency for the Evaluation of Medicinal Products; 2006. Available at: www.eudra.org/enmea.html.

61. Smith DA, Ackland MJ, Jones BC. Properties of cytochrome P450 isoenzymes and their substrates: Part 2. Properties of cytochrome P450 substrates. *Drug Discov Today*. 1997;2:479–486.

62. Ingelman-Sundberg M. The human genome project and novel aspects of cytochrome P450 research. *Toxicol Appl Pharmacol*. 2005;207(2 suppl): 52–56.

63. Mizutani T. PM frequencies of major CYPs in Asians and Caucasians. *Drug Metab Rev*. 2003;35:99–106.
64. PDR® Electronic Library™. Available at: www.thomsonhc.com/pdrel/librarian.
65. Honig PK, Wortham DC, Zamani K, Conner DP, Mullin JC, Cantilena LR. Terfenadine–ketoconazole interaction: pharmacokinetic and electrocardiographic consequences *J Am Med Assoc*. 1993;269:1513–1518.
66. Chu I, Favreau L, Soares A, Lin CC, Nomeir AA. Validation of higher-throughput high-performance liquid chromatography/atmospheric pressure chemical ionization tandem mass spectrometry assays to conduct cytochrome P450s CYP2D6 and CYP3A4 enzyme inhibition studies in human liver microsomes. *Rapid Commun Mass Spectrom*. 2002;14:207–214.
67. Nelson DL, Cox MM, Lehninger AL. *Principles of Biochemistry*, 4th ed. New York: W.H. Freeman; 2005.
68. Silverman RB. *Mechanism-Based Enzyme Inactivation: Chemistry and Enzymology*. Boca Raton, FL: CRC Press; 1988.
69. Wang RW, Newton DJ, Liu N, Atkins WM, Lu AYH. Human cytochrome P-450 3A4: in vitro drug–drug interaction patterns are substrate dependent. *Drug Metab Dispos*. 2000;28:360–366.
70. Walsky RL, Obach RS. Validates assays for human cytochrome P450 activities. *Drug Metab Dispos*. 2004;32:647–660.
71. Bu HZ, Knuth K, Magis L, Teitelbaum P. High-throughput cytochrome P450 (CYP) inhibition screening via cassette probe-dosing strategy: III. Validation of a direct injection/on-line guard cartridge extraction-tandem mass spectrometry method for CYP2C19 inhibition evaluation. *J Pharm Biomed Anal*. 2001;25:437–442.
72. Dierks EA, Stams KR, Lim HK, Cornelius G, Zhang H, Ball SE. A method for the simultaneous evaluation of the activities of seven major human drug-metabolizing cytochrome P450s using an in vitro cocktail of probe substrates and fast gradient liquid chromatography tandem mass spectrometry. *Drug Metab Dispos*. 2001;29:23–29.
73. Testino SA Jr, Patonay G. High-throughput inhibition screening of major human cytochrome P450 enzymes using an in vitro cocktail and liquid chromatography–tandem mass spectrometry. *J Pharm Biomed Anal*. 2003;30: 1459–1467.
74. Turpeinen M, Uusitalo J, Jalonen J, Pelkonen O. Multiple P450 substrates in a single run: rapid and comprehensive in vitro interaction assay. *Eur J Pharm Sci*. 2005;24:123–132.
75. Newton DJ, Wang RW, Lu AYH. Cytochrome P450 inhibitors: evaluation of specificities in the in vitro metabolism of therapeutic agents by human liver microsomes. *Drug Metab Dispos*. 1995;23:154–158.
76. Nomeir AA, Palamanda J, Favreau L. Identification of CYP mechanism-based inhibitors. In: Yan Z, Caldwell G, eds. *Optimization in Drug Discovery: In vitro Methods*. Totowa, NJ: Humana Press; 2004: 245–262.
77. Wrighton SA, Schuetz EG, Thummel KE, Shen DD, Korzekwa KR, Watkins PB. The human CYP3A subfamily: practical considerations. *Drug Metab Rev*. 2002;32:339–361.

78. Jenkins KM, Angeles R, Quintos MT, Xu R, Kassel DB, Rourick RA. Automated high throughput ADME assays for metabolic stability and cytochrome P450 inhibition profiling of combinatorial libraries. *J Pharm Biomed Anal*. 2004;34:989–1004.

79. Obach RS, Walsky RL, Venkatakrishnan K. Mechanism-based inactivation of human cytochrome P450 enzymes and the prediction of drug–drug interaction. *Drug Metab Dispos*. 2007;35:246–255.

80. Venkatakrishnan K, Obach RS. Drug–drug interactions via mechanism-based cytochrome P450 inactivation: points to consider for risk assessment from in vitro data and clinical pharmacologic evaluation. *Curr Drug Metab*. 2007;8:449–462.

81. Grime KH, Bird J, Ferguson D, Riley RJ. Mechanism-based inhibition of cytochrome P450 enzymes: an evaluation of early decision making in vitro approaches and drug–drug interaction prediction methods. *Eur J Pharm Sci*. 2009;36:175–191.

82. Nishiya Y, Hagihara K, Ito T, et al. Mechanism-based inhibition of human cytochrome P450 2B6 by ticlopidine, clopidogrel, and the thiolactone metabolite of prasugrel. *Drug Metab Dispos*. 2009;37:589–593.

83. Lin JH. CYP induction-mediated drug interactions: in vitro assessment and clinical implications. *Pharm Res*. 2006;23:1089–1116.

84. Hewitt NJ, de Kanter R, LeCluyse E. Induction of drug metabolizing enzymes: a survey of in vitro methodologies and interpretations used in the pharmaceutical industry—do they comply with FDA recommendations? *Chem Biol Interact*. 2007;168:51–65.

85. Hewitt NJ, LeCluyse EL, Ferguson SS. Induction of hepatic cytochrome P450 enzymes: methods, mechanisms, recommendations, and in vitro–in vivo correlations. *Xenobiotica*. 2007;3:1196–1224.

86. Kliewer SA, Moore JT, Wade L, et al. An orphan nuclear receptor activated by pregnanes defines a novel steroid signaling pathway. *Cell*. 1998;92:73–82.

87. Lehmann JM, McKee DD, Watson MA, Willson TM, Moore JT, Kliewer SA. The human orphan nuclear receptor PXR is activated by compounds that regulate CYP3A4 gene expression and cause drug interactions. *J Clin Invest*. 1998;102:1016–1023.

88. Hewitt NJ, Lechón MJ, Houston JB, et al. Primary hepatocytes: current understanding of the regulation of metabolic enzymes and transporter proteins, and pharmaceutical practice for the use of hepatocytes in metabolism, enzyme induction, transporter, clearance, and hepatotoxicity studies. *Drug Metab Rev*. 2007;39:159–234.

89. Lin JH, Lu AY. Interindividual variability in inhibition and induction of cytochrome P450 enzymes. *Annu Rev Pharmacol Toxicol*. 2001;41:535–567.

90. El-Sankary W, Gibson GG, Ayrton A, Plant N. Use of a reporter gene assay to predict and rank the potency and efficacy of CYP3A4 inducers. *Drug Metab Dispos*. 2001;29:1499–1504.

91. Luo G, Cunningham M, Kim S, et al. CYP3A4 induction by drugs: correlation between a pregnane X receptor reporter gene assay and CYP3A4 expression in human hepatocytes. *Drug Metab Dispos*. 2002;30:795–804.

92. Ripp SL, Mills JB, Fahmi OA, et al. Use of immortalized human hepatocytes to predict the magnitude of clinical drug–drug interactions caused by CYP3A4 induction. *Drug Metab Dispos*. 2006;34:1742–1748.

93. Martin H, Sarsat JP, de Waziers I, et al. Induction of cytochrome P450 2B6 and 3A4 expression by phenobarbital and cyclophosphamide in cultured human liver slices. *Pharm Res*. 2003;20:557–568.
94. Lake BG, Charzat C, Tredger JM, Renwick AB, Beamand JA, Price RJ. Induction of cytochrome P450 isoenzymes in cultured precision-cut rat and human liver slices. *Xenobiotica*. 1996;26:297–306.
95. LeCluyse EL. Human hepatocyte culture systems for the in vitro evaluation of cytochrome P450 expression and regulation. *Eur J Pharm Sci*. 2001;13:343–368.
96. Madan A, Graham RA, Carroll KM, et al. Effects of prototypical microsomal enzyme inducers on cytochrome P450 expression in cultured human hepatocytes. *Drug Metab Dispos*. 2003;31:421–431.
97. Bjornsson TD, Callaghan JT, Einolf HJ, et al. The conduct of in vitro and in vivo drug–drug interaction studies: a Pharmaceutical Research and Manufacturers of America (PhRMA) perspective. *Drug Metab Dispos*. 2003;31:815–832.
98. Kojima K, Nagata K, Matsubara T, Yamazoe Y. Broad but distinct role of pregnane X receptor on the expression of individual cytochrome P450s in human hepatocytes. *Drug Metab Pharmacokinet*. 2007;22:276–286.
99. Egnell AC, Houston B, Boyer S. In vivo CYP3A4 heteroactivation is a possible mechanism for the drug interaction between felbamate and carbamazepine. *J Pharmacol Exp Ther*. 2003;305:1251–1262.
100. Graves NM, Holmes GB, Fuerst RH, Leppik IE. Effect of felbamate on phenytoin and carbamazepine serum concentrations. *Epilepsia*. 1989;30:225–229.
101. Taft DR. The isolated perfused rat kidney model: a useful tool for drug discovery and development. *Curr Drug Discov Technol*. 2004;1:97–111.
102. Ghibellini G, Leslie EM, Brouwer KL. Methods to evaluate biliary excretion of drugs in humans: an updated review. *Mol Pharm*. 2006;3:198–211.
103. Chandra P, Brouwer KL. The complexities of hepatic drug transport: current knowledge and emerging concepts. *Pharm Res*. 2004;21:719–735.
104. Hoffmaster KA, Turncliff RZ, LeCluyse EL, Kim RB, Meier PJ, Brouwer KL. P-glycoprotein expression, localization, and function in sandwich-cultured primary rat and human hepatocytes: relevance to the hepatobiliary disposition of a model opioid peptide. *Pharm Res*. 2004;21:1294–1302.
105. Maurice M, Rogier E, Cassio D, Feldmann G. Formation of plasma membrane domains in rat hepatocytes and hepatoma cell lines in culture. *J Cell Sci*. 1988;90:79–92.
106. Liu X, Brouwer KL, Gan LS, et al. Partial maintenance of taurocholate uptake by adult rat hepatocytes cultured in a collagen sandwich configuration. *Pharm Res*. 1998;15:1533–1539.
107. LeCluyse EL, Audus KL, Hochman JH. Formation of extensive canalicular networks by rat hepatocytes cultured in collagen-sandwich configuration. *Am J Physiol*. 1994;266: C1764–C1774.
108. Dunn JC, Yarmush ML, Koebe HG, Tompkins RG. Hepatocyte function and extracellular matrix geometry: long-term culture in a sandwich configuration. *FASEB J*. 1989;3:174–177. Erratum in: *FASEB J*. 1989; 3: 1873.

109. Liu X, Chism JP, LeCluyse EL, Brouwer KR, Brouwer KL. Correlation of biliary excretion in sandwich-cultured rat hepatocytes and in vivo in rats. *Drug Metab Dispos*. 1999;7:37–44.

110. Liu X, LeCluyse EL, Brouwer KR, et al. Biliary excretion in primary rat hepatocytes cultured in a collagen-sandwich configuration. *Am J Physiol*. 1999;277: G12–G21.

111. LeCluyse EL, Bullock PL, Parkinson A, Hochman JH. Cultured rat hepatocytes. *Pharm Biotechnol*. 1996;8:121–159.

112. Liu X, LeCluyse EL, Brouwer KR, Lightfoot RM, Lee JI, Brouwer KL. Use of Ca^{2+} modulation to evaluate biliary excretion in sandwich-cultured rat hepatocytes. *J Pharmacol Exp Ther*. 1999;289:1592–1599.

113. McRae MP, Lowe CM, Tian X, et al. Ritonavir, saquinavir, and efavirenz, but not nevirapine, inhibit bile acid transport in human and rat hepatocytes. *J Pharmacol Exp Ther*. 2006;318:1068–1075.

114. Ghibellini G, Vasist LS, Leslie EM, et al. In vitro–in vivo correlation of hepatobiliary drug clearance in humans. *Clin Pharmacol Ther*. 2007;81:406–413.

115. Mei H, Korfmacher W, Morrison R. Rapid in vivo oral screening in rats: reliability, acceptance criteria, and filtering efficiency. *AAPS J*. 2006;8: E493–E500.

116. White RE, Manitpisitkul P. Pharmacokinetic theory of cassette dosing in drug discovery screening. *Drug Metab Dispos*. 2001;29:957–966.

117. Christ DD. Cassette dosing pharmacokinetics: valuable tool or flawed science? Commentary. *Drug Metab Dispos*. 2001;29: 935.

118. Manitpisitkul P, White RE. Whatever happened to cassette-dosing pharmacokinetics? *Drug Discov Today*. 2004;9:652–658.

119. Smith NF, Raynaud FI, Workman P. The application of cassette dosing for pharmacokinetic screening in small-molecule cancer drug discovery. *Mol Cancer Ther*. 2007;6:428–440.

120. Raynaud FI, Fischer PM, Nutley BP, Goddard PM, Lane DP, Workman P. Cassette dosing pharmacokinetics of a library of 2,6,9-trisubstituted purine cyclin-dependent kinase 2 inhibitors prepared by parallel synthesis. *Mol Cancer Ther*. 2004;3:353–362.

121. Proksch JW, Ward KW. Cassette dosing pharmacokinetic studies for evaluation of ophthalmic drugs for posterior ocular diseases. *J Pharm Sci*. 2007;19:1–11.

122. He K, Qian M, Wong H, et al. *N*-in-1 dosing pharmacokinetics in drug discovery: experience, theoretical and practical considerations. *J Pharm Sci*. 2007;3:1–13.

123. Janser P, Neumann U, Miltz W, Feifel R, Buhl T. A cassette-dosing approach for improvement of oral bioavailability of dual TACE/MMP inhibitors. *Bioorg Med Chem Lett*. 2006;16:2632–2636.

124. Watanabe T, Schulz D, Morisseau C, Hammock BD. High-throughput pharmacokinetic method: cassette dosing in mice associated with minuscule serial bleedings and LC/MS/MS analysis. *Anal Chim Acta*. 2006;559:37–44.

125. Smith NF, Hayes A, Nutley BP, Raynaud FI, Workman P. Evaluation of the cassette dosing approach for assessing the pharmacokinetics of geldanamycin analogues in mice. *Cancer Chemother Pharmacol*. 2004;54:475–486.

126. Kuo BS, Van Noord T, Feng MR, Wright DS. Sample pooling to expedite bioanalysis and pharmacokinetic research. *J Pharm Biomed Anal*. 1998;16:837–846.

127. Cox KA, Dunn-Meynell K, Korfmacher WA, et al. Novel procedure for rapid pharmacokinetic screening of discovery compounds in rats. *Drug Discov Today*. 1999;4:232–237.

128. Korfmacher WA, Cox KA, Ng KJ, et al. Cassette-accelerated rapid rat screen: a systematic procedure for the dosing and liquid chromatography/atmospheric pressure ionization tandem mass spectrometric analysis of new chemical entities as part of new drug discovery. *Rapid Commun Mass Spectrom*. 2001;15:335–340.

129. van de Waterbeemd H, Gifford E. ADMET in silico modelling: towards prediction paradise? *Nat Rev Drug Discov*. 2003;2:192–204.

130. Hou T, Wang J, Zhang W, Wang W, Xu X. Recent advances in computational prediction of drug absorption and permeability in drug discovery. *Curr Med Chem*. 2006;13:2653–2667.

131. Hou T, Wang J, Li Y. ADME evaluation in drug discovery: 8. The prediction of human intestinal absorption by a support vector machine. *J Chem Inf Model*. 2007;47:2408–2415.

132. Huisinga W, Telgmann R, Wulkow M. The virtual laboratory approach to pharmacokinetics: design principles and concepts. *Drug Discov Today*. 2006;11:800–805.

133. Norinder U, Bergström CA. Prediction of ADMET properties. *ChemMedChem*. 2006;1:920–937.

134. Smith DA. Hello Drug Discovery, I am from In silico, take me to your president. *Drug Discov Today*. 2002;7:1080–1081.

135. Lipinski CA, Lombardo F, Dominy BW, Feeney PJ. Experimental and computational approaches to estimate solubility and permeability in drug discovery and development settings. *Adv Drug Deliv Rev*. 1997;23:3–25.

136. Lipinski CA. Drug-like properties and the causes of poor solubility and poor permeability. *J Pharmacol Toxicol Methods*. 2000;44:235–249.

137. Ekins S, Boulanger B, Swaan PW, Hupcey MA. Towards a new age of virtual ADME/TOX and multidimensional drug discovery. *J Comput Aided Mol Des*. 2002;16:381–401.

138. Tetko IV, Bruneau P, Mewes HW, Rohrer DC, Poda GI. Can we estimate the accuracy of ADME-Tox predictions? *Drug Discov Today*. 2006;11:700–707.

139. Liu X, Tu M, Kelly RS, Chen C, Smith BJ. Development of a computational approach to predict blood–brain barrier permeability. *Drug Metab Dispos*. 2004;32:132–139.

140. Jensen BF, Vind C, Padkjaer SB, Brockhoff PB, Refsgaard HH. In silico prediction of cytochrome P450 2D6 and 3A4 inhibition using Gaussian kernel weighted *k*-nearest neighbor and extended connectivity fingerprints, including structural fragment analysis of inhibitors versus noninhibitors. *J Med Chem*. 2007;50:501–511.

141. O'Brien SE, de Groot MJ. Greater than the sum of its parts: combining models for useful ADMET prediction. *J Med Chem*. 2007;48:1287–1291.

142. Sakiyama Y, Yuki H, Moriya T, et al. Predicting human liver microsomal stability with machine learning techniques. *J Mol Graph Model*. 2008;26:607–615.

143. Nicholson JK, Lindon JC, Holmes E. "Metabonomics": understanding the metabolic responses of living systems to pathophysiological stimuli via multivariate statistical analysis of biological NMR spectroscopic data. *Xenobiotica*. 1999;29:1181–1189.

144. Lindon JC, Holmes E, Nicholson JK. Metabonomics in pharmaceutical R&D. *FEBS J*. 2007;274:1140–1151.

145. Claudino WM, Quattrone A, Biganzoli L, Pestrin M, Bertini I, Di Leo A. Metabolomics: available results, current research projects in breast cancer, and future applications. *J Clin Oncol*. 2007;25:2840–2846.

146. Ryals J. Metabolomics: an important emerging science. Business Briefing. *Pharmatech*. 2004; 51–54. Available at: www.touchbriefings.com.

147. German JB, Hammock BD, Watkins SM. Metabolomics: building on a century of biochemistry to guide human health. *Metabolomics*. 2005;1:3–9.

148. Morvan D, Demidem A. Metabolomics by proton nuclear magnetic resonance spectroscopy of the response to chloroethylnitrosourea reveals drug efficacy and tumor adaptive metabolic pathways. *Cancer Res*. 2007;67:2150–2159.

149. van Ravenzwaay B, Cunha GC, Leibold E, et al. The use of metabolomics for the discovery of new biomarkers of effect. *Toxicol Lett*. 2007;172:21–28.

150. Dettmer K, Aronov PA, Hammock BD. Mass spectrometry–based metabolomics. *Mass Spectrom Rev*. 2007;26:51–78.

151. Weljie AM, Dowlatabadi R, Miller BJ, Vogel HJ, Jirik FR. An inflammatory arthritis-associated metabolite biomarker pattern revealed by ^{1}H NMR spectroscopy. *J Proteome Res*. 2007;6:3456–3464.

152. Goodacre R, Vaidyanathan S, Dunn WB, Harrigan GG, Kell DB. Metabolomics by numbers: acquiring and understanding global metabolite data. *Trends Biotechnol*. 2004;22:245–252.

153. van Doorn M, Vogels J, Tas A, et al. Evaluation of metabolite profiles as biomarkers for the pharmacological effects of thiazolidinediones in type 2 diabetes mellitus patients and healthy volunteers. *Br J Clin Pharmacol*. 2007;63:562–574.

154. Jordan KW, Cheng LL. NMR-based metabolomics approach to target biomarkers for human prostate cancer. *Expert Rev Proteomics*. 2007;4:389–400.

155. Zhen Y, Krausz KW, Chen C, Idle JR, Gonzalez FJ. Metabolomic and genetic analysis of biomarkers for peroxisome proliferator-activated receptor alpha expression and activation. *Mol Endocrinol*. 2007;21:2136–2151.

3

PREDICTION OF PHARMACOKINETICS AND DRUG SAFETY IN HUMANS

PETER L. BULLOCK

3.1 INTRODUCTION

ADME (absorption, distribution, metabolism, and excretion) and toxicology failures cost drug sponsors up to $2 billion annually, resulting in extensive attempts to develop efficient approaches during drug discovery and early drug development, which can predict such failures successfully. The major strategy with these approaches is to identify potentially problematic compounds as soon as possible, thereby increasing the likelihood of success for those compounds that enter into clinical development.

The primary goal of this chapter is to describe the application and limitations of models, methods, techniques, and processes available to predict human pharmacokinetics and possible safety issues of potential drug candidates during drug discovery and development. In addition, relatively new and/or untested methods for predicting issues related to pharmacokinetics and safety are included but do not receive a thorough discussion, as many are untested beyond a small number of compounds. Some of the methodologies described are also discussed in other chapters, but the focus here is on the predictability of such tests to human subjects under the conditions of the therapeutic regimen targeted.

Typically, in small and medium-sized innovator companies, lead optimization depends heavily on in vitro models and less on in vivo and in silico methods, due to resource limitations. This may not be the case in big pharma companies, which generally have the resources to use all the methods discussed here. In

Early Drug Development: Strategies and Routes to First-in-Human Trials, Edited by Mitchell N. Cayen

fact, accurate prediction of the outcome of interactions between complex biological systems and xenobiotics is nearly an unattainable goal. Modeling these interactions to forecast or estimate disposition and adverse effects is perhaps the best that one can expect. Therefore, it is important to note that all models provide inaccurate predictions, but some models can be very useful. Modern pharmaceutical scientists drawn from several disciplines use these in vitro, in vivo, and in silico tools to create hypotheses about specific chemical–biological interactions and then generalize to other circumstances. In this chapter we demonstrate the rational application and limitations of these approaches and, whenever possible, emphasize the importance of evaluating pharmacokinetics and safety data from multiple sources. Typically, a winning strategy begins with a preliminary product profile as early as possible in drug discovery, which is a consensus document that should function as a well-conceived, living document through nonclinical programs. Moreover, the scope of the nonclinical program and the complexity of predictions should be matched to the intended therapeutic application of the candidate drug.

The development of new in vitro and in vivo/ex vivo models and methods of varying sophistication has facilitated the early investigation of dispositional behavior and cellular toxicity of new compounds very early in lead optimization. However, three major challenges are associated with using some of the more biologically or computationally advanced techniques:

1. The creation, organization, search, and integration of enormous databases in a user-friendly manner
2. Interpretation of the results based on our imperfect understanding of the different ways that biological systems react and interact
3. The relationship between these techniques, which is frequently based on nonhuman biology and outcomes obtained in human volunteers and patients

Ultimately, the responsibility of pharmaceutical scientists is to reduce the risk and cost of failure by collecting sufficient evidence on the nature and consequences of chemical–biological interactions to estimate or postulate the potential behavior of drug candidates confidently in human subjects. The value of these methods and models in predicting pharmacokinetic behavior and safety has changed over time. For example, the results of early large and complex toxicogenomics and metabolomics studies in nonhuman species using well-characterized reference xenobiotics were difficult to interpret because what we truly understand about biology is only a fraction of what there is to know. Early practitioners of these studies had difficulty comprehending the context and significance of the data and struggled with relating it to human safety concerns. However, as our collective experience applying these tools and databases accumulates and our genomic and proteomic knowledge expands, the emerging results have more significance and their predictive value has increased. The maturation of these very complex technologies has been accelerated by cooperation between scientists from academia, industry, and government.

On the contrary, some simpler biological models have been applied to questions of pharmacokinetics and safety for many years, becoming integrated into optimization algorithms and sometimes undergoing refinements during that time. Examples of these models include the use of human liver microsomes and hepatocyte suspensions to determine the hepatic clearance, kinetics of metabolism, and potential for drug interactions of candidate compounds with existing medications and the application of Caco-2 and other cell monolayers to investigate human intestinal drug absorption (Chapter 2). These models have historical value, permitting us to maintain comparability, if not complete continuity, between results obtained over dozens of years of research. The sequence of predictive studies generally proceeds from simple protocols to complex, lower to higher cost, not necessarily in vitro/ex vivo to in vivo. Two decades ago, many of the investigations now conducted during drug discovery were not carried out until a commitment was made to begin a nonclinical program (e.g., metabolism-based drug interactions, enzyme induction, and intestinal absorption). Typically, the most complex studies, such as toxicogenomic or metabolomic evaluations for safety, are often used to address questions arising from experimental studies, the answers to which frequently lie on the critical path for further development.

This chapter is organized according to the application of these three types of predictive methods, first to pharmacokinetic behavior and subsequently to the prediction of drug safety. Experimental methods in vitro take advantage of simple protocols using new biological tools, including subcellular fractions, recombinant proteins, immortalized cell lines, and primary cells, as well as a number of sensitive and specific analytical tools and methods. Methods based on in vivo experiments use biological matrices harvested from animal studies and form the basis of toxicogenomic and metabolomic/metabonomic investigations. In the final sections, in silico methods used to predict pharmacokinetics and safety are reviewed.

The selection of specific combinations of these in vitro, in vivo, and in silico methods for use in any lead optimization program will depend on the resources available to the program. Well-resourced programs conducted by large innovator companies tend to use most or all of the methods described in this chapter, whereas more modest programs tend to rely on in vitro and in vivo techniques to arrive at nomination of NCEs for further development.

3.2 PREDICTION OF HUMAN PHARMACOKINETIC BEHAVIOR

Some of the pharmacokinetic and ADME models discussed in this section have been described in Chapter 2. However, the focus in this chapter is the application of these models in the prediction of the pharmacokinetics of the drug candidate during therapeutic treatment of human subjects.

3.2.1 In Vitro Models for Predicting Intestinal Absorption, Intrinsic Hepatic Clearance, and Drug Interactions

The pharmacokinetic behavior (i.e., bioavailability, clearance, etc.) of xenobiotics after oral administration is a function of four processes traditionally encompassed by the acronym ADME. This simplification understates the complexity and elasticity of the biological processes involved in determining the final pharmacokinetic picture. There are several formidable biochemical barriers that function to limit the absorption of orally administered xenobiotics in the gastrointestinal tract [1]. The majority of small-molecule drugs cross the intestinal barrier by passive diffusion through the apical lipid membrane of enterocytes, which are joined by tight junctions. The intestinal absorption, and thus the bioavailability, of many drugs are limited by poor permeability. Permeability is a kinetic variable, which depends in part on lipophilicity. It is one of two important pharmaceutical properties included in the Biopharmaceutics Classification System (BCS) for the purpose of predicting the bioavailability and bioequivalence of orally administered, immediate-release medicinal compounds [2]. Figure 3.1 summarizes the four classes, which are based on these two independent properties of medicinal compounds. The other important pharmaceutical property considered in the BCS is aqueous solubility, a thermodynamic property whose effect on pharmacokinetic behavior is discussed later in the chapter. The relative importance of poor solubility and poor permeability to oral absorption depends on the approach used for lead generation [3].

Until a decade ago, the liver was thought to be the only important site of first-pass metabolism for orally administered drugs, but many reports have been published in the interim concerning the important role of the small intestine in influencing the bioavailability of many xenobiotics [4]. Drug-metabolizing enzymes are widely distributed throughout the body in humans, especially at sites of drug absorption (e.g., the gastrointestinal tract and liver) or compartments that require protection (e.g., the blood–brain barrier). Expression of these enzymes is relatively high in mammalian liver, but also in skin, the entire respiratory system, kidney, and the intestinal epithelium. Although the liver remains an important site of drug metabolism, duodenal and jejeunal enterocytes express several enzymes belonging to the important CYP450, as well as glutathione-*S*-transferase [5] and UDP-glucuronosyltransferase superfamilies [6]. Lower levels of expression have been observed in the eye, adrenal, pancreas, spleen, heart, brain, testis, ovary,

Class I High Permeability – High Solubility	Class II High Permeability – Low Solubility
Class III Low Permeability – High Solubility	Class IV Low Permeability – Low Solubility

FIGURE 3.1 The four major biopharmaceutical classes with respect to bioavailability and bioequivalence based on drug permeability and solubility.

TABLE 3.1 Relative Expression Levels of CYP450 Enzymes in Human Tissues

Organ	Level of Expression (nmol CYP450/mg tissue)
Liver	0.25–1.5
Lung	0.05–0.25
Small intestine	0.02–0.15
Brain	<0.1

placenta, and blood cells. Table 3.1 illustrates the relative expression levels of CYP450 enzymes observed in four metabolically important human tissues.

Drug interactions that affect pharmacokinetic behavior occur at several sites within the body, including in the gastrointestinal mucosa and the liver, and at drug-binding sites on plasma proteins. Drug interactions appear to be changes in the rate or extent of absorption as a result of changes in the function of drug transporters, alterations in the metabolism of compounds by way of inhibition or induction of metabolic enzymes and changes in the plasma concentration of one drug by competition with another for plasma protein binding (Chapter 2). During the past decade, the commercial availability of human biological products (e.g., liver microsomes, hepatocytes, recombinant enzymes, transporters) has helped improve predictions of pharmacokinetic behavior and reduced the previous uncertainty associated with using the nonhuman analogs of these tools.

Intestinal Absorption Certain physical and chemical properties of compounds affect their permeability through the intestinal barrier. Lipinski's rule of five was developed to predict passive intestinal permeability based on elementary physical and chemical properties. It was derived from a decade of experience with very large data sets of proprietary compounds and from testing the permeability of more than 300 marketed medications and proprietary compounds in Caco-2 (human colon adenocarcinoma cell line) monolayers [7]. Its predictive value appears to be very high, as the majority of pharmaceutical chemists incorporate these considerations when designing and selecting new compounds to synthesize. The rule of five suggests that poor absorption or permeability is more likely when a drug molecule (1) contains more than five hydrogen bond donors, (2) has a molecular weight above 500 Da, (3) has a log P value greater than 5, and (4) contains more than 10 hydrogen bond acceptors. Figure 3.2 shows the structure of a lead compound accompanied by its rule of five values, all of which are within the specified limits, with the exception of molecular weight, which exceeds 500 Da. However, this compound was well absorbed, despite the excessive mass.

To predict the pharmacokinetic behavior of orally administered medicinal compounds, some information needs to be generated as to how well the compounds cross the human intestinal barrier. Prior to 1989, in situ rodent intestinal perfusion models were used almost exclusively to estimate the absorption of

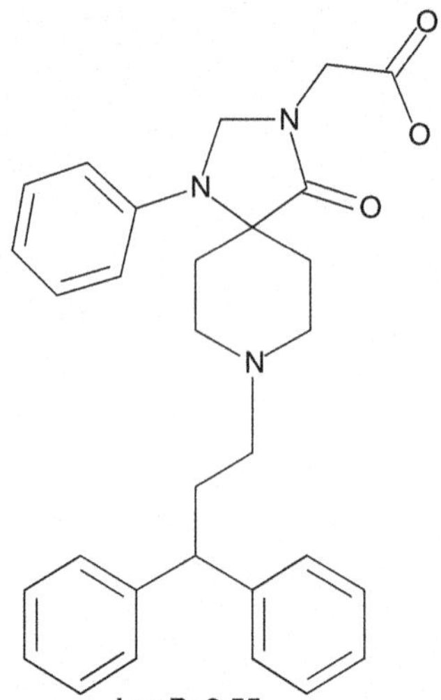

LogP: 3.55
MW: 551
Hydrogen bond donors: 2
Hydrogen bond acceptors: 6

FIGURE 3.2 Structure of a lead compound and the values for the rule of five as it pertains to permeability.

new compounds. After 1990, the apparent permeability coefficient (P_{app}), that is, the rate at which compounds traverse a cell monolayer, began to be widely adopted as an index of permeability. The value of P_{app} of compounds tested in Caco-2 monolayers model provided a reasonable prediction of human intestinal absorption [8,9]. The relationship between P_{app} and fraction absorbed appeared to suggest that when $P_{app} > 2 \times 10^{-6}$ cm/s, that fractional human intestinal absorption was going to be nearly complete ($\geq 90\%$) [10]. However, the relationship between P_{app} and fractional absorption is very steep and suggests that compounds can be reliably characterized only as either well or poorly absorbed. The value of P_{app} represents the net apical (luminal) to basolateral (serosal) movement of solute across the monolayer, that is, the human intestinal barrier, and is frequently the sum of several influences. This prediction works best to rank-order relative absorption or compounds within a series of chemical analogs, all with similar solubility in the cell culture medium. Table 3.2 illustrates the differences in Caco-2 permeability and intestinal absorption predicted for three potential lead candidates within a series of potential candidates for a novel anti-infective medication. Clearly, compound 02 will probably be much more permeable across the intestinal barrier, as the value of its P_{app} in the apical-to-basal (A-to-B) direction is at least an order of magnitude greater than the values exhibited by the other two test compounds shown. In fact, when all three compounds were orally administered to rats as a solution (20% hydroxyl-β-propylcyclodextran in water), compound 02 had much better bioavailability than the other two compounds.

TABLE 3.2 Differences in the Apparent Permeability (P_{app}), Efflux Ratio, and Absorption Potential of Three Chemical Analogs Tested in Caco-2 Cell Monolayers Cultured in 24-Well Transwell Plates

Test Compound ID	Direction[a]	Initial Donor Concentration (μM)	Recovery (%)	Mean P_{app} (10^{-6} cm/s)	Efflux Ratio	Absorption Potential	Significant Efflux
02	A-to-B	6.83	56	6.56	0.5	High	No
	B-to-A	7.07	54	3.27			
	Cell free	6.60	71	7.60			
29	A-to-B	6.21	54	0.87	1.3	Low	No
	B-to-A	6.31	60	1.11			
	Cell free	5.85	63	1.67			
40	A-to-B	7.11	63	0.59	1.0	Low	No
	B-to-A	6.64	57	0.56			
	Cell free	6.62	64	1.11			

[a] A-to-B, apical-to-basolateral direction; B-to-A, basolateral-to-apical direction; cell free, apical-to-basolateral direction measured in the absence of cell monolayers.

Many of the original reference compounds used to establish this method were quite soluble, in contrast to the current situation, where poor solubility and high lipophilicity appear to be common and significant problems. Therefore, the recovery of a test article is important in deciding the validity of results. Furthermore, these monolayers express drug-metabolizing enzymes and membrane-bound transporters that may complicate the interpretation of the results when the value of P_{app} is low. When the output of medicinal compounds began to rise around 1995 as a result of combinatorial synthesis and chemical "libraries," new in vitro models with increased testing capacity were required. Accordingly, this model was optimized for higher-throughput screening, and currently most of the permeability screening is conducted during drug discovery for the purpose of lead selection. However, the Caco-2 monolayer retains some value as a method of predicting the answers to mechanistic questions concerning absorption or drug interactions that arise during clinical testing. This prediction of absorption of immediate-release drugs by measuring permeability in vitro has been incorporated into the BCS. This protocol has been incorporated, along with measurements of aqueous solubility and dissolution of the product, into the U.S. Food and Drug Administration (FDA) bioequivalence guideline [11,12]. A drug substance is considered highly soluble when the highest dose strength is soluble in 250 mL of water over the pH range 1.0 to 7.5. A drug substance is considered highly permeable when the extent of absorption in humans is determined to be greater than 90% (e.g., $P_{app} > 1 \times 10^{-5}$ cm/s). Finally, a drug substance may be considered rapidly dissolving when greater than 85% of the labeled amount dissolves within 30 minutes using *U.S. Pharmacopeia* apparatus I or II in a volume of 900 mL or less. In fact, this paradigm for predicting bioequivalence by considering solubility and permeability is slowly being accepted globally after having been used to test its validity on 123 immediate-release products from the World Health Organization [12,13]. In addition, nongovernmental collaborations have extended the number of products evaluated by this method [14].

Intrinsic Hepatic Clearance In a recent review, it was noted that 75% of the top 200 drugs prescribed in the United States are cleared by metabolism in the liver, and two-thirds of these are metabolized by one or more CYP450 enzymes [15]. Therefore, the prediction of hepatic intrinsic clearance becomes important in the selection and optimization of most lead candidates. It is possible to estimate the contribution of any metabolic pathway by determining the intrinsic clearance (CL'_{int}) of that particular reaction by calculating the ratio V_{max}/K_m by monitoring the formation of each metabolite. However, during drug discovery, including lead optimization, it is more likely that simpler methods will be selected. In fact, human CL_{int} may be estimated by measuring the in vitro half-life of compounds in incubations with pooled human liver microsomes or human hepatocyte suspensions. This approach was originally suggested in 1975 [16] and was extended later [17]. It was not until much later, after the recognition that drug discovery required acceleration and predictions needed improvement, that robust microsomal methods were worked out and new techniques using hepatocytes were added [18]. The equation used for the microsomal procedure is

$$CL'_{int} = \frac{0.693 \cdot \text{liver weight}}{\text{in vitro } t_{1/2} \cdot \text{ liver in incubation } \cdot f_{u(\text{inc})}}$$

where $f_{u(\text{inc})}$ represents the unbound fraction of drug in microsomal incubations. Here, the value of liver weight is 21 g/kg for humans, the value of liver in incubation is based on 45 mg of microsomal protein per gram of tissue, and $f_{u(\text{inc})}$ is the unbound fraction in microsomal incubations. For practical purposes the latter term is typically omitted during lead selection and included during lead optimization. The unbound fraction of drug can, in part, influence the accuracy of the prediction [19]. The fidelity of this technique depends to some degree on whether the compound in question is basic, neutral, or acidic, based on the degree of nonspecific binding to microsomal material [20]. The parallel equation when suspensions of isolated human hepatocytes are used is

$$CL'_{int} = (0.693/t_{1/2}) \cdot (\text{mL/million cells} \cdot \text{million cells/g liver} \cdot \text{g liver/kg})$$

Here, the value of cells per gram of liver is 1.35×10^6. The variable in this case is the number of cells per milliliter selected for any given experiment. It appears that the use of hepatocyte suspensions yields somewhat more accurate predictions than the microsomal method. In addition, the microsomal method works well to predict CL'_{int} when the test compounds are metabolized primarily by CYP450 enzymes.

Drug–Drug Interactions The evaluation of the potential of an NCE to be involved in clinical drug–drug interactions and the possible impact of such an interaction on its pharmacokinetic behavior are an integral part of the drug development process and regulatory review prior to market approval [21]. Four fundamental questions require consideration:

1. Will established drugs alter the plasma exposure to the new drug?
2. Will the new drug change plasma exposure to other drugs?
3. Should exposure alterations occur, will this result in changes in the safety and/or efficacy of either drug?
4. Most important, will these interactions alter the exposure, safety, and/or efficacy significantly enough to require dose adjustment of the new drug or other, coadministered medicines?

In vitro metabolic studies are now widely accepted as a critical step in candidate drug selection and early drug development, as the results of these studies can be used to establish the need for subsequent in vivo assessment of potential drug–drug interactions. Our understanding of the in vitro–in vivo correlations regarding drug interactions and the ability to predict possible interactions has improved significantly during the past decade. However, the biological tools used for the identification of substrates, inhibitors, and inducers of drug transporters, and the ability to predict potential transporter-mediated drug interactions are much less advanced than those for drug-metabolizing enzymes such as those of the CYP450 system.

Role of Drug-Metabolizing Enzymes in Drug Interactions Since 1997 the FDA and other regulatory agencies have emphasized the importance of documenting the potential of new oral drug candidates to be involved in metabolism-based pharmacokinetic drug interactions with coadministered medicines before the candidates reach FIH studies. Many of these interactions have received considerable attention because some successful drugs (e.g., terfenadine, cisapride) caused severe adverse effects when coadministered with certain anti-infectives.

Human liver contains about a dozen of these enzymes, which exhibit broad and overlapping substrate specificity. As mentioned previously, CYP450 enzymes are very important in this context because of their involvement in the metabolic elimination of the majority of marketed drugs. Six of these microsomal CYP450 enzymes are considered clinically important: CYP3A4, CYP2D6, CYP2C9, CYP2C19, CYP2C8, and CYP2B6. Due to this broad specificity, it is possible that two or more CYP450 enzymes can contribute to the metabolism of a single candidate compound and that many therapeutically unrelated drugs can be metabolized by the same enzyme. When multiple CYP450 enzymes metabolize the same compound, their relative contribution is determined by the ratio V_{max}/K_m and the intrinsic clearance (e.g., oxycodone, CYP2D6, CYP3A4). When a single CYP450 enzyme determines the rate of elimination of many drugs, they typically exhibit very different affinities and rates of reaction (e.g., serotonin reuptake inhibitors, CYP2D6).

Human in vitro systems are commercially available to investigate drug interactions for the purpose of predicting if new compounds could be involved in clinically significant CYP450-related pharmacokinetic interactions, by assisting in the design of meaningful and cost-effective clinical drug interaction studies [22–24]. These tools include characterized human liver microsomes and enzyme-selective probe substrates and inhibitors combined with rapid and sensitive analysis via liquid chromatography (LC)–mass spectrometry (MS)/MS. Predictions of potential pharmacokinetic drug interactions are derived from two types of in vitro studies. Enzyme identification and inhibition studies using pooled human liver microsomes are employed to determine if a candidate drug is capable of inhibiting interacting with any of the clinically relevant CYP450 enzymes and to what degree. The results of enzyme induction studies, conducted in human liver microsomes and/or cultured hepatocytes, are typically used to predict the effect of a test compound on the level of expression of clinically relevant CYP450s. Consensus recommendations for appropriate experimental protocols used for CYP450 inhibition studies have been refined and published [25–27], and an example used in a big pharma company is presented in Chapter 2. These include recommendations for CYP450-selective probe substrates with which to measure the activity of each enzyme and for potent and selective reference inhibitors with which to compare the results of the candidate compound, and methods for carrying out required experiments. Table 3.3 summarizes the relative importance of the major human liver CYP450 enzymes and includes CYP450-selective probe substrate reactions and preferred reference inhibitors (positive controls) for use in inhibition studies. In a typical protocol for this type of study, a test compound is incubated with human liver microsomes at pH 7.4 in the presence of the probe substrate, which is present at a concentration that approximates the K_m value for the reaction. The reactions are started with the addition of NADPH and the mixture is incubated at 37°C. Typically, in the absence of pharmacokinetic data, the test compound is included at one to three concentrations of the compound undergoing evaluation. Negative controls contain no compound other than the organic solvent in which the compound was dissolved. No such recommendations have been proposed for conducting human CYP450 induction studies in vitro.

Pharmacokinetic Interactions Mediated by Enzyme Inhibition It is important to remember that if an NCE is metabolized by a particular CYP450 enzyme, it can inhibit that enzyme to a degree that depends on the affinity of the drug for the catalytic site of the enzyme (K_m) and the concentration of the compound under investigation. Conversely, however, a compound is not necessarily metabolized by a CYP450 enzyme merely because it inhibits that enzyme. An excellent example of this apparent contradiction is quinidine, which is a potent inhibitor of CYP2D6 but is metabolized by other CYP450 enzymes, including CYP3A4 [28].

TABLE 3.3 Characteristics of Human Liver CYP450 Enzymes and Their Probe Substrates

CYP450	Typical Proportion in Human Liver (%)	Proportion of Drugs Affected (%)	Preferred/Acceptable Reactions	Preferred Inhibitor
CYP3A	30	52	Testosterone 6β-hydroxylation and midazolam 1-hydroxylation	Ketoconazole
CYP2C9	12	11	Tolbutamide methyl-hydroxylation or diclofenac 4′-hydroxylation	Sulfaphenazole
CYP1A2	12	5	Phenacetin O-deethylation or 7-Ethoxyresorufin O-deethylation	Furafylline
CYP2C8	7	1	Taxol 6-hydroxylation or amodiaquine N-deethylation	Quercetin
CYP2E1	7	4	Chlorzoxazone 6-hydroxylation	Diethyldithio-carbamate
CYP2B6	3	25	Bupropion hydroxylation or efavirenz hydroxylation	Ticlopidine
CYP2D6	1.5	30	Bufuralol 1′-hydroxylation or dextromethorphan O-demethylation	Quinidine
CYP2C19	0.2	4	*S*-Mephenytoin 4′-hydroxylation or omeprazole hydroxylation	Ticlopidine

When they occur, metabolism-based pharmacokinetic interactions involving enzyme inhibition can cause a large increase in exposure to one of the drugs administered, by acting as an alternate substrate or an inhibitor, which frequently leads to the onset of adverse rather than therapeutic effects [22]. This type of interaction most frequently arises from the competition between two compounds for the specific CYP450. These interactions can also occur via noncompetitive (allosteric) interactions or by metabolic inactivation of an enzyme by one of the drugs. Metabolic interactions can occur in the small intestine. Thus, the purpose of investigating drug candidates as CYP450 inhibitors in vitro is to qualitatively predict their potential to change pharmacokinetic behavior. For example, if polymorphically expressed CYP2D6 is inhibited strongly by a candidate compound, the following are factors that must be considered when the possible in vivo human significance of the inhibition is predicted:

- The extent to which the candidate is cleared by CYP2D6
- The potential for saturating the metabolic capacity of CYP2D6 (easier in poor metabolizers than in extensive metabolizers)

- The pharmacokinetic behavior of the candidate drug (the potential inhibitor)
- The possible magnitude and potential consequences of alterations (typically, increases) in the pharmacokinetic behavior of other CYP2D6 substrates, specifically exposure [the area under the plasma or serum concentration–time curve (AUC)]
- The likelihood that the candidate drug will be administered with other medications that are CYP2D6 substrates during therapeutic treatment of the target population

The first factor links reaction phenotyping (enzyme identification) and enzyme inhibition studies. As an example, for a given in vivo concentration of a potential inhibitor, as the fraction of the coadministered medication cleared by metabolism (f_m) increases, the AUC will increase nonlinearly, until at $f_m = 0.99$, the exposure, expressed as the AUC, can typically increase 35-fold [22]. This was the case for terfenadine exposure when it was coadministered with normal doses of ketoconazole, a potent CYP450 inhibitor [29]. After conducting an extensive analysis of the utility of these enzyme inhibition studies, Obach et al. concluded that CYP450 in vitro inhibition data are valuable in designing clinical drug–drug interaction study strategies and can be used to predict the magnitude of these interactions [30].

To complete a semiquantitative prediction of the effect of a candidate drug on the pharmacokinetic behavior of an established drug, it is important to determine K_i, the inhibition rate constant, of the candidate compound for each of the major human liver CYP450 enzymes. K_i is an intrinsic inhibition constant that defines the affinity of the test compound (as opposed to the probe substrate) for the enzyme in question. The value of K_i is much more reproducible from one laboratory to another than IC_{50}, which is specific to a given set of experimental conditions. Currently, the FDA recommends that the ratio $[I]/K_i$ should be used to qualitatively predict the probability of significant pharmacokinetic interactions [21], where [I] represents the mean steady-state C_{max} value for total drug (bound + unbound) following administration of the highest clinical dose proposed. For example, given a marketed drug with $f_m = 0.70$, if $[I]/K_i = 0.1$ for the candidate drug, the AUC ratio will be 3.2. However, if $f_m = 0.99$, if $[I]/K_i = 0.1$ the AUC ratio will be 36.5. Figure 3.3 illustrates this point. However, if $[I]/K_i = 1.0$, the AUC ratio will be approximately 1.6 and when $[I]/K_i = 1000$, the AUC ratio would be approximately 3.99. Figure 3.4 summarizes this effect. The FDA position on the value of $[I]/K_i$ in predicting the significance of interactions is that if its value is 1.0 or more, it is likely that clinically relevant pharmacokinetic interactions will occur and that appropriate clinical drug–drug interaction studies need to be planned. As f_m increases, however, the rise in $[I]/K_i$ will cause greater increases in AUC.

In contrast to the CYP450 enzymes, the human hepatic UDP-glucuronosyltransferase enzymes (UGTs) participate in the clearance of only 15% of the top 200 drugs [15]. In addition, in reports describing drug interactions involving

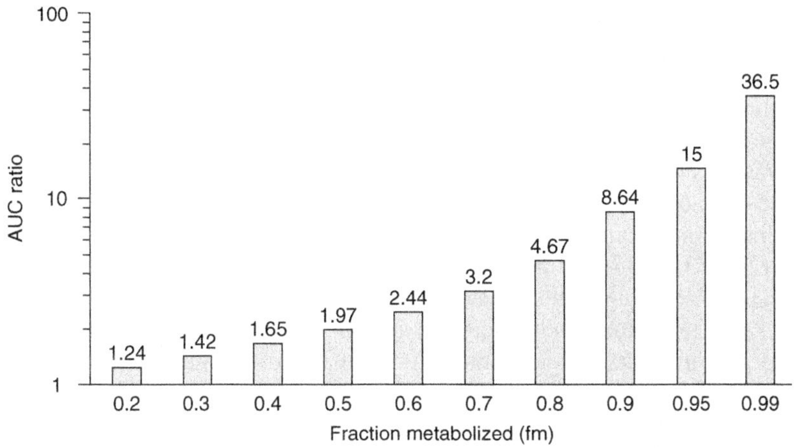

FIGURE 3.3 Dependence of AUC ratio on the fraction of dose eliminated by hepatic metabolism when [I] = 6 μg/mL and K_i = 0.1 μg/mL.

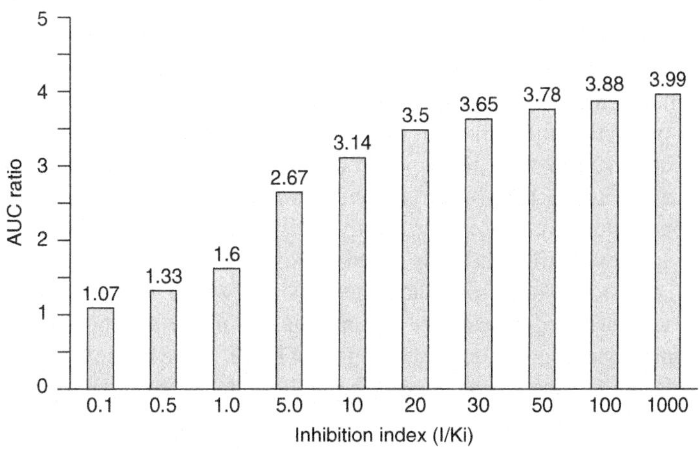

FIGURE 3.4 Dependence of AUC ratio on the inhibition index ([I]/K_i) when f_m = 0.75.

UGT substrates, increases in the exposure to the aglycone of the NCE were rarely greater than twofold.

Drug–Drug Interactions Mediated by Enzyme Induction Drug–drug interactions can also result from an increase in the expression of individual drug-metabolizing enzymes, particularly the hepatic CYP450 enzymes. The expression of most of the clinically relevant microsomal CYP450 enzymes in human liver are under the control of xenobiotic-activated nuclear receptors and may be induced by exposure to xenobiotics, such as drugs, components of food, herbal supplements, and occupational and environmental contaminants. The notable exception to this generalization is CYP2D6. Many marketed drugs are capable of inducing one or more CYP450 enzymes at therapeutic doses. The effect of enzyme induction is to reduce the exposure to drugs which are substrates for the enzyme(s) undergoing induction by increasing the metabolic clearance. In this way, an inducer may change the pharmacokinetic behavior of a second drug or it may increase its own rate of clearance (autoinduction). The resulting diminution of exposure can reduce efficacy or eliminate desired therapeutic effects.

Hepatic microsomal CYP450 induction is subject to important species-related differences [31,32] such that induction studies conducted with nonhuman species can yield misleading results, making accurate human predictions risky. Furthermore, induction studies conducted in nonhuman species tend to be expensive and require a substantial amount of test compound. However, these difficulties have been overcome by the development of robust human hepatocyte culture methods and the general availability of fresh and cryopreserved cells for this purpose [33]. The constitutive expression of CYP450 genes in cultured hepatocytes invariably falls for the first 48 to 72 hours after seeding regardless of culture conditions. However, the responsiveness of these genes to appropriate inducers is preserved if culture conditions are selected carefully [34–36] These culture conditions permit the hepatocytes to exhibit near-normal cellular physiology, gene expression, intercellular contacts, and bile canaliculi formation [37]. Thus, primary cultures of human hepatocytes serve as a selective and sensitive model for predicting the induction of CYP450. Retrospective studies suggest that induction observed in vivo can be reproduced in vitro [33]. Care must be taken, however, when using high inducer concentrations because the induction effect may disappear due to cell toxicity. Cell toxicity, de-differentiation, and poor solubility of the test compound may yield false negatives. For these reasons it is very important to include reference inducers for which reproducible induction has been demonstrated repeatedly. When cultured under appropriate conditions, human hepatocytes appear to respond to CYP450 inducers consistent with the clinical effects of those inducers, and the magnitude of the response is generally consistent with the activities observed in vivo [35].

Enzyme induction may be measured in several ways. After exposure of human hepatocyte cultures to pharmacologically relevant concentrations of test compound, or vehicle, for two to three days, CYP450-specific mRNA and protein are typically measured and compared. Monitoring enzyme activity against CYP450-specific substrates, directly in cultures or in microsomes harvested from cultures, may also be used to detect enzyme induction [33].

In the best case, there is a clear relationship between nominal test compound concentration and the fold increase in CYP450. In this model, β-naphthaflavone, phenobarbital, and rifampin are considered potent prototypical human CYP450 inducers against which the effect of a test compound is compared. For example, typically, β-naphthaflavone induces the expression of CYP1A2, phenobarbital induces CYP2B6, and rifampin induces CYP3A4 and CYP2C19. Figure 3.5 illustrates the typical magnitude of induction of human CYP450s in sandwich-cultured human hepatocytes by these compounds. Phenobarbital and rifampin

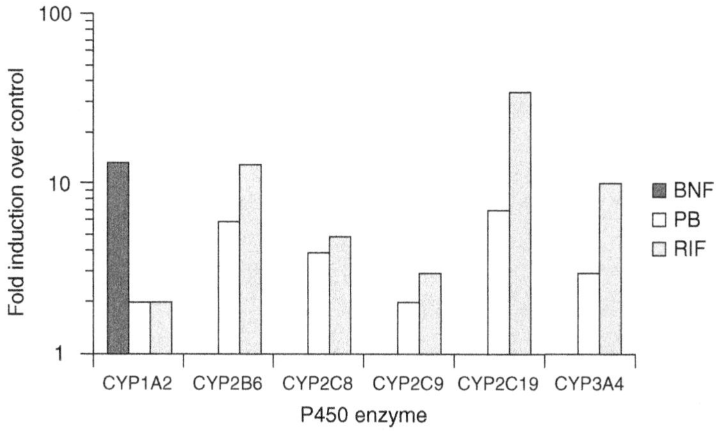

FIGURE 3.5 Typical magnitude of induction of cytochrome P450 enzymes achievable in cultured human hepatocytes by 30 μM β-naphthoflavone (BNF), 100 μM phenobarbital (PB), or 30 μM rifampin (RIF).

are also capable of inducing members of the CYP2C and CYP2E subfamilies. However, there is crosstalk between the nuclear receptors that regulate these enzymes, which may result in a pleiotropic response to some inducers [35]. The best example of this is the effect of phenobarbital on liver function and CYP450 induction [38]. In many cases the demonstration of CYP450 induction in vitro provides an explanation for changes in pharmacokinetic behavior observed in patients receiving the drug in question. Although the human hepatocyte model is sensitive and specific, it does not predict the magnitude of pharmacokinetic changes in vivo consistently and accurately because of the multitude of other factors that can alter drug disposition. However, one method has been suggested for quantitatively predicting the effect of CYP450 induction on pharmacokinetic behavior based on results from in vitro experiments using cultured human hepatocytes [39]. The resulting in vitro–in vivo relationship for eight drugs characterized as inducers of CYP1A and CYP3A enzymes and several enzyme-selective substrates suggested that the ratio E_{max}/EC_{50} for induction determined in cultured human hepatocytes correlated moderately well ($r = 0.768$, $p < 0.05$) with the change in intrinsic hepatic clearance calculated from pharmacokinetic data before and after administration of the inducing drug. This represents a respectable prediction, however imperfect.

More recently, the activation and translocation of the nuclear receptors that control the transcription of these enzymes have been used as indicators of induction [40,41]. These receptors include AhR (aryl hydrocarbon receptor), CAR (constitutive androstane receptor), and PXR (pregnane X receptor). PXR is the most promiscuous of these [42] and it frequently functions as part of a heterodimer with CAR. Once in the nucleus, these xenosensors bind to xenobiotic-responsive elements (proximal and distal promoter sequences) on the target genes and cause an increase in transcription. The heterodimerization of these transcription factors is responsible for the crosstalk observed in CYP450 induction. Although our understanding of these molecular events involved in induction continues to evolve, it is still early in the process of developing a practical method using this phenomenon to predict the magnitude human liver CYP450 induction and its effect on pharmacokinetic behavior. One reason for this delay is that hepatocyte culture conditions must support the near-normal expression of these nuclear receptors, and no consensus opinion exists on ideal or optimal culture conditions. For example, the expression of PXR is under the influence of the glucocorticoid receptor [38].

Drug–Drug Interactions Mediated by Drug Transporters Many human tissues, including the small intestine, liver, kidney, and central nervous system, express a wide variety of drug transporters. These can act as potential sites for the interaction of two or more drugs, which can alter pharmacokinetic behavior significantly, similar to the interactions involving drug-metabolizing enzymes discussed previously. Solute carrier transport (SLC) proteins are typically located on a basolateral membrane of cells (e.g., hepatocyte sinusoidal membrane), and ATP-binding cassette (ABC) transporter proteins are typically located on the apical membrane (e.g., biliary canalicular membrane, duodenal enterocyte membrane, renal distal tubule membrane). Pharmaceutical compounds that happen to be good substrates for the export transporters may exhibit poor or variable pharmacokinetic behavior, including limited or unpredictable bioavailability and altered elimination. The export transporters may also alter trough plasma drug concentrations and the disposition of substrates to peripheral tissues and compartments, thereby changing the dose–response relationship and altering therapeutic effects.

The multidrug export transporter P-glycoprotein (P-gp) is the most extensively studied member of the ABC transporter family and is an important site for potential transporter-mediated drug–drug interactions. It is present in the small intestine, blood–brain barrier, distal renal tubule, and placenta. Generally, understanding of P-gp and the biological and chemical tools with which to study its contribution to drug interaction potential are more advanced than are other transporters of the ABC and SLC families.

PHARMACOKINETIC INTERACTIONS MEDIATED BY INHIBITION OF P-GLYCOPROTEIN Like many of the human hepatic microsomal CYP450 enzymes, the substrate specificity of P-gp is very broad, which makes the prediction of P-gp–mediated drug–drug interactions from in vitro studies quite difficult. Compounds that interact with P-gp may be organized into three classes, based on their ability to stimulate the ATPase activity of P-gp and whether they are substrates or inhibitors [43–46]. These classes include unambiguous nonsubstrates (e.g., methotrexate), unambiguous substrates (e.g., ritonavir), possible inhibitors (e.g., testosterone), and nontransported substrates (e.g., midazolam) [43].

New chemical entities (NCEs) may be tested to determine if they are P-gp substrates or inhibitors by conducting a bidirectional permeability study in monolayers of polarized cells expressing P-gp. These include Caco-2 cells, MDR1-transfected Madin–Darby canine kidney cells, LLC-PK1 and MDR1-transfected LLC-PK1 cells. These experiments include reference substrates that exhibit low to moderate passive membrane permeability (2.0 to 30 × 10^{-6} cm/s) and a net flux ratio of at least 2.0, and inhibitors that exhibit low values of K_i or IC_{50} (<10 μM). Examples of acceptable reference substrates with which to compare new compounds include digoxin, loperamide, and vinblastine, and examples of suitable reference inhibitors include cyclosporin A and elacridar [47]. Unfortunately, multiple efflux transporters may be expressed in model cell systems and some compounds may inhibit multiple transporters, so further experiments should be conducted. However, if the efflux ratio of the new compound is greater than 2.0 and two or three known P-gp inhibitors reduce the net flux ratio significantly, the compound is likely to be a P-gp substrate. If a significant proportion of the efflux activity in not inhibited by reference P-gp inhibitors, other efflux transporters may contribute to the efflux activity. Table 3.4 summarizes the absence of an interaction with P-gp, as the efflux ratios all fell below a value of 2.0 and the presence of PGP inhibitors cyclosporin and ritonavir did not increase the $P_{\mathrm{appA-B}}$ significantly. Presently, the results described in the latter case are somewhat difficult to interpret, as our understanding of the many other human efflux transporters is quite limited relative to P-gp. The results of studies designed to identify new compounds as P-gp substrates may be used to design in vivo studies for the exploration of P-gp interactions. Clinical examples of P-gp–related drug interactions include altered pharmacokinetics of digoxin caused by quinidine as well as altered fexofenadine pharmacokinetics caused by ketoconazole and erythromycin [47]. Clearly, the involvement of drug transporters can have a significant effect on pharmacokinetic behavior [48].

Pharmacokinetic Interactions Mediated by Induction of P-glycoprotein The expression of P-gp in the intestinal epithelium is moderated by the same nuclear receptor, the pregnane X receptor (PXR), which regulates the expression of CYP3A4. Therefore, repeated oral administration of agents such as rifampin or St. John's wort can result in an increase in the efflux of P-gp substrates, thereby changing pharmacokinetic behavior by reducing the bioavailability of substrate drugs and reducing therapeutic effects. However, structurally, the ligand-binding domains among animal species are quite divergent from each other and from the human PXR. Furthermore, the Caco-2 cell monolayers, so useful in estimating intestinal permeability and absorption, is not suitable for this purpose, possibly due to a lack of human PXR activity in this cell line. However, one may use the human cell adenocarcinoma cell LS180/WT, and its adriamycin-resistant (LS180/AD) or vinblastine-resistant (LS180/V) sublines have been used to study P-gp induction. However, in general, methods for

TABLE 3.4 Apparent Permeability Coefficient (P_{app}) and Efflux Ratio of a New Lead Candidate Measured in MDR1-MDCK Cell Monolayers in the Absence and Presence of Two Recognized P-Glycoprotein Inhibitors

Inhibitor	Direction[a]	Recovery (%)	Mean P_{app} (10^{-6} cm/s)	Efflux Ratio
None	A-to-B	20	15.1	
	B-to-A	36	14.4	1.0
	Cell free	23	10.8	
Cyclosporin (10 μM)	A-to-B	29	20.4	
	B-to-A	50	14.5	0.7
	Cell free	39	13.8	
Ritonavir 0.5 μM	A-to-B	31	30.7	
	B-to-A	48	14.3	0.5
	Cell free	37	13.2	
1.0 μM	A-to-B	28	21.3	
	B-to-A	51	17.0	0.8
	Cell free	38	14.1	
2.0 μM	A-to-B	31	28.9	
	B-to-A	55	15.5	0.5
	Cell free	39	16.0	

[a] A-to-B, apical-to-basolateral direction; B-to-A, basolateral-to-apical direction; cell free, apical-to-basolateral direction measured in the absence of cell monolayers.

in vitro evaluation of P-gp induction and for predicting the effect of this phenomenon on pharmacokinetic behavior are not well established. In addition, it is very difficult to predict the magnitude of the effect P-gp induction will have on pharmacokinetic variables such as bioavailability. However, it is possible to identify new pharmaceutical compounds that are likely to be good P-gp substrates and therefore susceptible to changes in their pharmacokinetic behavior due to changes in the level of P-gp expression.

Physicochemical Properties At least four physicochemical properties of pharmaceutical compounds influence their pharmacokinetic behavior: (1) aqueous solubility, (2) lipophilicity, (3) charge state, and (4) dissolution rate of the substance (as opposed to the specific formulation of a compound, i.e., the drug product). Aqueous solubility is, to some degree, a function of the other three properties listed. Poor solubility has been cited in an increasing number of papers published on pharmaceutical compounds from 1975 to 2005, and the number of papers mentioning poor solubility began to rise precipitously in the mid-1990s. Compounds having aqueous solubility below 100 μg/mL often present a limitation to absorption [49]. Several methods are used to predict the solubility of compounds in the gastrointestinal (GI) tract, including (1) equilibrium, (2) apparent, (3) kinetic, (4) thermodynamic, and (5) intrinsic solubility. These terms and the various methods used to measure solubility are described in detail elsewhere [50]. However, due to the existence of a pH gradient along the length of the GI tract, the relationship between solubility and pH of the medium is extremely important when making predictions of the solubility in vivo [51]. This pH–solubility profile of mono acids and mono bases may be predicted by calculating the intrinsic equilibrium solubility ($S_{\mathrm{eq,int}}$), which depends on the values of the equilibrium solubility of the dissociated species ($S_{\mathrm{eq,ion}}$), the dissociation constant of the compound (K_a), and the hydrogen ion concentration.

Frequently, the rate-limiting step to absorption of drugs from the GI tract is often dissolution. The dose-to-solubility ratio of the compound provides an estimate of the volume of fluid required to dissolve an individual dose. When this volume exceeds 1 L, dissolution is often problematic. In addition, the surface area of the compound depends on its particle size. Therefore, dissolution rate of the unformulated compound has an impact on absorption and the AUC. This rate must be less than or equal to the transit time of the upper GI tract. In fasted humans, the transit time through the stomach and the small intestine is approximately 12 minutes and 3 to 4 hours, respectively. Should the time required for complete dissolution of a given dose exceed this window, absorption will be incomplete and the plasma AUC could be less than predicted. This dissolution rate may be predicted by the Nernst–Brunner equation [52,53], which incorporates the amount of undissolved solid, the surface area of this solid, and the diffusion coefficient of the drug [50].

3.2.2 In Vivo Models for Predicting Pharmacokinetic Behavior

Formulation Selection and Pharmacokinetic Predictions The prediction of the pharmacokinetic behavior of lead compounds in human subjects during optimization is frequently highly dependent on the way in which the compound is formulated in the liquid vehicle or suspension used to orally dose nonhuman species. There is probably no single vehicle that has proven to be suitable for all, or even a majority, of pharmaceutical compounds. In this modern age of drug discovery, one is typically working to improve the absorption of poorly soluble lipophilic compounds without including vehicle components that may be toxic to the intestinal barrier. Furthermore, it is most appropriate to formulate test compounds as solutions rather than suspensions of fine particles. Table 3.5 summarizes some general recommendations for the most useful components of aqueous vehicles used for this purpose, and some of their limitations. These are generic in nature and have been drawn from a consideration of the biochemical, pharmacokinetic, and toxicological effects of the major components. They represent one consensus opinion derived from the accumulated experience of several biopharmaceutical scientists. They do not, however, represent regulatory guidelines. It is desirable to select simple vehicles for this purpose, as opposed to using complex formulations that might require elaborate preparatory procedures. In addition, it is important to select vehicle components that have little or no toxicity in nonhuman species and are compatible with human health when used in repeated short-term dosing.

TABLE 3.5 General Guidelines for Selecting Liquid Dosing Vehicles Used for Oral Administration of NCEs

Vehicle	Current Guideline (Maximum Concentration)	Recommendation (Maximum Concentration and Volume)
Cremophor EL	10%	10% @ 5 mL/kg
Dimethylacetamide	10%	10% @ 4 mL/kg
Ethanol	20% @ 1 mL/kg	50% @ 1 mL/kg in rat and mouse; 25% @ 10 mL/kg for monkey
Glycerol	50% @ 5 mL/kg	50% @ 5 mL/kg in rat and mouse; 1 mL/kg in dog and monkey
2-Hydroxy-β-cyclodextrin	50%	50% @ 5 mL/kg
Hydroxymethylcellulose	0.25–0.50%	1% @ 10 mL/kg in rat, mouse, and dog; 2% @ 10 mL/kg in monkey
Poloxamer 188	2%	15% @ 10 mL/kg in rat and mouse; 5 mL/kg in dog and monkey
Polyethylene glycol 400	100%	100% @ 2 mL/kg in rat and mouse; 25% @ 2 mL/kg in dog; 25% @ 5 mL/kg in monkey
Propylene glycol	80%	50% @ 5 mL/kg in rat and mouse; 50% @ 1 mL/kg in dog and monkey
Sorbitol	70%	50% @ 2 mL/kg in rat and mouse; 20% @ 2 mL/kg in dog and monkey
Tween 80	100%	50% @ 5 mL/kg in rat and mouse; 25% @ 5 mL/kg in rat and mouse; 25% @ 5 mL/kg in monkey[a]
Vegetable oils	100%	100% @ 5 mL/kg in rat and mouse; 100% @ 2 mL/kg in dog and monkey

[a]Not recommended for use in dog.

Accordingly, aqueous solutions of cyclodextrins are very useful for this application [54,55]. Hydrophobic, hydrophilic, and ionic derivatives of cyclodextrins are available. They typically form inclusion complexes or noncovalent conjugates with pharmaceutical compounds and thereby can enhance absorption [56] and improve bioavailability by increasing apparent water solubility [57]. One of the most useful of these is hydroxypropyl-β-cyclodextrin (HPβCD). It is tolerated by nonhuman species as well as human subjects, with the main adverse effect being mild diarrhea [58]. In addition, it is an acceptable vehicle for repeatedly dosing of humans for up to two weeks, which would make it an appropriate formulation for first-in-human (FIH) pharmacokinetic studies.

Figure 3.6 illustrates the results of a series of pharmacokinetic studies recently conducted in adult cynomolgus monkeys for the purpose of comparing the relative exposure (dose-normalized AUC) of a lead compound administered orally in several liquid formulations. Fortunately, the cynomolgus monkey appears to be a reasonable model for this type of study, as monkeys appear to be a good predictor of the fraction of drug absorbed (F_a) in humans but only a moderately good predictor of human bioavailability. Furthermore, the gastric pH of unfed monkeys is similar to that of fasting humans, so monkeys are a good model to use for studies on the gastric emptying of drug-containing liquids after fasting, and food intake has little or no effect on the oro-cecal transit time of liquids in either monkeys or humans [60–62]. Higher reported metabolic clearances and hepatic enzyme activity in monkeys may account for this difference [59–62]. This compound is a BCS class II drug that exhibits acceptable permeability and poor solubility. Therefore, it was thought that the cynomolgus monkey was a reasonable model for a comparison of formulations. In the left half of the figure (the first six bars), the reference formulation is 10% HPβCD in water, and the total dose in every case is 50 mg per animal. Clearly, the AUC of this compound varies as much as fourfold between the six formulations shown. In addition, the strength of the dosing solution (12.5 to 50 mg/mL) has a significant effect on the AUC; that is, the more concentrated the dosing solution, the lower the resulting AUC. These results are typical of solubility-limited exposure. The right-hand side of the figure illustrates that the solubility limitation also has an effect on the AUC

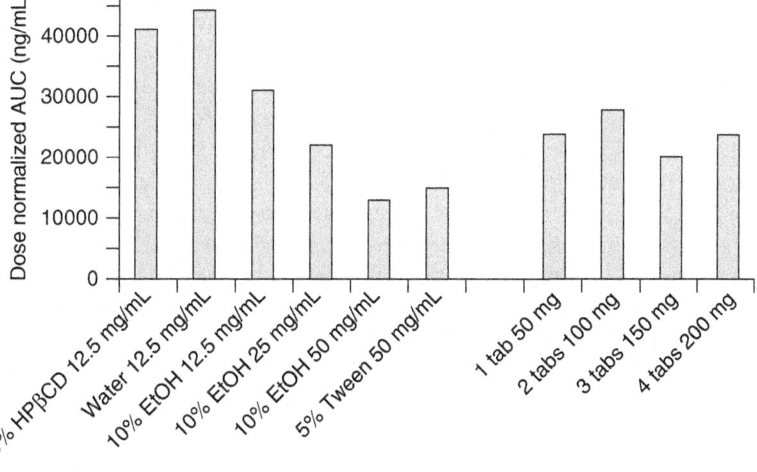

FIGURE 3.6 Dose-normalized AUC in cynomolgus monkeys of a new, solubility-limited lead candidate as a function of the nature and concentration of dosing solutions containing 50 mg and as total dose (50 to 200 mg), administered as one to four tablets.

of the drug when given in increasing doses (50 to 200 mg) in the form of one to four tablets, revealing nonlinear bioavailability. As it turned out, the result for the liquid formulations containing 10% HPβCD and only water at 12.5 mg/mL also yielded the highest exposure in human subjects. Furthermore, the effect of solution strength on AUC was also observed in humans. This 18-month study also yielded a solid dosage formulation that was significantly superior in monkeys and humans.

Another approach to evaluation of the relative bioavailability of an NCE in different formulations is to conduct an exploratory IND directly in human subjects. This is discussed in Chapter 11.

Physiologically Based Pharmacokinetic Modeling and Allometric Scaling During lead optimization one must depend on in vitro and in vivo data generated in small mammals, such as mice and rats, and rarely dogs and monkeys, to predict the pharmacokinetic variables of lead candidates in humans in order to help plan the specifics of an FIH study. However, these animal species do not accurately represent small humans with respect to their physiology [63], so direct extrapolations for the purposes of predicting human pharmacokinetics are almost always inaccurate. One method originally used to address these inaccuracies is to develop mathematical models for the calculation of human pharmacokinetics based on the results of animal testing.

Physiologically based pharmacokinetic (PBPK) models have been used for many years to predict human pharmacokinetics. PBPK models function by using mass balance equations to link tissue compartments by way of the plasma compartment. These simulate the absorption, distribution, and elimination of xenobiotics, including plasma exposure. They are based on physiologic mechanisms and can be used over a large range of doses and multiple routes of administration [64]. Bioavailability is incorporated into PBPK models by mechanistically describing oral absorption rates and the first-pass metabolism that occurs presystemically. PBPK models may be used to calculate individual dosing regimens for drugs with small therapeutic indices, such as theophylline, or when there are severe alterations in patient physiology, such as in pediatric patients or during pregnancy [65]. Empirical models are developed by applying experimental data, and it is these data alone that define the complexity of the model. This type of model is used primarily to describe and interpolate rather than explain observations for specific compounds. Conversely, whole-body PBPK overlays drug-specific data onto an essentially independent structural model consisting of tissues and organs connected and perfused by the vascular system [66]. One advantage of this type of model is that its structure is essentially common to all mammalian species, thereby facilitating interspecies scaling. Furthermore, the possibility exists for efficient use of limited drug-specific data in order to make reasonably accurate predictions with respect to the pharmacokinetics of specific compounds, both within and between species under a variety of conditions. In its simplest form, a model is reduced to predicting steady-state behavior characterized by clearance and volume of distribution. The drug-specific data include tissue affinity, plasma protein binding, membrane permeability, and enzymatic activity and transporter involvement.

In addition to compound-specific PBPK models developed to address the needs of individual lead optimization programs, there have been efforts to compile generic models that might be employed for predicting pharmacokinetic behavior in rats from in vitro data alone [67]. If validated adequately, this approach could be applied across many optimization programs. In an extension of this work, this type of model has been parameterized for human physiology and used to evaluate recently published predictive methods that involve allometric scaling from in vivo animal data. This requires the evaluation of a training set of in vivo pharmacokinetic data from the literature and validated with a separate test set of published in vivo data [67]. Inputs to these models include physicochemical properties of the compounds in question and the volume of distribution at steady state [68]. It appears that general PBPK models and those focused on a single compound or a chemical series can be a very useful tool for predicting human pharmacokinetics as long as validation by teaching and test sets of compounds is rigorous. One of the best examples of this technique is the application of PBPK modeling to the angiotensin-converting enzyme inhibitors ramipril and ramiprilat, which have complex and poorly characterized pharmacokinetics [69].

Originally, these models gained sophistication during the 1960s from contributions by the chemical engineering community as computing power increased. They have become relatively well accepted in the field of risk assessment by the chemical industry and for environmental protection. However, application to pharmaceutical research has remained relatively academic to date. As a practical matter, PBPK models may be applied at various points in the drug development continuum with varying success. It is now more feasible to predict overall pharmacokinetic behavior by coupling in silico computations with relevant in vitro data relating to absorption, intrinsic clearance, plasma free fraction, intestinal permeability, and the impact of drug transporters during lead selection and optimization using mechanistically based models. This would contribute to a systematic and rational approach to identification of the critical properties of a compound that should be defined in early development. Allometric scaling has traditionally been the dominant method for interspecies scaling during nonclinical testing. However, the use of this approach alone has come under close scrutiny for predicting FIH strategy because of its failure to account for active processes that affect pharmacokinetic behavior, such as first-pass metabolism and transport. It is clear that the PBPK approach can account for the effects of active processes when used in an iterative manner, particularly for a series of structurally related compounds.

Currently, the common practice when estimating pharmacokinetic parameters from plasma concentration–time studies is to drop the whole-body PBPK approach upon entry into human studies in favor of empirical approaches such as the fit of a sum of exponentials or a compartmental model to the existing data. There is some benefit in having models that are as physiologic as possible, incorporating physical aqueous spaces and plasma-free fraction. However, there have been relatively few published applications of the PBPK approach in regulatory decision making to date. Perhaps the best example is the application of PBPK modeling to the exposure of fetuses to all-*trans* retinoic acid [74], which was requested by the FDA.

The take-home message on PBPK modeling should be that after decades of existence, it remains an evolving technique that still requires validation through repeated use and additional regulatory experience, despite the fact that several databases are available that contain reliable values for relevant human physiologic parameters. Furthermore, this approach is not for inexperienced persons and perhaps should not be used exclusively to predict FIH pharmacokinetic behavior.

Allometric (interspecies) scaling is an alternative but related method used to predict, or extrapolate to, human pharmacokinetic behavior from information derived from nonhuman species. This concept of correlating pharmacokinetic variables with body weight and other data from different animal species has become a useful tool in drug development and may be used as early as lead optimization. This method is based on a power function in which the body weight of the species in question is related to the pharmacokinetic variables of interest. CL/*F*, the volume of distribution, and the elimination half-life are the three most frequently extrapolated pharmacokinetic variables [70]. Of these variables, oral clearance is one of the most important pharmacokinetic variables, as it plays a role in the selection of a safe and tolerable dose for FIH studies. One of the problems associated with this method is the large overpredictions of human clearance (vertical allometry) for many drugs [71,72]. A comparison of four different methods, including simple allometry, the rule of exponents, the unbound CL/*F* approach, and the unbound fraction corrected intercept method showed that the most successful predictions of CL/*F* were obtained using the unbound CL/*F* approach in combination with the maximum life span potential or the brain weight as correction factors based on the rule of exponents [73]. As is the case of many predictive models, this approach has exhibited various degrees of success using different methods for various drugs, and no single model may be applicable to all lead compounds. Furthermore, the fidelity of pharmacokinetic predictions depends on the quality of the data used to develop the models. Although allometric scaling for the purpose of predicting pharmacokinetics requires further refinements, this approach exhibits potential to predict human pharmacokinetic behavior.

In Silico Methods for Predicting Human Pharmacokinetics The generation of high-quality in vitro and in vivo ADME data is an absolute requirement for the development of in silico methods of predicting human pharmacokinetic behavior. Furthermore, applying computational methods to the prediction of human pharmacokinetics has had a relatively short history and has developed in parallel with the evolution of computing power during the past 30 years. These methods developed during the 1950s and 1960s using small sets of in vivo ADME data. Following this, during the 1970s and 1980s, in vitro ADME data were incorporated as substitutes for in vivo information, which promoted an increase in various proprietary [74] and commercially available in silico packages for this purpose. In both cases, the cost and time required to develop and validate these programs are substantial, and proprietary programs are often too expensive for medium-sized and small innovators. Finally, during the last two decades, human in vitro data for intrinsic clearance, intestinal absorption, drug interactions, SLC and ABC drug transporters, and blood–brain barrier penetration have been included, all of which have strengthened these predictive tools [75]. These software programs integrate many different algorithms [76] and in this modern era have taken advantage of artificial neural networks to improve predictions [77–79]. Currently, there is a plethora of commercially available programs, but they, too, can be cost-prohibitive for most small pharmaceutical companies.

The most important factor in determining the value of the results of in silico predictions is the quality of the data used to develop and validate the algorithms embedded in the software, and as in the case of PBPK modeling and allometry, any one software package may not be applicable to the entire chemical inventory space represented by realistic drug candidates and successful pharmaceutical compounds.

3.3 PREDICTION OF DRUG SAFETY

The prediction of drug safety for the purpose of risk assessment is one of the most elusive goals related to drug discovery and development. This is especially true during lead optimization, which does not typically incorporate detailed evaluations of potential adverse effects of exposure to NCEs. A number of drugs have been withdrawn or have required special labeling due to adverse effects observed postmarket. During the last decade two out of three withdrawals of these market withdrawals were caused by hepatotoxicity or cardiovascular toxicity [80]. Drug toxicity is the leading cause of acute liver toxicity in the United States [81,82]. In fact, acetaminophen was the second most common cause of acute liver failure in 2007, and antimicrobials led the list of nonacetaminophen causes of drug-induced liver injury [83]. In fact, more than 600 drugs currently on the market have the potential to cause liver injury [84]. In addition, although perhaps less frequent, cardiovascular toxicity has been associated with a number of drugs distributed across several drug classes, including nonsedating antihistamines and gastrointestinal prokinetics [85], statins [86], anticancer medicines [87], and anti-inflammatory agents [88].

The human body is obviously comprised of many tissue and cell types, all of which exhibit different susceptibilities to drug exposure and most of which are exposed to different drug concentrations, as influenced by the drug's pharmacokinetic behavior. That safety is related to dose and/or exposure is a biological phenomenon that has been well documented. However, this is not always the case, as evidenced by the repeated appearance of "idiosyncratic toxicity" that occurs some time after the medicine in question was last taken and the involvement of reactive drug metabolites and immune factors as causes of this phenomenon [89]. For example, although acute liver failure is rare, 13 to 17% of all such cases are attributable to idiosyncratic drug reactions [90].

It is clearly impossible to predict drug safety accurately, even in the late stages of development, as rare adverse events will occur only after the drug has been administered to a sufficient numbers of patients. Therefore, accurate prediction of human drug safety requires resources and time to clearly define important toxic mechanisms and corresponding risk factors. This record of repeated predictive failures has prompted a great deal of effort to improve in vitro, ex vivo, in vivo, and in silico methods and systems available for this purpose. Whenever possible, the all four methods should be considered during the development continuum.

3.3.1 In Vitro Approaches for Predicting Drug Safety

An in vitro approach to the prediction of drug safety is probably the most widespread strategy used during lead optimization by most sponsors with modest resources at their disposal. The development of in vitro models for the prediction of acute drug toxicity began in earnest during the 1980s with the improvement of primary culture systems in which the cells retained differentiated functions and responses observed in intact tissues and the identification of markers of toxicity in primary cultures of heart, liver, and kidney cells [91–93]. However, the study of toxicity in vitro has historically been complicated by the persistent difficulties of maintaining cells in culture due to a lack of understanding of the humoral and matrix requirements [94]. Many of the problems of maintaining relatively normal gene expression and biochemical responses to xenobiotic exposure in cultured primary cells have been resolved to some degree [33], but there remain many issues that arise from differences between the dynamic homeostatic systems in vivo and the static systems used to model these in vitro.

Beginning in the 1980s, the Scandinavian Society of Cell Toxicology initiated a program entitled the Multicenter Evaluation of In Vitro Cytotoxicity [95] with the goal of elucidating toxic mechanisms of chemicals and validating in vitro models for use in acute toxicity testing. This work has continued since that time, using a wide variety of cells in culture, including rat hepatocytes [96], mouse fibroblasts [97], and rat hepatoma–derived Fa32 cells [98,99]. The development of an in vitro test battery for the estimation of acute human systemic toxicity is the most significant outcome of this work [100]. Unfortunately, many of the compounds tested were not pharmaceuticals. In addition, the work of these researchers has been paralleled by efforts by the Scientific Group on Methodologies for the Safety Evaluation of Chemicals [101]. The large and sustained collaborative efforts on behalf of in vitro methods for safety predictions have had mixed results, however, and they have demonstrated that the prediction of drug safety with in vitro systems continues to be difficult [102]. Furthermore, in vitro systems are inadequate for the prediction of chronic toxicity resulting from repeated administration of drugs over many weeks or months. If only in vitro methods such as cultured hepatocytes are used to estimate toxicity, it will be important to measure several possible pathways or mechanisms responsible for cell damage or death.

One area in which in vitro systems have essentially failed to improve predictions of drug safety is the prediction of idiosyncratic drug toxicity. Idiosyncratic drug toxicity is a serious and rare event (<1 in 5000), and it is an event that is specific to humans (from the observational perspective) which cannot be studied in animal models. Generally, the major determinants associated with this effect are the chemical properties of the compound, the level of exposure, environmental factors, the presence of CYP450 inducers, and the clinically relevant pharmacokinetic interactions with other drugs [103]. However, at this time it is impossible to predict which new pharmaceutical compounds will cause unexpected, unusual, or exaggerated toxicity that in most cases is delayed and which is not related to dose magnitude or dose rate [104]. The peculiar character of these events has made mechanistic studies extremely problematic [105,106]. Several specific hypotheses have been developed to explain the onset of these events, including the danger hypothesis, which is taken from the study of immunology [107], specifically the interaction between chemically reactive metabolites and lymphocytes. Furthermore, these events may be related to specific HLA genes. Examples of this phenomenon include the association between isoniazid and the onset of lupus erythrematosus [108], as well as aminopyrine and agranulocytosis [109]. Finally, the role of mitochondrial permeability transition in the onset of idiosyncratic toxicity has been suggested. It is possible that gradually accumulating and initially silent mitochondrial damage eventually causes mitochondrial swelling, leakage of calcium ions, and mitochondrial membrane depolarization, and the oxidation of NADPH and protein thiols may be involved [110,111]. In vitro models of drug toxicity such as cultured rat hepatocytes are useful for studying these individual effects.

The generation of electrophilic, reactive metabolites from pharmaceutical compounds has also been implicated in the pathogenesis of drug-induced hepatotoxicity [112,113]. These metabolites are able to bind to nucleophilic macromolecules in exposed tissues, resulting in chemical modifications that alter protein function, producing a cascade of effects on cell signaling, regulation, defense, function, and viability [114]. The most recent and interesting example of a drug so implicated is troglitazone. This compound, already withdrawn from the market, is metabolized to two major reactive metabolites that form glutathione conjugates, but the role of these metabolites in toxicity remains somewhat controversial. Mitochondrial dysfunction, particularly mitochondrial permeability transition, is probably a pathological event. However, other potentially toxic events, such as apoptosis due to calcium dysregulation, PPAR-γ-dependent steatosis and cholestasis attributable to bile salt export pump inhibition caused by the sulfate conjugate, have also been observed [115].

New and sometimes very novel in vitro methods for the assessment of drug safety continue to be developed, as they provide a relatively rapid and inexpensive means to roughly estimate the risk of drug exposure. Some of these represent modifications to existing methods, including integrated discrete multiple-organ cell culture, an extension of primary cell co-culture [116] and flow cytometry for the determination of basal toxicity in immortalized HepG2 cells [117]. Alternative original methods have been developed and will require validation with reference pharmaceutical compounds, including the application of microfluidic cell biochips [118] and liver stem cells that provide a continual and readily available source of hepatic parenchymal cells for culture [119]. The application of these new and relatively untested methods of estimating different aspects of toxicity are currently restricted to what one might designate as exploratory toxicology. In fact, all in vitro methods of forecasting toxicity will require extensive validation and must be tested exhaustively to determine if a reproducible in vitro–in vivo correlation exists, as the estimation of risk for the purpose of drug approval and registration is very highly regulated and the focus of nonclinical and clinical studies. Furthermore, under the very best circumstances, in vitro systems used to forecast the risk of toxicity have, in many cases, failed to provide adequate and appropriated information, which has led to compound failure during clinical studies and in the postmarketing period.

3.3.2 In Vivo and Ex Vivo Methods for Predicting Drug Safety

Predictions from In Vivo Studies Generally, in vivo methods of safety prediction find limited application during lead optimization in most innovator companies, primarily because of resource limitations and the financial and scientific pressures inherent in drug discovery. However, before the "modern" era of drug discovery that incorporates the widespread use of in vitro methods (before 1985), the use of these in vivo methods was considered standard practice. Even before this contemporary era there were attempts to analyze the validity and usefulness of predictions arising from animal studies. These studies were frequently focused on determining safe doses for FIH pharmacokinetics (phase I) studies by measuring tolerable and toxic doses in rats, dogs, and monkeys [120]. The results of these analyses typically suggested that if the starting dose in phase I trials was selected by calculating one-third of the maximum dose tolerated in the most sensitive nonhuman species, the trials could be initiated safely. Alternatively, calculating the lethal doses for 10% and 90% of normal mice could also yield good quantitative prediction of human toxicity.

The predictive value of animal studies for human safety has since been reevaluated retrospectively in the case of 130 pharmaceutical agents from multiple sponsors. The conclusions of this particular review suggested that the prediction rate of animal models for human toxicity was 69% and that results from dog and primate species have reasonable potential to identify human toxicity across multiple therapeutic classes [121]. Nevertheless, there is concern that normal, healthy animals might be poor models in certain cases because underlying disease in patients may be an important influence in the susceptibility to adverse effects. This is particularly true in the immune response to biotherapeutic candidates, systemic toxicity, and idiosyncratic drug reactions [122]. Once again, it is idiosyncratic reactions to drug exposure that are problematic when it comes to predicting human drug safety. The characteristics of these outcomes and the likely involvement of immune factors are certainly complicating factors. Unfortunately, human idiosyncratic reactions are also idiosyncratic in animals; that is, they are rare, exhibit delayed onset, and the response does not typically track with dose. Unfortunately, at this time only a small number of models of idiosyncratic reactions are available. These include sulfamethoxazole-induced hypersensitivity in beagle dogs, penacillamine-induced autoimmunity in brown Norway rats, and propylthiouracil-mediated hypersensitivity in cats, all of which are similar to reactions observed in human subjects [123,124].

One new in vivo model for predicting human drug safety and drug metabolism is the chimeric mouse, which is equipped with a humanized liver. In this case, human hepatocytes are transplanted into a urokinase-type plasminogen activator (+/+)/severe combined immunodeficient transgenic mouse line. This may be useful because the liver is frequently the site of drug biotransformation and toxicity [125]. Like other new models used for prediction, this will require sustained testing and validation.

Predictions from Ex Vivo Studies Ex vivo methods are also available for the prediction of drug safety—methods that analyze tissues, tissue extracts, or fluids from animals previously exposed to lead candidates and the comparison of these results to those derived from untreated animals. Examples of these approaches include various "omics" disciplines: metabolomics/metabonomics, proteomics, toxicogenomics/transcriptomics. However, these methods are very expensive and time consuming to develop and validate and require significant computational power for the purpose of data collection, storage, and analysis, as well as database management and interrogation.

The term *metabolomics* refers to the systematic study of the unique chemical fingerprints that specific cellular processes leave behind, that is, the end products of gene expression [126]. The term *metabonomics* refers to the quantitative measurement of the dynamic, multiparametric metabolic response of living systems to pathophysiological stimuli or genetic modifications [127]. Although the difference is somewhat subtle, metabolomics places greater emphasis on comprehensive metabolic profiling under "normal" conditions, and metabonomics is used to describe multiple metabolic changes caused by biological disturbances (e.g., after drug exposure). In this case, the term *metabolite* refers to the intermediates and products of the metabolism of endogenous compounds, not of xenobiotics. Urine and plasma are the most common, but not the only, sources of these metabolites. Therefore, metabonomics may be more applicable to the prediction of drug safety than metabolomics [128]. However, the metabolomic database is the foundation on which biochemical changes, detected by metabonomics, are interpreted [129,130]. Essentially, metabolomics functions as a link between genotype and phenotype [131]. Metabolomics may also be used to improve our understanding of the biochemical basis of diseases [132]. However, consensus needs to be reached on the interpretation of experimental results of metabonomic studies, and standards for reporting the results of metabolomic and metabonomic studies still need to be standardized [133]. Although these techniques have been included in a section describing ex vivo methods of predicting drug safety, they depend on sophisticated statistical analysis and significant computing power.

In a way that parallels metabolomics, transcriptomics, or gene expression profiling, describes the genome-wide measurement of messenger RNA expression levels, most frequently using DNA microarray techniques [134]. The term *toxicogenetics* is the large-scale identification of genetic polymorphisms in order to understand the genetic basis for individual differences in response to potential toxicants [135]. Furthermore, toxicogenomics is a form of analysis whereby the activity of a particular xenobiotic on organs or tissues can be identified based on a profiling of its effects on genetic material, which parallels the application of metabonomics to changes in metabolites. Therefore, strictly speaking, transcriptomics is a technique used to understand results from toxicogenetic and toxicogenomic studies. In this regard, toxicogenetics could be helpful in understanding the reasons for interindividual differences in responses to xenobiotics, as pharmacogenetics is used to elucidate differences in drug metabolism by CYP450 enzymes.

In the context of this chapter, transcriptomics has been applied to mechanistic and predictive toxicology [136,137] in evaluating changes in the expression of toxicologically relevant genes [138]. These techniques have also been applied to the understanding of genetic and epigenetic mechanisms of toxicity [139]. Toxicogenomics as a method to predict drug safety is still early in its development and validation, although there are high expectations for its ability to reduce the uncertainties associated with respect to toxicity predictions and risk assessment [140–145]. Similar to the application of metabonomics, the interpretation of toxicogenomic studies requires large-scale databases that are species specific [146].

Two very important points require clarification. The first is that the value of individual techniques described previously might be enhanced by the integration of these methods into a systems toxicology approach to predictions of drug safety, because each method has its advantages and limitations [147]. It is possible that toxicogenomics could reveal the crucial steps and sequence of events at the molecular level and might be studied to provide insights into mechanisms of toxic action. This technique could provide more sensitive and earlier detection of adverse effects in nonhuman studies. However, these mechanistic data are generated in vitro or ex vivo in inbred animal models that may not be especially relevant in predicting the risk to human subjects. Furthermore, where metabolic activation is required to cause changes in gene expression, species differences may result in spurious associations between exposure and effect. Second, as these techniques became more widely adopted into pharmaceutical research, there was speculation that more classical methods of risk assessment would become superfluous and that they would help classify compounds early in drug development, perhaps during lead optimization, saving animals, time, and money in nonclinical programs. In addition, it began to appear that the molecular mechanisms of underlying toxicity would be revealed in this way [148]. However, as professional and responsible pharmaceutical research scientists, we always need to be skeptical and cautious and adhere closely to the scientific method that is the foundation of our work.

In light of that admonition, one novel adaptation of these techniques is the application of toxicogenomics to drug-induced toxicity using the widely adopted model of sandwich-cultured hepatocytes [149], which has proven useful in the prediction of changes in pharmacokinetic behavior resulting from CYP450 induction, described previously. However, under the best culture conditions, animal and human hepatocytes rapidly lose the expression of drug-metabolizing enzymes, leaving this system useful only for the determination of basal toxicity.

3.3.3 In Silico Methods for Predicting Drug Safety

The development and application of large computer programs were set in motion during the 1980s to address concerns about the potential carcinogenic and mutagenic potential of chemicals released into the environment, many of which originated in workplaces as effluent. These early programs were based on pattern recognition [150] and quantitative structure–activity relationships (QSARs) between molecular structure or substructure and biological effects. They were moderately effective in classifying xenobiotics as active (toxic) or inactive, but the results were qualitative only when it came to the nature of the consequent predictions. Modern equivalents, including commercial products such as Ecosar and Biowin, employ linear regression to predict ecotoxicity and biodegradability based on molecular fragments and molecular weight [151]. As pharmaceutical research moved into the modern era in the mid-1980s and pressure mounted to screen larger numbers of compounds accurately and to reduce the failure of otherwise appealing compounds, these programs were adapted to the evaluation of NCEs arising from pharmaceutical research. The chemical space occupied by environmental contaminants and industrial chemicals is quite different from that occupied by medicinal compounds, so the software required profound modifications. Although the prediction of carcinogenicity and mutagenicity remained a central goal, the programs were modified to account for effects such as the electrophilic attack of chemicals on biological molecules [152], a feature of genotoxic carcinogens. However, at that time they did poorly at predicting carcinogenic effects of epigenetic carcinogens, such as tumor promoters. Unfortunately, the predictive value of many of these programs was limited to specific chemical classes [153]. As the interest in predictions of drug toxicity intensified, the number of commercially available rule- or knowledge-based QSAR programs increased dramatically and came to include products such as Derek, Meteor, StAR, and Topkat. Currently, modern predictive programs have a mechanistic or empirical basis and exhibit varying degrees of success under specific circumstances. However, these programs are designed to be used by knowledgeable experts, and their application can be counterproductive in the hands of inexperienced researchers. Even so, the results of applying these programs are probably no substitute for carefully generated experimental data, upon which they actually depend. Comparisons of these products to determine their relative actual performance continue [154,155], and both commercially available and proprietary programs are continually updated by expanding teaching and test sets of relevant medicinal compounds.

One novel approach for the prediction of potential adverse drug reactions of an NCE is to search for its interaction with adverse drug reaction–associated proteins. This is the basis of Invdock, a new commercial software program. To date it has been tested on 11 marketed anti-HIV drugs, and in an initial report this in silico approach achieved a success rate of 60 to 90% in predicting adverse effects, based on data culled from the scientific literature [156]. However, this feasibility study requires follow-up, and the approach requires further extensive validation.

The challenges involved in forecasting human drug safety are obviously considerable; reliable and accurate predictions may be nearly impossible with current technology. However, the quality of predictions may certainly be enhanced by adopting a comprehensive approach, by integrating some of the methods described in this chapter as well as those from other scientific disciplines. An integrated approach should include all of the following considerations [157]:

1. Possible toxicity due to interactions with unintended targets or with targets in unintended tissues
2. Chemical scaffolds or chemical substituents about which there is already concern regarding possible toxicity
3. Toxicity in animals and in relevant cultured animal or human cells
4. Pharmacokinetic behavior, including ADME, as well as drug–drug interactions and induction of metabolism
5. Physiological, genetic, and environmental factors that lead to interindividual differences between patients

Integration of these considerations also implies that the in vitro, in vivo–ex vivo, and in silico methods described here should be used whenever considered relevant or possible, recognizing that most of us are trying to do more with less and that some of the in silico techniques available are not affordable under any circumstances [158].

3.4 CONCLUSIONS

Interestingly, the term *lead optimization*, as it is used in the context of this chapter, does not appear in a Medline search before 1995. However, by this point it should be clear that methods of predicting pharmacokinetic and drug safety have evolved during the past four decades in parallel with the increasing demand for speed and accuracy. As the degree of competition within the pharmaceutical industry has intensified, the cost of developing new medicines has soared and the consequences of late stage failure have grown in parallel. The in vivo–ex vivo methods that were employed originally have acted as the foundation on which modern in vitro techniques were developed. Furthermore, the in silico techniques described herein have arisen from the results of thousands of in vitro and in vivo experiments conducted through the intervening years. Although predictions of human pharmacokinetics are generally accurate, if less than perfect, we should also recognize that there are toxicity results of drug exposure that will remain difficult to predict for some time to come. The best, or worst, examples of these remaining obstacles are embodied in idiosyncratic drug reactions.

REFERENCES

1. Letendre L, Scott M, Dobson G, Hidalgo I, Aungst B. Evaluating barriers to bioavailability in vivo: validation of a technique for separately assessing gastrointestinal absorption and hepatic extraction. *Pharm Res*. 2004;21(8):1457–1462.
2. Lennernäs H, Alrahamsson B. The use of biopharmaceutic classification of drugs in drug discovery and development: current status and future extension. *J Pharm Pharmacol*. 2005;57(3):273–285.
3. Lipinski CA. Drug-like properties and the causes of poor solubility and poor permeability. *J Pharmacol Toxicol Methods*. 2000;44(1):235–249.
4. Kaminski LS, Zhang Q-Y. The small intestine as a xenobiotic-metabolizing organ. *Drug Metab Dispos*. 2003;31:1520–1525.
5. Coles BF, Chen G, Kadlubar FF, Radominska-Pandya A. Interindividual variation and organ-specific patterns of glutathione *S*-transeferase alpha, mu and pi expression in gastrointestinal tract mucosa of normal individuals. *Arch Biochem Biophys*. 2002;403(2):270–276.
6. Fisher MB, Paine MF, Strelevitz TJ, Wrighton SA. The role of hepatic and extrahepatic UDP-glucuronosyltransferases in human drug metabolism. *Drug Metab Rev*. 2001;33(3–4):273–297.
7. Lipinski CA, Lombardo F, Dominy BW, Feeny PJ. Experimental and computational approaches to estimate solubility and permeability in drug discovery and development settings. *Adv Drug Deliv Rev*. 2001;46:3–26.
8. Hidalgo IJ, Raub TJ, Borchardt RT. Characterization of the human colon carcinoma cell line (Caco-2) as a model system for intestinal epithelial permeability. *Gastroenterology*. 1989;96(3):736–749.
9. Artursson P. Epithelial transport of drugs in cell culture: I. A model for studying the passive diffusion of dugs over intestinal absorptive (Caco-2) cells. *J Pharm Sci*. 1990;79(6):476–482.
10. Artursson P, Karlson J. Correlation between oral drug absorption in humans and apparent drug permeability coefficients in human intestinal epithelial (Caco-2) cells. *Biochem Biophys Res Commun*. 1991;175(3):880–885.
11. Löbenberg R, Amidon GL. Modern bioavailability, bioequivalence and biopharmaceutics classification system: new scientific approaches to international regulatory standards. *Eur J Pharmacol Biopharm*. 2000;50(1):3–12.
12. Kasim NA, Whitehouse M, Ramachandran C, et al. Molecular properties of WHO essential drugs and provisional biopharmaceutical classification. *Mol Pharmacol*. 2004;1(1):85–96.

13. Lindenberg M, Kopp S, Dressman JB. Classification of orally administered drugs on the WHO model list of essential medicines according to the biopharmaceutics classification system. *Eur J Pharmacol Biopharm*. 2004;58(2):265–278.
14. Takagi T, Ramachandran C, Bermejo M, Yamashita S, Yu LX, Amidon GL. A provisional biopharmaceutical classification of the top 200 oral drug products in the United States, Great Britain, Spain, and Japan. *Mol Pharmacol*. 2006;3(6):631–643.
15. Williams JA, Hyland R, Jones BC, et al. Drug–drug interactions for UDP-glucuronosyltransferase substrates: a pharmacokinetic explanation for typically observed low exposure (AUC_I/AUC) ratios. *Drug Metab Dispos*. 2004;32(11): 1201–1208.
16. Wilkinson GR, Shand DG. Commentary: a physiological approach to hepatic drug clearance. *Clin Pharmacol Ther*. 1975;18(4):377–390.
17. Pang KS, Rowland M. Hepatic clearance of drugs: I. Theoretical considerations of a well-stirred model and a parallel model: influence of hepatic blood flow, plasma and blood cell binding, and the hepatocellular enzymatic activity on hepatic drug clearance. *J Pharmacokinet Biopharm*. 1977;5(6):625–653.
18. Ito K, Houston JB. Comparison of the use of liver models for predicting drug clearance using in vitro kinetic data from hepatic microsomes and isolated hepatocytes. *Pharm Res*. 2004;21(5):785–792.
19. Obach RS. Nonspecific binding to microsomes: impact on scale-up of in vitro intrinsic clearance to hepatic clearance as assessed through examination of warfarin, imipramine and propranolol. *Drug Metab Dispos*. 1977;25(12):1359–1369.
20. Obach RS. Prediction of human clearance of twenty-nine drugs from hepatic microsomal intrinsic clearance: an examination of in vitro half-life approach and non-specific binding to microsomes. *Drug Metab Dispos*. 1999;27(11):1350–1359.
21. Huang S-M, Strong JM, Zhang L, et al. New era in drug interaction evaluation: US Food and Drug Administration update on CYP enzymes, transporters and the guidance process. *J Clin Pharmacol*. 2008;31(Mar 31).
22. Bertz FJ, Granneman GR. Use of in vitro and in vivo data to estimate the likelihood of metabolic pharmacokinetic interactions. 1997;32(3):210–258.
23. Lin JH, Lu AY. Inhibition and induction of cytochrome P450 and the clinical implications. *Clin Pharmacokinet*. 1998;35:361–390.
24. Obach RS, Walsky RL, Venkatakrishnan K, Gaman EA, Houston JB, Tremaine LM. The utility of in vitro cytochrome P450 inhibition data in the prediction of drug–drug interactions. *J Pharmacol Exp Ther*. 2006;316:336–348.
25. Lu AYH, Wang RW, Lin JH. Cytochrome P450 in vitro reaction phenotyping: a re-evaluation of approaches used for P450 isoform identification. 2003;31: 345–350.
26. Bjornsson TD, Callaghan JT, Einolf HJ, et al. The conduct of in vitro and in vivo drug–drug interaction studies: a Pharmaceutical Research and Manufacturers of America (PhRMA) perspective. *Drug Metab Dispos*. 2003;31(7):815–832.
27. Yuan R, Madani S, Wei X-X, Reynolds K, Huang S-M. Evaluation of cytochrome P450 probe substrates commonly used by the pharmaceutical industry to study in vitro drug interactions. *Drug Metab Dispos*. 2002;30(12):1311–1319.
28. Guengerich FP, Muller ED, Blair IA. Oxidation of quinidine by human liver cytochrome P-450. *Mol Pharm*. 1986;30:287–295.

29. Honig PK, Worham DC, Zamani K, Conner DP, Mullin JC, Cantilena LR. Terfenadine–ketoconazole interaction: pharmacokinetic and electrocardiographic consequences. *J Am Med Assoc*. 1993;269(12):1513–1518.

30. Obach RS, Walsky RL, Venkatakrishnan K, Houston JB, Tremaine LM. In Vitro cytochrome P450 inhibition data and the prediction of drug–drug interactions: qualitative relationships, quantitative predictions, and the rank-order approach. *Clin Pharmacol Ther*. 2005;78(6):582–592.

31. Lu C, Li AP. Species comparison in P450 induction: effects of dexamethasone, omeprazole, and rifampin on P450 isoforms 1A and 3A in primary cultured hepatocytes from man, Sprague–Dawley rat, minipig, and beagle dog. *Chem Biol Interact*. 2001;134:271–281.

32. Nishimura M, Koeda A, Suganuma Y, Satoh T, Narimatsu S, Naito S. Comparison of inducibility of CYP1A and CYP3A mRNAs by prototypical inducers in primary cultures of human, cynomolgus monkey, and rat hepatocytes. *Drug Metab Pharmacokinet*. 2007;22(3):178–186.

33. Hewitt NJ, Lechón MJG, Houston JB, et al. Primary hepatocytes: current understanding of the regulation of metabolic enzymes and transporter proteins, and pharmaceutical practice for the use of hepatocytes in metabolism, enzyme induction, transporter, clearance, and hepatotoxicity studies. *Drug Metab Rev*. 2007;39:159:343–368.

34. LeCluyse EL. Human hepatocyte culture systems for the in vitro evaluation of cytochrome P450 expression and regulation. *Eur J Pharm Sci*. 2001;13:343–368.

35. Madan A, Graham RA, Carroll KM, et al. Effects of prototypical microsomal enzyme inducers on cytochrome P450 expression in cultured human hepatocytes. *Drug Metab Dispos*. 2003;31:421–431.

36. Hewitt NJ, de Kanter R, LeCluyse E. Induction of drug metabolizing enzymes: a survey of in vitro methodologies and interpretations used in the pharmaceutical industry—do they comply with FDA recommendations? *Chem Biol Interact*. 2007;168(1):51–65.

37. LeCluyse EL, Andus KL, Hochman JH. Formation of extensive canalicular networks by rat hepatocytes cultured in collagen-sandwich configuration. *Am J Physiol*. 1994;266(6pt 1): C1764–2774.

38. Handschin C, Meyer UA. Induction of drug metabolism: the role of nuclear receptors. *Pharmacol Rev*. 2003;55:649–673.

39. Kato M, Chiba K, Horikawa M, Sugiyama Y. The quantitative prediction of in vivo enzyme-induction caused by drug exposure from in vitro information on human hepatocytes. *Drug Metab Pharmacokinet*. 2005;20(4):236–243.

40. Hewitt NJ, LeCluyse EL, Ferguson SS. Induction of hepatic cytochrome P450 enzymes: methods, mechanisms, recommendations, and in vitro–in vivo correlations. *Xenobiotica*. 2007;37:1196–1224.

41. Staudinger JL, Madan A, Carol KM, Parkinson A. Regulation of drug transporter gene expression by nuclear receptors. *Drug Metab Dispos*. 2003;31(5):523–527.

42. Lim Y-P, Huang J-D. Interplay of pregnane X receptor with other nuclear receptors on gene regulation. *Drug Metab Pharmacokinet*. 2008;23(1):14–21.

43. Polli JW, Wring SA, Humphreys JE, et al. Rational use of the in vitro P-glycoprotein assays in drug discovery. *J Pharmacol Exp Ther*. 2001;299:620–628.

44. Schwab D, Fischer H, Tabatabaei A, Poli S, Huwyler J. Comparison of in vitro P-glycoprotein screening assays: recommendations for their use in drug discovery. *J Med Chem*. 2003;46:1716–1725.
45. Balimane PV, Han Y-H, Chong S. Current industrial practices of assessing permeability and P-glycoprotein interaction. *Am Assoc Pharm Sci*. 2006;8(1): E1–E13.
46. Rautio J, Humphreys JE, Webster LO, et al. In Vitro P-glycoprotein inhibition assays for assessment of clinical drug interaction potential of new drug candidates: a recommendation for probe substrates. *Drug Metab Dispos*. 2006;34: 786–792.
47. Zhang L, Strong JM, Qiu W, Lesko LJ, Huang S-M. Scientific perspectives on drug transporters and their role in drug interactions. *Mol Pharm*. 2006;3(1):62–69.
48. Mizuno N, Niwa T, Yotsumoto Y, Sugiyama Y. Impact of drug transporter studies on drug discovery and development. *Pharmacol Rev*. 2003;55:425–461.
49. Hörter D, Dressman JB. Influence of physicochemical properties on dissolution of drugs in the gastrointestinal tract. *Adv Drug Deliv Rev*. 2001;46:75–87.
50. Sugano K, Okazaki A, Sugimoto S, Tavornvipas S, Omura A, Mano T. Solubility and dissolution profile assessment in drug discovery. *Drug Metab Pharmacokinet*. 2007;22(4):225–254.
51. Hendriksen BA, Sanchez-Felix M, Bolger MB. The composite solubility versus pH profile and its role in intestinal absorption prediction. *AAPS PharmSci*. 2003;5:1–15.
52. Nernst W. Theory of reaction velocity in heterogeneous systems. *Z Phys Chem*. 1904;47:52–55.
53. Brunner E. Velocity of reaction in non-homogeneous systems. *Z Phys Chem*. 1904;47:56–102.
54. Uekama K. Design and evaluation of cyclodextrin-based drug formulation. *Chem Pharm Bull*. 2004;52:900–915.
55. Challa R, Ahuja A, Ali J, Khar RK. Cyclodextrins in drug delivery: an updated review. *AAPS PharmSciTech*. 2005;6:E329–E357.
56. Sharma P, Varma MV, Chawla HP, Panchhagnula R. Absorption enhancement, mechanistic and toxicity studies of medium chain fatty acids, cyclodextrins and bile salts as peroral absorption enhancers. *Farmaco*. 2005;60:884–893.
57. Brewster ME, Loftsson T. Cyclodextrins as pharmaceutical solubilizers. *Adv Drug Rev*. 2007;59:645–666.
58. Gould S, Scott RC. 2-Hydroxypropyl-beta-cyclodextrin: a toxicology review. *Food Chem Toxicol*. 2005;43:1451–1459.
59. Chiou WL, Buehler PW. Comparison of oral absorption and bioavailability of drugs between monkey and human. *Pharm Res*. 2002;19:868–874.
60. Kondo H, Shinoda T, Nakashima H, Watanabe T, Yokohama S. Characteristics of the gastric profiles of unfed and fed cynomolgus monkeys as pharmaceutical product development subjects. *Biopharm Drug Dispos*. 2003;24:45–51.
61. Kondo H, Takahashi Y, Watanabe T, Yokohama S, Watanabe J. Gastrointestinal transit of liquids in unfed cynomolgus monkeys. *Biopharm Drug Dispos*. 2003;24:131–140.

62. Kondo H, Watanabe T, Yokohama S, Watanabe J. Effect of food on gastrointestinal transit of liquids in cynomolgus monkeys. *Biopharm Drug Dispos*. 2003;24:141–151.
63. Martinez NM. Interspecies differences in physiology and pharmacology: extrapolating preclinical data to human populations. In: Rogge MC, Taft DR, eds. *Preclinical Drug Development*. New York: Taylor & Francis; 2005.
64. Riviere JE. *Comparative Pharmacokinetics: Principles, Techniques and Applications*. Ames, IA: Blackwell Publishing; 1999.
65. Bjorkman S. Prediction of drug disposition in infants and children by means of physiologically based pharmacokinetic modeling: theophylline and midazolam as model drugs. *Br J Clin Pharmacol*. 2004;59:691–704.
66. Rowland M, Balant L, Peck C. Physiologically based pharmacokinetics in drug development and regulatory science: a workshop report. *AAPS PharmSci*. 2004;6:1–12.
67. Brightman FA, Leahy DE, Searle GE, Thomas S. Application of a generic physiologically based pharmacokinetic model to the estimation of xenobiotic levels in human plasma. *Drug Metab Dispos*. 2006;34:94–101.
68. De Buck SS, Sinha VK, Fenu LA, Nijsen MJ, Mackie CE, Glissen RA. Prediction of human pharmacokinetics using physiologically bases modeling: a retrospective analysis of 26 clinically tested drugs. *Drug Metab Dispos*. 2007;35:1766–1780.
69. Levitt DG, Schoemaker RC. Human physiologically based pharmacokinetic model for ACE inhibitors: ramipril and ramiprilat. *BMC Clin Pharmacol*. 2006;6:1–27.
70. Mahmood I. Allometric issues in drug development. *J Pharm Sci*. 2000;88:1101–1106.
71. Tang H, Mayerson M. A novel model for prediction of human drug clearance by allometric scaling. *Drug Metab Dispos*. 2005;33:1297–1303.
72. Tang H, Mayerson M. On the observed large interspecies overprediction of human clearance (vertical allometry) of UCN-01; further support for a proposed model based on plasma protein binding. *J Clin Pharmacol*. 2006;46:398–400.
73. Sinha VK, De Buck SS, Fenu LA, et al. Predicting oral clearance in humans: How close can we get with allometry? *Clin Pharmacokinet*. 2008;47:35–45.
74. Subramanian K. truPK: human pharmacokinetic models for quantitative ADME prediction. *Expert Opin Drug Metab Toxicol*. 2005;1:555–564.
75. Ekins S, Waller CL, Swaan PW, Cruciani G, Wrighton SA, Wikel JH. Progress in predicting human ADME parameters in silico. *J Pharmacol Toxicol Methods*. 2000;44:251–572.
76. Clark DE, Grootenhuis PD. Progress in computational methods for the prediction of ADMET properties. *Curr Opin Drug Discov Dev*. 2002;5:382–390.
77. Brier ME, Aronoff GR. Application of artificial neural networks to clinical pharmacology. *Int J Clin Pharmacol Ther*. 1996;34:510–514.
78. Schneider G, Coassolo P, Lavé T. Combining in vitro and in vivo pharmacokinetic data for prediction of hepatic drug clearance in humans by artificial neural networks and multivariate statistical techniques. *J Med Chem*. 1999;42:5072–5076.
79. Turner JV, Maddalena DJ, Cutler DJ. Pharmacokinetic parameter prediction from drug structure using artificial neural networks. *Int J Pharmacol*. 2004;270:209–219.

80. Schuster D, Laggner C, Langer T. Why drugs fail: a study on side effects in new chemical entities. *Curr Pharm Des*. 2005;11(27):3545–3559.
81. Chang CY, Schiano TD. Review article: drug hepatotoxicity. *Aliment Pharmacol Ther*. 2007;25(10):1135–1151.
82. Shapiro MA, Lewis JH. Causality assessment of drug-induced hepatotoxicity: promises and pitfalls. *Clin Liver Disease*. 2007;11(3):477–505.
83. Norris W, Paredes AH, Lewis JH. Drug-induced injury in 2007. *Curr Opin Gastroenterol*. 2008;24(3):287–297.
84. Ostapowicz G, Fontana RJ, Schiødt FV, et al. Results of a prospective study of acute liver failure at 17 tertiary care centers in the United States. *Ann Intern. Med*. 2002;137(12):947–54.
85. Paakkari I. Cardiotoxicity of new antihistamines and cisapride. *Toxicol Lett*. 2002;127(1–3):279–284.
86. Sirvent P, Mercier J, Lacampagne A. New insights into mechanisms of statin-associated myotoxicity. *Curr Opin Pharmacol*. 2008;31 [Epub ahead of print].
87. Sereno M, Brunello A, Chiappori A, et al. Cardiac toxicity: old and new issues in anti-cancer drugs. *Clin Translat Oncol*. 2008;10(1):35–46.
88. Brophy JM. Cardiovascular effects of cyclooxygenase-2 inhibitors. *Curr Opin Gastroenterol*. 2007;23(6):617–624.
89. Ju C, Uetrecht JP. Mechanism of idiosyncratic drug reactions: reactive metabolite formation, protein binding and the regulation of the immune system. *Curr Drug Metab*. 2002;3(4):367–377.
90. Hussaini SH, Farrington EA. Idiosyncratic drug-induced liver injury: an overview. *Expert Opin Drug Saf*. 2007;6(6):673–684.
91. Ekwall B, Acosta D. In Vitro toxicity of selected drugs and chemicals in HeLa cells, Chang liver cells and rat hepatocytes. *Drug Chem Toxicol*. 1982;5(3): 219–231.
92. Acosta D, Sorensen EM, Anuforo DC, et al. An in vitro approach to the study of target organ toxicity of drugs and chemicals. In Vitro *Cell Dev Biol*. 1985;21(9):495–504.
93. Davila JC, Lenherr A, Acosta D. Protective effect of flavanoids on drug-induced hepatotoxicity in vitro. *Toxicology*. 1989;57(3):267–286.
94. Farkas D, Tannenbaum SR. In Vitro methods to study chemically-induced hepatotoxicity: a literature review. *Curr Drug Metab*. 2005;6(2):111–125.
95. Bondesson I, Ekwall B, Hellberg S, Romert L, Stenberg K, Walum E. MEIC: a new international multicenter project to evaluate the relevance to human toxicity of in vitro cytotoxicity tests. *Cell Biol Toxicol*. 1989;5(3):331–347.
96. Shrivastava R, Delomenie C, Chevalier A, et al. Comparison of in vivo acute lethal potency and in vitro cytotoxicity of 48 chemicals. *Cell Biol Toxicol*. 1992;8(2):157–170.
97. Rasmussen ES. Cytotoxicity of MEIC chemicals Nos.11–30 in 3T3 mouse fibroblasts with and without microsomal activation. In Vitro *Mol Toxicol*. 1999;12(3):125–132.
98. Dierickx PJ. Cytotoxicity of the MEIC reference chemicals in rat hepatocytes in rat hepatoma-derived Fa32 cells. *Toxicology*. 2000;150(1–3):159–169.

99. Dierickx PJ, Scheers EM. Neutral red uptake inhibition in adhered and adhering rat hepatoma-derived Fa32 cells to predict human toxicity. *J Appl Toxicol*. 2002;22(1):61–65.

100. Clemendson C, Nordin-Anderson M, Bjerregaard HF, et al. Development of an in vitro test battery for the estimation of acute human systemic toxicity: an outline of the EDIT project. Evaluation-guided development of in vitro test batteries. *Altern Lab Anim*. 2002;30(3):313–321.

101. Spielman H, Bochkov NP, Costa L, et al. 13th Meeting of the scientific group on methodologies for the safety evaluation of chemicals (SGOMSEC): an alternative testing methodologies for organ toxicity. *Environ Health Perspect*. 1998;106(suppl 2):427–439.

102. Suter W. Predictive value of in vitro safety studies. *Curr Opin Chem Biol*. 2006;10(4):362–366 [Epub July 3, 2006].

103. Li AP. A review of the common properties of drugs with idiosyncratic hepatotoxicity and the "multiple determinant hypothesis" for the manifestation of idiosyncratic drug toxicity. *Chem Biol Interact*. 2002;142(1–2):7–23.

104. Uetrecht J. Prediction of a new drug's potential to cause idiosyncratic reactions. *Curr Opin Drug Discov Dev*. 2001;4(1):55–59.

105. Uetrecht J. Idiosyncratic drug reactions: current understanding. *Annu Rev Pharmacol Toxicol*. 2007;47:513–539.

106. Uetrecht J. Idiosyncratic drug reactions: past, present and future. *Chem Res Toxicol*. 2008;21(1):84–92.

107. Seguin B, Utrecht J. The danger hypothesis applied to idiosyncratic drug reactions. *Curr Opin Allergy Clin Immunol*. 2003;3(4):235–242.

108. Hofstra AH, Li-Muller SM, Uetrecht JP. Metabolism of isoniazid by activated leucocytes: possible role in drug-induced lupus. *Drug Metab Dispos*. 1992;20(2):205–210.

109. Uetrecht JP. Reactive metabolites and agranulocytosis. *Eur J Haematol*. 1996;60:83–88.

110. Masubichi Y, Nakayama S, Horie T. Role of mitochondrial permeability transition in diclofenac-induced hepatocyte injury in rats. *Hepatology*. 2002;35(3):544–551.

111. Boelsterli UA, Lim PL. Mitochondrial abnormalities: a link to idiosyncratic drug hepatotoxicity? *Toxicol Appl Pharmacol*. 2007;220(1):92–107.

112. Park BK, Kitteringham NR, Maggs JL, Pirmohamed M, Williams DP. The role of metabolic activation in drug-induced hepatotoxicity. *Annu Rev Pharmacol Toxicol*. 2005;45:177–202.

113. Baillie TA. Future of toxicology—metabolic activation and drug design: challenges and opportunities in chemical toxicology. *Chem Res Toxicol*. 2006;19(7):889–893.

114. Williams DP. Toxicophores: investigations in drug safety. *Toxicology*. 2006;226(1):1–11.

115. Masubuchi Y. Metabolic and non-metabolic factors determining troglitazone hepatotoxicity: a review. *Drug Metab Pharmacokinet*. 2006;21:347–356.

116. Li AP. In Vitro evaluation of human xenobiotic toxicity: scientific concepts and the novel integrated discrete multiple cell co-culture (IdMOC) technology. *ALTEX*. 2008;25(1):43–49.

117. Tuschl H, Schwab CE. Flow cytometry methods used as screening tests for basal toxicity of chemicals. *Toxicol In Vitro*. 2004;18(4):483–491.
118. Baudoin R, Corlu A, Griscom L, Legallais C, Leclerc E. Trends in the development of microfluidic cell biochips for in vitro hepatotoxicity. *Toxicol In Vitro*. 2007;21(4):535–544.
119. Dan YY, Yeoh GC. Liver stem cells: a scientific and clinical perspective. *J Gastroenterol Hepatol*. 2008;23(5):687–698.
120. Goldsmith MA, Slavik M, Carter SK. Quantitative prediction of drug toxicity in humans from toxicology in small and large animals. *Cancer Res*. 1975;35:1354–1364.
121. Olson H, Betton G, Stritat J, Robinson D. The predictivity of the toxicity of pharmaceuticals in humans from animal data: an interim assessment. *Toxicol Lett*. 1998;102–103:535–538.
122. Dixit R, Boelsterli UA. Healthy animals and animal models of human disease(s) in safety assessment of human pharmaceuticals, including therapeutic antibodies. *Drug Discov Today*. 2007;12(7–8):336–342.
123. Shenton JM, Chen J, Uetrecht JP. Animal models of idiosyncratic drug reactions. *Chem Biol Interact*. 2004;150(1):53–70.
124. Uetrecht J. Role of animal models in the study of drug-induced hypersensitivity reactions. *AAPS J*. 2006;7(4):E914–921.
125. Katoh M, Tateno C, Yoshizato K, Yokoi T. Chimeric mice with humanized liver. *Toxicology*. 2008;246:9–17.
126. Daviss B. Growing pains for metabolomics. *Scientist*. 2005;19(8):25–28.
127. Nicholson JK, Lindon JC, Holmes E. Metabonomics: understanding the metabolic responses of living systems to pathophysiological stimuli via multivariate statistical analysis of biological NMR spectroscopic data. *Xenobiotica*. 1999;29(11):1181–1189.
128. Lindon JC, Holmes E, Nicholson JK. Metabonomics in pharmaceutical R&D. *FEBS J*. 2007;274:1140–1151.
129. Wishart, DS, Tzur D, Knox C, et al. HMDB: the human metabolome database. *Nucleic Acids Res*. 2007;35:D521–D526.
130. Browne M, Dunn WB, Ellis DI, et al. A metabolome pipeline: from concept to data to knowledge. *Metabolomics*. 2005;1(1):39–51.
131. Fiehn O. Metabolomics: the link between genotypes and phenotypes. *Plant Mol Biol*. 2002;48(1–2):155–171.
132. Salek RM, Maguire ML, Bentley E, et al. A metabolomic comparison of urinary changes in type 2 diabetes in mouse, rat and human. *Physiol Genom*. 2007;29(2):99–108.
133. Fiehn O, Kristal B, van Ommen B, et al. Establishing reporting standards for metabolomic and metabonomic studies: a call for participation. *OMICS*. 2006;10(2):158–163.
134. Gomase VS, Tagore S. Transcriptomics. *Curr Drug Metab*. 2008;9(3):245–249.
135. Orphanides G, Kimber I. Toxicogenetics: applications and opportunities. *Toxicol Sci*. 2003;75:1–6.
136. Fielden MR, Zacharewski TR. Challenges and limitations of gene expression profiling in mechanistic and predictive toxicology. *Toxicol Sci*. 2001;60:6–10.

137. Storck T, von Brevern MC, Beherns CK, Scheel, Bach A. Transcriptomics in predictive toxicology. *Curr Opin Drug Discov Dev*. 2002;5(1):90–97.
138. Kier LD, Neft R, Tang L, et al. Applications of microarrays with toxicologically relevant genes for the evaluation of chemical toxicants in Sprague–Dawley rats in vivo and human hepatocytes in vitro. *Mutat Res*. 2004;549(1–2):101–113.
139. Burchiel SW, Knall CM, Davis JW, Paules RS, Boggs SE, Afshari CA. Analysis of genetic and epigenetic mechanisms of toxicity: potential roles of toxicogenomics and proteomics in toxicology. *Toxicol Sci*. 2001;59:193–195.
140. Nuwaysir EF, Bittner M, Trent J, Barrett JC, Afshari CA. Microarrays and toxicology: the advent of toxicogenomics. *Mol Carcinogen*. 1999;24(3):153–159.
141. Meyer UA, Gut J. Genomics and the prediction of xenobiotic toxicity. *Toxicology*. 2002;181–182:463–466.
142. Castle AL, Carver MP, Mendrick DL. Toxicogenomics; a new revolution in drug safety. *Drug Discov Today*. 2002;7(13):728–736.
143. Hong Y, Muller UR, Lai F. Discriminating two classes of toxicants through expression analysis of HepG2 cells with DNA arrays. *Toxicol In Vitro*. 2003;17(1):85–92.
144. Boverhof DR, Zacharewski TR. Toxicogenomics in risk assessment: applications and needs. *Toxicol Sci*. 2006;89(2):352–360.
145. Maggioli J, Hoover A, Weng L. Toxicogenomic analysis methods for predictive toxicology. *Pharmacol Toxicol Methods*. 2006;53(1):31–37.
146. Kiyosawa N, Shiwaku K, Hirode M, et al. Utilization of a one-dimensional score for surveying chemical-induced changes in expression levels of multiple biomarker gene sets using a large-scale toxicogenomics database. *J Toxicol Sci*. 2006;31(5):433–448.
147. Heijne WH, Kienhuis AS, van Ommen B, Stierum RH, Groten JP. Systems toxicology: applications of toxicogenomics, transcriptomics, proteomics and metabolomics in toxicology. *Expert Rev Proteom*. 2005;2(5):767–780.
148. Luthe A, Suter L, Ruepp S, Singer T, Weiser T, Albertini S. Toxicogenomics in the pharmaceutical industry: hollow promises or real benefit? *Mutat Res*. 2005;575(1–2):102–115.
149. Kienhuis AS, Wortelboer HM, Hoflack J-C, et al. Comparison of coumarin-induced toxicity between sandwich-cultured primary rat hepatocytes and rats in vivo: a toxicogenomics approach. *Drug Metab Dispos*. 2006;34(12):2083–2090.
150. Wold S, Dunn WJ, Hellberg S. Toxicity modeling and prediction with pattern recognition. *Environ Health Perspect*. 1985;61:257–268.
151. Hulzebos E, Sijm D, Traas T, Posthumus R, Maslankiewicz L. Validity and validation of expert (Q)SAR systems. *SAR QSAR Environ. Res*. 2005;16(4):385–401.
152. Benigni R, Zito R. Designing safer drugs: (Q)SAR-based identification of mutagens and carcinogens. *Curr Top Med Chem*. 2003;3(11):1289–1300.
153. Dearden JC. In silico prediction of drug toxicity. *J Comput Aid Mol Des*. 2003;17(2–4):119–127.
154. Greene N. Computer systems for the prediction of toxicity: an update. *Adv Drug Deliv. Rev*. 2002;54(3):417–431.
155. Greene N, Judson PN, Langowski JJ, Marchant CA. Knowledge-based expert systems for toxicity and metabolism prediction: DEREK, StAR and METEOR. *SAR QSAR Environ Res*. 1999;10(2–3):299–314.

156. Ji ZL, Wang Y, Yu L, Han LY, Zheng CJ, Chen YZ. In silico search of putative adverse drug reaction related proteins as a potential tool for facilitating drug adverse effect prediction. *Toxicol Lett*. 2006;164(2):104–112.
157. Li AP. A comprehensive approach for drug safety assessment. *Chem Biol Interact*. 2004;150(1):27–33.
158. Richard AM. Future of toxicology—predictive toxicology: an expanded view of "chemical toxicity." *Chem Res Toxicol*. 2006;19(10):1257–1262.

4

BIOANALYTICAL STRATEGIES

CHRISTOPHER KEMPER

4.1 INTRODUCTION

4.1.1 Bioanalysis: The Primary Basis for Pharmacokinetic and Pharmacodynamic Evaluations

The generation of pharmacokinetic and pharmacodynamic data in support of drug discovery and development is dependent on the best estimation of analyte concentrations in biological matrices. The purpose of this chapter is to outline the processes that can be put into place to obtain reliable and rapid drug (and, if deemed necessary, metabolite) concentrations in biological matrices in support of studies conducted prior to the first-in-human (FIH) trial. These data can then be used to support drug discovery, to bridge animal safety data to humans, to optimize dosage forms in discovery and development, and to develop proper dosing regimens to elicit optimum drug performance with a minimum of toxicological risk. The issue of the assay of compounds used as biomarkers, although vitally important, will be mentioned but not pursued.

In addition to literature references, considerable material from discussion groups and symposia are cited. Some specific products and processes will be mentioned, even though there may be acceptable alternatives. Although technical issues are discussed, it is the mission of this chapter not to delve too deeply into the technical details but to describe the processes utilizing current technologies for improved and more efficient early stage drug development, as well as meeting international regulatory expectations.

Most of the discussion will center on molecules that can be assayed using mass spectral (MS) detection, which usually means for compounds with molecular weights less than 2000 Da. Degradation techniques have promise of expanding

Early Drug Development: Strategies and Routes to First-in-Human Trials, Edited by Mitchell N. Cayen

that range in the future. Most, if not all, newly developed small-molecule methods use MS. Currently, large-molecule analyses are required for most biopharmaceuticals and need some sort of ligand-binding assay (LBA). This field is growing as assays become more robust. However, the constraints of ligand-binding assays are far greater than for chromatographic MS methods. Most are based on the availability of an antibody receptor. Development of such an antibody is expensive in time and cost. It can take as much as nine months to a year to develop, and the skills required are extremely high. Therefore, the bioanalytical support in discovery and early development of biopharmaceuticals during the pre-FIH stage of development is limited.

Although the focus of this chapter is on regulated bioanalytical work, there will be some discussion of fit-for-purpose assays that are scientifically valid but do not fill all the requirements enumerated in the U.S. Food and Drug Administration (FDA) regulations [1,2], bioanalytical validation guidance [3], or the white papers written as commentary to the various FDA/American Association of Pharmaceutical Scientists (AAPS)-sponsored meetings [4–7]. Opinions vary as to what is good science and what is "fit for purpose" [8]. The case for biomarker validation is also not well defined. The basic question is just what level of risk should be taken by using methods that are not fully validated in order to accelerate studies early in discovery and development.

4.1.2 Regulatory Initiatives in Bioanalysis

Criteria for acceptable method validation for bioanalysis were highly variable until the first Bioanalytical Method Validation Workshop hosted by FDA/AAPS in Arlington, Virginia (Crystal City) on validation harmonization was held in 1990. A history of the three "Crystal City" conferences may be found in Shah [9]. The 1990 meeting established a common approach for the criteria to be used to evaluate method validation and sample analysis [4]. Although statistical approaches were forwarded, the 4 : 6 : 15 rule was established as being a reasonable compromise among competing mindsets. This rule refers to the following: "Of 6 (or more) quality control (QC) samples (at three concentrations), at least 4 (or 2/3rds) must be within 15% of the nominal concentration." At least 50% of the QCs within one concentration must also pass. Many statistical paradigms have been forwarded throughout the years [9], but none has gained universal acceptance.

A follow-up meeting was held in 2000 [5] and an FDA guidance was issued in May 2001 [3]. The guidance addresses validation criteria for IND-, NDA-, and ANDA-track studies, and therefore applies to all GLP (nonclinical)- and GCP (clinical)-related studies that support drug submissions. The guidance was reviewed at a meeting in Arlington in 2006 (Crystal City III) and a white paper was issued [6]. In practice, the guidance forms the basis for regulatory review of bioanalytical work presented to the FDA and most other regulatory authorities worldwide. The white paper from the 2006 meeting may be considered as an amendment to the guidance. Although the FDA has not expressed specific approaches to deal with the issues in the white paper, individual inspectors have wide latitude on compliance. These inspectors have expressed their ideas through a series of FDA form 483s. Details of this important guidance and associated white papers are presented later in the chapter.

4.2 BASIC BIOANALYTICAL TECHNIQUES AND METHOD DEVELOPMENT

There are many excellent texts that deal with bioanalytical processes and techniques [10–26]. Although some of these references may appear to be a bit aged, they contain information that will never be outdated. For example, the Snyder et al. and Shugar and Ballinger books [23,24] are particularly useful. The reader is also urged to obtain a free subscription to *Liquid Chromatography/Gas Chromatography* (see Table 4.1 for the web address); back issues are available online. The AAPS Web site is also a good site for emerging bioanalytical perspectives; access to *Pharmaceutical Contract Research* and the *AAPS Journal* requires membership in AAPS, which is a good investment. Other sites are listed that can provide valuable information at minimal cost.

While chromatographic techniques such as gas chromatography (GC) and nonchromatographic techniques such as ligand-binding assays (LBAs) are important components in discovery and early development, the role of liquid chromatography (LC)-MS has special relevance. The bulk of the discussion herein will therefore focus on this technique. The recent Korfmacher book [18] is a treasure trove of LC-MS information and is strongly recommended. Some commercial courses are also useful.

4.2.1 Sample Preparation

Knowing how the target analyte(s) behave chemically and how they interact with the matrix of interest is the first challenge facing an analytical chemist. Most physicochemical information on the drug substance is obtained during the chemical characterization process. Metabolite characteristics emerge later. However, as discussed in Chapters 2 and 8, with the exception of prodrugs, it is often not critical to develop and validate bioanalytical assays for a metabolite at the pre-FIH development stage.

Lipophilicity, pK_a values, and water solubility can give an indication of what sample preparation techniques will optimally clean a sample and give an indication of what chromatographic options may be employed. Clean samples yield robust methods. The degree of sample cleanup should be a function of the needs of the method at the stage of nonclinical development. Requirements may increase as development goes from non-GLP (good laboratory practices) animal studies to GLP toxicology support to the assay to be used in the FIH study.

There are five basic types of sample preparation procedures for plasma, serum, urine, or a tissue extract: (1) dilute and shoot, (2) crash and shoot, (3)

TABLE 4.1 Web-Based Resources for the Bioanalytical Scientist[a]

Resource	Web Site
Accium	www.acciumbio.com/
Analytical Techniques in Immunochemistry	books.google.com/books?id=kPLyt8b_44gC&dq=immunochemistry&printsec=frontcover&source=web&ots=pJ-ROc33Td&sig=gqbLIaGRjpWY4ir6BBPgcT6o7fg&PPP1,M1
Central Drugs Standard Control	cdsco.nic.in/index.html
Chromatography Forum	www.sepsci.com/chromforum/index.php
Chromatography Online	chromatographyonline.findanalytichem.com/lcgc
Chrom Manager	www.acdlabs.com/products/chrom_lab/chrom_manager/
ChromSword Group	iristech.net/
CPSA (and Milestone Development)	www.milestonedevelopment.com/index.html
Engineering Statistics (including MIL 105D)	www.itl.nist.gov/div898/handbook/
European Bioanalytical Forum	www.bioanalysis-forum.com
Immunochemistry Basics	books.google.com/books?id=BZAUZGNAhRAC&dq=immunochemistry&printsec=frontcover&source=web&ots=fk1GgwQtaw&sig=0qLVWZ2AAasnDJmNJLFGaQ0RF-Q&PPA4,M1
Liquid Chromatography/Gas Chromatography	www.chromatographyonline.com
LC Resources	www.lcresources.com
Linde Gas	hiq.lindegas.com/international/web/lg/spg/likelgspg.nsf/docbyalias/anal_gaschrom
Mass Spectrometry Interest Group of the NCI at Frederick	msig.ncifcrf.gov/default.asp
Mass Spectrometry Society of Japan	www.mssj.jp/
Meso Scale Discovery	www.mesoscale.com
Millipore: Immunochemistry	www.millipore.com/immunodetection/id3/immunochemistryhome
Millipore: Tutorial	www.millipore.com/immunodetection/id3/antibodiestutorial
North Jersey ACS Mass Spec Discussion Group	www.njacs.org/msdg/index.html
Novatia	www.enovatia.com/; www.enovatia.com/structure_elucidation)
OECD GLP	www.oecd.org/department/0,3355,en_2649_34381_1_1_1_1_1,00.html
Outsourcing Pharma	outsourcing-pharma.com/
PerkinElmer	las.perkinelmer.com/

TABLE 4.1 *(Continued)*

Resource	Web Site
Pharmaceutical Contract Research	www.business.com/directory/pharmaceuticals_and_biotechnology/research_and_development/contract_research/
Pharsight, general	www.pharsight.com/main.php
Research Triangle Park Drug Metabolism Discussion Group	www.rtpnet.org/rtpdmdg/
Sam Houston State U. (GC/MS)	www.shsu.edu/~chemistry/primers/gcms.html
Thermo–Turboflow site	www.cohesivetech.com/technologies/turboflow/index.asp
ThermoFisher (home page)	www.thermo.com
Waters	www.waters.com/watersdivision/
Watson–ThermoFisher	www.thermo.com/com/cda/product/detail/0,1055,10120349,00.html
Xceleron	www.xceleron.com

[a]Additional sites are listed in Appendix 3 at the end of the book.

liquid–liquid extraction, (4) solid-phase extraction (SPE), and (5) direct injection. Newer techniques, such as MALDI (matrix-assisted laser desorption/ionization), have emerged that allow direct input into the mass spectrometer.

When preparing plasma, ethylenediaminetetracetic acid (EDTA) as an anticoagulant appears to be superior to heparin, in that it is more effective than heparin in the prevention of thrombin clots. Regardless of how carefully samples are handled, there will always be a finite amount of systematic and random error regarding plasma composition, which can affect accuracy and/or precision. The microenvironment of each sample will also be a little different (e.g., samples taken after a meal) and may affect the assay. A critical way of reducing these errors is to add an internal standard to the sample as soon as possible. Ideally, this standard will behave chemically in exactly the same way as the analyte(s) of interest. Stable label internal standards, with substitutions of several (usually, four or more) of the natural ^{12}C and/or ^{14}N atoms of the analyte(s) of interest with stable ^{13}C and ^{15}N atoms, respectively, are considered the gold standard. However, these may not be readily available, especially in drug discovery and early development, and depending on the location of substitutions and availability of precursor reagents, they can be very expensive. The use of deuterium atoms is also common, but care must be taken to ensure that the chemical site of the hydrogen atom substitutions are not subject to exchange with surrounding water. Close chemical analogs are also used as internal standards in discovery and frequently in early development. Regrettably, the use of internal standards for ligand-binding assays is not yet possible, which accounts for the wider acceptance limits for those assays and analyzing samples in replicates [1]. It is recommended that stable label internal standard(s) be used for all GLP studies, and their use is strongly recommended for all human studies, including FIH.

Dilute and Shoot This technique involves taking an aliquot of the sample, adding the internal standard, and diluting the aliquot with water, buffer, or another, cleaner matrix (e.g., stripped plasma). A dilution with a protein solution may be necessary to maintain solubility. The method, frequently used in ligand-binding assays, has the advantages of being fast and inexpensive, with minimal sample manipulation. Disadvantages include no cleanup and no enrichment. Chromatographic techniques typically do not involve this approach, except, notably, when urine is the matrix. Without endogenous proteins and other solubilization agents, analytes in urine can fall out of solution or bind to sample storage containers. Recovery needs to be monitored closely during method development for urine assays.

Crash and Shoot In this method a solution or solvent is added to a sample, precipitating proteinaceous material. The sample is centrifuged and the supernatant is injected onto a chromatograph. Precipitation reagents include acids (e.g., trichloroacteic acid, hydrochloric acid); organic solvents (acetonitrile, acetone, ethanol, and methanol are commonly used), and zinc and copper salts. The following is a typical method:

1. Add 100 μL of internal standard solution to 100 μL of plasma.
2. Shake the sample vigorously.
3. Add 300 μL of acetonitrile (shake).
4. Centrifuge.
5. Transfer the sample to a chromatograph autosampler.

A 3 : 1 acetonitrile precipitation is perhaps the most common. Other methods may be laborious to prepare (the salt solutions) or reactive (methanol, the acids). Advantages include speed, cost, and minimal sample manipulation. Disadvantages are minimal cleanup, no enrichment (dilution rather than concentration of the sample), loss due to entrapment in the precipitate, and dilution effects. The sample still has a considerable load of unwanted materials, so chromatographic column lifetimes may be shortened. It is recommended that a diversion valve be used to prevent overloading the interface with nonvolatile sample residues. Although high-performance liquid chromatography (HPLC) is discussed in a later section, Figure 4.1 shows a basic system. The diversion valve would be placed between the column and the detector.

Liquid–Liquid Extraction Liquid–liquid extraction is an old technique that has had a resurgence in popularity in the last few years. It is simple, flexible, reproducible, amenable to automation, and relatively inexpensive. Sample manipulation can be minimized with the use of 96-well extraction plates and robots [27]. The basic premise is: "Like will dissolve into like" (i.e., polar compounds into polar media; nonpolar compounds into nonpolar media). This is a method that rewards the thorough understanding of analyte chemistry mentioned above.

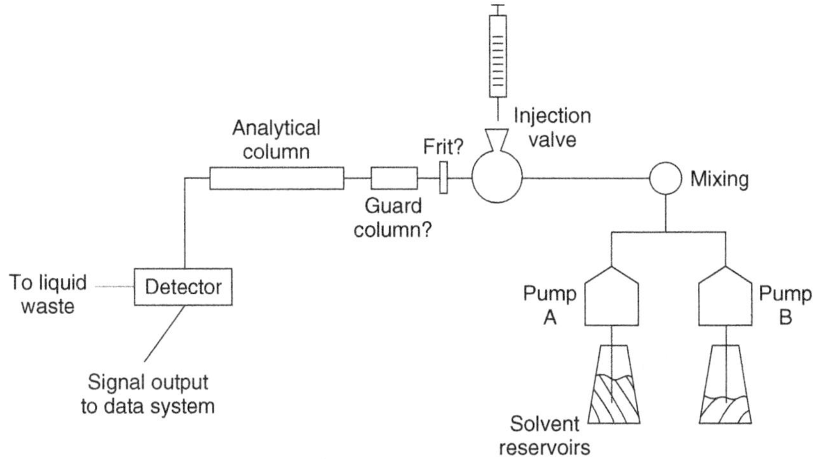

FIGURE 4.1 Basic high-performance liquid chromatograph. (Courtesy of Richard LeLacheur, Taylor Technology.)

The relative polarity of various molecular functional groups is provided by Snyder et al. [23]. Typically, a sample is pH-adjusted and extracted into an organic solvent such as butyl chloride, which is transferred to another tube and evaporated. The sample is then reconstituted in the injection solvent, usually similar to the HPLC mobile phase. Care has to be taken to prevent mismatches between the injection solvent and the mobile and solid phases of the HPLC. If the analyte has a high affinity for the injection solvent, a portion of the sample may be split and eluted in the solvent peak that precedes actual analyte separation, resulting in unrecorded analyte and a negative bias for the method.

Extraction solvents include ethyl acetate (good for polar analytes, but extracts can be dirty), methyl *tert*-butyl ether (which is less polar but cleaner than ethyl acetate), and many chlorinated solvents (e.g. methylene chloride, which is nonpolar and heavier than water). Butyl chloride has the advantage of being lighter than water, thereby simplifying automated sample handling. One possible disadvantage with chlorinated solvents is their potential toxicity. There are also environmental concerns, making proper discarding of waste solvent expensive.

A typical extraction could proceed as follows:

1. Combine 300 μL of plasma with 100 μL of internal standard.
2. Mix the sample vigorously.
3. Add 300 μL of borate buffer (pH 9.2) and mix the sample.
4. Add 1 mL of butyl chloride, mix, and centrifuge.
5. Transfer the butyl chloride.
6. Evaporate to dryness.
7. Reconstitute in 100 μL of injection solvent.

An additional back extraction can be done to improve sample cleanup. Advantages are that the method is selective, materials are inexpensive, and the technique is (usually) highly reproducible. There is also the potential for sample enrichment, which can improve sensitivity. For example, in the procedure described above, a 300 – μL sample is reduced in volume to 100 μL of injection solvent, a three-fold increase in concentration, assuming complete recovery. Increasing the plasma volume could increase this ratio but could also reduce the cleanliness of the sample, increasing the potential for unwanted interferences. Disadvantages with this method are that it can be time consuming and may require extensive sample manipulation. Use of robots for automated sample handling [e.g., Janus (formally Mutiprobe II, PerkinElmer), Tomtec (Tomtec), and Hamilton Star (Hamilton Robotics)] have alleviated these disadvantages markedly. Web addresses for these vendors may be found in Table 4.1. Despite the age of the basic technique (at least 100 years, perhaps millennia), liquid extraction remains a major bioanalytical tool in drug discovery and development support.

Solid-Phase Extraction SPE has become a popular cleanup technique in recent years. A variety of SPE columns (stationary phases) are available, ranging from ion exchange to reversed phase to mixed phase. The most popular are the silica reversed-phase columns. The basic column chemistry of the latter consists of a solid particle support with a hydroxylated silica surface (support–Si—OH). A certain percentage of the hydroxyls are reacted with a silicon-based reactant to form silicon ethers with a hydrophobic group such as C8 or C18.

In a typical SPE procedure, a liquid sample (e.g., plasma with a buffer and internal standard) is loaded onto the top of a column, the other side of the column is attached to a vacuum, and the liquid is pulled through the column by the vacuum (the eluant) and discarded. With a properly designed assay, the analytes of interest should remain on the column. A solvent that does not elute the analytes is loaded and some of the contaminants on the column are washed in a similar manner through the column to waste. A solvent that will desorb the analytes is loaded and the column washed again (but this time the eluant is collected), leaving more strongly retained materials behind. Because a milliliter or more of sample can be loaded, samples can be enriched.

SPE cartridges are available as individual columns or in a 96-well format for use with robots. In general, one should use an SPE stationary phase that is "orthogonal" (e.g., is different chemically) to the analytical column (analytical columns are discussed later). For example, if a C18 column is used on the LC, a mixed-bed or ion-exchange SPE cartridge might be chosen. It is important not to lose sight of the fact that SPE is the same as an HPLC column but is much less efficient than analytical columns. The same principles of solvent strength, pH, and retention apply. An example of such an extraction follows.

- Condition the SPE column twice with 1 mL of methanol (MeOH), then 1 mL of water.
- Add 500 μL of plasma +100 μL of internal standard and mix vigorously.

- Add 300 μL of borate (pH 9.2); vortex.
- Add 500 μL of the mix to an SPE cartridge.
- Wash with 1 mL of NH_4HCO_3 (pH 9).
- Elute with 1 mL of NH_4OH/MeOH (5/95% v/v).
- Evaporate and reconstitute in injection solvent.

Direct Injection (Online Preparation) Online sample preparation techniques have been available for some time [28]. In the simplest model, a smaller version of the HPLC column (called a *guard column*) is used instead of a loop on a sample injection valve in standard HPLC. The sample is loaded on the guard column, with components of interest sticking on the column and more polar materials eluted to waste. The valve controlling the injection is then switched in line with the analytical column and the components of interest are released from the cleanup column with a stronger solvent. Many laboratories use this technique routinely with very satisfactory results. Advantages include selectivity and sample enrichment, since the entire sample is on the column. Disadvantages are more complex apparatus, reduced column lifetime, differential extraction, and an increase in analysis time.

Another useful technology is the ThermoFisher/Cohesive TurboFlow system, which allows direct injection of biological samples into an MS/MS system. When the mobile phase flows through the TurboFlow column, high linear velocities are created which are 100 times greater than what is typically observed with HPLC columns. The large interstitial spaces between the column particles and the high linear mobile-phase velocity create turbulence within the TurboFlow column. Since small-molecular-weight molecules diffuse faster than those with large molecular weight, the small sample compounds diffuse into the particle pores. The turbulent flow of the mobile phase quickly flushes the large sample compounds through the column to waste before they have an opportunity to diffuse into the particle pores. Of the sample molecules that enter the pores, those that have an affinity to the chemistry inside the pores bind to the column particles' internal surfaces (Figure 4.2). The small sample molecules, which have a lower binding affinity, quickly diffuse out of the pores and are flushed to waste. TurboFlow columns are available with a variety of column chemistries to accommodate different analyte types. A mobile-phase change then elutes the small molecules that were bound by the TurboFlow column to the mass spectrometer or to a second analytical column for further separation.

4.2.2 Component Separation

While HPLC dominates the area of chromatographic separations, gas-phase chromatography (GPC, or now just GC) still has many uses. These techniques are discussed in more depth in the following sections. Although HPLC can theoretically deal with any biomolecule, in some cases the superiority of GC sensitivity

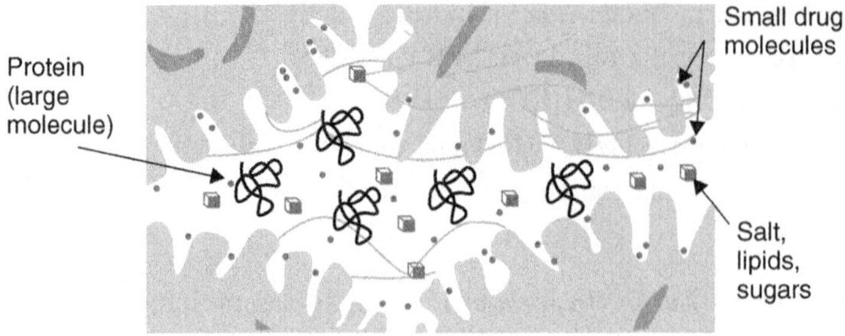

FIGURE 4.2 Cohesive system particle chemistry binds small molecules, while large molecules such as protein flow to waste. (Courtesy of ThermoFisher.)

and selectivity makes it an attractive alternative. Small, volatile molecules and molecules that can easily be volatized by derivatization can be targets for GC methodology. Metabonomic biomarkers that are endogenous, such as steroids and prostaglandins, which at low inherence concentrations require high sensitivity as well as high selectivity, may be particularly well suited using GC. However, for ease of use, HPLC is usually the method of choice.

Chromatography

High-Performance Liquid Chromatography After a sample has been prepared, the analyte of interest must be detected without interference by the other components within the sample. A typical HPLC setup is shown in Figure 4.1. An HPLC column is an inert metal tube packed with very fine (<5 μm) uniform particles. Although very similar, the particles are generally smaller and more uniformly sized than the SPE particles described above. Like SPE, using the reversed-phase chemistry is a popular approach. If SPE is used, the chemistry should be as different as possible. As above, separation is achieved by the difference in affinity between the components of the sample and the particle packing (the stationary phase) and the fluid moving through the column (the mobile phase). More details on the theoretical aspects of HPLC are provided by Snyder et al. [23].

After selecting several likely column types for further development, the next step in the bioanalytical LC-MS/MS assay development process is to select the LC method. Many published methods have critical missing specifications and/or procedures, without which it is not possible to meet current acceptable scientific and regulatory standards. However, these methods can provide clues and guidance for the basis of bioanalytical assays for new chemical entities (NCEs) under early development (e.g., the appropriate column type and the general mobile phase conditions) and can provide a head start on the new method, which can be appropriately validated.

There is still a large element of art rather than science in matching the column with the column conditions. Although proper use of literature tools such as PubMed is essential, even published methods for specific compounds may not fill the analyst's needs. Complete understanding by the analyst of the chemistries involved is necessary (more on that later). Courses such as those offered by LCResources can be useful in developing method development skills. Modeling programs such as ChromSword, ChromManager, and DryLab can also be useful. Much of the basis for these programs may be found in Snyder et al. [23]. A compatible pair of stationary- and mobile-phase systems needs to be identified. The effects of changing the pH, the organic component of the mobile phase, and the column temperature can then be determined. The data could be downloaded to a product like DryLab and DryLab used to determine the optimum separation and retention of the analytes of interest. It should be noted that columns should always be jacketed and heated, even if just a few degrees above ambient. It is sometimes possible for two analytes to switch elution order because of temperature variations caused by laboratory heating and cooling cycles from working hours to off-hour conditions.

Of course, to be able to obtain any data, detector conditions have to be set appropriately to generate a signal. The determination of MS conditions is described later in the chapter. At the LC development stage, initial conditions are best found with standards diluted in mobile phase or another suitable solvent. There are many possible chromatographic modes that can be used for LC-MS [22]. Reversed phase, the most common chromatographic mode, is the most compatible with both electrospray (ESI) and atmospheric pressure chemical ionization (APCI).

Standard columns for routine LC-MS/MS are 2.1 $\times$ 30 mm or 50-mm columns packed with 3-, 3.5-, or 5-μm silica particles. Either of the 2.1-mm columns can usually generate acceptable separations. Larger-diameter columns (e.g., 4.6 mm) require more solvent, which results in a greater burden on the MS interface. Smaller-diameter columns may challenge the plumbing of the system and give marginal gains. The flow rate should be scaled with the square of the column diameter. A 4.6-mm-internal-diameter column has five times the cross-sectional area of a 2.1-mm column, and therefore the 4.6-mm column run at 1.5 mL/min generates a linear velocity equivalent to that of a 2.1-mm column operated at 0.3 mL/min. Smaller particles are less sensitive to flow rate changes, so flow rates up to about 0.5 mL/min often can be used without compromising the separation. A sample chromatogram is shown in Figure 4.3.

A new development (but actually a relatively old concept) that has appeared in the field of HPLC is ultrahigh-performance liquid chromatography [called simply ultra-performance LC (UPLC)]. Columns that had similar characteristics (called microbore columns in the 1980s) had reduced pressure requirements and tended to clog. The benefit of UPLC systems is higher resolving power, increased sensitivity, and reduced run time. Although not standard in the pharmaceutical industry at this writing, the performance of UPLC has been sufficiently good that more laboratories are converting to this system, especially in drug discovery, where speed, sensitivity, and selectivity are at a premium. Of course, these systems can also be used for drug development studies that require GLP analysis [3].

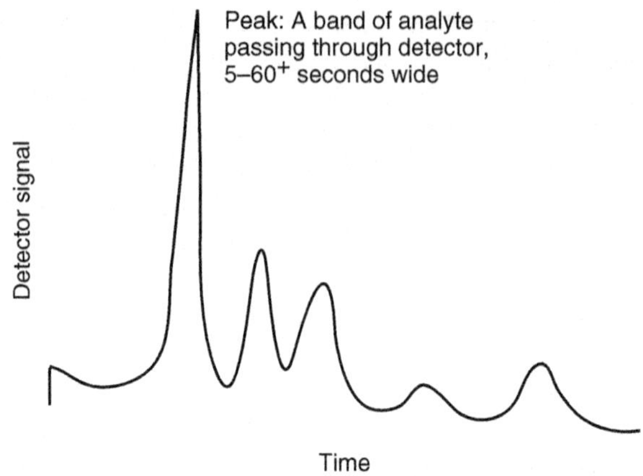

FIGURE 4.3 Sample HPLC chromatogram. (Courtesy of Richard LeLacheur, Taylor Technology.)

There is much debate about LC-MS methods regarding the relative merits of isocratic or gradient elutions. Isocratic runs are simple, because no mobile-phase mixing during a run is required. Isocratic runs can be fast if the peaks elute early and within a narrow region. However, if the peaks are spread out and retention times are long, isocratic runs can be more time consuming than gradients. Not having to reequilibrate the column between runs is an advantage of isocratic runs, but this may be countered with problems created by late-eluting compounds. Many isocratic methods use a flush after the peaks of interest elute so that strongly retained materials are removed from the column.

Gradients are more flexible than isocratic runs and can deal with a wider range of analyte polarities. Peaks tend to be narrower with gradients, which can translate to better detection limits. The gradient finishes with a strong solvent that flushes the column between each run. This can result in less interference of desired analytes by other components or contaminants in the sample. Because column reequilibration must be accomplished, gradients can sometimes be longer than their isocratic equivalents, but if the isocratic method uses a postrun flush, the difference is eliminated.

Gas Chromatography Like HPLC, gas chromatography separates chemical substances by relying on differences in partitioning behavior between a flowing mobile phase (a gas) and a stationary phase [29]. The sample is carried by a moving gas stream through a tube or column (Figure 4.4), the interior of which is lined with a film of a liquid. Because of its simplicity, sensitivity, and effectiveness in separating components of mixtures, GC is one of the most important analytical tools in chemistry. It is widely used for quantitative and qualitative analysis of mixtures, for the purification of compounds, and for the determination of such thermochemical constants as heats of solution and vaporization and vapor pressure. A typical chromatogram is shown in Figure 4.5.

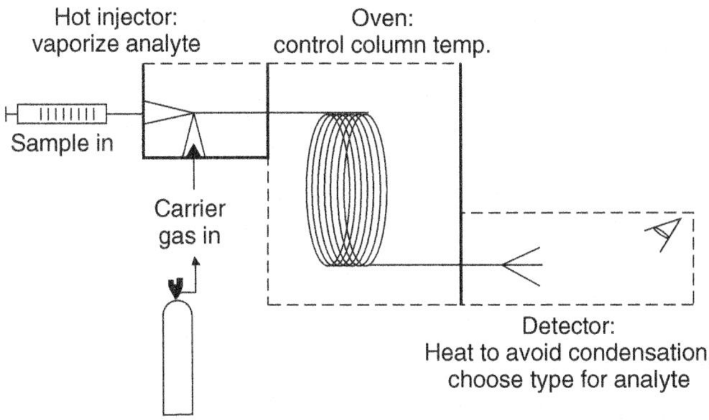

FIGURE 4.4 Basic components of a gas chromatograph. (Courtesy of Richard LeLacheur, Taylor Technology.)

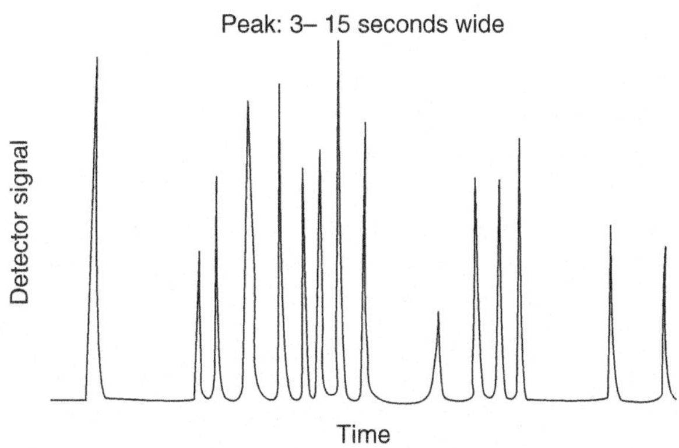

FIGURE 4.5 Typical GC chromatogram. (Courtesy of Richard LeLacheur, Taylor Technology.)

The method consists of introducing the test mixture or sample into a stream of an inert gas (commonly helium, nitrogen, hydrogen, argon, or even CO_2) that acts as a carrier. Liquid samples are vaporized before injection into the carrier stream. The gas stream is passed through the packed column, through which the components of the sample move at velocities that are influenced by the degree of interaction of each constituent with the stationary nonvolatile phase. The substances having the greater interaction with the stationary phase are retarded to a greater extent and consequently separate from those with smaller interaction. As the components elute from the column, they can be quantified by a detector and/or collected for further analysis.

Because of limitations in mobile-phase selection and sample volatility, GC techniques were predicted to disappear with the advent of commercially available

HPLCs in the early 1970s [30]. However, at about the same time, a new technique was being developed: open tubular or glass capillary GC [31]. Instead of having particles resting in an open tube, the tube itself was coated with a liquid stationary phase. The tube dimensions were radically different: from an internal diameter of about 1 mm for packed columns to less than 0.25 mm for capillary columns, and for length, from 2 to 4 m for packed columns to 50 m for capillary columns. Selectivity could be increased 10-fold or run time decreased 10-fold, or there could be a compromise between the two. When flexible silica replaced glass as the tube material, GC applications increased rapidly, although not to their previous heights.

The choice of carrier gas depends on the type of detector that is used and the components that are to be determined. Carrier gases for chromatographs must be of high purity and chemically inert with the sample. The carrier gas system can contain a molecular sieve to remove water or other impurities. The most common injection systems for the introduction of gas samples are the gas sampling valve and injection with a syringe. Both gaseous and liquid samples can be injected with a syringe. In the simplest form the sample is first injected into a heated chamber, where it is vaporized before being transferred to the column. When packed columns are used, the first part of the column often serves as the injection chamber, heated separately to an appropriate temperature. For capillary columns, a separate injection chamber is used from which only a small part of the vaporized or gaseous sample is transferred to the column, called *split injection*. This is necessary in order not to overload the column with a high sample volume.

When trace amounts of analyte(s) are expected in the sample, on-column injection can be used for capillary GC. The liquid sample is injected directly into the column with a syringe. The solvent is thereafter allowed to evaporate and a concentration of the sample components takes place. If the sample is gaseous, the concentration is achieved by cryofocusing. The sample components are concentrated and separated from the matrix by condensation in a cold trap before the chromatographic separation. Loop injection is often used in process control, where gaseous or liquid samples flow continuously through the sample loop, which is filled in an off-line position with a syringe or an automatic pump. Thereafter, the loop is connected in series with the column and the sample is transferred by the mobile phase. Sometimes a concentration step is necessary.

4.2.3 Detection

Mass Spectrometry A mass spectrometer is an instrument that measures the masses of individual molecules that have been converted into ions (i.e., molecules that have been electrically charged). A mass spectrometer does not actually measure the molecular mass directly but, rather, the mass-to-charge ratio of the ions formed from the target molecule. The charge on an ion is denoted by the integer number z as the fundamental unit of charge, and the mass-to-charge ratio m/z represents the mass (in daltons) per fundamental unit of charge. In many cases, the ions encountered in mass spectrometry have just one charge ($z = 1$),

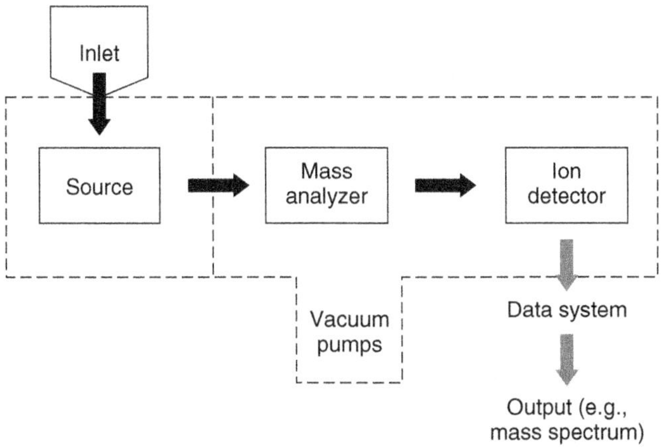

FIGURE 4.6 Components of a mass spectrometer. (Courtesy of Richard LeLacheur, Taylor Technology.)

so the *m*/*z* value is numerically equal to the molecular (ionic) mass in daltons. For large molecules and biomolecules, multiple ionization sites are possible and the response from a single molecule can result in multiple ratios and therefore multiple mass peaks.

The sample, which may be a solid, liquid, or vapor, must enter the mass spectrometer as a collection of gas-phase ions. The gas phase is generated by a combination of heat and low pressure (Figure 4.6). The gas-phase ions are sorted in the mass analyzer according to their mass-to-charge (*m*/*z*) ratios and then collected by a detector. In the detector, the ion stream is converted to a proportional electrical current. The data system records the magnitude of these electrical signals as a function of *m*/*z* and converts this information into a mass spectrum. For quantitative bioanalysis, coupling two stages of mass analysis (MS/MS) or tandem mass spectrometry is the routine approach (Figure 4.7). From a mixture of ions, those of a particular *m*/*z* value are selected in the first stage of mass analysis (quadrupole 1). These *parent* or *precursor ions* are

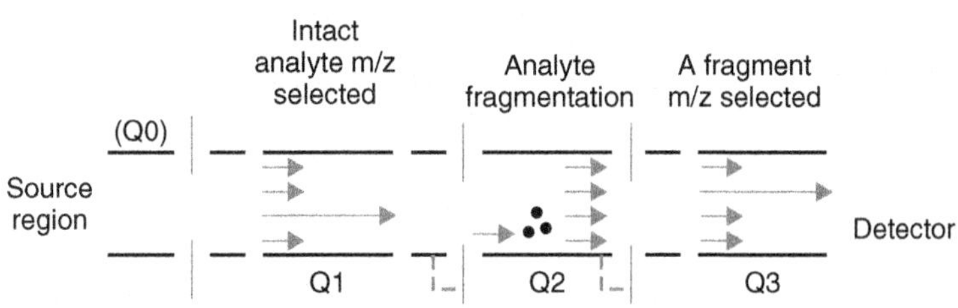

FIGURE 4.7 Expanded diagram of a triple-quadrupole LC-MS/MS system. (Courtesy of Richard LeLacheur, Taylor Technology.)

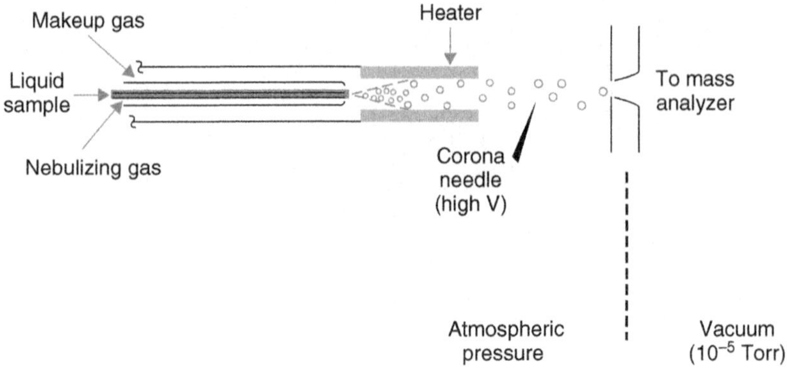

FIGURE 4.8 Atmospheric pressure chemical ionization. (Courtesy of Richard LeLacheur, Taylor Technology.)

fragmented in quadrupole 2 and then the product *daughter ions* resulting from the fragmentation are analyzed in a second stage of mass analysis (quadrupole 3). If a single compound is eluting at the time the mass spectrum is obtained, additional information can be obtained about the structure of the compound, which is helpful in identifying metabolites.

The two techniques generally used in biomarker and pharmacokinetic quantification are atmospheric pressure chemical ionization (APCI; Figure 4.8) and electrospray ionization (ESI; Figure 4.9) [32]. In both approaches, the ions produced can be positive or negative. A typical mass spectrum is shown in Figure 4.10. A starting point would be to infuse a solution of the analyte(s) into the MS, starting with 1 μg drug/mL at 300 to 500 μL/h in a solution of 50/50 methanol/0.1% formic acid at a rate of 0.2 mL/min. ESI should be attempted, in

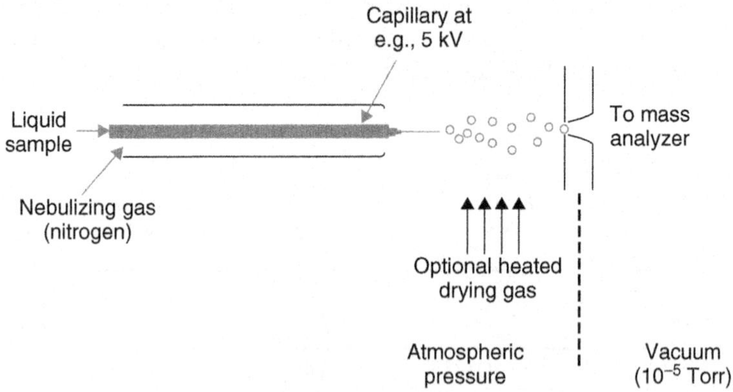

FIGURE 4.9 Electrospray source ionization. (Courtesy of Richard LeLacheur, Taylor Technology.)

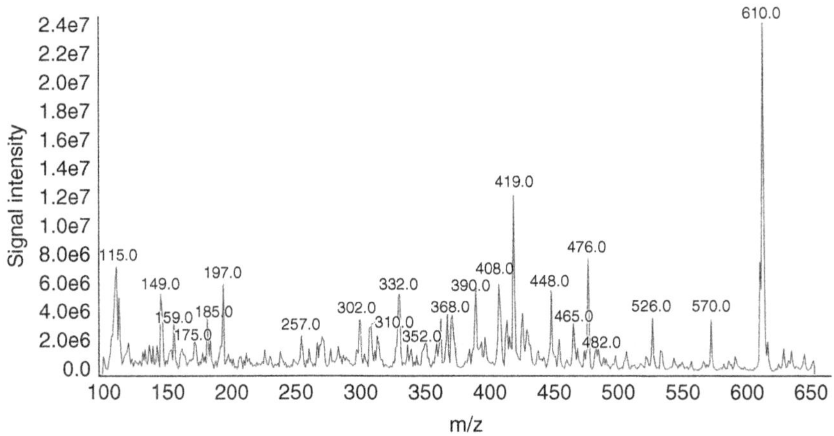

FIGURE 4.10 Typical mass spectrum. (Courtesy of Richard LeLacheur, Taylor Technology.)

both positive and negative mode, then APCI. The ions and then their general MS conditions are determined. Once the MS is set up to detect the ions of interest, the LC development work can begin in earnest [33].

Matrix Effects When materials co-elute with the analyte(s) or internal standard(s) of interest into the ion source, either reduced (suppressed) or increased (enhanced) signal may result, due to changes in source efficiency. With LC methods, it is desirable to have sufficient retention such that the unwanted material at the solvent front does not interfere with the target analyte. Suppressed ionization can lead to nonlinearity and inaccurate quantification [34].

One facile way to check for ion suppression is to infuse a constant concentration of a standard into the mobile-phase stream after the column. Once the baseline stabilizes, an extracted matrix blank is injected on the column. At the solvent front a negative dip will usually be seen as ionization-suppressing materials elute and reduce the baseline signal (Figure 4.11a). When the baseline returns to normal, many (but not all) of these suppressing agents have passed through the detector. Just as analyte peaks can elute anywhere in the run, ion suppression can occur anywhere, so it is very important to run the ion-suppression experiment to assure that ion suppression will not compromise the method. Sample cleanup can reduce this suppression considerably, as shown in the chromatogram in Figure 4.11b.

Carryover Contamination, carryover (material from a previous sample interfering with the current sample), or blank response from a matrix or reagents can affect the accuracy and precision of quantification at all concentrations [35]. However, the relatively lower concentration samples are most at risk. Care should be taken to minimize interference from all putative contamination factors, and

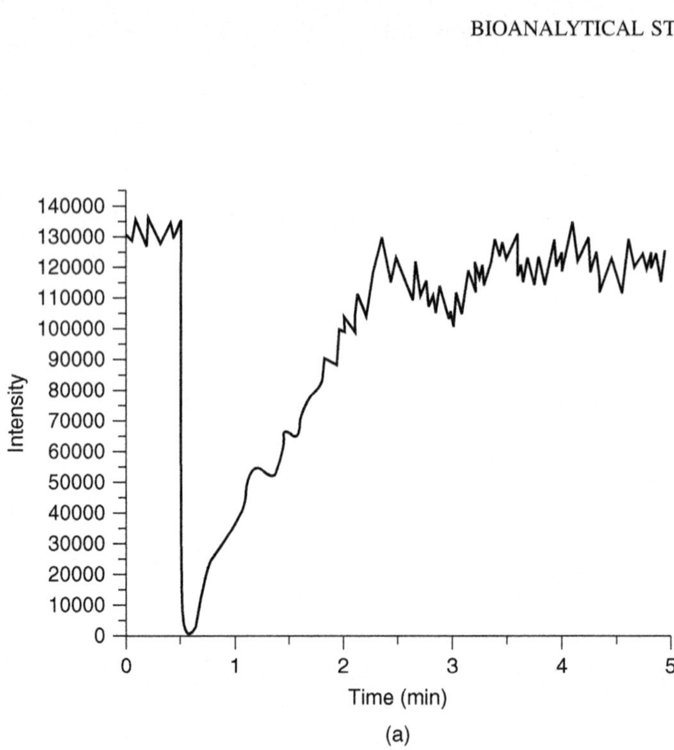

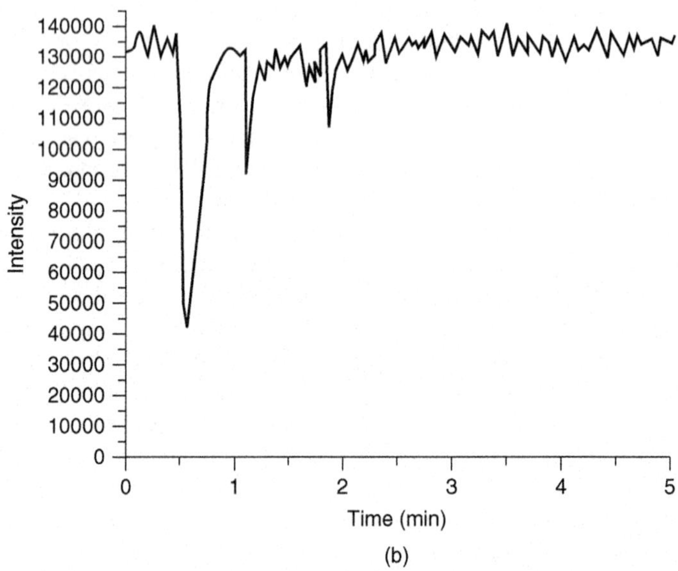

FIGURE 4.11 Ion suppression chromatographs: (a) with a crash and shot sample preparation step; (b) with SPE purification. (Courtesy of ThermoFisher.)

the interference should not significantly affect the accuracy and precision of the assay. The following points about carryover should be noted.

- Carryover does not necessarily involve just consecutive samples in the analysis sequence. In fact, carryover from late-eluting residues on columns may affect chromatograms several samples later.
- Carryover from residues in rotary sampling/switching valves often appears later in the samples.
- Carryover should be assessed during validation by injecting one or more blank samples following a high-concentration sample or standard. The injector should be flushed with appropriate solvents to minimize carryover.
- If carryover is unavoidable for a highly retained compound, specific procedures should be provided in the method to handle known carryover. This could include injection of blanks after certain samples or even after each sample.
- Randomization of samples should be avoided, since it may interfere with the assessment of carryover problems.
- Carryover should be addressed in validation and minimized, and an objective determination should be made in the evaluation of analytical runs.
- Interestingly, there is no standard acceptable magnitude of carryover for passing a bioanalytical run.

Precautions should be taken to avoid contamination during sample collection and preparation. Contamination can be assessed by monitoring blank response in the presence of high-concentration samples or standards. The assay platform (manual or automated), configuration of sampling, and extraction method (manual, automated, online or solid phase, etc.) in the assay should be taken into consideration when ascertaining carryover.

Matrix effects and carryover have been emphasized here because of their major impact on the credibility of laboratories that ignore or minimize these considerations. Scientific and regulatory issues are involved and at least one major bioanalytical laboratory is known to have suffered severe consequences for deficiencies in this area.

4.2.4 Ligand-Binding Assays

LBA is a term commonly used for macromolecule assays in general. However, ligand binding to its receptor is a very specific type of biological process used only a fraction of the time as the basis for an immunochemistry assay as compared to the more frequently used antigen–antibody assays. As the general technique matures and biopharmaceuticals become more frequent as candidate drugs, the nomenclature should improve. Although the terms *immunochemistry assays* and *biological assays* are more common in many scientific circles, they could exclude ligand-binding assays.

Basic Principles General immunochemistry concepts [36,37] and methods regarding validation procedures for biopharmaceuticals [8, 39–42] have been well reviewed. Millipore offers several excellent tutorials on ligand-binding assays at their Web site (Table 4.1). The basic principle of any immunochemical technique is that a specific antibody will combine with its specific antigen to produce an exclusive antibody–antigen complex. An *antigen* is defined as any foreign substance that elicits an immune response (e.g., the production of specific antibody molecules) when introduced into the tissues of a susceptible animal and is capable of combining with the specific antibodies formed. Antigens are generally of high molecular weight and commonly are proteins or polysaccharides. Polypeptides, lipids, nucleic acids, and many other materials can also function as antigens.

Immune responses may also be generated against smaller substances, called *haptens*, if these are coupled chemically to a larger carrier protein, such as bovine serum albumin. A variety of molecules, such as drugs, simple sugars, amino acids, small peptides, phospholipids, and triglycerides, may function as haptens. Thus, given enough time, just about any foreign substance will be identified by the immune system and evoke specific antibody production. However, this specific immune response is highly variable and depends heavily on the size, structure, and composition of antigens. Antigens that elicit strong immune responses are said to be *strongly immunogenic*.

Antibodies are a class of immunological proteins [or immunoglobulins (Ig's)] produced by β-cells and are antigen specific. They are composed of two heavy chains and two light chains with disulfide bonds holding them together (see Figure 4.12). There are several types of antibodies:

- *IgM:* occur in blood and are involved in complement-fixation reactions
- *IgA:* are secreted across epithelial surfaces into gut, intestines, and mammary gland
- *IgG:* neutralize toxins and prevent infections by blocking bacterial and viral entry into cells
- *IgE:* are involved in allergic reactions

The small site on an antigen to which a complementary antibody may specifically bind is called an *epitope*. This usually comprises one to six monosaccharides or five to eight amino acid residues on the surface of the antigen. Because antigen molecules exist in space, the epitope recognized by an antibody may be dependent on the presence of a specific three-dimensional antigenic conformation (e.g., a unique site formed by the interaction of two native protein loops or subunits), or the epitope may correspond to a simple primary sequence region. Such epitopes are described as *conformational* and *linear*, respectively. The range of possible binding sites is enormous, with each potential binding site having its own structural properties derived from covalent bonds, ionic bonds, and hydrophilic and hydrophobic interactions.

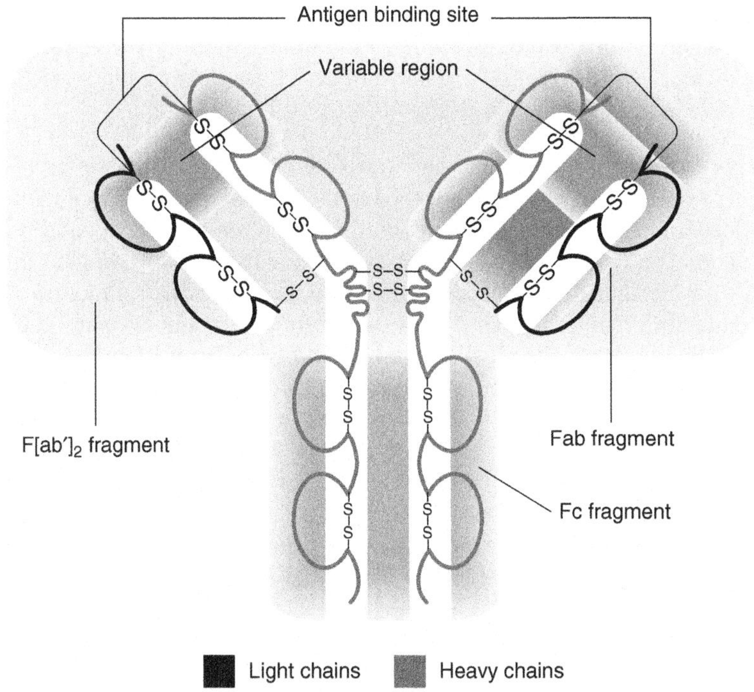

FIGURE 4.12 Antibody structure. (Courtesy of Millipore.)

For efficient interaction to occur between the antigen and the antibody, the epitope must be readily available for binding. If the target molecule is denatured (e.g., through fixation, reduction, pH changes, or during preparation for gel electrophoresis), the epitope may be altered, and this may affect its ability to interact with an antibody. For example, some antibodies are ineffective in Western blot but very effective in immunohistochemistry because in the latter procedure, a complex antigenic site might be maintained in the tissue, whereas in the former procedure the process of sample preparation alters the protein conformation sufficiently to destroy the antigenic site and hence eliminate antibody binding. Thus, the epitope may be present in the antigen's native, cellular environment, or may be exposed only when denatured. In their natural form they may be cytoplasmic (soluble), membrane associated, or secreted. The number, location, and size of the epitopes depend on how much of the antigen is presented during the antibody-making process.

If a gene product of interest is present in extremely low concentrations, one may choose to use known nucleotide sequence information to derive a corresponding peptide for generating sequence-specific antibodies. In some instances, peptide antigens have advantages over whole protein antigens in that the antibodies generated may be targeted to unique sequence regions. This is especially useful when investigating proteins that belong to families of high sequence homology.

Enzyme-Linked Immunosorbent Assays (ELISAs) ELISAs are arguably the most common of the ligand-binding assays currently in use. Four ELISA formats are sandwich, competitive, direct, and bridge. A diagram of the sandwich and competitive methods is shown in Figure 4.13.

Sandwich Format One primary antibody (the capture antibody) is purified and bound to a solid phase, typically attached to the bottom of a plate well. Antigen is then added and allowed to complex with the bound antibody. Unbound products are then removed with a wash, and a labeled secondary antibody, which has linked to it an enzyme such as horseradish peroxidase, is allowed to bind to the antigen, thus completing the "sandwich." A second "primary" antibody may be used, as shown in Figure 4.13. The assay is then quantified by measuring the amount of labeled second antibody bound to the matrix, through the use of a substrate for the enzyme that will change color or luminescence (see below) upon reaction. The major advantages of this technique are that the antigen does not need to be purified prior to use, and that these assays are very specific. One disadvantage is that not all antibodies can be used. Monoclonal antibody combinations must be qualified as *matched pairs*, meaning that they can recognize separate epitopes on the antigen so that they do not hinder each other's binding.

Competitive Format An unlabeled purified primary antibody is coated onto the wells of a 96-well microtiter plate. This primary antibody is then incubated with unlabeled standards or unknowns. After this reaction is allowed to equilibrate, an enzyme-labeled antigen is added. This conjugate will bind to the primary antibody wherever its binding sites are not already occupied by unlabeled standards or unknowns. Thus, the more immunogen in the sample or standard, the lower the amount of conjugated immunogen bound. The plate is then developed with substrate and a color or luminescence change is measured.

Radioimmunoassays In radioimmunoassay, a fixed concentration of labeled tracer antigen is incubated with a constant amount of antiserum such that the concentration of antigen-binding sites on the antibody is limiting; for example, only 50% of the total tracer concentration may be bound by antibody. If unlabeled antigen is added to this system, there is competition between labeled tracer and unlabeled antigen for the limited and constant number of binding sites on the antibody, and thus the amount of tracer bound to antibody will decrease as the concentration of unlabeled antigen increases. This can be measured after separating antibody-bound from free tracer and counting the bound fraction, the free fraction, or both. A calibration or standard curve is set up with increasing amounts of known antigen, and from this curve the amount of antigen in the unknown samples can be calculated. Thus, the four basic necessities for a radioimmunoassay system are:

1. An antiserum to the compound to be measured
2. The availability of a radioactively labeled form of the compound

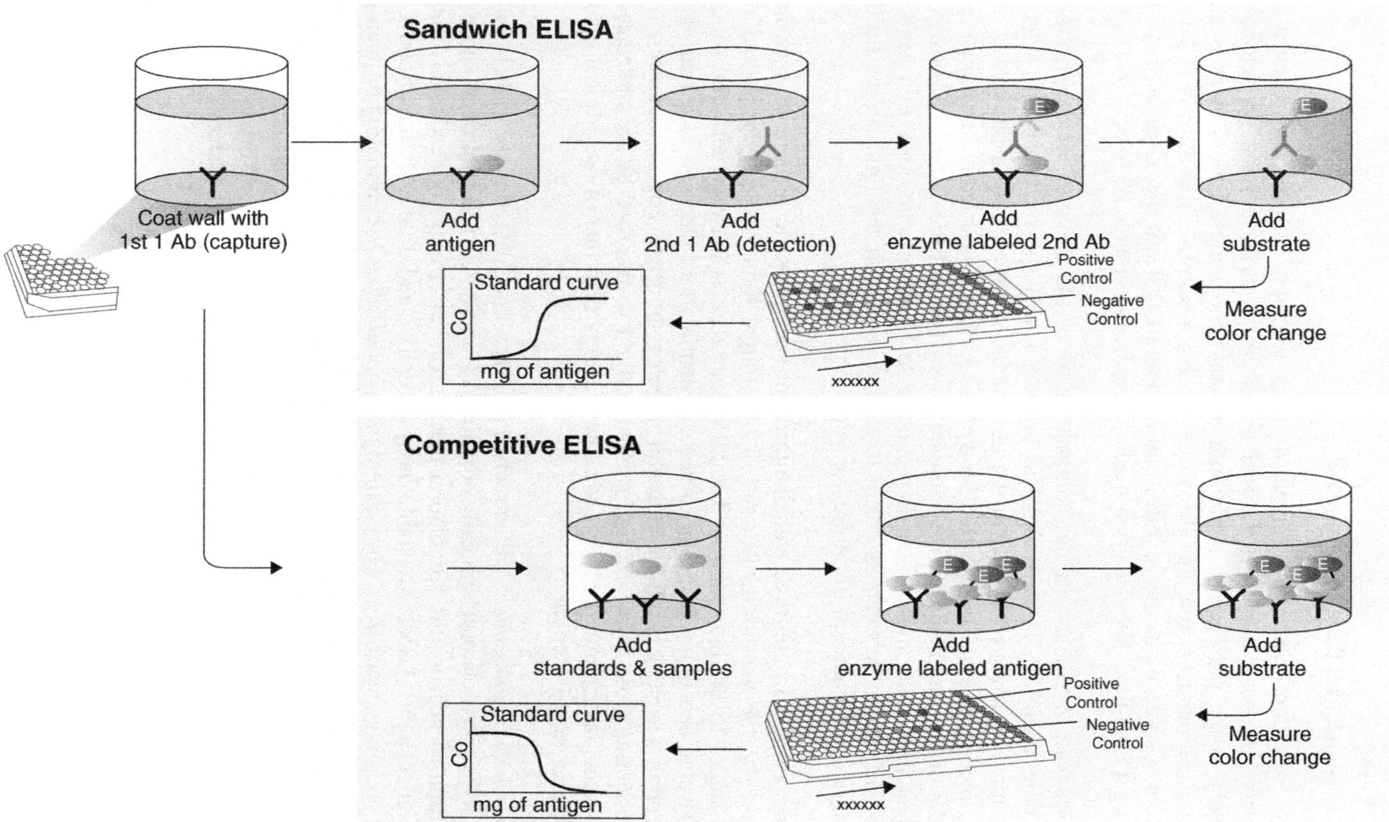

FIGURE 4.13 ELISA assays. (Courtesy of Millipore.)

3. A method whereby antibody-bound tracer can be separated from unbound tracer
4. A standard unlabeled compound

Types of Detection for Ligand-Binding Assays Once an exclusive antibody–antigen complex is formed within the matrix, it must be detected uniquely in the presence of a plethora of other molecules. Unless there is an additional separation step, the ultraviolet–visible absorption spectrum is of little help since some molecules exhibit chromphore(s) that are the same as that of the target complex. The detection method requires assurance of selectivity.

Colorimetric Detection If the complex alone or the complex in conjugation with other chemicals in the sample can produce a very specific color shift, selectivity may be achieved by measuring the change in absorption in the visible or ultraviolet spectrum. The inherent limitation to using this detection technique is that the drug being analyzed is quantified on the basis of the difference between incident light with and without the sample. At low concentrations, this would be the difference between two very large numbers, with the light source itself having a certain amount of "noise" or variability.

Fluorescence In contrast, with luminescent spectrometric techniques such as fluorimetry, the measurement is not of transmitted light but of light emitted at right angles to the light source. The difference then is between zero and some small value and is not as prone to noise contamination. One can vary both the absorption wavelength and the emission wavelength, decreasing interferences. In fluorescence, some of the energy of incident light is absorbed by the molecules present and later emitted, always at a lower energy than that of the original light and higher in wavelength.

Electrochemiluminescence Electrochemiluminescence detection uses labels that emit light when electrochemically stimulated (Figure 4.14). Background signals are minimal because the stimulation mechanism (electricity) is decoupled from the signal (light). Labels are stable, nonradioactive, and offer a choice of convenient coupling chemistries. They emit light at about 620 nm, eliminating problems with color quenching. Few compounds interfere with electrochemiluminescent labels; thus, large, diverse libraries can be used with confidence. Multiple excitation cycles of each label amplify the signal to enhance light levels and improve sensitivity. Commercial ECL systems are based on the use of organometallic ruthenium complexes; the basic chemical processes used to generate electrochemiluminescence from these labels are shown in Figure 4.14.

4.2.5 Integration of Method Development Components: Example with LC-MS/MS

Method development and qualification/validation is not a static process. The analysis will need to integrate dry lab research, sample preparation,

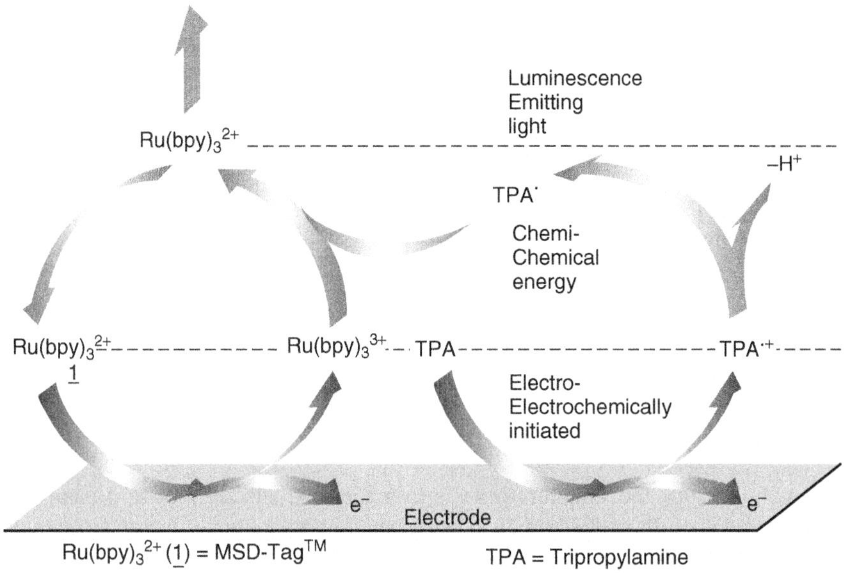

FIGURE 4.14 LBA assay using electrochemiluminescence as the detection moiety. (Courtesy of Meso Scale Discovery. Copyright © 2010 Meso Scale Discovery, a division of Meso Scale Diagnostics, LLC. All rights reserved.)

component separation, detector response, data capture [e.g., laboratory information management system (LIMS)], and report preparation/review [18,22,23]. The LC Resources Web site (www.lcresources.com) is a source of guidance. The first step in developing an LC-MS/MS method is to identify the molecular ion. A literature search should be made to ensure that no previous MS work has been conducted with the NCE or similar compound. If any strongly basic sites (e.g., amines) are present on the molecule, the most appropriate molecular ion will probably have positive polarity, and the interface to start with will be electrospray. If the molecule is not basic but contains electronegative atoms (e.g., oxygen), the best interface to try may be APCI. The MS would be set for continuous infusion.

A continuous infusion into the detector, with the concentration of the analyte remaining constant, will allow adjustments to be made to the various voltages of the detector. This can also be done with the LC system running and the mobile phase adjusted to the approximate concentrations expected at the time of analyte elution. The mass analyzer is then optimized. The next step would be to adjust the LC conditions: column type and temperature, mobile phase composition, and so on. The LC-MS/MS interface is then optimized. For example, the turbo ion spray interface for the PE Sciex instrument has seven adjustable variables: LC eluant flow, nebulizer gas flow, auxiliary gas flow, curtain gas flow, auxiliary gas heater temperature, spray voltage, and probe position. The goal is the highest sensitivity possible consistent with a stable signal. Optimizing mobile-phase flow feeds back to the LC conditions. The gas flow depends on the mobile-phase flow; changing one usually means changing the other. The voltage–current signal tends to rises rapidly to a plateau above some critical value. The lowest temperature should be selected consistent with good signal and peak shape.

At this point the instrumentation is optimized for the NCE. A set of analyte samples should be run at concentrations bracketing the concentration range expected. Response should be linear with concentration, and the signal should be significant at low concentrations. Method qualification or validation is the next step. The extent of validation is dependent on the phase of discovery and development.

4.3 BIOANALYTICAL METHOD VALIDATION

4.3.1 Introduction to Validation

Although later in the chapter there is considerable discussion of bioanalytical "qualification" with characteristics less stringent than those currently expected by the FDA [a fit-for-purpose approach in support of drug discovery and non-GLP (good laboratory practices) studies], ultimately a bioanalytical assay must be fully validated according to specific scientific and regulatory criteria. The first studies that require such fully validated assays are in support of the toxicokinetic data conducted during the GLP-regulated pre-FIH toxicity studies. Even though the GLPs (Chapter 9) are frequently cited for describing the practice and oversight of bioanalytical studies, it is the bioanalytical method validation (BMV) guidance [1,5,6] that applies specifically to most assay methods currently used in drug development: GC; LC; "hyphenated" techniques such as LC-MS, LC-MS/MS, and GC-MS; ligand-binding assays [39,44,45]; and cell-based assays. These assays measure drugs and/or metabolites in biological matrices. The assay must be shown to be sensitive and selective enough to detect pharmacologically and toxicologically relevant concentrations of analytes in appropriate matrices. Clinical studies come under the good clinical practice (GCP) regulations, not GLP. Reports describing clinical studies that have bioanalytical components should indicate that the bioanalytical portion was conducted using the BMV for guidance, not the GLP.

The primary metrics required to determine bioanaltytical assay suitability are (1) accuracy, (2) precision, (3) selectivity, (4) sensitivity, (5) reproducibility, and (6) stability. A specific, detailed description of the bioanalytical method should be written. This can be in the form of a protocol (usual in the United States) or a study plan [in OECD (Organization for Economic Cooperation and Development) countries]. The components of a study plan are shown in Table 4.2. Methods are frequently described in a separate standard operating procedure (SOP) or test method. Results are described in a formal report. Any claims or conclusions about the method should be included in this report.

Requirements for the six parameters listed above as well as secondary parameters (such as incurred sample reanalysis) apply to chemical-based assays as

TABLE 4.2 Study Plan Components[a]

Administration	
Title	Sponsor and contact information[b]
Protocol information	Date plan approval
Drug product	Approval signatures, including regulatory guidelines
Principal investigator	Table of contents
Internal project number	
Body of Text	
Introduction	
Tentative time schedule	Determination of assay carryover
Study personnel	Incurred sample reproducibility
Experimental	Reporting
Method summary	Raw data review
Reference standards	Quality control check
Sample analysis details	Quality assurance review
Assay interference check	Sample storage and disposal
Batch acceptance criteria	Archives
System suitability	References

[a] The study plan is composed of an administrative section, including approvals, followed by the body of text detailing the bioanalytical study.
[b] Applicable regarding the interaction between a drug sponsor and a bioanalytical CRO. All other components are relevant whether or not the sponsor and bioanalytical laboratory are within the same institution.

well as ligand-binding assays and are described in the FDA bioanalytical method validation guidance and in supplemental white papers [1,5,6]. Requirements for chemical assays are listed in Table 4.3. The initial key requirement for a successful method validation is the acquisition of suitable reference standards. Standard analytes require a certificate of analysis or recertification of purity or stability for the time of use. Internal standards (ISs) do not require a certificate of analysis. Suitable and well-characterized small-molecular-weight compounds are generally available at the time of method validation which can be selected as internal standards. For ligand-binding assays, the critical reagents are typically an antibody or a pair of antibodies for immunoassays. Although these requirements must be met for regulated studies, assays for discovery or pharmacodynamics/pharmacokinetics (PD-PK) studies may require less stringent criteria. This "risk-based" approach is described in Section 4.7.

4.3.2 The Primary Metrics: Acceptance Criteria

- *Accuracy:* within ±15% of nominal
- *Precision:* within ±15% of nominal

TABLE 4.3 Routine Drug Analysis Process and Run Acceptance Criteria

<table>
<tr><th>Process or Criteria</th><th>Chromatographic Assays</th><th>Ligand-Binding Assays</th></tr>
<tr><td>1. Preparation of standards and QC samples</td><td colspan="2">Standards and QC samples can be prepared from the same spiking stock solution, provided that the solution stability and accuracy have been verified. A single source of matrix may also be used, provided that selectivity has been verified.</td></tr>
<tr><td>2. Placement of samples</td><td colspan="2">Standard curve samples, blanks, QCs, and study samples can be arranged as appropriate within the run, and support detection of assay drift over the run.</td></tr>
<tr><td>3. Number of calibration standards in a run</td><td>Include with each analytical batch:
Blank matrix (sample without IS)
Zero standard (matrix sample with IS)
Nonzero calibration standards: a minimum of six standard concentrations</td><td>Include with each analytical batch or microtiter plate:
Blank matrix
Nonzero calibration standards: a minimum of six concentrations; can include anchor points (below LLOQ or above ULOQ in the asymptotic low- and high-concentration end of the standard curve)</td></tr>
<tr><td>4. Acceptance criteria for calibration standards</td><td>Residuals (absolute difference between the back-calculated and nominal concentration) for each calibration standard should meet the following limits:
LLOQ standard <20%
All other standards <15%</td><td>Residuals for each calibration standard should meet the following limits:
LLOQ and ULOQ standards <25%
All other standards <20%
If used, anchor points are not to be included in the acceptance criteria above.</td></tr>
<tr><td></td><td colspan="2">A minimum of 75% standards (at least six nonzero points) should be within the limits noted above for the analytical run to qualify. Values falling outside these limits can be discarded, provided that they do not change the established model.</td></tr>
</table>

5. Number of QC samples in a batch	Include QC samples at the following three concentrations (within the calibration range) in duplicate with each analytical batch: Low: near the LLOQ (up to 3× LLOQ) Medium: midrange of calibration curve High: near the high end of the range	QC samples at the following three concentrations (within the calibration range) in duplicate should be added to each microtiter plate: Low: above the second non-anchor point standard, approx. 3× LLOQ Medium: midrange of the calibration curve High: below the second non-anchor point high standard at about 75% of ULOQ
	Each analytical batch should contain six or a minimum of 5% of the total number of unknown samples. Add QCs in multiples of three concentrations (low, medium, high) when needed.	
6. Acceptance criteria for QC samples[a]	Allowed % deviation from nominal values: QCs prepared at all concentrations greater than LLOQ<15% Low QC (if prepared at LLOQ)<20%	Allowed % deviation from nominal values: QCs prepared at all concentrations other than LLOQ and ULOQ<20% Low and high QC (if prepared at LLOQ or ULOQ)<25% Wider acceptance criteria may be justified (e.g., when total error during assay validation approaches 30%)
	At least 67% (four out of six) of the QC samples should be within the limits above. 33% of the QC samples (not all replicates at the same concentration) can be outside the limits. If there are more than two QC samples at a concentration, 50% of that concentration should pass the limits of deviation above.	

(*Continued overleaf*)

TABLE 4.3 ***(Continued)***

Process or Criteria	Chromatographic Assays	Ligand-Binding Assays
7. Replicate analysis	In general, samples may be analyzed with a single determination without replicate analysis if the assay method has acceptable variability as defined by the validation data. Duplicate or replicate analysis may be performed for a difficult procedure when high precision and accuracy might be difficult to obtain.	Accuracy can generally be improved by replicate analysis; therefore, duplicate analysis is recommended. If replicate analysis is performed, the same procedure should be used for samples and standards.
8. Multiple analytes in a run[b]	Samples involving multiple analytes in a run should not be rejected based on the data from one analyte failing the acceptance criteria.	
9. Rejected runs	The data from rejected runs need not be documented, but the fact that a run was rejected and the reason for failure should be reported.	

[a]Monitoring the effect of sample dilution is referred to in the FDA guidance [3].

[b]Although the guidance [3] indicates that a run should not be rejected for the remaining analytes if one fails, it does not address how to assess and report all analyte concentrations upon reanalysis of the failed "metabolite." In this regard, concentrations from the first run accepted should be reported, and if this analyte is repeated in simultaneous assays when analyzing for different analytes, it is not necessary to quantitate the analytes already reported.

- *Selectivity:* lower limit of quantification (see below) five fold greater than blank response
- *Sensitivity:* lowest calibrator standard that meets other criteria
- *Reproducibility:* two-thirds of incurred samples reanalyzed within ±20%
- *Stability:* >85 to 90% of nominal

Accuracy The FDA guidance definition of *accuracy* is: "the degree of closeness of the determined value to the nominal or known true value under prescribed conditions. This is sometimes termed trueness." A metaphor for accuracy comes from target shooting with the classic "bull's eye" or concentric ring pattern. How close to the bull's eye you are with every shot (or, in our case, how close the concentration value determined by the assay is to the nominal concentration) is a measure of accuracy. The guidance continues: "The accuracy of an analytical method describes the closeness of mean test results obtained by the method to the true value (concentration) of the analyte. Accuracy is determined by replicated analysis of samples containing known amounts of the analyte. Accuracy should be measured using a minimum of five determinations per concentration. A minimum of three concentrations in the range of expected concentrations is recommended. The mean value should be within 15% of the actually value except at the lower limit of quantification (LLOQ), where it should not deviate by more than 20%. The deviation of the mean from the true value serves as the measure of accuracy." Accuracy is thus determined by replicate analyses of calibration and quality control (QC) samples. The metric determined is the deviation from nominal concentration.

Precision The FDA guidance defines *precision* as "the closeness of agreement (degree of scatter) between a series of measurements obtained from multiple sampling of the same homogeneous sample under prescribed conditions." Again using the target-shooting metaphor, how much the shots are scattered is a measure of the precision of the shooter. The guidance states further that "precision should be measured using a minimum of five determinations per concentration."

Thus, precision is also determined by replicate analyses of calibration and QC samples. The metric at each concentration is the coefficient of variation. Precision is subdivided into intra- and inter-run variability. General practice has been to enlarge the number of QCs for one run to obtain an intrarun value. Although not statistically appropriate, a total precision number is determined by using all three runs of QC samples for the inter-run accuracy and precision estimates instead of an analysis of variance (ANOVA) approach. An example of the relationship between the % coefficient of variation (%CV) and the log of a set of standard concentrations is shown in Figure 4.15. In this example, the %CV is relatively constant and acceptable above 16 ng/mL. At this point it increases rapidly with decreasing concentration.

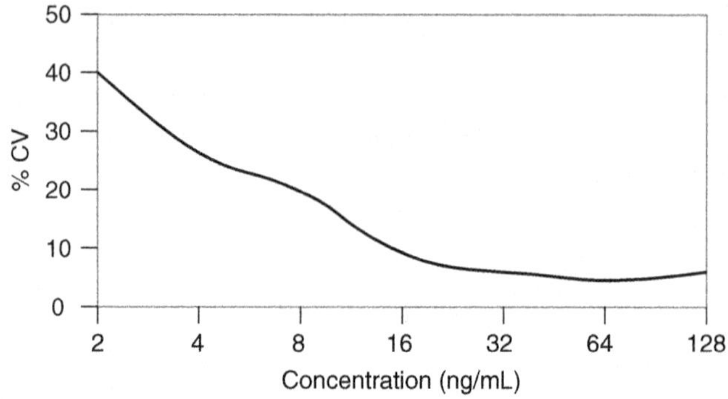

FIGURE 4.15 Theoretical plot of the heteroscedascity of a chemical-based assay. The plot is relatively flat at concentrations greater than 16 ng/mL when the %CV starts to increase to above acceptable levels.

Selectivity The FDA guidance defines *selectivity* as "the ability of the bioanalytical method to measure and differentiate the analytes in the presence of components that may be expected to be present. These could include metabolites, impurities, degradants, or matrix components." The guidance elaborates: "For selectivity, analyses of blank samples ... should be tested to ensure that there is no interference." Interferences can originate from endogenous matrix components, metabolites, decomposition products of the analyte and metabolites, concomitant medications (and their metabolites), and other xenobiotics. During validation, the operator should assess the analyte response due to blank matrix while eliminating or minimizing other contaminants. The analyte response at the LLOQ should be at least five times the response due to blank matrix. For immunoassays, and if the analyte is also present endogenously in the matrix, the blank response can exceed 20% of LLOQ, but the contribution should not interfere with the accuracy required in measurement of the LLOQ. In such cases, specific procedures should be provided in the method used to handle blank matrix response.

Sensitivity While the FDA bioanalytical guidance does not define *sensitivity*, it is generally recognized as the lower limit of quantification. The guidance does state that the LLOQ is the lowest concentration of the standard curve that can be measured where "the analyte response at the LLOQ should be at least 5 times the response compared to [a] blank response [and] analyte peak (response) should be identifiable, discrete, and reproducible with a precision of 20% and accuracy of 80–120%."

In Figure 4.15 the concentration correlating with 20%CV is 8 ng/mL. It should be noted that any assay right at the edge of the acceptance criteria is a weak assay and is likely to produce a high number of failed runs. Although "number of failed runs" is not an official metric and the percentage of failed runs that constitutes an unofficial metric has not been determined uniformly, the expectation of any reviewing body, whether regulatory, client (internal or external), or management, is that this number needs to be very low (5 to 10%), if it exists at all.

The highest standard that conforms to the guidance acceptance criteria will define the upper limit of quantification (ULOQ) of an analytical method. If a sample is found to be beyond the ULOQ, it is acceptable practice to dilute the sample and try again, provided that dilution samples are tested during validation. Together, the concentrations between the LLOQ and ULOQ constitute the dynamic range of the assay. For current MS assays, 2.5 to 3 orders of magnitude generally is the widest that an assay range can be stretched. However, chip-based nanoelectrospray MS technology may allow four to six orders of magnitude [46]. For ligand-binding assays, the range is frequently only one order of magnitude, necessitating one or more dilution steps for values estimated to be above the ULOQ.

Reproducibility *Reproducibility* in the FDA guidance is defined as "the precision between two laboratories. It also represents precision of the method under the same operating conditions over a short period of time." Presumably, this means the same laboratory over time.

In practice, at least three comparable consecutive runs are usually performed on consecutive days. Although it may be more efficient to conduct the runs on the same day, the ultimate point of the validation is to mimic the conditions under which the actual samples will be analyzed. Although it is conceivable that nonclinical samples could be run in one day, FIH samples almost certainly will take several days. Three concentrations of QC samples—low, medium, and high—are quantified in the same matrix and species as the putative study samples. If plasma is the matrix from different species, plasma from each target species must be evaluated separately, as potential interferences can be species specific. In practice, the low concentration should be three times the LLOQ, and the high is generally about 80% of the ULOQ. Various paradigms for the middle concentration are: one-half the projected $C_{\max}$, the geometric mean, or the median of the calibration standard range. Ideally, half the incurred samples should be above and half below the middle QC concentration. During actual sample analysis, if 90% or more of the samples observed are below the middle QC, another QC is frequently prepared and run with the remaining samples. The previous samples do not need to be reanalyzed. There are multiple opinions about whether an additional QC sample is needed if the dilution was tested during the first validation and, if an additional QC is added, whether an additional partial, one-day validation is required. These samples are distributed throughout the next run.

Stability The FDA guidance cites *stability* simply as "the chemical stability of an analyte in a given matrix under specific conditions for given time intervals." The guidance elaborates as follows:

- "The stability of the analyte (drug and/or metabolite) in the matrix during the collection process and the sample storage period should be assessed, preferably prior to sample analysis."

- "For compounds with potentially labile metabolites, the stability of analyte in matrix from dosed subjects (or species) should be confirmed."
- "The stability of the analyte in biological matrix at intended storage temperatures should be established. The influence of freeze–thaw cycles (a minimum of three cycles at two concentrations in triplicate) should be studied."
- "The stability of the analyte in matrix at ambient temperature should be evaluated over a time period equal to the typical sample preparation, sample handling, and analytical run times."

The stability of an NCE in a study sample needs to be accounted for from the collection-to-detector response, including solutions used to prepare calibrator and QC samples [47]. This is species and matrix specific, and studies must involve appropriate analyte-free, interference-free biological matrix. For pre-FIH bioanalytical assay validation, the species studied are those used for toxicological evaluation the toxicity species (typically, the rodent and nonrodent selected) as well as humans, so that the validated assay is in place to support the actual FIH trial. The analyte is typically the parent drug only, unless the drug substance is a prodrug, or early studies have uncovered a major and/or active metabolite that is considered necessary for monitoring at this early development stage. Pursuant to the guidance, the following stability determinations on the appropriate analyte(s) should be performed at the pre-FIH stage of development:

1. Stock solutions for as long as the intended use, generally at room temperature for at least 6 hours as well as in the refrigerator.
2. Long-term stability of study samples at the storage temperatures anticipated, generally −20 and −70°C. Note: Stability experiments for both temperatures are needed, as stability at −20°C does not necessarily translate into stability at −70°C, especially for biopharmaceuticals, which can be prone to denaturation at the lower temperature. Enough sample should be available for analysis on three separate occasions. Stability testing should encompass the maximum anticipated storage time of study samples.
3. Short-term stability (benchtop, room temperature): three aliquots at low and high QC concentrations thawed at processing temperature (usually, room temperature) from 4 hours benchtop to the maximum duration that samples would be thawed during the course of a study. Replicating the lifetime of the samples intact or in process is the object of these experiments.
4. Freeze–thaw stability: three cycles, three replicates, 24 hours frozen at storage temperature, thawed at room (or appropriate thawing) temperature, refrozen for 12 to 24 hours, rethawed. Note: Unmixed or incomplete thawing can result in erroneous results. Concentration gradients can form during thawing. Unless the sample is remixed completely, an aliquot for analysis may not reflect the true analyte concentration in the sample.

5. Preparative and post-preparative stability (normal and interrupted processing) in autosampler solvent.
6. Emerging issues of incurred sample stability and reproducibility are discussed later.

4.3.3 Additional Validation Criteria

Recovery The FDA guidance defines *recovery* as "the extraction efficiency of an analytical process, reported as a percentage of the known amount of an analyte carried through the sample extraction and processing steps of the method." Thus, recovery is the amount of analyte that can be accounted for at the end of an assay. This parameter is generally measured by comparing the detector response with an extracted blank sample spiked with the analyte just before the detector step to a blank sample spiked at the beginning of sample preparation. Concentrations at the low, middle, and high QC levels should be used. Although recovery need not be 100%, the recovery of the analyte and the IS (essential) should be consistent, precise, and reproducible.

The attitude of the bioanalytical community towards recovery is not consistent. Many feel that it is unimportant. This author disagrees, even when stable label internal standards are used. The lower the recovery, the greater the potential for micro changes in the sample treatment to produce relatively large changes in results. There is no consensus about how much difference in analyte recovery between study samples and the ISs becomes problematic. This author believes that the analyte(s) of interest recovered should be no more than a few percentage points different from the ISs. The IS chemistry needs to be as close as possible to the analyte. A difference in recovery would clearly show a mismatch in chemistries. As far as stable label internal standards are concerned (where the chemistries should be identical), an unofficial auditor review (be it regulatory, client, or management) should include variability of detector response of the ISs over time. Even assuming that an IS compensates for differences in the recovery of the analyte of interest, if the IS detector response is variable, the auditor may question the reliability of the assay.

Parallelism Most references to parallelism deal with ligand-binding assays and the necessity to dilute samples because of their inherently narrow dynamic range. In this context, *parallelism* is defined as the "determination of whether an assay's accuracy depends on the analyte concentration in the sample used" [48]. This concept also applies to the necessity, for both pharmacokinetic and biomarker analyses, of using matrices for QCs and calibration standards that are different from the matrices actually analyzed. This applies to rare matrix samples (e.g., fetal rat blood) and samples where the analyte is endogenous (e.g., steroid hormones). The QCs and standards need to be made with "stripped" matrix, frequently plasma or serum treated with charcoal. Matrix diluted with phosphate-buffered saline is also frequently used. Herein, analyses are conducted before and after dilution of a spiked or incurred sample. In validation, the analyte is added to the matrix at multiple concentrations across the analytical range expected. If the results are parallel to but not coincident with undiluted samples, a "quasiquantitative interpretation" [8] would be needed where a correction factor may need to be applied.

Standards and QCs for rare matrices may need to be prepared in a closely related matrix, for example nonpregnant female or male rat plasma. In this sense "parallelism documents that the concentration–response relationship of the analyte in the sample matrix from the study population is sufficiently similar to that in the substitute matrix" [8].

For a rare matrix or endogenous analytes, a test using a variation of the *method of addition* can be used [49]. In a validation for a rare matrix, the analyte is added to the true matrix at multiple concentrations across the analytical range expected. A similar set of samples in the matrix to be used for calibration standards and QCs are prepared across the same range. The results are evaluated in a manner similar to the diluted samples above. For endogenous substrates, a similar approach can be employed, but the calibration standard and QC range is expanded downward to LLOQ. However, there is no uniform experimental protocol to deal with these issues.

Calibration Standards (QCs) Calibration standards (QCs) are used to define the relationship between concentration and the detector response, and need to be prepared in the same species/matrix as the study samples. Exceptions can be made for rare matrices that are difficult to acquire. For replacement/surrogate matrices, parallelism would need to be determined. Generally, the following QC standards are prepared: (1) a blank sample, (2) a zero sample (a blank sample processed with internal standard), and (3) six to eight samples with concentrations ranging from the LLOQ to the ULOQ, in generally logarithmic order (e.g., 1, 3, 10, 30, 100, 300, 1000 ng/mL for a 1 to 1000 ng/mL curve). One set of samples is run at the beginning of the run, another at the end.

All assessments must be made in the unmodified target matrix unless the matrix is rare or the analyte endogenous. The key to method development and formal validation is to conceptualize each step in the analysis and then determine its effect on the analyte(s) and what the impact might be on the six primary validation metrics. It is also important to consider the intended use of the assay, whether for biomarker determination or pharmacokinetcs. The criteria for bioanalytical validation for pharmacokinetic or toxicokinetic regulated studies are fairly well established. On the other hand, there are no specific guidelines for biomarker assays. Comparison of the criteria for successful method development of assays for pharmacokinetics, biomarker in support of drug development, and biomarkers for diagnostics may be found in Lee et al. [8]. This paper also has a nice fit-for-purpose table relating parameter assay elements to various stages of drug development. The use of blank matrix for QC and calibrators of the same type and species is critical. As mentioned above, there can be exceptions but only as a last resort.

Although conducted infrequently, sample collection stability, including the stability of analytes in whole blood, should be assessed, especially if the analyte and/or its metabolite(s) are known to be unstable. Blood and urine samples are frequently not processed immediately after collection. Samples may be at room temperature for a finite period of time in a clinical setting. One approach is to split a select number of samples: half are processed on wet ice, plasma separated using a refrigerated centrifuge, frozen, and stored immediately; the other half are allowed to remain at room temperature for select intervals before processing. Portions are taken after 0.5, 1, and 2 hours and processed as above. An alternative approach is to spike fresh, blank blood with the target analyte(s), allow time for distribution, sample at one or more intervals thereafter, and then process immediately. An extended study would be called for if the analyte concentration continues to decrease. The samples are considered stable if the percent of deviation compared to the 0-hour sample is less than $\pm 15.0\%$ without red blood cell distribution [50].

Matrix Effects and Ion Suppression To quote from the Crystal City III white paper [6]: "The quantitative measure of matrix effect can be termed as Matrix Factor and defined as a ratio of the analyte peak response in the presence of matrix ions to the analyte peak response in the absence of matrix ions"; that is,

$$\text{matrix factor} = \frac{\text{peak response in presence of matrix ions}}{\text{peak response in absence of matrix ions}}$$

A matrix factor of unity signifies no matrix effects. A value of less than unity suggests ionization suppression. A matrix factor >1 may be due to ionization enhancement and can also be caused by analyte loss in the absence of matrix during analysis. The IS normalized matrix factor is the matrix factor of analyte divided by that of the IS. The IS-normalized matrix factor can also be obtained by substituting peak response with peak response ratio (analyte/internal) in the foregoing equation. The internal standards in MS-based assays can help minimize the impact of matrix effects by a normalization phenomenon. Stable isotope-labeled IS minimizes the influence of matrix effects most effectively since the physicochemical properties of the analyte and its stable isotope are virtually identical. Analog internal standards may also compensate for matrix effects; however, the stable isotope-labeled internal standards are the most effective and should be used whenever possible.

An absolute or IS normalized matrix factor of about unity is not necessary for a reliable bioanalytical assay. The white paper stated that when using stable isotope internal standards, it was not necessary to determine the IS normalized matrix factor in the six different lots. However, use of a stable label IS is not a panacea for normalizing matrix effects. Jemal et al. [51] showed an example of a matrix effect problem that was observed even with such an IS.

4.4 SPECIAL ISSUES WITH LIGAND-BINDING ASSAYS

Although many of the concepts of chemical assays are shared with ligand-binding assays, the latter has several different characteristics [41].

4.4.1 Characterization

Unlike small molecules, which can be synthesized and characterized within a mass unit, biopharmaceuticals generally have a range of masses and structures that can complicate both the development of the drug product and the bioanalysis. Even so, acceptable variability of reference materials needs to be established and key reagents such as antibodies, binding proteins, receptors, tracers, and matrix should be characterized appropriately and stored under well-controlled conditions. An additional and important complication with assays that use ligand-binding technology is that internal standards of any kind are usually impossible to apply, increasing the influence of systemic and random error on the results.

4.4.2 Selectivity Issues

The core principle of most ligand-binding assays is based on the affinity of the analyte for an antibody. This antibody binding can be promiscuous, and cross-reactivity by endogenous substances, metabolites, other medications, and so on, occurs with many assays. For example, it was shown that radioimmunoassays (RIAs) for estradiol elicited apparent concentrations that were three- to four-fold higher than the more selective assays, such as a recombinant ultrasensitive bioassay using HeLa cells and GC-MS/MS [52]. This suggests that nonestrogen interferences influenced the RIA assay.

Interferences can occur from two sources: compounds that are chemically similar to the analyte(s) and matrix effects that are independent of substances related to the analyte [1]. Although the chances for selectivity issues are greater for ligand-binding assays, the issue is dealt with in much the same way as small-molecule selectivity. Multiple lots (six to ten) of blank matrix are analyzed, as are samples generated from a matrix pool that are spiked at or near the LLOQ [41]. When available, incurred samples should be spiked using the method of addition mentioned above to determine dilutional linearity and to detect study/patient-related interferences and changes that might be introduced with a change in the lot of the antibody. Although not stated specifically in the guidance, like small molecules, blanks should be less than 20% of the LLOQ. Smolec et al. [41] recommends that at least 80% of the spiked samples be 20 to 25% of the nominal concentration. The gold standard for selectivity is a comparison with a validated chromatographic method such as LC-MS/MS.

4.4.3 Matrix Effects

Although matrix effects have been acknowledged only recently as being a major issue with MS methods, their influence on ligand-binding assays has been appreciated since their inception. The basic assay premise is that an analyte is in equilibrium between a free and an antibody-bound state. Any number of factors can influence these binding equilibria (e.g., matrix composition, use of buffers, type of glassware/plasticware), and results can vary. Cross-checks are essential. The standard curve in biological fluids should be compared with standard in buffer. Parallelism of diluted samples should be evaluated, and nonspecific binding should be determined.

4.4.4 Quantification Issues

In addition to the nonlinear relationship between detector response and concentration, the response and error relationship for ligand-binding assay standard curves is not a constant function of the mean response (see Figure 4.16 compared with the plot for chromatographic systems in Figure 4.15). For chromatographic systems, there is, for the most part, a linear relationship between the %CV and the standard concentration above the LLOQ. A different mathematical model must be employed for ligand-binding assays, with anchor points above the ULOQ and below the LLOQ.

4.5 PARTIAL AND CROSS-VALIDATIONS

The FDA guidance recommends that full validations be conducted when "developing and implementing a bioanalytical method for the first time, for a new drug entity, or/and if metabolites are added to an existing assay for quantification." In practice, full validations as described above are conducted routinely for most changes in the bioanalytical method. Partial validations can involve as little as one run (as opposed to three runs in full validations). The list in the guidance [1] is shown in Table 4.4. It is important to note, independent of where the assay

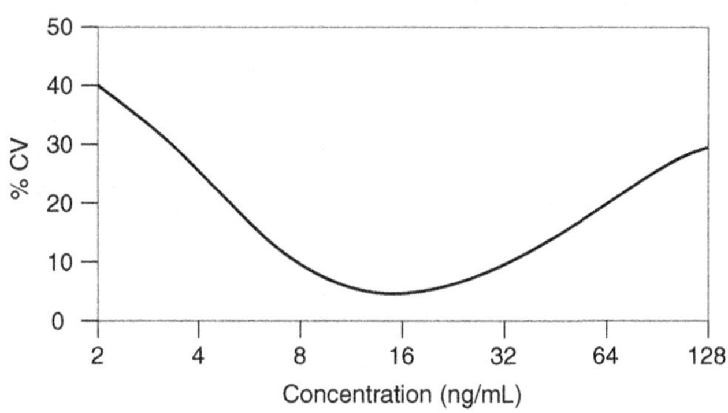

FIGURE 4.16 Theoretical plot of the heteroscedascity of an LBA-based assay. The useful analytical range is truncated due to increasing %CV values at the high and low concentration ranges.

TABLE 4.4 Conditions Under Which Partial Validations May Be Acceptable

Bioanalytical method transfers between laboratories[a] or analysts	Change in relevant concentration range
Change in analytical methodology (e.g., change in detection systems)	Changes in instruments and/or software platforms
Change in anticoagulant	Limited sample volume (e.g., pediatric study)
Change in matrix within species (e.g., human plasma to human urine)[a]	Rare matrices (e.g., fetal rat plasma)
Change in sample processing procedures[a]	Selectivity demonstration of an analyte in the presence of concomitant medications
Change in species within matrix (e.g., rat plasma to mouse plasma)	Selectivity demonstration of an analyte in the presence of specific metabolites

Source: Adapted from [3].
[a]In practice, full validations are usually run.

is run, all the data obtained from a full validation, including stability data, have to be at the bioanalytical assay site for a particular study. With the exception of stability and matrix interference, which are not site specific, a transfer of a method from one laboratory to another (e.g., from a pharma company to a CRO) generally requires revalidation of the method. It is also good practice to analyze incurred samples at the second site and compare the results with those from the first laboratory, if possible.

Cross-validations are conducted to determine the method parameters when two or more methods are used to analyze data from the same study or when the comparison of results from multiple studies is critical for product development. This includes analyzing samples from the same study across different sites or laboratories. Basically, samples are split and run at each laboratory during the course of a full validation. It is strongly recommended that these be incurred samples. Generally, a cross-validation is conducted when one assay has been used over time and serves as a reference for other assays developed that are fundamentally different but may have desirable properties Generally, this is not an issue in early development up to FIH and is therefore beyond the scope of this chapter.

4.6 APPLICATION OF VALIDATED METHODS TO SAMPLE ANALYSES: SOME PERSPECTIVES

The bioanalytical method validation guidance [1,5,6] also applies to routine drug analysis of biological samples. While the validation procedures described should mimic the actual analysis of samples from regulated nonclinical and clinical studies, there are some issues that are specific to sample analysis.

4.6.1 Stability

Sample stability is a key issue (maybe *the* key issue) in sample analysis. Samples generated in the course of nonclinical and clinical studies are rarely if ever analyzed within a short period (e.g., one day) after acquisition, but are usually stored refrigerated at −20°C, −70°C, or on dry ice (sublimation temperature −78.5°C) for extended periods. All assays for these samples need to be completed within the time frame determined explicitly in stability experiments and at the conditions used during those experiments. Storage at −20°C does not imply stability at −70°C. There has been considerable discussion and debate within the bioanalytical community about the differences in sample composition or decomposition at the two temperatures; the reasons for such potential differences are not intuitively clear. It may be that a lower temperature increases protein denaturation, and such a subtle alteration in sample integrity may produce a substantial change in the results of sample analysis.

All environments the samples are exposed to need to be taken into account. Generally, samples need only be analyzed once if the variability of the measurement is acceptable. Ligand-binding assays, with a higher, heteroscedasic variability and lower accuracy without compensating internal standards may require analyses in duplicate. However, the relatively short turnaround due to the limited amount of sample preparation and analyte detection times allow duplicate or even triplicate analyses to be efficient.

The stability of parent drug and/or prodrug and/or metabolite must be demonstrated in all target matrices for each species. Rodent esterases, for example, have high ex vivo metabolic activity, and thus ester drugs can undergo hydrolysis in plasma after blood withdrawal. Differences in fresh versus aged matrix have been seen. If samples are unstable, prodrug or metabolite stabilization may be necessary to avoid conversion of metabolite back to parent (e.g., glucuronides, N-oxides, thiols (disulfides), lactone–hydroxy acid interconversion) and to ensure accurate measurement of metabolites. However, the stabilization medium may affect the integrity of the matrix. Stabilization of the analyte may result in destabilization of the matrix and enhance or suppress ionization (interference). Jemal et al. [51] described strategies to handle metabolites that can convert to the parent drug during various stages preceding introduction of the sample into the LC-MS/MS system and/or in the source of the mass spectrometer. The metabolites listed are acylglucuronides, lactones, hydroxy acids, O-glucuronides, O-sulfates, N-glucuronides, N-oxides, disulfides, and S-oxides.

Stabilization can be achieved by the use of enzyme inhibitors added to the matrix or by pH adjustment. Examples of enzyme inhibitors are diisopropyl fluorophosphate (DFP) [53], phenylmethylsulfonylfluoride (PMSF) [54], and sodium fluoride [55] (also an anticoagulant). Low-pH buffers afford optimum chemical stabilization of esters, can denature enzymes, and affect protein conformation/binding and viscosity. 1-O-acyl glucuronides [56–61] tend to be labile in base, even at the physiological normal plasma pH of 7.4. Keeping samples acidic is essential during sample processing. On the other hand, many sulfoxides are labile in acid, and thus samples with such analytes need to be kept alkaline.

4.6.2 Calibration Curves

Calibration curves should be created that mimic the validation curves, with one set at the beginning of the run, another at the end. There should be no fewer than six concentrations that cover the range of the assay, including a blank (without the IS) and a zero standard (a blank with an IS). There has been the question of whether multiplate assays (i.e., assays where samples are in 96- or 384-well plates) constitute one run or multiple runs. In one run, conceivably only one standard curve would need to be on each plate, with the exception of the last plate. General practice limits one run to one plate. Each calibrator can be spiked with one or more analytes as long as the validation data support this practice. It should be noted that the number of failed runs, a measure of the robustness of the method, seems to increase factorially for many assays: two analytes, twofold failure; three analytes, sixfold failures; four analytes, 24-fold failures; and so on. As mentioned above, there is no universally accepted number of failed runs that would indicate an unreliable or insufficiently robust assay. Certainly, more than 10% failures would indicate a weak method, unless mitigating circumstances are discovered by investigation and documented. Extrapolation of concentrations above the assay range is not acceptable. As mentioned before, for ligand-binding assays, the error function is nonlinear and increases exponentially beyond the limits of the assay (Figure 4.16). Samples above the ULOQ would need to be diluted or the standard curve should be repeated at a higher concentration. Any change in the calibration curve that affects the basic regression equation would require partial validation. If diluted, the samples involved would need to be run with a dilutional QC during a study (see below) unless a dilutional QC is run during validation. It is also good practice to run all samples for a given subject in one analytical run.

4.6.3 Quality Control Samples

As surrogates for incurred samples, the use of QC samples is essential in monitoring the continued precision and accuracy of a bioanalytical method. As discussed in Section 4.3.6, QC samples should be prepared at low, middle, and high concentrations. Preferably, these should be prepared before or just as study samples are initially prepared or received. After preparation, QC samples should be stored with the study samples. A minimum of two QCs per concentration level per run is required. The QCs should be placed throughout a sample analysis run so as to determine the assay reproducibility during the entire run. There should be a minimum of six total QC samples or 5% of the number of unknown samples.

4.6.4 Analytical Notes

The order of samples analyzed in a run should be in a sequence of low to high concentration or in the time order in which the samples were obtained for each subject. A random assortment of samples in a run should be avoided due to crossover issues. Standards and QCs should be prepared in blank matrix of the type and species studied. Changes in assay responses during a study, including major changes in response (e.g. 50%), indicate problems and should be investigated. A standard operating procedure (SOP) should be developed to that end. Standards and QCs can be prepared from the same stock solutions, assuming that there is sufficient stability to justify the stock solution use for the intended period of time. The stability of reference material does not affect the duration of the stability of a stock solution. Stock solutions prepared any time from day 1 to the limit of stability determined for the reference material are acceptable. For example, a stock solution may have an established stability of six months, and the reference material of one year. The stock solution has a stability lifetime of six months even if it was prepared on the last day the reference material has been documented as being stable.

4.6.5 Acceptance Criteria

The 2007 Crystal City III white paper [6] contains a table outlining routine drug analysis process and run acceptance criteria and is reproduced in Table 4.3. A run is acceptable when 75% (or a minimum of six standards) of the back-calculated values of the calibration samples fall within 15% of the nominal value. The exception is the acceptance at the LLOQ, which is 20%. Values falling outside the range 15 to 20% may be discarded if they do not change the model established for data analysis. For chemical assays, this is a generally a weighted regression; for ligand binding, a 4P model.

For QCs, the run is accepted if two-thirds of the QCs are within 15% of their nominal concentrations and there is an acceptable QC at each concentration level. In multiple analyte assays, the run for one analyte may fail while a second passes. The analyte values that passed may be reported. Samples may be rerun for the failed analyte. The data for the analyte from the repeat run originally passed must be archived but does not have to be reported. All failed runs must be reported. Repetition of sample analysis for reasons other than calibrator or QC failure or analytical failures (e.g., automatic injector failure) can be made. The reasons for repetition due to pharmacokinetic considerations must be clearly documented. Criteria for pharmacokinetic repeats should be clearly outlined in an a priori SOP. Only the pharmacokineticist responsible for the study can make the decision to repeat a determination, although the analyst may flag some samples for immediate attention. The generation of an a posteriori SOP for repeat pharmacokinetic determinations is not recommended.

If an assay failure has been identified, the second, repeat value obtained is reported as the value for that sample. For pharmacokinetic repeats, reporting is more complicated. The most common reason for requesting a repeat analysis for pharmacokinetic reasons is that the samples for two adjacent values in a plasma concentration curve profile look like they have been switched sometime in their handling, causing an "under, then over sawtooth" profile. This sort of problem is ordinarily impossible to prove. The sawtooth profile may be unrealistic from a pharmacokinetic model viewpoint, and repeats are considered. There is no universal way to deal with these data. If the repeats are within a certain percentage of the original value (e.g., 20%), the mean is reported. If the repeats are different by more than a certain percentage, the second value is generally reported. Another approach is to have a double repeat analysis for the samples of interest. If one or both of the repeats are within a certain percentage of the original value, the median is reported. If both values are beyond the accepted percentage, their mean is reported.

No approach for pharmacokinetic repeats is universally accepted by regulatory agencies, clients, and/or laboratory managers. Some laboratories have banned pharmacokinetic repeats outright because there are too many issues when dealing with them and the repeats may not have a significant influence on the interpretation of the study. In general, failed runs and sample repeats are considered major measures of the viability of an assay, and investigation of root causes for these failures is necessary. The BMV guidance recommends reassays should be done in triplicate if sample volume allows, although this approach is rarely used.

4.6.6 Repeat Analyses of Incurred Samples

The use of incurred samples to determine the reproducibility and accuracy of an analytical method was mandated by the FDA/AAPS meeting in February 2008 on incurred sample reanalysis [7]. There has been a lively discussion on the topic for the past several years. The basic issue is an old one: Calibration and QC standards are prepared by adding known analytes to a blank target matrix, usually plasma or serum obtained in bulk from normal, healthy volunteers. The volunteer and the phlebotomist are under no real time pressures. The volunteer is catheterized once and is allowed to lie down undisturbed for the time it takes to acquire 500 mL of blood. The blood is processed in an unhurried environment.

Samples obtained during the course of a study, however, are different. These are obtained a few milliliters at a time over the course of many hours or days from multiple needle sticks or catheters. Phlebotomy stations have to be organized carefully to obtain the proper samples from multiple, well-identified subjects at prescribed times after dosing. Sometimes the samples are not processed immediately or properly (see above on sample collection stability). Subjects may be from healthy populations or from populations that have abnormal matrix compositions due to, for example, hepatic or renal insufficiency. Endogenous compound compositions can differ due to population variability or from drug-modulated differences in concentration or activity. Fasting states could cause similar variability. Formulation components can cause matrix effects or degrade to conversion products that can elicit interferences. As mentioned earlier, both accuracy and interday precision may be affected by metabolite instability, which can interfere with analyte determination.

The issue was first discussed at Crystal City in 1990 and mentioned in the follow-up report [4]. Although not an FDA concern at the time, the concept was supported by Health Canada. In 1992, a Health Canada Guideline required the following: "In general, single sample analysis will suffice. When single assays are performed, 15 percent of the incurred samples must be randomly selected and re-assayed. (Studies in which the sample of blood is insufficient for duplicate analysis should include a pre-study verification with incurred samples.)" At Crystal City III it was stated that this requirement was revoked in 2003 because Health Canada did not have a strategy for interpretation of the data. More recently, the FDA noted that 50% of their audits had significant deficiencies, and whereas validations were acceptable (QC 6% CV), study runs were frequently found to differ at C_{max} by 30 to 80%. There could also be a 350% difference between original and repeat sample values. The overall frequency was not determined. Investigators at Hoffmann LaRoche [62] noted that of 110 approved data sets analyzed over several years, three were fully rejected and three partially rejected for lack of reproducibility.

How to implement a program to determine the accuracy and reproducibility of a bioanalytical method was not addressed at the Crystal City III meeting and remains a controversial subject. A meeting solely on incurred sample reanalysis (ISR) was held at Crystal City in 2008, and a white paper was published [7]. A subsequent meeting of the Delaware Valley Drug Metabolism Discussion Group was held on this topic, and some points that emerged are discussed below.

What has generally been accepted is that if the primary study goal is toxicokinetics or pharmacokinetics, incurred sample reanalysis must be considered. For those laboratories that have already implemented reanalysis programs, incurred sample reanalysis, guided by an SOP, reinforces confidence in the method by its consumers that the assay is valid and reproducible. If a reanalysis test fails, an investigation needs to be made, preferably guided by an SOP, and the analytical portion of a study should be placed on hold until the investigation is carried out and follow-up action is completed.

Incurred sample reanalysis should involve individual samples, not a pool of samples. There is a better chance of finding anomalous samples or subjects if more subjects with fewer samples are used. One paradigm is to take one sample at C_{max} and one near the end of elimination (to capture metabolite effects) for multiple subjects during each study period. Samples previously requested for toxicokinetic or pharmacokinetic repeats that have already been reanalyzed in duplicate should not be used. Data should be placed in study reports and appended to assay validation reports.

For nonclinical GLP studies, one study per species per method per lab should be tested using ISR, usually the first subchronic toxicity study where samples are available. Given the low number of nonclinical samples or species, this could be part of the validation of the method [6]. For clinical studies, incurred sample reanalysis should be done for all bioequivalence studies and for selected healthy volunteer, patient population, and small-molecule drug–drug interaction studies as appropriate. Samples from patients with disease should be tested. ISR tests should be conducted as soon as possible in the study to verify that the results obtained from the rest of the study are valid. Long-range studies may have multiple tests throughout the study.

It should be stated that failure of the incurred sample reanalysis does not result in acceptance or rejection of the bioanalytical assay but only indicates that an investigation and follow-up are necessary. For small molecules, if two-thirds of the difference between original and reanalyzed results divided by the mean of original and reanalyzed results are within 20%, the test passes. For large molecules, acceptance is within 30%. No results are excluded except for demonstrable bioanalytical reasons.

There are other approaches that may be used, such as:

1. Bioequivalence criteria, which employ the confidence interval (CI) ANOVA approach (also known as a two one-sided *t*-test) [63].
2. Regression analysis, where the metric is the slope with an expected value of 1. The slope is evaluated using a 95% CI. The regression would be between the repeat (dependent) variable and the reference value, and if the CI value is between 80 and 125%, the test is successful [64,65].
3. U.S. Military Standard 105D [66].

The two-thirds method, which is derived from the 4–6–15% approach currently being used for quality assurance (QA) acceptance, is preferred until more data can be accumulated and analyzed. While the topic is still being debated, 5% (for large studies) to 10% (for small studies) of the samples in a study should be repeated for ISR, with a minimum of 20 samples. The dividing line between small and large studies has not been determined, but many laboratories consider studies with more than 1000 samples to be large studies.

4.6.7 Sample Stability and Incurred Samples

Neither the bioanalytical method guidance nor the Crystal City meetings specified the use of incurred samples for stability experiments. The white paper [6] did specify that "drug stability experiments should mimic conditions under which samples are collected, stored and processed, as closely as possible." The differences between QCs prepared from a blank matrix and reference and incurred samples were discussed above. Although stability tests with incurred samples are not yet mandated, such tests may be appropriate. Potential stability tests are outlined in Table 4.5. One approach to demonstrate stability would be to assay pooled samples from day 1 at three or more concentration levels (e.g., low, middle, and high). Intraday precision of a representative sample could then be determined. Acceptance criteria for $n = 6$ replicates would be <15% CV. The pooled samples would be stored and reassayed at later time points (e.g., at two weeks). Such a two-week value would be compared to two-week stability in validation (normal QC). An additional time point at the longest sample storage time would also be compared to the ongoing long-term stability standard (normal QC). A comparison at the end of the study may be needed for late pharmacokinetic repeats. Samples would be evaluated as unstable if the difference is >15.0% or by acceptance criteria defined by assay variance.

TABLE 4.5 Stability Experiment Evaluations

Stability Experiment	Normal QC Evaluation	Incurred QC Evaluation
Stock solution	Test to nominal	Not applicable
Reinjection integrity and autosampler stability	Test to nominal	Test to time zero
Room temperature	Test to nominal	Test to time zero
Freeze/thaw	Test to nominal	Test to time zero
Long term	Test to nominal	Test to time zero

Source: Adapted from [50].

4.6.8 Scientific Versus Production Issues

In the realm of bioanalysis, there are scientific issues concerning method development and validation, and there are the "day in, day out" sample analysis issues involving the efficient assay of perhaps thousands of samples from multiple studies over the lifetime of the development of a drug product. These scientific and "production" issues go hand in hand and change as drug screening and discovery matures into full-fledged drug development.

Initially, little is known about the chemistry of a drug candidate. In fast-track drug discovery, the analyst at a contract research organization (CRO) may not even know the structure, only the platform on which the compound series is based. If a group of samples appears at the door on an "as available, on submission, by-project" basis and are not part of a projected structural series, the generic method developed for the platform is probably not going to be appropriate and the "as available" samples will not "fit the mold" of the assay. Whereas it is natural from a scientific point of view to think in terms of a "by project" grouping of compounds for screening, from an analytical production view, it is not efficient. It is entirely sequential, with each compound in its own miniexperiment. Batching and automation options may not present themselves until a batch exceeds one plate's worth, usually 60 to 70 samples in a 96-well plate.

What is efficient, and can represent major throughput improvements, is grouping compounds by analytical characteristics having a library of basic assays that are tailored for common characteristics, and applying a triage process that pairs methods with compounds. Since compounds should be grouped early in the process by their biopharmaceutic drug classification [67,68] and Lipinski's rule of five [69,70] (Chapter 3), such a grouping can be synergistic with other drug metabolism/pharmacokinetic and pharmacodynamic activities. As an analytical grouping, the analyst can batch samples that optimize the performance of the automation systems in place and can keep equipment running close to capacity.

A proposed triage approach has been presented with the following grouping rules [71]:

1. Review the molecular weight and potential of fragments from one compound to interfere with those of another.

2. Check the ionization response with group APCI and ESI, both positive and negative. If there is no response, remove from the group.
3. Check the retention time. If it is 0.3 to 2.3 min, it is okay.
4. Arrange compounds as close as possible in groups.

The compounds that do not fit into these "factory/production" rules need to be dealt with by the "scientific/lab" function. It must be remembered that science is done in the laboratory and manufacturing is done in the factory. The latter can deal with routine assays to yield data to drive decisions. New and challenging science, new theories, and observations come from the laboratory. Although the equipment may be the same and the lab and the factory often have to coexist, the processes are fundamentally different.

Emerging from the screening and discovery mode, the factory side takes on more importance as the chemistry of a drug candidate is better understood, experience with an assay increases, and the assay becomes more routine. The FDA has produced guidance [72] from the current good manufacturing practices (cGMP) world that may provide some suggestions on dealing with out-of-specification results in this phase of drug development. The guidance emphasizes extensive documentation, especially of investigation events, identifying the root cause for an out-of-specification event, and determining the impact of that event. Errors are rare in a properly run analytical factory. Frequent errors can suggest insufficient resources, poor analyst training or attitude, and/or poor equipment maintenance.

The laboratory side may have a major impact on the out-of-specification investigation and a means of remediation. The causes listed above are systemic, and caused by deficiencies in the production assay group across programs. As exemplified by the FDA's recent posture toward the necessity of repeating the assay of study samples, subtle or not so subtle differences in process, people, equipage (e.g., SPE cartridges), equipment, matrix (e.g., plasma from renally impaired subjects), metabolite distribution (e.g., HIV changes in the 2D6 phenotype), and so on; there is always the potential that yesterday's assay may not fill the needs of every study.

The world is awash in production management paradigms. One that seems particularly suited to the laboratory is Goldratt's *Theory of Constraints* [73–75]. This approach stresses improvement of a system as opposed to each individual process. A system is actually an interdependent chain of processes. Improving most of the links will do little if the weakest link is not improved. That weakest link is the constraint in the system. By managing that link, the highest probability of managing the chain is achieved. By modulating the slowest or constraining process, the entire system can be monitored and adjusted by speeding it up or slowing it down.

4.6.9 Documentation

Analytical equipment is ordinarily associated with laboratory information management systems (LIMS) that transform raw data into concentration values.

Depending on the sophistication of the LIMS, these data can be paired with sample inventory and protocol information to yield pharmacokinetic data organized by patient, treatment, and/or other groupings, such as gender or age. There may also be advanced statistical features that would allow discrimination between groupings. The most popular LIMS system is Watson by ThermoFisher. This software can perform basic pharmacokinetic and toxicokinetic analysis. More extensive pharmacokinetic and pharmacodynamic analysis and modeling can be done using WinNonLin software. Data can then be transferred to a sophisticated statistical program such as SAS Stat. Links to Watson, WinNonLin, and SAS Stat can be found in Table 4.1, as can links to their parent companies: ThermoFisher, Pharsight, and the SAS Institute. There is considerable overlap in capabilities between these products. There are also many other fine products with similar features. An investigator should review their requirements and evaluate what software meets their needs.

Documentation issues are dealt with extensively in the bioanalytical method validation guidance and the Crystal City III white paper. As stated in the white paper, "records generated during the course of method validation and study sample analysis are source records and should be retained to demonstrate the validity of the method under the conditions of use, and to support the statements made in the report. This is necessary to enable the reconstruction of the laboratory events as they occurred since the information generated by the individual laboratory might differ from what the sponsor includes in the application." A table is supplied in the white paper that outlines the details of documentation (Table 4.6). References are made to standards, stock solutions, calibrators and QCs, run acceptance criteria, assay procedure, sample tracking, analysis details and documentation, failed runs, reintegration, deviations from SOPs and methods, reassays, and communications among analysts, managers, and sites. Although the details of final validation and sample analysis reports vary, the basic components are relatively constant.

4.6.10 Resources

The ultimate goal of a bioanalytical laboratory intending to support an investigational new drug (IND)/clinical trial application (CTA) submission is to have the resources necessary to conduct assays compliant with GLP and the relevant regulatory guidelines. These resources should be physically separated from the nonregulated discovery resources as best as possible. Such a separation removes the need to validate and document equipment, equipage, and (perhaps) personnel used in discovery processes and limits the scope of instrumentation, operation, and performance qualification.

The following discussion is an example about resource organization for a GLP laboratory; this has also been well described by others [76,77]. Much of the discussion pertains to setting up a GLP system within a bioanalytical CRO and thus can provide a checklist regarding a due-diligence review of such a CRO by a putative sponsor. However, it should be noted that the components of a GLP bioanaltyical laboratory can be appropriately tailored to sponsor companies

TABLE 4.6 Details of Documentation Desirable at the Bioanalytical Site and in Validation and Bioanalytical Reports

Item	Bioanalytical Site	Validation Report	Validation Report Appendix	Bioanalytical Report	Bioanalytical Report Appendix
Standard	Certificate of analysis, purity, stability for analyte Record of receipt and storage Lack of interference between IS and analyte	Batch/lot no., purity, and manufacturer stability at time of use		Batch/lot no., purity and manufacturer stability at time of use	
Stock solution preparation	Records of preparation Storage location and condition				
Calibrator and QC preparation	Records of preparation Freezer log (sample ingress/egress, temperature)	Preparation dates Storage conditions		Storage conditions	
Run acceptance criteria	SOPs for calibrators, QCs, chromatographic interferences	Short description	SOP (optional)	Short description	SOP (optional)
Assay procedure	SOP for the method	Brief description of extraction and analysis	SOP (optional)	Brief description	SOP (optional)

Sample tracking	Sample receipt, condition on receipt, and location of storage Tracking of QC, calibrators, and study samples; freezer logs	Storage condition and location		Dates of receipt of shipments and contents Sample condition on receipt Storage location and condition	
Analysis	Dates of extraction and analysis and instrument identification (ID) for each run Identity of QCs, calibrators, and study samples Documentation of processing of calibrators, QCs, and study samples for each run Documentation of instrument settings and maintenance Run summary sheets 100% chromatograms LIMS and Mode of integration Extraction dates	Table of runs, instrument ID, and analysis dates Table of calibrator results of all runs with accuracy and precision Tables of within- and between-run QC results (accuracy and precision). Bench-top, freeze–thaw, long-term, and postpreparative and stock solution stability data Extraction recovery and matrix effect	Representative chromatograms Cross-validation, if applicable Additional validation, if any Long-term stability appended or written in a separate report	Table of all runs and analysis dates Table of calibrator results of all passed runs with mean and %CV Tables of QC results of all passed runs with accuracy and precision; OK to include QC results of the failed runs	Chromatograms from 5–20% of subjects for ANDA and representative chromatograms for NDA submissions

(*Continued overleaf*)

TABLE 4.6 (*Continued*)

Item	Bioanalytical Site	Validation Report	Validation Report Appendix	Bioanalytical Report	Bioanalytical Report Appendix
Failed runs	Same as in "Analysis"	Identify runs, assay date, and reason for failure		Identify runs, assay dates, and reason for failure	
Reintegration	Audit trail: original and reintegration Reason for reintegration Mode of reintegration				SOP (optional)
Deviations from SOPs/method	Documentation of deviations and unexpected events Investigation of unexpected events Impact assessment	Description of deviations Impact on study results Description and supporting data of significant investigations		Description of deviations Impact on study results; description and supporting data of significant investigations	
Reassay	Refer to "Analysis" SOP for reassay criteria		SOP (optional)	Table of sample IDs, reason for reassay, original and reassay values, and run IDs	SOP
Commun-ication	Between analytical site and clinical site/sponsor				

with dedicated resources. (As an aside, the term the "spirit of GLP" has been employed for some studies, but regulatory authorities recommend that this be avoided.) The creation of a GLP laboratory is an immense undertaking, the number of details stunning and a triage approach should followed, starting with oversight and control by QA. A master plan should be developed and followed dealing with the site, personnel, equipment (critical and noncritical), equipage and reagents, LIMS and information technology, chain of custody, science and production, QC, documentation, and archiving.

SOPs and Quality Assurance The first task in the creation of a GLP bioanalytical laboratory is the employment of full or part-time personnel, or on a consulting basis, in a team of well-trained, experienced QA professionals. Becoming a member of the Society of Quality Assurance (SQA) gives access to the resources of their Web site (www.sqa.org/) to help in the selection process. Creating a full library of integrated operating procedures is a huge task. For example, a possible list of SOPs from a fully functional bioanalytical laboratory is shown in Table 4.7. A balance needs to be struck with SOPs. They need to be specific enough to provide guidance but general enough to give a scientist latitude to deal with specific problems. A minimalist approach to SOPs is strongly recommended.

Bioanalytical Site Although a de novo, built-for-purpose site is always desired, various commercial spaces and pharmaceutical companies can also be refitted. A financial and capacity budget needs to be drawn up for electrical, waste, and ventilation requirements. Components should include, but not be limited to, the following:

- Nuclear Regulatory Commission (NRC) license: radioactive sample analysis capability (if needed)
- Biosafety level 2 laboratory hoods
- Secure freezer storage room with walk-in -20°C unit
- Natural gas backup generator and individual uninterrupted power supply systems
- Archive and network rooms equipped with HFC227-ea fire suppression systems
- Drug Enforcement Agency (DEA)-registered facility for schedule 2, 3, 3N, 4, and 5 controlled substances
- Continuous (24/7, 365) monitoring of sample storage conditions

Infectious agents may require more than level 2 hoods, but hepatitis and HIV samples can be handled in them safely. NRC licenses can be titrated, depending on the isotopes used in the laboratory.

Personnel Despite automation and specific methods with MS detection, there will never be a substitute for scientists, analysts, and backup personnel who are highly capable, experienced, and well trained. Although automation has vastly

TABLE 4.7 SOPs Recommended for a Fully Functional Bioanalytical Laboratory

General	
Administration	Records
Computer/information technology (IT)	Reporting
Data analysis	Safety
Data management	Sample storage
Equipment	System suitability
Facility	Test methods
Reagents	
Specific	
96-Well drier	Long-term stability evaluation
Analysis lists	Maintenance of study protocols by QA
Analytical balance	Management responsibility for GLPs
Analytical materials	Master schedule
Analytical system	Method training and qualification
Archives	Method validation
Archiving of computerized information generated by analytical instruments	Notebook control
	Organization
Biohazard safety	OSHA inspections
Calibration manager	Periodic review of IT systems
Carryover	pH meter calibration
Centrifuge maintenance	Pipette calibration
Chain of custody	QA reports
Change control for computer systems	QA responsibilities
Chemical acceptance procedures	QA statement
Chromatographic reintegration	QC storage
Cold storage	Raw data documentation
Computer system administration	Reagent and solution control
Computer system time administration	Record retention
Confidentiality	Repeat analysis
Contingency plan for materials requiring cold storage	Report process
	Role of principal investigator
Control of laboratory equipment	Sample handling
Deviation documentation	Security of computerized systems
Documentation correction codes	Setting resolution and calibration of quadrupole mass spectrometers
Documentation of requests for analysis	
Electronic signatures	Facility inspections
Employee training	Significant figures and rounding in the display and calculation of sample results
External communication for GLP studies	
FDA inspections	
Guidelines for reporting reassay results	Stability of analytical solutions
Incubator use and maintenance	Standard operating procedures
In-process inspections	Study archiving operations
Investigation procedures	Study audits
Laboratory hood maintenance	Validation of computer systems

improved productivity, problems can occur when a trained observer is not present during a process step. Examples include peak retention drift to outside the data acquisition range, incomplete thawing, and the angle of IS introduction into the wells of a 96-well plate. Task specialization, although attractive from an efficiency point of view, can be problematic when it comes time to hand off samples between steps in an analytical process. The bulk of the problems and delays that this author has observed or heard about have been due to some communication failure between analysts transferring samples to the next step. Communication between "silos" can break down.

The education and training of scientists and analysts can never be too great and can never stop. Care must be taken not to let experienced analysts become bored and/or complacent. For all the supposed inefficiencies of humans, the need for analysts to develop into "complete chemists" is still essential, not only for knowing basic chemistry and techniques, but for higher-end data analysis. There are multiple benefits to maintaining the minimum number of people working on a given batch of samples, preferably to just one: minimal communication handoff errors, detection of mistakes or trends on the spot, and most important, ownership of the assay.

A hypothetical organization for the bioanalytical team (whether at a CRO or within a sponsor company) responsible for every aspect of sample analysis, from sample receipt to report generation, is shown below.

1. Principal bioanalytical investigator
   a. Primary client contact
      - Coordinates study schedules and client requirements
   b. Senior scientist
      - Directs method development, validation, and sample analysis
   c. Project management
      - Manages resources (time lines, equipment, staff)
2. Analysts
   - Perform method development and validation
   - Perform sample analysis, including extraction and instrumental analysis
   - Perform initial data processing
3. Report coordinators
   a. Client sample information managers
      - Receipt to study completion
      - Study design
      - Sample identification and discrepancies
   b. Client report experts
      - Report formats and templates
      - Data transfer
   c. Database experts

4. Laboratory support personnel
   a. Sample management group
      - Manage samples, freezers, and reference materials
   b. Laboratory and system support group
      - Provide expert equipment qualification and validation
      - Provide expert equipment repair, including MS
   c. Quality control group (separate from QA)
      - Review data for proper assembly
   d. Facilities group
      - Manage the facility, including purchasing
5. Quality assurance auditors
   - Handle in-process sample receipt and extraction and analysis procedures
   - Handle data and data and report release
   - Develop SOPs and processes
   - Supervise relevant facility activities
6. Archivist/document control administrator

LIMS and Information Technology There are two basic approaches to a laboratory information management system (LIMS) and information technology:

1. Create a staff of developers and network and support personnel for in-house development of data acquisition, analysis, and storage needs. The LIMS and databases could be built on a customizable kernel such as Oracle or 4D. This would provide the ability to respond rapidly to client needs. It would also require personnel infrastructure and the development of tools to customize processes for the LIMS and a database for QA audits, deviations, scheduling, and tracking training. This approach would maximize flexibility and speed at the cost of maintaining a relatively large overhead in information technology.

2. Acquire a commercially available LIMS. The mostly widely used product is Watson (see Table 4.1 for the Web site). Watson uses a central Oracle database and offers a point-and-click graphical interface. It is compliant with GLP regulations and the 21 CFR Part 11 guidance [2], and has system security and audit trails. It is also capable of handling standard and complex study protocols, providing audit trails to track deviations and amendments to each study. Although it has an attractive suite of features and a minimum of overhead, this approach is not as flexible, especially for custom requirements.

Chain of Custody of Bioanalytical Samples Generally, an independent sample management group is responsible for the physical management of samples, freezers, and reference materials. Samples should be received at a primary receiving area that is manned when samples are expected to be received. Coordination between the laboratory generating the samples, sample shippers, and this management group is critical. If the chain of custody is broken and there is a period during which the storage conditions cannot be accounted for, the samples may be declared "nonevaluable" (i.e., ruined). Samples are shipped in a thoroughly sealed, cold storage container (generally, Styrofoam) with dry ice. When samples are received, if there is still intact dry ice, the samples are considered still evaluable. Some laboratories require a temperature recorder. Typically, in-life study sites are asked by the bioanalytical laboratory to ship samples to the lab on a Monday, Tuesday, or Wednesday to avoid the possibility of defrosting over a weekend. However, given the increasing number of distant clinical sites and the necessity for ultrafast turnaround (e.g., for an ascending dose human study), weekend receipt is no longer uncommon. Bioanalytical labs today are generally amenable to weekend delivery if notified in advance.

Once samples are received, inventory should be conducted on the same day, certainly within 24 hours. Bar coding with direct LIMS input has greatly improved both the speed and accuracy of sample receipt and can allow discrepancies to be identified almost immediately. Discrepancies should be resolved immediately with the shipper. Sample management is then responsible for sample storage conditions. Analysts typically submit a list of samples to a sample management coordinator who retrieves just the sample requested. LIMS systems are generally designed so that the period from the time that samples are removed from the freezer to the time they are returned is recorded automatically. The LIMS compares these data to the established stability limitations, and the samples flagged if those limitations preclude the analysis of those samples.

QC and QA Even for a relatively small facility, QC needs justify the services of full-time employees. The QC scientist maintains a checklist system approved by a quality assurance unit (QAU) regarding documentation. Personnel should be experienced GLP bioanalyst(s) whose sense of project ownership and accountability is fully developed. To maintain a connection to the process, the QC scientist should also perform some benchwork in addition to his or her QC responsibilities.

All GLP studies require a protocol, a study director, and a QAU. Without a QAU, a GLP group cannot exist as stated in 21 CFR Part 58 [3], the code dealing with GLP. The development of a QAU must be independent of existing GLP-like or GMP structures. The complex and rapidly evolving nature of GLP bioanalysis requires structure and personnel technically oriented and highly specific to deal with the component systems. These include but are not limited to freezers and refrigeration, detectors, an LC/GC/LBA system, LIMS, and acquisition software. An external auditor should be engaged prior to launching the QAU to perform a gap analysis.

Documentation and Archival Processes Brockman and Wu [77] summarize key considerations for a documentation system. They used a three-ring binder system to file the approved, official, tracked forms issued by their documentation group. In addition, they added an SOP for a rigorous file nomenclature and archival system to facilitate the use of raw electronic data. They elected to use protocols to drive validation, and a portion of the validation report constitutes a bioanalytical procedure used during sample analysis. Electronic records are acquiring increased importance, and how they are handled requires special care. Some mechanism is needed to access these records even when the technology is outdated. For example, tape and old floppy disk readers would need to be stored as well as the media on which the records are stored. One common practice is to convert all records to pdf format, the format most commonly used by regulatory agencies, including the FDA. This concern will increase when generally useful electronic notebooks are available.

4.7 RISK-BASED PARADIGMS: DISCOVERY AND DEVELOPMENT SUPPORT

The criteria for bioanalytical assay development and validation in support of discovery and early (pretoxicology support) development vary among drug sponsors. Zhang and Banks [78] discussed screening strategies and Chaudhary et al. [79] presented a risk-based approach. In most companies, there is almost a quantum leap in the assay expectations between these early phases and toxicology/clinical support studies (candidate evaluation). At the discovery and optimization level, bioanalytical support needs to be as fast as possible, but with sufficient emphasis on sensitivity, ruggedness, and documentation. Candidate evaluation support requires high sensitivity and rugged bioanalytical methods that conform to regulatory guidelines with the concomitant documentation. The ideal approach would be a gradual transition between discovery and candidate evaluation, with adherence to *good bioanalytical practices* (GBPs) [79]. GBPs would morph into GLPs when studies are conducted that would be part of the safety package provided for IRB (institutional review board) and regulatory approval. Studies that may come under the GBP umbrella are shown in Table 4.8. Since the bioanalytical method validation guidance states that acceptance criteria need to be set in advance, it is recommended that a SOP be established for GBPs.

The basic theme is the "need for speed" in discovery and early development [18,80]. Although there is still discussion of when monitoring of metabolites should begin (some members of the community think no earlier than FIH), there may be value in monitoring metabolites in discovery pharmacokinetic studies if metabolite data can aid in the interpretation of pharmacodynamic observations [81]. There are fundamental differences between the development of small-molecule assays and the ligand-binding assays that are at the heart of most macromolecule (>5000 amu) bioanalytical development. Whether the phrase *fit-for-purpose method development* or *good bioanalytical practices* is used, some

TABLE 4.8 Examples of Bioanalytical Studies which May Be Conducted Using GBP (Good Bioanalytical Practices) Instead of Full GLP or GCP

Nonclinical	Clinical
Pilot pharmacokinetics/toxicokinetics	—
Metabolite quantification[a]	Metabolite quantification[a]
Support of safety pharmacology	—
Tissue penetration (e.g., brain)	PET ligand studies
Protein binding	Protein binding
Biomarker quantification	Biomarker quantification
PK/PD modeling	PK/PD modeling
—	Proof of concept (POC) support

[a]For initial non-GLP or non-GCP studies.

generalizations can be made. One possible program, with some general parameters, is shown in Table 4.9. A specific fit-for-purpose program for ligand-binding assays was discussed by Lee et al. [8].

For the purposes of developing an LC-MS/MS program, assay qualifications can be divided into three broad categories: (1) drug screening, (2) non-GLP method development, and (3) regulated development. For drug screening, the purpose is to rank-order compounds with desirable pharmacokinetic characteristics using a bioanalytical method that can be considered "semiquantitative." Once a subset of compounds has been identified for further evaluation, a more qualified method may be necessary but still does not require a full GLP-level validation.

A semiquantitative bioanalytical method supporting drug screening or discovery may take only a few hours to develop and might consist of the following: (1) a "crash and shoot" sample preparation with a plasma sample and 2 volumes of acetonitrile, (2) a "universal" ballistic gradient HPLC method, and (3) detection on a triple-quadrupole mass spectrometer with a wide MS detection range.

4.7.1 Logistics and Discovery

The goal of bioanalytical support of discovery and early development is speed, so as to be synchronized with other disciplines involved in candidate selection. Rapid turnaround of bioanalytical and thus pharmacokinetic data is critical for coordination with such in vivo pharmacokinetic screens as the Rapid Rat [82] (Chapter 2) or similar screens in larger animals, wherein groups of compounds are processed in a semiautomated manner, including compound purity assessment [83], dosing, sample processing, bioanalysis, and data dissemination (usually, on Excel spreadsheets). One of the key necessities is the development of a bioanalytical method in a very short time frame (usually, one day) and analyzing the samples expediously. Typically, method development and sample analysis are combined and conducted non-GLP. Automation for this type of work is improving. Integrated systems such as the BASi Culex automated blood sampler are

TABLE 4.9 Fit-for-Purpose Approach to Bioanalytical Qualification or Validation 4.9

	Criterion or Specification		
Characteristic	Screening (Semiquantitative)	Non-GLP Development	Regulated Development
Certified reference material	No	Yes	Yes
Sample preparation	Protein precipitation or liquid–liquid extraction	Same as screening	Any method, including solid-phase extraction
Internal standard	Yes, probably an analog	Same as screening	Yes, preferably the analyte with a >M + 4 stable label
Standard set	Beginning and end of a run	Same as screening	Same as screening
Zero standard	Run but not included in standard curve	Same as screening	Response needs to be less than 20% of LLOQ
Standard curve range	100-fold range (e.g., 25, 250, 2500 ng/mL)	Up to 5000-fold range (e.g., 1 to 5000 ng/mL)	Up to 5000-fold
Standard curve concentrations	10-fold apart	6 to 13 levels (approx. log distance) at the beginning and end of a run	Same as non-GLP development
QCs	No	Yes	Yes
QC replication and concentration	Not applicable (n/a)	At least three concentrations in duplicate	Same as non-GLP development
QC acceptance	n/a	2/3 <25% of nominal value	2/3 <15% of nominal value
Dilutional QC	n/a	Yes	Yes
Final range	Pick one decade (e.g., 25 to 250 ng/mL)	Selected (see below); at least five consecutive concentrations	Full range of calibration standards
Data analysis	Unweighted regression	Weighted or unweighted regression; power fit; $R^2 > 0.95$	Weighted regression; $R^2 > 0.95$

Qualification/validation runs	1	1	3
Calibration standard and QC acceptance	±27% of back-calculated value	No change	Precision, accuracy <20% at LLOQ; <15% for LLOQ
Standard acceptance rate	75%	75%	75%
LLOQ	May be as low as 0.4 times the lowest standard; >3 times the back-calculated value for zero standards; signal/noise >3	Same as screening	Lowest acceptable standard
Samples below the LLOQ	Reported as "0" or BLOQ	Reported as "0" or BLOQ	Reported as "0" or BLOQ
ULOQ	Highest standard used	Highest standard used	Highest standard used
Samples reportable as multiple of ULOQ	2× (if linear); otherwise, diluted	1×; otherwise, diluted	Same as non-GLP development
Stability	4-h room-temperature (RT) matrix stability; otherwise, assumed unless loss exceeds 25%	4-h RT; overnight at −20°C; one freeze–thaw cycle; multiple-day and benchtop stability	Benchtop, short- and long-term storage; autosampler
QA oversight	No	No	Yes
QA'd validation report	No	No	Yes

Note:

1. Until formal validation, LC-MS/MS is usually the methodology of choice.
2. Standard curve calibrators and QC standards are from separate stocks. Weighings are separate after correcting the reference standard for salt, water content, impurity factors, and so on.
3. Until regulated method validation guidelines are applied, the screening and non-GLP assays are conditionally qualified, not validated.
4. The calibrant and samples should be prepared on the same day. QC standards should be treated as surrogate samples and prepared as soon as samples are acquired. They should be stored with the samples. Spiking solutions may be stored as long as stability data are available. Reference material expiration dates are independent of the expiration dates of the spiking solutions assuming that the latter are prepared before reference material expiration.
5. Placement of QCs: one near the ULOQ (typically, 80% of LLOQ), one near the middle (e.g., $\frac{1}{2}C_{\max}$, geometric mean or the median of expected or observed sample concentrations), and one at 3× LLOQ.

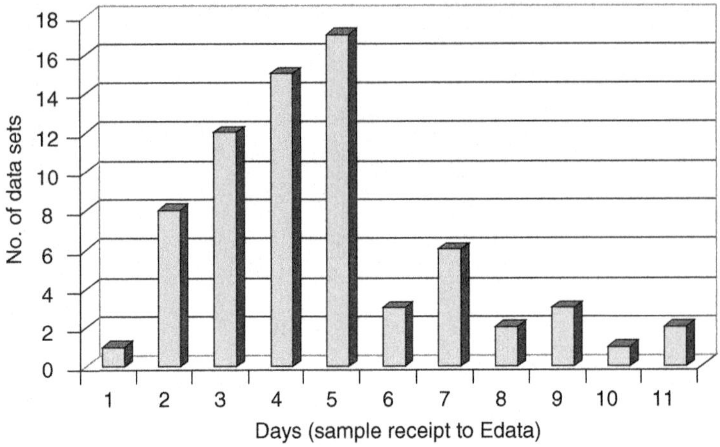

FIGURE 4.17 Bioanalytical data turnaround during accelerated PK screening. This does not include the in-life portion of the study (Courtesy of Thomas Oglesby and Micheal Koleto, Taylor Technology.)

being used more extensively. Figure 4.17 shows a profile of delivery by one laboratory. Although the bulk of the data sets are typically available within three to five days following receipt of the samples, the turnaround time can sometimes be shorter if all components of a study are conducted in a single organization, or longer for those compounds that may require bioanalytical challenges. Clearly, seamless collaboration among the various disciplines (medicinal chemistry, in vivo laboratory, bioanalytical laboratory, pharmacokinetics, coordinating scientist, etc.) is a requirement for the generation of results as rapidly as is technically possible.

4.7.2 Early Involvement of Consultants and CROs

Earlier we discussed various issues associated with starting a GLP laboratory. A critical feature was the utilization of trained and seasoned personnel to develop SOPs and oversee the fundamentals involved in the creation of a site, the installation of site utilities [gas, electric, water and wastewater, and HVAC (heating, ventilation, and air conditioning)], equipment, analytical processes, and so on. Few laboratories, especially at new sites, have the requisite infrastructure to create a GLP laboratory. One option used by many pharmaceutical companies is to utilize the services of external consultants. Corporate mergers have eliminated "redundant" services. These industry trends have produced a cadre of highly skilled and experienced scientists now offering their services on a freelance basis. The American Association of Pharmaceutical Scientists (AAPS), PhRMA (Pharmaceutical Research and Manufacturers Association), and Contract Pharma Web sites can provide initial contact information. Mass spectrometry, chromatography, and drug metabolism discussion groups have frequent meetings with consultants as speakers.

Another alternative is to outsource work to a contract research organization (CRO), even in the discovery phase. Although most bioanalytical CROs prefer to support larger, late-stage projects since they are easier to manage and deemed more profitable, many have discovery and early-phase programs staffed with high-level scientists. These laboratories can generally be identified as having specific drug discovery and early development programs already established. They should have a basic philosophy of establishing a relationship with a sponsor laboratory early in drug development. Contact information on bioanalytical CROs can be found on the Contract Pharma Web site (see Table 4.1). Some advantages and considerations regarding interactions of drug sponsors with CROs in general are discussed in Chapter 1.

4.7.3 Metabolites: Bioanalytical Issues Pre-FIH

An FDA guidance entitled "Safety Testing of Drug Metabolites" [84] [from the Metabolites in Safety Testing (MIST) initiative] was issued in 2008. The subject was part of the Crystal City III meeting, the white paper [6] from which states the following: "There is general support from the pharmaceutical community for the idea that a more extensive characterization of the pharmacokinetics of unique and/or major human metabolites would provide greater insight into the connection between metabolites and toxicological observations. This information would be best generated by the use of rugged, bioanalytical methods applied at appropriate times in drug development."

A tiered approach to bioanalytical methods validation was recommended, with the "specifics of this tiered validation process driven by scientifically-appropriate criteria, established a priori." That said, there is no set validation process or fit-for-purpose approach (outlined in Table 4.9) that could be applied to metabolites. Full validation is usually limited by the lack of reference materials noted above. Samples from early toxicology studies can be employed to conduct "exploratory" metabolite work. Although the use of radiolabeled materials is still the gold standard for detecting compounds that are drug derived, modern MS methods can allow detection and characterization of metabolites (Chapter 2) [18,85]. The Novatia Web site also offers case studies on structure elucidation (Table 4.1).

Once metabolites have been identified, a decision needs to be made as to whether to monitor them during early drug development. Only under special circumstances are more than one or two metabolites monitored during the early phases of drug development. Several laboratories have a policy that none are monitored prior to the FIH trial. It is imperative, however, that the metabolites be identified early in drug development. Failure to ensure that the species used for safety assessment are exposed to the same drug-derived materials as humans can affect the interpretation of toxicity studies (Chapters 2 and 7). In most instances the bioanalytical support of the pre-FIH toxicity studies involves the measurement only of parent drug in the circulation and demonstration of dose-related exposure (Chapter 8). One of the main themes of the metabolite guidance [84] is that if the concentration of any circulating metabolite in plasma exceeds 10% of that of parent drug, consideration should be given as to whether this metabolite has been examined appropriately in nonclinical safety studies. However, such clinical data are not generated until after or during the FIH study; thus, the toxicity studies that would be considered for metabolite evaluation would be those which are longer term (i.e., post-FIH). On the other hand, based on the results of the early ADME (absorption, distribution, metabolism, and excretion) and pharmacokinetics studies in support of discovery and candidate selection (Chapter 2), it may be deemed prudent to develop and validate an assay for parent drug and/or metabolite(s) in plasma (or serum) of the rodent and nonrodent toxicity species in support of the pre-FIH safety evaluations. In such instances, all validation criteria described in this chapter must pertain to all analytes, including potential interference in the quantification of one analyte by the presence of another.

4.7.4 Racemic Mixtures

It is no longer in vogue to develop drugs that are racemic mixtures due to the well-known characteristic that the component enantiomers can have different pharmacokinetic and pharmacodynamic properties within the chiral environment of biological systems. However, for whatever reason, in those rare instances when a racemate is selected for development, it is highly recommended that a chiral bioanalytical assay in support of all toxicity (including pre-FIH) and clinical (including FIH) studies be developed and fully validated for quantification of the individual stereoisomers in the target matrices. In this manner, any stereoselective differences in the metabolic fate and pharmacokinetics of the component enantiomers can be determined as early as possible in development, and appropriate interpretations generated.

4.8 THE ROAD TO "FIRST IN HUMAN"

Some common questions scientists involved in bioanalytical drug development ask in support of their first set of in vivo studies are (1) Which analyte(s) should be monitored? and (2) What is the concentration range to be monitored? The dynamic range of the assay is a little more complicated. In discovery and early development, the range is standardized since no pertinent data are available pending further examination. Adjustments are relatively easy at that stage since it is not necessary to conduct a formalized validation. By the time formal safety studies are being conducted, a fully validated method with a well-defined dynamic range is required. At this point, the analyst and the relevant biological disciplines need to integrate the available pharmacological, ADME, and pharmacokinetic data across species. In many cases, a model can then be constructed that can provide a strategy for the starting FIH dose and the targeted drug concentrations in plasma. The bioanalytical challenge is to assure that the validation encompasses the range of analyte concentrations anticipated in both the nonclinical safety assessment program and the clinical evaluations throughout the entire development program. As discussed above, changes may be dictated based on emerging data, such as the identification of a major or significant human metabolite that will require monitoring. However, at the pre-FIH stage, it is advisable to plan as wisely as possible so as to minimize the number of changes to the validation process at later stages of the program.

With new bioanalytical tools, an additional option has been made available recently: exploratory INDs [86] (Chapter 11), a strategy that enables the performance of studies in humans with a low dose(s) of the NCE without a full IND or IRB package. The challenge is to develop a method that can detect drug concentrations with such a low dose. Recent advances in LC-MS and GC-MS technology allow concentrations in the sub-picogram/mL range to be detected. Frequently, this is not sensitive enough. Theoretically, the relatively new technique of accelerator mass spectrometry (AMS) [25] allows detection of zeptograms (10^{-21} g) of material, roughly the equivalent of measuring a particular drop of water in the ocean. Not only can concentrations of potential analytes be determined, but potential metabolites could be identified as well. Metabolite characterization in humans generally requires a radiolabeled study using significant amounts of labeled drug (usually, 100 μCi ^{14}C or tritium) after an animal dosimetry study and IRB and NRC approval. Although AMS requires ^{14}C material, the trace amount (e.g., 200 nCi) required is below the threshold that would require lengthy approval. Compared to methods such as LC-MS/MS, which would be used for higher doses, the use of AMS has been reported to produce acceptable levels of accuracy, precision, and parallelism.

4.8.1 Clinical Collaboration Prior to Initiation of the FIH Trial

While clinic personnel involved in early stage development with healthy normal volunteers normally understand the phase I study processes fairly well, it is strongly recommend that detailed instructions for sample handling be crafted and at least one face-to-face meeting be held between clinical and analytical personnel before initiation of a FIH study. This is especially important if the two groups of personnel have not worked together previously. Nothing is more frustrating to bioanalytical sample coordinators than to receive a shipment of samples that is incomplete, poorly documented, or, worse, not evaluable. Ordinarily, mishaps can be avoided if a close communication link between clinical and bioanalytical sites is created and maintained, even if both functions are within the same company. Sample acquisition and shipment dates (with inventories), courier, and expected sample receipt dates by the bioanalytical laboratory must be transmitted to the laboratory by the clinic. Bar-coded samples keyed to an electronic database are highly recommended. Creation of sample kits by the analytical lab, with clear labels (and bar codes) and clear sample handling and shipping instructions, is very effective at reducing mistakes. Such a prestudy collaboration should be implemented at the protocol generation stage.

4.9 INTERNATIONAL PERSPECTIVES

The international organization that most influences bioanalytical requirements is the Organization for Economic Cooperation and Development (OECD). The forerunner of the OECD, the Organisation for European Economic Cooperation (OEEC), was formed in 1947 to administer American and Canadian aid under the Marshall Plan for the reconstruction of Europe following World War II. The OECD took over from the OEEC in 1961. Since then, its mission has been to help its member countries achieve sustainable economic growth and employment and to raise the standard of living in member countries while maintaining financial stability. Although most members are European, the Pacific Rim countries of Australia, Japan, Korea, and New Zealand are signatories, as well as Canada and the United States. Two of the former Eastern Block countries (the Czech and Slovak republics) have also signed. The primary objective of the OECD Principles of GLP is to ensure the generation of high-quality, reliable test data related to the safety of industrial chemical substances and preparations in the framework of harmonizing testing procedures for the mutual acceptance of data [87,88]. However, specific requirements are mandated by each member country (Chapter 9). There is no equivalent of the FDA bioanalytical method validation guidance, but the current 30 members of the OECD as well as many nonmembers tend to abide by the FDA bioanalytical precepts. ICH has also been working on bioanalytical procedures [89,90], but their recommendations do not have the force of law or of regulatory agency expectations.

Although the FDA has been subject to criticism from industry and public sources in the United States, its bioanalytical assay validation guideline has become the de facto standard throughout the world. As discussion regarding the FDA guidance and the 2007 white paper from the 2006 Crystal City meeting escalates, more worldwide pharmaceutical companies and regulatory agencies are adapting to the recommendations described therein. The source of this acceptance is the belief that the FDA has encouraged a collaborative approach with industry and CROs to fashion its requirements.

4.9.1 European Union

The European Medicines Agency (EMEA) is a decentralized body of the European Union with headquarters in London. Its mission is to foster scientific excellence in the evaluation and supervision of medicines for the benefit of public and animal health. The EMEA is the European Union body responsible for coordinating the existing scientific resources put at its disposal by member states for the evaluation, supervision, and pharmacovigilance of medicinal products [91] (Table 4.1). The agency provides its member states and the institutions of the EU with scientific advice on any question relating to the evaluation of the quality, safety, and efficacy of medicinal products for human or veterinary use referred to it, in accordance with the provisions of EU legislation relating to medicinal products. Its 2006 "Procedure for Coordinating GLP Inspections" [92] specified that inspections be assessed as to compliance with OECD GLP principles.

As with the OECD, the EMEA has no guidance for bioanalytical method validation. Recent meetings of the European Bioanalytical Forum (EBF) have indicated that the recommendations in the FDA guidance and Crystal City III white paper will generally be followed. As the chair of the EBF has said: "It is time to go into the cold water." Although the EBF is composed of European pharma, they do not yet have any intention to prepare a European version of the method validation guidelines. They have, however, planned to publish any consensus they have reached, in the same manner as does the AAPS. The EBF plans on creating a new large-molecule focus group as well.

4.9.2 Japan

The Japanese have extensive experience with de novo drug development. New drug approvals for manufacturing or importing drugs in Japan are reviewed by Japan's Ministry of Health, Labor, and Welfare (MHLW) [93]. Japan's Drug Organization (Kiko) functions to improve the safety and quality of new drugs. Kiko, a half-public, half-private organization supervised by the MHLW, focused originally on monitoring adverse drug reactions of drugs during clinical trials, promoting the research and development of new drugs, and performing selective reviews of some drugs, generics, and cosmetics. Now, however, Kiko is cooperating with the Japanese Evaluation Center to ensure compliance with safety and review standards, is performing raw data checks, and is giving advice to companies on clinical development and trials. Raw bioanalytical data in paper format are submitted to Kiko for inspection. The data must be consistent with the standards in the MHLW ordinances, such as GLPs, GCPs, and standards for the reliability of application data, which cover bioanalytical method validation.

Japan is a member of the OECD. The Japanese pharmaceutical industry is divided roughly into two constituencies: multinationals and traditional national companies. The former take a global and more liberal view, while the latter tend to be more conservative in their approach. The results of the May 2006 Crystal City III [6] meeting are being reviewed at the time of this writing. It is likely that both groups will model their validation approaches on the FDA's bioanaltyical assay validation guidance and the related white paper.

4.9.3 India

Drug regulatory authority in India is governed by the Drug Controller General of India. The biopharmaceutical industry has matured rapidly from a strictly generic structure to a group with a pharmaceutical innovation focus [94]. With this shift has come an increasing toxicological awareness and its associated challenges. This has resulted in the implementation of international quality management systems, such as GLPs, and industry has taken the initiative. Although the GLP guidance was formulated in 1978, major progress was not made for a decade because of the lack of mobilization of adequate resources. However, more recently, Indian government agencies have taken action to ensure that laboratories are able to comply with GLP standards [94]. With this increase in drug development focus and the Indian desire to expand its reach, the FDA has established a presence in India, where inspections on product development processes are encouraged.

4.10 CONCLUSIONS

The past years have been labeled the Golden Age of Drug Discovery [82] based primarily on five phenomena that have converged at the present moment in history that will never occur again:

1. The human genome has been mapped.
2. Computational advances allow us to find targets in the genome and model the associated proteins.
3. Combinatorial chemistry allows us to explore vast areas of "chemical space" to find new leads.
4. Many unexploited targets still exist, and many serious diseases remain poorly treated.
5. A robust pharmaceutical industry, aided by universities and the National Institutes of Health, is pursuing these targets aggressively.

Early stage bioanalysis will have its chance to contribute. Current technologies allow high-sensitivity, high-throughput drug discovery support for pharmacokinetic profiling and metabolite elucidation. An offshoot of this effort is the determination of reactive metabolites early in development, allowing changes in drug structure before development resources are drained on potentially toxic products doomed to failure. Tissue imaging techniques will improve and allow localization of drug and drug-derived compounds in tissues and cellular components without the delays, costs, and limitations of using labeled materials. The emergence of the importance and utility of biomarkers is due largely to the improvement in bioanalytical techniques for their identification and monitoring. The field of bioanalysis has come a long way in the past 100 years, but there are still unmet medical needs and the field has a long way to go. It should be an exciting trip.

Acknowledgments

This chapter would have been impossible to prepare without the talents and effort of Richard LeLacheur, Taylor Technology (TTI), who provided many of the figures and reviewed the text; Rohan Thakur of TTI, who provided much advice about the international aspects of bioanalysis; Anthony Jones of TTI, who reviewed the quality assurance and regulatory issues; Thomas Jupile of LCResources, who generously provided his notes from the LCResources lectures on bioanalysis; and Adam Brochman, Shire Pharmaceuticals, whose insights into laboratory organization and whose work with the BSAT/APA meetings gave me much valuable information on this immense field.

REFERENCES

1. Guidance for Industry: Bioanalytical Method Validation. U.S. Department of Health and Human Services, Food and Drug Administration, Center for Drug Evaluation and Research, Center for Veterinary Medicine; 2001.
2. Electronic Records; Electronic Signatures. *Code of Federal Regulations*, 21 CFR Part 11. U.S. Department of Health and Human Services, Food and Drug Administration, Center for Drug Evaluation and Research; Feb. 23, 2003.
3. Good Laboratory Practice for Nonclinical Laboratory Studies. *Code of Federal Regulations*, 21 CFR Part 58. U.S. Department of Health and Human Services, Food and Drug Administration, Center for Drug Evaluation and Research; Dec. 22, 1978; amended 1999.
4. Shah VP, Midha KK, Dighe S, et al. Analytical methods validation: bioavailability, bioequivalance and pharmacokinetic studies. *Pharm Res*. 1992;9:588–592.
5. Shah VP, Midha KK, Findlay JWA, et al. Bioanalytical method validation: a revisit with a decade of progress. *Pharm Res*. 2000;17:1551–1557.
6. Viswanathan CT, Bansal S, Booth B, et al. Quantitative bioanalytical methods validation and implementation: best practices for chromatographic and ligand binding assays. *AAPS J*. 2007;(1):art 004.
7. Fast DM, Kelley, M, Viswanathan CT, et al. Workshop Report and Follow-Up—AAPS Workshop on Current Topics in GLP Bioanalysis: Assay Reproducibility for Incurred Samples—Implications of Crystal City Recommendations. *AAPS J*. (published online) 2009; Apr 21.
8. Lee JW, Devanarayan V, Barrett YC, et al. Fit-for-purpose method development and validation for successful biomarker measurement. *Pharm Res*. 2006;23(2):312–328.
9. Shah VP. The history of bioanalytical method validation and regulation: evolution of a guidance document on bioanalytical methods of validation. *AAPS J*. 2007;9: E43–E47.
10. Chamberlain J. *The Analysis of Drugs in Biological Fluids*, 2nd ed. Boca Raton, FL: CRC Press; 1995.
11. Ahuja A, ed. *Ultratrace Analysis of Pharmaceuticals and Other Compounds of Interest*. New York: Wiley; 1986.
12. Bidlingmeyer BA. *Practical HPLC Methodology and Applications*. New York: Wiley; 1992.
13. Cunico RL, Gooding KM, Wehr T. *Basic HPLC and CE of Biomolecules*. Richmond, CA: Bay Bioanalytical Laboratory; 1998.
14. Dolan JW, Snyder LR. *Troubleshooting LC Systems*. Totowa, NJ: Humana Press; 1989.

15. Dux JP. *Handbook of Quality Assurance for the Analytical Chemistry Laboratory*. New York: Van Nostrand Reinhold; 1986.
16. de Hoffmann E, Stroobant V. *Mass Spectrometry: Principles and Applications*. Wiley, Chichester, UK; 2007.
17. Kenkel J. *Analytical Chemistry for Technicians*. Ann Arbor, MI: Lewis Publishers; 1994.
18. Korfmacher, WA, ed. *Using Mass Spectrometry for Drug Metabolism Studies*. Boca Raton, FL: CRC Press; 2005.
19. Krstulovic AM, Brown PR. *Reversed-Phase High Performance Liquid Chromatography*. New York: Wiley; 1982.
20. Lee MS. *Integrated Strategies for Drug Discovery Using Mass Spectrometry*. Hoboken, NJ: Wiley; 2005.
21. McMaster M, McMaster C, eds. *GC/MS: A Practical User's Guide*. Wiley-VCH, Weinheim, Germany; 1998.
22. Niessen WMA. *Liquid Chromatography–Mass Spectrometry*, 3rd ed. Boca Raton, FL: CRC Press; 2006.
23. Snyder LR, Kirkland JJ, Glajch, JL. *Practical HPLC Method Development*, 2nd ed. New York: Wiley; 1997.
24. Shugar GJ, Ballinger JT, eds. *Chemical Technicians' Ready Reference Manual*, 3rd ed. New York: McGraw-Hill; 1990.
25. Tuniz C, Bird JR, Fink D, Herzog GF. *Accelerator Mass Spectrometry*. Boca Raton, FL: CRC Press; 1998.
26. Venn RF, ed. *Principles and Practice of Bioanalysis*. New York: Taylor & Francis; 2000.
27. Peng SX, Branch TM, King SL. Fully automated 96-well liquid–liquid extraction for the analysis of biological samples by liquid chromatography with tandem mass spectrometry. *Anal Chem*. 2001;73:708–714.
28. Ayrton J, Dear GH, Leavens WJ, Mallett DN. Optimisation and routine use of generic ultra-high flow-rate liquid chromatography with mass spectrometric detection for the direct on-line analysis of pharmaceuticals in plasma. *J Chromatogr A*. 1998;828:199–207.
29. Grob RL, Barry EF, eds. *Modern Practice of Gas Chromatography*, 4th ed. Hoboken, NJ: Wiley; 2004.
30. Majors RE. The rise and fall of expertise in gas chromatography. *LCGC North Am*. 2006;24(5). Available at the LC/GC Web site.
31. Jennings WG. *Applications of Glass Capillary Gas Chromatography*. New York: Marcel Dekker; 1981.
32. Gilber JD, Olah TV, McLoughlin DA. High-performance liquid chromatography with atmospheric pressure ionization in tandem mass spectrometry as a tool in quantitative bioanalytical chemistry. In: Snyder AP, ed., *Biochemical and Biotechnical Applications of Electrospray Ionization Mass Spectrometry*. ACS Symposium Series, Washington, DC: American Chemical Society; No. 619. 1998: 330–350.
33. Feng WY. Mass spectrometry in drug discovery: a current review. *Curr Drug Discov Technol*. 2004;1:295–312.

34. Nelson MD, Dolan JW. Ion supression in LC/MS/MS: a case study. *LCGC North Am.* 2002;20(1):24–33. Available at the LC/GC Web site.
35. Hughes NC, Wong EY, Fan J, Bajaj N. Determination of carryover and contamination for mass spectrometry–based chromatographic assays. *AAPS J.* 2007;9(3): E353–E360.
36. van Oss CJ, van Regenortal MHV, eds. *Immunochemistry*. New York: Marcel Dekker; 1994.
37. Johnstone A, Turner MW, eds. *Immunochemistry: A Practical Approach*. New York: Oxford University Press; 1997.
38. Miller KJ, Bowsher RR, Celniker A, et al. Workshop on bioanalytical method validation for macromolecules: summary report. *Pharm Res.* 2001;18:1373–1383.
39. Kelley M, DeSilva B. Key elements of bioanalytical method validation for macromolecules. *AAPS J.* 2007;9(2): E156–E163.
40. Mire-Sluis AR, Barrett YC, Devanarayan V, et al. Recommendations for the design and optimization of immunoassays used in the detection of host antibodies against biotechnology products. *J Immunol Methods*. 2004;289(1–2):1–16.
41. Smolec J, DeSilva B, Smith W, et al. Bioanalytical method validation for macromolecules in support of pharmacokinetic studies. *Pharm Res.* 2005;22(9).
42. Crowther JR. *The ELISA Guidebook*. Totowa, NJ: Humana Press; 2000
43. Destefano AJ, Takigiku R. Bioanalysis in a regulated environment. In: *Pharmacokinetics in Drug Development: Regulatory and Development Paradigms*, Vol. 2. Arlington, VA: AAPS Press; 2004: 105–125.
44. Findlay JWA, Smith WC, Lee JW, et al. Validation of immunoassays for bioanalysis: a pharmaceutical industry perspective. *J Pharm Biol Anal.* 2000;21:1249–1273.
45. Findlay JWA, Dillard RF. Appropriate calibration curve fitting in ligand binding assays. *AAPS J.* 2007;9(2): E260–E267.
46. Chaudhary AK. Chip-based nanoelectrospray MS as a bioanalysis tool: an objective assessment. Presented at the BSAT/APA Meeting, Boston, Sept. 12–16, 2005.
47. Mikkelsen SR, Corton E. *Bioanalytical Chemistry*. Hoboken, NJ: Wiley; 2004.
48. Nowatzke W, Woolf E. Best practices during bioanalytical method validation for the characterization of assay reagents and the evaluation of analyte stability in assay standards, quality controls, and study samples. *AAPS J.* 2007;9(2): E117–E122.
49. Peters DG, Hayes JM, Hieftje GM. *Chemical Separations and Measurements*. Philadelphia: W.B. Saunders; 1974.
50. Unger S. The effect of sample stability on bioanalytical methods and its impact on accuracy and reproducibility of incurred samples. White paper presented at the DVDMDG Symposium on the Crystal City III, Apr. 17, 2007.
51. Jemal M, Ouyang Z, Powell ML. A strategy for a post-method: validation use of incurred biologicial samples for establishing the acceptability of a liquid chromatography/tandem mass-spectrometric method for quantitation of drugs in biological samples. *Rapid Commun Mass Spectrom.* 2002;16(16):1538–1547.
52. Santen R. Measurement of plasma estradiol as biomarker for determining risk of breast cancer. Presented at the BioScience Forum, "Biomarkers and Their Application to the Drug Discovery and Development Process," June 2004.

53. Zeng J, Onthank D, Crane P, et al. Simutaneous determination of a selective adenosine 2A agonist, BMS-068646, and its acid metabolite in human plasma by liquid chromatography–tandem mass spectrometry: evaluation of the esterase inhibitor, diisopropyl fluorophosphate, in the stabilization of a labile ester-containing drug. *J Chromatogr B*. 2007;1(852):77–84 [Epub].

54. Takatori T, Yamaoka A. Effects of phenylmethylsulphonylfluoride on activities of cholesterol ester synthesis and hydrolysis in testes of rats, and on serum testosterone and LH levels. *J Reprod Fertil*. 1979;55(10):69–74.

55. Los LE, Welsh DA, Herold EG, Bagdon WJ, Zacchei AG. Gender differences in toxicokinetics, liver metabolism, and plasma esterase activity: observations from a chronic (27-week) toxicity study of enalapril/diltiazem combination in rats. *Drug Metab Dispos*. 1996;24(1):28–33.

56. Compernolle F, Van Hees GP, Blanckaert N, Heirwegh KP. Glucuronic acid conjugates of bilirubin-IXalpha in normal bile compared with post-obstructive bile: transformation of the 1-O-acylglucuronide into 2-, 3-, and 4-O-acylglucuronides. *Biochem J*. 1978;171(1):185–201.

57. Shipkova M, Schütz E, Armstrong VW, Niedmann PD, Oellerich M, Wieland E. Determination of the acyl glucuronide metabolite of mycophenolic acid in human plasma by HPLC and Emit. *Clin Chem*. 2000;46(3):365–372.

58. Baba A, Yoshioka T. Synthesis of 1-beta-O-acyl glucuronides of diclofenac, mefenamic acid and (*S*)-naproxen by the chemo-selective enzymatic removal of protecting groups from the corresponding methyl acetyl derivatives. *Org Biomol Chem*. 2006;4(17):3303–3310.

59. Li C, Benet LZ, Grillo MP. Studies on the chemical reactivity of 2-phenylpropionic acid 1-O-acyl glucuronide and *S*-acyl-CoA thioester metabolites. *Chem Res Toxicol*. 2002;15(10):1309–1317.

60. Liu JH, Smith PC. Predicting the pharmacokinetics of acyl glucuronides and their parent compounds in disease states. *Curr Drug Metab*. 2006;7(2):147–163.

61. Boelsterli UA. Xenobiotic acyl glucuronides and acyl CoA thioesters as protein-reactive metabolites with the potential to cause idiosyncratic drug reactions. *Curr Drug Metab*. 2002;3(4):439–450.

62. Bansal S. Repeat analysis according to the Guidance and beyond... Presented at the DVDMDG Symposium, "The Bioanalytical Validation Guidance: Past, Present, and Future," Feb. 22, 2006.

63. Midha KK, Rawson MJ, McKay G, Hubbard JW. Exposure measures applied to the bioequivalence of two sustained release formulations of bupropion. *Int J Clin Pharmacol Ther*. 2005;43(5):244–254.

64. Walpole RE, Myers RH. *Probability and Statistics for Engineers and Scientists*, 2nd ed. New York: Macmillan; 1978.

65. Kleinbaum DG, Kupper LL. *Applied Regression Analysis and Multivariable Methods*. Boston: Duxbury Press; 1978.

66. Prins J. Process or product monitoring and control in NIST/SEMATECH. In: e-Handbook of Statistical Methods. Gaithersburg, MD: National Institute of Standards and Technology; 2007. Available at: www.itl.nist.gov/div898/handbook/pmc/section2/pmc231.htm.

67. Amidon GL, Lennernäs H, Shah VP, Crison Jr. A theoretical basis for a biopharmaceutic drug classification: the correlation of in vitro drug product dissolution and in vivo. bioavailability. *Pharm Res*. 1995;12(3):413–420.

68. Wu CY, Benet LZ. Predicting drug disposition via application of BCS: transport/absorption/elimination interplay and development of a biopharamaceutics drug disposition classification system. *Pharm Res*. 2005;22(1):11–23.

69. Lipinski CA. Drug-like properties and the causes of poor solubility and poor permeability. *J Pharmacol Toxicol Methods*. 2000;44(1):235–249.

70. Lipinski CA, Lombardo F, Dominy BW, Feeney PJ. Experimental and computational approaches to estimate solubility and permeability in drug discovery and development settings. *Adv Drug Deliv Rev*. 2001;46(1–3):3–26.

71. King R. A triage approach to industrialized bioanalysis. Presented at the BSAT/APA Conference, Boston, Sept. 17–21, 2007.

72. Guidance for Industry: Investigating Out-of Specification (OOS) Test Results for Pharmaceutical Production. U.S. Department of Health and Human Services, Food and Drug Administration; 2006.

73. Goldratt, EM, Cox J, Whitfield D. *The Goal: A Process of Ongoing Improvement*, 3rd ed. Croton-on-Hudson, NY: North River Press; 2004.

74. Goldratt, EM. *What Is This Thing Called Theory of Constraints and How Should It Be Implemented?* Croton-on-Hudson, NY: North River Press; 1990.

75. Dettmer HW. *Goldratt's Theory Constraints: A Systems Approach to Continuous Improvement*. Milwaukee, WI: ASQC Press; 1997.

76. James CA, Hill HM. Procedural elements involved in maintaining bioanalytical data integrity for good laboratory practices studies and regulated clinical studies. *AAPS J*. 2007;9(2): E123–E127.

77. Brockman A, Wu JT. How to build a GLP bioanalytical lab. *LCGC North Am*. Available at the LC/GC Web site. Accessed Oct. 2006.

78. Zhang L, Banks M. Screening strategy for lead optimization. *Am Drug Discov*. 2006;1(1):6–11.

79. Chaudhary AK, Wickremsinhe ER, Berna MJ, Ackermann BL. A risk-based approach to bioanalytical methods validations and sample analyses during drug discovery and development. *Am Drug Discov*. 2006;1(1):34–42.

80. Xu X, Lan J, Zhou Q, Tucker G, Jean J, Korfmacher WA. Designing LC-MS/MS methods that are good enough to provide bioanalytical support for new drug discovery assay. *Am Drug Discov*. 2007;2(3).

81. Tiller PR, Romanyshyn LA. Liquid chromatography/tandem mass spectrometric quantification with metabolite screening as a strategy to enhance the early drug discovery process. *Rapid Commun Mass Spectrom*. 2002;16(12):1225–1231.

82. White R. Drug discovery and development: current challenges and future trends. Presented at the BSAT/APA Conference, Boston, Sept. 17–21, 2007.

83. Kerns EH, Di L. Strategy for integrity and purity assessment in early discovery. Presented at the BSAT/APA Meeting, Boston, Sept. 12–16, 2005.

84. Guidance for Industry: Safety Testing of Drug Metabolites. U.S. Department of Health and Human Services, Food and Drug Administration; 2008.

85. Chowdhury SK. Identification and quantification of drugs, metabolites and metabolizing enzymes by LC-MS. In: *Progress in Pharmaceutical and Biomedical Analysis*, Vol. 6. New York: Elsevier; 2005.
86. Guidance for Industry: Exploratory IND Studies. U.S. Department of Health and Human Services, Food and Drug Administration; 2006.
87. OECD Series on Principles of Good Laboratory Practice and Compliance Monitoring, No. 1. Organization for Economic Co-operation and Development; 1997. Available at: www.oecd.org.
88. Good Laboratory Practice: The Application of the OECD Principles of GLP to the Organization and Management of Multi-site Studies. Organization for Economic Co-operation and Development; 2001. Available at: www.oecd.org.
89. ICH Quality Guideline: Validation of Analytical Procedures: Text and Methodology. ICH Q2 (R1). International Conference on Harmonization; 1996. Available at: www.ich.org.
90. Technical Requirements for Registration of Pharmaceuticals for Human Use. Validation of Analytical Procedures: Methodology. International Conference on Harmonization; 1996. Available at: www.ich.org.
91. Note for Guidance on Validation of Analytical Procedures: Methodology. European Agency for the Evaluation of Medicinal Products; June 18, 1997. Available at: www.emea.europa.eu/.
92. Procedure for Coordinating GLP Inspections. European Agency for the Evaluation of Medicinal Products; Aug. 15, 2006. Available at: www.emea.europa.eu/.
93. Chow SC, ed. *Encyclopedia of Biopharmaceutical Statistics*. New York: Informa Healthcare; 2003.
94. Mukerji B, Cherian KM. Good laboratory practice in India. *Qual Assur J*. 2000;4:15–21.

PART III

BRIDGING FROM DISCOVERY TO DEVELOPMENT

5

CHEMISTRY, MANUFACTURING, AND CONTROLS: THE DRUG SUBSTANCE AND FORMULATED DRUG PRODUCT

Örn Almarsson and Christopher J. Galli

5.1 INTRODUCTION

Our aim in this chapter is to provide a practical and goal-oriented treatise on chemistry, manufacturing, and controls (CMC) development in support of investigational new drug applications (INDs) in the United States and analogous European clinical trial authorization (CTA) submissions to regulatory agencies. We discuss technical and strategic concepts and provide references to appropriate regulations and guidance documents. Although the chapter is organized by development stage in roughly chronological fashion, the aim is to raise awareness of parallel and ongoing CMC activities that feed a program as it advances from discovery into toxicological and clinical evaluation. Ultimately, the goal is to help demystify the CMC area by showing how the chemistry, materials science, analytics, and phase-appropriate interpretation of regulations for drug substance and formulation create a vital link between a new active molecule and a potential medicine as a program enters clinical evaluation.

Although not always obvious to discovery personnel or development partners, long-term value opportunities such as pharmaceutical developability, which can be a critical differentiating factor for product development, emerge when a molecule or group of molecules have gained sufficient interest to be considered as possible development candidates. Hence, CMC-related work *before* declaration of

Early Drug Development: Strategies and Routes to First-in-Human Trials, Edited by Mitchell N. Cayen

the new chemical entity (NCE) as a new drug candidate is covered in the chapter, along with the efforts required to support good laboratory practice (GLP) toxicology formulation and clinical trial materials (CTMs) development. Although focus is placed primarily on small-molecule pharmaceutical compounds, a section on biopharmaceuticals is included, complementing Chapter 12. Two case studies on the interactions of CMC development with other functions are provided to shed some light on specific applications of the concepts presented. One case study involves a marketed product, an oral antiviral drug, while the other is an injectable development candidate with the hybrid character of a small molecule and a biopharmaceutical. Finally, a brief foray is made into projecting the future of the drug development process, with the objective of exploring likely implications of acceleration and customization of studies as the process evolves to enhance the industry's productivity.

5.2 PRE-NCE ACTIVITIES AND CMC DEVELOPMENT

5.2.1 Rationale for CMC Involvement in Discovery

Prior to any application being filed with regulatory authorities, and indeed before any formal and regulated testing is initiated for such an application, the active pharmaceutical ingredient (API) must be identified. Occasionally, the API will be a known entity (or combination of known entities), but often it will be a new agent with as yet unknown actions. As outlined in Chapters 1 to 3, the effort to identify and select an NCE relies largely on close interaction between the discovery groups and ADME (absorption, distribution, metabolism, and excretion) experts. NCEs nominated for development without input from development scientists do not benefit from the broad, multidisciplinary evaluation, which can uncover differentiating properties and mitigate risk. The rationale is based on the idea that linking CMC insight with late lead optimization and ADME evaluation provides a way to address risk related to the material properties (i.e., chemical and physical attributes, which are referred to collectively as *pharmaceutical properties*). It is known that unfavorable pharmaceutical properties can seriously hinder developmental progress. Similarly, a major challenge in chemical synthesis can, at least initially, provide a significant barrier to entry to clinical studies of a compound. Figure 5.1 illustrates the concept of adding CMC expertise, both process chemistry input and pharmaceutical insights relating properties and biopharmaceutics (oral absorption and bioavailability), into the late lead optimization stage of drug discovery.

In essence, Figure 5.1 speaks to a co-optimization of process chemistry and pharmaceutical/material properties at the late lead optimization stage overlaid onto discovery, ADME, and early toxicological (non-GLP) evaluations to select the optimal candidate. Interactions of process chemistry with medicinal chemistry are particularly helpful at a point when the selection of a compound from a series of closely related analogs is imminent. The challenge is to take a medicinal

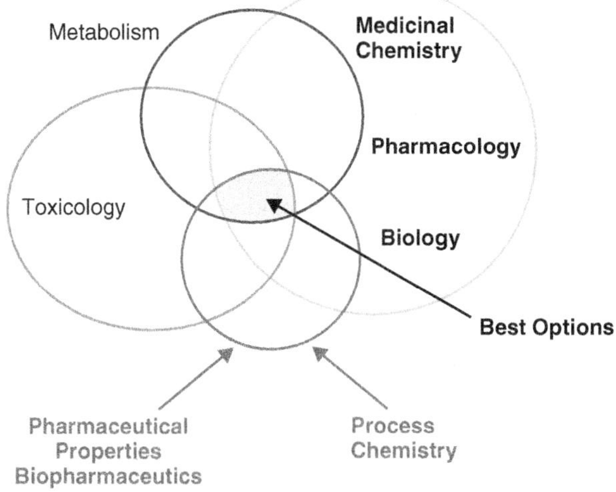

FIGURE 5.1 Input regarding process chemistry and pharmaceutical properties, in addition to potency, selectivity, and metabolism, can aid in the identification of best compounds in late discovery.

chemistry route, which is designed with access to a diversity of candidates in mind, and tailor or change it to suit a particular subset of candidates—ultimately to allow the most facile route possible to a specific compound that is to be named. Pharmaceutical science input can occur even earlier than process chemistry input to rank the diversity of possible candidate compounds. In some cases it may be advantageous to employ criteria of pharmaceutical properties, such as crystallinity, solubility, and formulation options to help focus selection within a particular compound series [1].

5.2.2 Pharmaceutical Properties

In some discovery programs, pharmaceutical properties of candidates are generally favorable. This means that compounds are crystalline, aqueous solubility is high relative to anticipated doses, and the physicochemical stability profile is good. Key and additional criteria are summarized in the next section. Table 5.1 provides examples of compounds that exhibit a range of pharmaceutical properties. As an illustration, acetaminophen (paracetamol; the active antipyretic in many drug products, such as Tylenol) is a compound with favorable properties. An example of a compound with reasonable crystallinity and solubility properties but showing some tendency for instability is acetylsalicylic acid (aspirin). A compound with a good stability profile but somewhat challenging solubility and dissolution for oral formulation is carbamazepine (Tegretol, Carbatrol, and other antiepileptic products). A final example is indinavir, a compound with marginal pharmaceutical properties and a challenging ADME profile. This compound is

TABLE 5.1 Summaries of Pharmaceutical Properties of Select Compounds

Compound	Aqueous Solubility (Room Temperature)	Stability	Biopharmaceutics	Ref.
Acetaminophen (paracetamol)	14 mg/mL, pH independent below pH 10	Excellent unless dissolved in acid or basic solution	Oral bioavailability not highly affected by formulation	[22]
Acetylsalicylic acid (aspirin and many others)	3 mg/mL, acid form	Loss of acetic acid in solid state and solution (pH dependent)	Oral bioavailability not highly affected by formulation	[22]
Carbamazepine (Tegretol, Carbatrol, others)	0.03 mg/mL (dihydrate form)	Suitable for solid dosage forms and suspensions at room temperature	Formulation dependent; hydrate dissolution limited	[23]
Indinavir (Crixivan)	0.02 mg/mL (free-base hydrate); >1 g/mL (sulfate salt)	Poor in acidic solution and amorphous solid state exposed to moisture	Absorption from acidic solutions or sulfate salt; major CYP interaction	[24]

considered further in the case studies section as an example of the synergies possible between discovery, ADME, and CMC experts.

What is the potential impact of linking CMC evaluation of pharmaceutical properties into late-stage discovery? In early development, aspects of stability and bioavailability are most commonly the CMC-related aspects at issue. Some challenges of either stability or bioavailability can be addressed proactively in discovery either to help select a new molecule or mitigate risk with the current molecule of interest. If a molecule is identified as having highly preferred biological and pharmacokinetic properties while presenting a challenge in terms of pharmaceutical properties, concessions may be necessary. Two brief examples are provided at the end of this section. In addition to the pharmaceutical aspects, sourcing the API can be a challenge, as stated earlier. The ultimate impact of early CMC interactions is on the toxicology program and on the acceptability of formulations for dosing to animals. Occasionally, there are implications for the dosage forms for humans as well. It is worthwhile to cultivate connections between investigators in discovery and CMC development such that the latter group can take early ownership and accountability for addressing delivery issues before a compound enters development. A recent monograph addresses the challenges of water-insoluble compound formulation [2].

Although some CMC issues can be addressed at an early stage with short-term fixes, it is nevertheless wise and strategically important to highlight possible downstream limitations to development should the compound survive the initial nonclinical safety studies. As a nonexhaustive list of examples, it is worth communicating clearly about risks in situations where:

- A medicinal chemistry synthesis route, due to hazards or other issues, can only be used to produce batches up to the size of a toxicology and first-in-human (FIH) pharmacokinetics
- Lack of a crystalline form suggests risks of physical and chemical instability as well as challenges with compound isolation and purification during drug substance synthesis
- A short-term formulation approach, limited by instability, tolerability, or manufacturability, can allow only the early definition of animal and human safety and pharmacokinetic parameters
- Long-term instability would probably lead to degradation products being present in the dosage form(s) envisioned for human studies
- Instability is sufficiently pronounced that a room-temperature storage option is not feasible in the long run

In some programs, chemical instability may be an unavoidable feature of the structure of the pharmacophore, as exemplified by the β-lactam antibiotics. In this class of compounds, the context in which a molecule is placed has a significant impact on chemical stability. Thus, formulations based on crystalline β-lactams typically have shelf lives at room temperature in the range 18 months to three years, whereas liquid preparations show unacceptable potency loss in days to a few weeks under the same storage conditions. A second example of chemically unstable compounds is the statin class (exemplified by simvastatin, lovastatin, atorvastatin, and pravastatin), which generally possess oxidative instability, especially in dissolved or noncrystalline forms. A third general example is prodrugs, which are designed for in vivo biochemical activation. The functionality involved in the formation of the prodrug must be assessed carefully to ensure shelf stability of the stored material while maintaining activity upon dosing. It is useful to elucidate and highlight a stability challenge at the earliest point possible, so that the risks and options for development strategy can be weighed properly.

Bioavailability challenges and hydrophobicity in new chemical entities are commonly discussed phenomena in recent years. We should consider that until about two decades ago, NCE discovery was based largely on in vivo pharmacology feedback. Historically, a compound intended for the oral route was dosed to an animal, a physiological response observed (along with a pharmacokinetic profile), and further testing was enabled by the very fact that exposure was achieved in the in vivo pharmacology experiments. In the last two decades, as a result of enhancement in cloning of biochemical targets and other technical developments, a dramatic shift has occurred toward in vitro pharmacology feedback as a guide to molecular discovery. On this basis, and in the face of increasing molecular complexity and the structural demands that some of the biological targets impose, the industry seems to be experiencing a greater incidence of challenge with CMC development on their NCE programs. Whether it is for reasons of philosophy or due to resource constraints, the approach of inserting CMC experts into the discovery arena is not practiced consistently among sponsor companies at the time of this chapter. The view expressed here is that it is useful to insert pharmaceutical science at the pre-NCE stage in order to expose material-related issues, and to allow for proactive input regarding options for synthesis and timely delivery of the substance in toxicology studies and in the clinic. Similar views presumably guided teams in the development of MK-591 and itraconazole. Involvement of pharmaceutical scientists in the former program, targeting leukotriene biosynthesis, led to the use of amorphous API in nonclinical and early clinical studies. Preparation of stabilized amorphous drug was achieved using a lyophilization process, and this material had significantly higher oral exposures than the crystalline materials, a property that proved vital to the elucidation of the toxicology profile of MK-591 [3]. In the case of itraconazole, the involvement of pharmaceutical science led to the use (and eventual development) of hydroxypropyl-β-cyclodextrin (HPβCD) solutions of the water-insoluble drug. HPβCD is a solubilizer used in formulations for both oral and parenteral administration. The initial application of HPβCD to give exposures in nonclinical studies was in fact followed by the approval of an oral solution of itraconazole (HPβCD in water with dilute HCl) as well as an injectable version of this highly hydrophobic antifungal agent. To make a solid dosage form available, Janssen Pharmaceuticals developed a coated bead in capsule formulation which contains the amorphous drug (Sporanox capsule) [4]. This product is an exception, given that the vast majority of solid dosage forms include crystalline drug substances, which in most cases would have been identified in nonclinical or early clinical stages.

5.2.3 CMC Interactions with Discovery at NCE Selection

The process of providing CMC interactions to move a compound from discovery into development status involves two main steps: (1) evaluation of the synthetic aspects and pharmaceutical profile of the NCE proposed, and (2) evaluation of options, quantitative to the extent possible, based on an intended delivery route for the compound in the toxicology and clinical studies. Table 5.2 lists some aspects to consider in supporting a discovery program in the throes of NCE selection. It is important to realize that "no one size fits all." For example, limited compound availability and/or low complexity of the delivery challenge can mean that either very little involvement is required, or a significant intervention of CMC is in order to solve a stability problem and/or develop approaches to enhance bioavailability. Occasionally, problems with bioavailability have their roots in presystemic metabolism (see Chapters 2 and 8). In such a case, it is important for a discovery group to know that formulation cannot overcome an intrinsic metabolic effect—the best one can hope for is amelioration of impact: for example, in the case of a CYP3A4 first-pass interaction. A first-pass metabolism effect, whether in the liver and/or in the gut, can yield nonlinear pharmacokinetics, and formulations that maximize availability of the compound in the intestine will help mitigate the effect, especially at higher doses, where saturation of the presystemic metabolism is possible. The case studies in this chapter help to illustrate the challenge scenarios outlined here.

Table 5.2 gives an idea of the dialogue and cross-training that are useful for CMC staff interfacing with discovery programs. Together, the combined discovery, ADME, clinical pharmacology, and CMC team can achieve the "best options" target of Figure 5.1, but only with seamless input and guidance from all contributors. Typical time frames and resource requirements for NCE support will vary with candidate and delivery complexities, so the estimates in Table 5.2 should be viewed with some caution. The following additional comments may prove useful:

- Ideally, for a given discovery program in late lead optimization, one CMC chemist with an organic chemistry background can be assigned part-time (perhaps alongside a development program or one or a couple of other discovery programs).
- From the time a target has a viable lead, it can take 3 to 12 months to select the first NCE; sometimes a longer time limit than 12 months is allowed; Seldom is a group able to advance a compound in less than 2 to 3 months from its identification to development status.

TABLE 5.2 Technical and Practical CMC Considerations in Pre-NCE Discovery Support

Consideration	Process Chemistry	Pharmaceutical Science
Type of early CMC support recommended	Understanding of chemistry routes for a type/class of compound	Consultation on formulation and physical properties
Ideal backgrounds for CMC scientist	Synthetic chemistry, chemical process technology experience	Physical–organic chemistry, materials science experience
Additional experience useful to CMC staff	Pharmaceutical properties, toxicology regulation awareness, etc.	Basic pharmacology, toxicology and metabolism understanding, etc.
Key questions to address in the pre-NCE stage	Can the current approach be used for initial synthesis in a process lab? Are there steps with major safety hazards? What scale limitations exist? Form of compound as is?	Bioavailability, delivery? What is the quantitative picture of chemical stability? What is the chemical and physical form of the compound as is? Form change needed? (If so, why?)
Estimate of effort prior to NCE selection	0.1–0.25 process chemists, 3–12 months	0.25–0.75 pharmaceutical chemists, 3–12 months

- Backup compounds for the same target can take 0 to 12 months, depending on luck and accessible molecular diversity in the program.
- The effort and time frames cited above do not take into account governance processes, which can add more time to the act of bringing a compound forward to NCE status.

Specifics of the types of CMC interactions that a discovery team requires and desires vary. As indicated earlier, the extent of process chemistry consultation will generally be less than that required by a pharmaceutical scientist. Process chemistry evaluations ideally form a section of a monograph that is provided at the NCE stage. A pharmaceutical portion of such a monograph would also be provided. Components of the latter are listed in Table 5.3.

Most compounds are targeted for oral or injection delivery. The mode of delivery determines to a certain extent the focus of pharmaceutical evaluation at the early stages. Clearly, solubility profiling in aqueous media should be undertaken in significant detail for a compound intended for injection. An oral compound also benefits from a detailed solubility profile, but use of the information is different from that in the case of injections: The pH dependence of solubility can, for example, be used along with pharmacokinetic data in animals to understand any influence of the physicochemical properties on biopharmaceutical performance.

Studying pharmaceutical properties and providing the material options for animal studies is a process that is occasionally shortchanged at the discovery–development interface. Such evaluation should not be overlooked, however, since it is a relatively inexpensive way to address risk related to materials that could slow progress in development once a compound is selected. Even when a known compound is being considered for a novel delivery method, route, or device, the relevance of properties and possible incompatibilities should be addressed prior to significant formulation development. Aspects of stability and solubility can be assessed proactively and quantitatively with small amounts of material (less than 500 mg is often all that is available prior to selection and scale-up of the compound into GLP toxicity studies). Outsourcing of activities at the preselection stage is not advisable, due to the essential requirement for interactive co-optimization (see Section 5.6.2).

5.2.4 Biopharmaceuticals

In the context of this chapter, a *biopharmaceutical* is defined loosely based on its relationship to a biopolymer (e.g., peptide, protein (such as an antibody), DNA, RNA, polysaccharide), or a hybrid of a biological substance with a nonbiological agent. An example of the latter is pegylated interferon, PEG-Intron, an injectable therapy for hepatitis C. Three principal practical CMC themes that distinguish biopharmaceuticals from small molecules are:

TABLE 5.3 Components of Pharmaceutical Evaluation Monographs for Compounds Entering NCE Status

Component	Examples of Techniques	Uses of the Information
Chemical form (free base, acid, salt, etc.)	HPLC, NMR, elemental analysis, thermogravimetric analysis, with MS detection of volatile components	Stoichiometry of compound components; stereopurity
Physical form, crystallinity	Optical and electron microscopy, powder x-ray diffraction, calorimetry	Form purity analysis, interpretation of solubility, and physical stability data
Solubility, aqueous media	Aqueous, pH-dependent (buffers): kinetic powder dissolution and thermodynamic solubility; typically quantified via spectrophotometrics; can be combined with separation technologies (e.g., HPLC)	Solvation and precipitation kinetics, thermodynamic solubility data
Solubility, nonaqueous	HPLC, shake flask technique at small scale, two temperatures	Help to synthetic chemistry for isolation, crystallization
Physical stability (hydrate, solvate, polymorphism)	Moisture sorption balance, differential scanning calorimetry, thermal microscopy, PXRD, and LC solubility of slurries of API	Expose handling challenges or hydrate forms, analysis of polymorphism potential, surface properties
Chemical stability, solid state	HPLC, selective for degradates, relies on forced degradation studies and reference samples	Quantitative stability over a wide temperature range to project stability of the solid
Chemical stability, aqueous solution	pH dependence (buffers) by HPLC, selective for degradates	Mechanisms of degradation, elucidation of any instability
Biopharmaceutics implications	PK in rats and a nonrodent, usually with likely toxicology species (collaboration with ADME/toxicology)	Early indications of ability to achieve exposures in GLP studies, prognosis on human dosage form(s)

- Challenges with sourcing of the API due to complexity of structure and/or processing
- Requirement for a sterile product (almost all products are injectable)
- Particulate matter issues (molecular size and aggregation potential)

TABLE 5.4 Main Techniques for Pharmaceutical Evaluation of Biopharmaceuticals[a]

Component	Examples of Techniques	Uses of the Information
Chemical identity	HPLC, NMR, MS (MS/MS, high-resolution techniques)	Chemical purity and salt form (if applicable)
Aggregation potential	Dynamic light scattering, GPC, Gel electrophoresis, NMR	Understand potential for aggregation, particulate formation
Size evaluation	Dynamic light scattering, microscopy, analytical and preparative (ultra)centrifugation	Tracking of size distribution of assemblies, aggregates, etc.

[a]These components and techniques are in addition to considerations in Table 5.3.

Considerations of toxicology and clinical applications for biopharmaceutical products are covered in Chapter 12. In terms of CMC, several of the additional techniques required to study the larger molecules are listed in Table 5.4.

Characterization of batch-to-batch variation in a biological material can be significantly more challenging than in a small-molecule campaign. In many cases, this means that the manufacturing process for the API is closely linked to the formulation and is more likely to be narrowed down at a very early stage compared to what happens with the production of a small-molecule API and its formulations.

5.3 CMC CONSIDERATIONS AT THE NCE STAGE

Hopefully, the compound is a well-behaved solid fit for development. How does a discovery group find such a favorable scenario?

5.3.1 Solid-State Compounds

The vast majority of APIs are solid-state materials. Most drug development candidates have sufficient molecular weight and chemically interacting functionality to be solids at standard conditions of temperature and pressure. Indeed, only a small fraction of biologically active compounds are gases (inhalation anesthetics such as isoflurane and nitrous oxide are examples) or liquids (the short-acting sedative/hypnotic propofol 2,6-diisopropyl phenol is a notable example, having a melting point around 17°C at 1 atm pressure). Accordingly, the evaluation of solid-state properties is central in the CMC studies of NCEs.

In the last decade or so, significant attention has been paid to the nature of crystalline pharmaceuticals and crystal polymorphism in pharmaceutical compounds. Polymorphism in crystals is the propensity of a particular chemical to

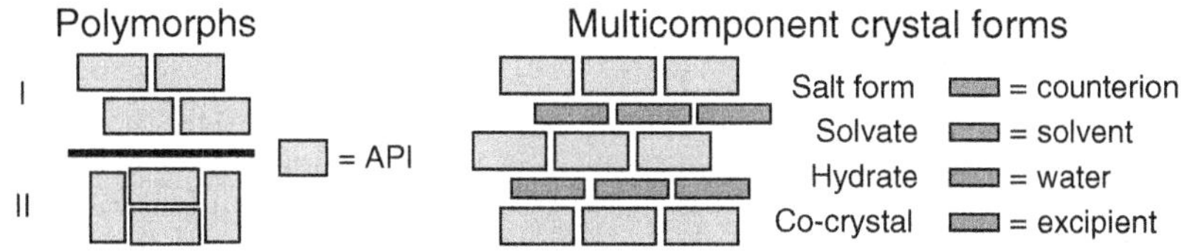

FIGURE 5.2 Possible types of compositions of API solid forms in pharmaceutical products.

appear in multiple crystalline forms (much as carbon can exist as graphite or diamonds or in other forms). A useful reference entitled *Polymorphism of Molecular Crystals* provides a broad and multifaceted introduction to the subject [5]. Polymorphism is fairly common in pharmaceutical compounds, as highlighted in the reference.

Polymorphs can affect the processing, stability, and occasionally, bioavailability of a compound, especially if it is poorly soluble in aqueous media. A profound effect on properties is often achieved when an API is converted from a free form to a salt. A simple example is that of acetic acid and sodium acetate. The former is a viscous liquid, generally containing some water, whereas the latter is a hygroscopic solid. For pharmaceutical compounds, the effect of salt-form change on properties is often significant with respect to solubility and stability. An excellent handbook was published on the topic of pharmaceutical salt forms [6], and this volume is an essential reference on the topic. Figure 5.2 illustrates schematically the types of solid-state compounds that might be encountered in development.

5.3.2 Selection of Development Form (Crystalline State)

As the proposed NCE advances to formal nomination status, it is essential to identify the form for development. For example, if a crystalline HCl salt of a basic API were used to perform pharmacological studies and the form is bioavailable and stable, it seems warranted to nominate the NCE specifically as the crystalline HCl salt. If, however, the same API, having low solubility as the basic form in water, were dosed from acidified solutions to achieve aqueous solubility for dosing, a discovery team has two main choices: (1) nominate the base compound and stipulate a short-term solution approach to dosing using suspensions of the base (if bioavailable) or acidified solutions as before, or (2) conduct form (e.g., salt) screening in order to identify a crystalline (salt) form for future development. The choices to use the base or to use another form are not mutually exclusive, but the precise choice of strategy depends on perceptions of risk and a sponsor's willingness to invest in the form selection process. Here, again, the value of early material evaluation can be expressed: If the constellation of options is understood prior to the selection stage, the proper choices can be made before NCE nomination as a candidate drug.

Options for outsourcing of form selection have evolved dramatically within the last decade. Whereas in the late 1990s there were few options for external form selection support, about a dozen companies offer fee-for-service crystallization and crystal form analysis. Companies such as SSCI (Aptuit), Solvias, Avantium (Crystallics), Wilmington Pharmatech, Polycrystalline, and others provide services related to study of crystal forms of pharmaceuticals. Some companies also provide process chemical support, such as catalyst evaluation for critical steps en route to the final API.

Examples of crystal forms in products are given in Table 5.5. The table includes rare examples of changes in chemical form after a compound has been developed or even marketed. Such changes are not ideal, due to costly reengineering and additional study requirements. The message should be one of "an ounce of prevention is worth a pound of cure." Early attention to a suitable development form can save significant time and cost in later development.

A change of chemical form between the enabling toxicity studies and initial clinical use, say from a salt to a free compound or from one salt to another, is not advisable and is likely to result in regulatory holds. Toxicity and exposure studies to compare forms are needed at a minimum, but each case of a potential switch of form requires attention to a bridging strategy that will satisfy scientific and regulatory needs. A couple of common scenarios can be highlighted in question–answer format to illustrate topics that may arise regarding form:

Q.: We used the amorphous HCl salt in development for an oral administration compound, but now we have realized that the crystalline free base is

TABLE 5.5 Examples of Crystal Form Properties and Issues for Some Marketed Drugs

Drug Product	Development Form	Comment[a]
Zantac	Ranitidine HCl	Polymorphs I and II were the subject of significant patent litigation and intrigue in the 1990s
Zoloft	Sertraline HCl	Polymorphic but otherwise well-behaved material
Tegretol	Carbamazepine form III	Polymorphic, unsolvated; problem of dihydrate appearance in products lowered oral bioavailability
Norvir capsules	Ritonavir form II	Disastrous polymorph change postmarket forced a formulation change and interruption in supply
Lipitor	Atorvastatin calcium trihydrate	Initial studies proceeded with an amorphous sodium salt, but calcium salt was ultimately chosen

[a] See Bernstein [5, p. 298].

suitable for development of the oral formulation. What bridging studies are required, if any?

A.: At a minimum, two things must be done and documented properly: (1) the purity profiles of the HCl salt and free base need to be compared with sensitive and selective analytical methods to determine what (if any) differences exist in purity and impurity levels between the HCl salt from toxicology studies and the proposed free-base form—there will be significant implications if any species previously untested are being introduced without proper toxicological qualification; and (2) biopharmaceutical properties need to be compared in animals, ideally a nonrodent absorption model such as a dog, to understand at a dose relevant to anticipated human therapeutic dose levels—it would be important to maintain the exposure pattern seen in previous studies to avoid complex bridging. Finally, if the change is being considered at a relatively early stage (e.g., phase I or IIa), qualification in the integrated toxicology program is under way and hence the new form should be introduced at a logical point, say at the start of a new study.

Q.: The form we have been using was amorphous but now it has crystallized. What are our options to continue the program?

A.: Crystallization is thermodynamically driven and you have just been reminded that nature is eventually going to show us all the lowest-energy state of things. Crystallization is also a purification process, so one would imagine that the impurity profile of your materials has changed. This is the good news. Hopefully, you have good news on the performance of the form in formulation: namely, that you have retained the requisite solubility and/or bioavailability—and bridging is therefore unnecessary and confined solely to the CMC processes. If the news is not good on these fronts, more complex bridging exercise may lie ahead, complete with a form change or a pharmaceutical process that involves trying to recreate and maintain the amorphous form. Remember that the act of making things amorphous in formulation increases the energy state of the material, and this in itself imposes risks of chemical and physical instability. The need for an amorphous formulation approach thus adds risk and possibly increases complexity and cost of CMC development.

Q.: A new, less soluble polymorph of our already poorly soluble compound has appeared in phase II testing. What can be done?

Q.: A less soluble polymorph is more stable and thus represents the preferred polymorph of the compound from this point forward. A physicochemical comparison with the previously known forms is of critical importance, along with a biopharmaceutical impact assessment. The latter can take place in animal models, although it may be most advisable to take forward a GMP- qualified formulation of the new polymorph to determine if any impact is felt in the drug product. The situation is complex and fluid, but can presumably be managed with added cost but perhaps without a major time line deviation. At this point, it becomes crucial to clarify and document which clinical and API supplies represent which polymorphic form.

Q.: We have a reasonable form (though not ideal) in phase I development. We are aware of better crystal forms; ones that have greater purity, improved handling characteristics, and retain the bioavailability attributes that we are seeking. Should we consider changing form, and if so, when?

A.: As long as there are no overwhelming technical or regulatory drivers for changing form, the question becomes one of preference and strategic fit. Pharmaceutical acceptability is one topic where technical and regulatory considerations intersect. If the preferred choice involves using a non-GRAS (generally regarded as safe) or other uncommon material with questionable acceptance in all regions or regulatory areas, it would hardly be advisable to make the change. A change from one acceptable material to another that is equally acceptable is more tricky to evaluate. It may be useful to reflect on the fact that there are numerous examples of good forms that are not perfect but nevertheless, are used successfully in pharmaceutical products: These cases illustrate the inertia inherent in changing CMC approaches significantly along the development pathway when there remains the risk that the compound can fail for non-CMC reasons (lack of efficacy, poor tolerability long term, or low market drive, for example). A strategic discussion must be facilitated to resolve the preferred approach, where the choices are laid out with pros and cons for each form identified in as objective a fashion as possible.

5.3.3 Characterization of Drug Substance (Preformulation)

In the development process of small molecules for therapeutic application, the term *drug substance* typically refers to a solid-state powder that is produced by chemical development scientists using a controlled synthetic process. As the program matures in development, the level of characterization and control of the synthetic process increases significantly in an effort to maintain the crystallinity, polymorphism, and impurity profile within an acceptable development space. The drug substance is generally stored for subsequent incorporation into a *drug product*, a formulated pharmaceutical dosage form that includes functional excipients promoting desirable stability, processing, and/or bioavailability properties.

Even at an early stage of development, the physical and chemical form of the drug substance comprises a significant part of CMC development and documentation,. Physicochemical data (including drug substance crystallinity, salt form, thermodynamic solubility, stability, etc.) relate to the toxicological and clinical programs directly, inasmuch the drug substance characteristics can affect both exposure in the GLP studies and the assessment of overall risk for the program. For example, water-insoluble compounds intended for oral administration occasionally show less-than-proportional increases in plasma exposure with increased dose in animals and humans as a result of insufficient dissolution or other physical dynamics of the material in the gastrointestinal tract. Early elucidation of such a challenge can facilitate problem solving at the nonclinical and clinical pharmacology interface to increase oral absorption by formulation approaches where this is possible.

Another example of risk mitigation is the early description of impurities and degradates of the compound, which may be present in the eventual drug product. Data-driven projections of future levels of related and unrelated substances in the drug product, with reference to the analytical results for materials used in toxicology studies with associated no-effect levels, should be made to help set initial specifications as well as to select appropriate storage and handling conditions. Appropriate forced degradation studies and other stability monitoring under stress can help in this regard.

Detailed attention to a pH–solubility profile is warranted as soon as a crystalline reference state has been identified. Solubility measurements are truly meaningful only if the solid phase that is in contact with saturated solutions is crystalline. When a compound is intended to be formulated as a solution, an understanding of solubility is crucial to ensure that stable solutions can be made without unpredictable precipitation or loss of solubility. Injections are ideally aqueous with minimal use of solubilizers or extremes of pH. A pH–solubility profile can also be helpful in understanding and predicting the state of an oral compound as it experiences variations in pH and surfactant content in the gastrointestinal tract.

A *preformulation* effort, detailed investigation and documentation of the physicochemical and biopharmaceutical properties of the drug substance lots, is an essential aspect of CMC development. The aspects exemplified in the preceding paragraphs are integral parts of the early stage CMC effort, and most sponsors elect to commission a preformulation report to collect the properties of the drug candidate. Contents and emphases vary, and there is no single agreed-upon template for such a report. Because many of the solid-state kinetic processes (e.g., annealing, spontaneous polymorphic conversion), as well as the chemical degradation processes exhibited by the drug substance, occur on a month or year scale, a well-defined and characterized initial state at declaration may be the only means of verifying and quantitating subsequent changes. Although the term *preformulation* is commonly used, it implies that all characterization of the drug substance is complete prior to formulation efforts, whereas in reality, formulation and drug substance characterization are overlapping activities. If any changes are encountered, such as polymorphism or particle engineering (e.g., milling, nanosizing), there should be cross-checking against the *pharmaceutical chemistry profile* (used here as a preferred term for preformulation). In essence, as a development program evolves, the challenge is to ascertain how changes made to dosage form or processing methods may affect the stability and bioavailability profiles of the drug substance.

Attendant naming and numbering conventions need to be addressed at this point if they have not been already. Because the definition, performance, and utility of the materials are now becoming evident, it is imperative to develop a suitable systematic naming convention to correlate unambiguously the body of data under discussion to specific lots and forms of the API. If code names are used to disguise the molecular entity, a method by which different lots and compositions (salt form, free form, polymorph, formulations, etc.) can be discerned aids communication and interpretation of evolving data and can save a lot of backtracking effort later. An efficient system might assign a number to the API, an extension indicating the salt or free form, a batch or lot number, indication of polymorph if necessary, and any other unique characteristic of the material.

5.4 NCE-TO-GLP TRANSITION (BRIDGING FROM DISCOVERY TO PRE-FIH DEVELOPMENT)

5.4.1 Drug Synthesis and Formulation for Toxicity Studies: Meeting the Delivery Objectives

Perhaps the most critical time in an NCE program is the period when a formal commitment has been made to begin development but the supply of the compound is insufficient or essentially nonexistent. A critical and rate-limiting activity is the generation of supplies for GLP toxicology. Two main options exist to achieve the goal of delivering material to GLP studies: (1) accelerate synthesis of a well-characterized substance in a process lab that is *not* qualified for good manufacturing practice (GMP) synthesis, or (2) develop a synthesis for ultimate scale-up and manufacture in a GMP-qualified laboratory. In this section we cover the requirements and regulations that play a part in surmounting the challenge of delivering the drug substance and suitable toxicology formulation to initiate drug development.

Drug Substance Requirements for GLP Studies Once a decision has been made to move forward toward clinical evaluation of a compound, drug substance synthesis and characterization for GLP toxicity studies (Chapters 7 and 8) are probably the "critical path" activities. The drug substance for GLP toxicity studies is covered in U.S. Food and Drug Administration (FDA) regulation 21 CFR Part 58, Section 105 (Test and Control Articles) [7], where emphasis is placed on documentation of characterization and stability to cover the duration of use. In effect, the identity, composition, strength (potency), and purity are key aspects that need to be characterized and documented. The goal of pre-FIH toxicity studies is to ensure that the cGMP (current good manufacturing practice) clinical material is safe over the intended dose range in phase I clinical studies [8] (i.e., the objective is dominated by the properties of the API). If it is anticipated that chemical conversion products of the API will be present in the cGMP clinical material to significant levels (greater than about 0.2%), the GLP toxicity studies must be designed to qualify the administration of these impurities. Although some sponsor companies elect to use the first cGMP drug substance lot for both

GLP toxicology and FIH clinical use, they pay a significant penalty in development time to do so. A science-based approach to GLP toxicological qualification includes a data-driven evaluation of the predicted levels of significant impurities at the end of clinical use, then inclusion of these impurities in the qualification. Doing so qualifies the active compound, the associated impurities, addresses the burden of cross-correlation or special qualification of the clinical material, and allows parallel execution of the two critical development activities: GLP toxicological qualification and cGMP drug substance production and release. Assuming that any further formulation does not alter the stability or purity profile in the clinical supplies relative to that present in GLP toxicology, the risk of additional qualification being required for the clinical supplies is low—the clinical supplies with its purity profile will be qualified by virtue of the GLP toxicology program that provides the margins for the first phase I study. Qualification of isolated impurities in drug products is covered in Chapter 7.

In addition, the chemical form of the drug substance should remain consistent between enabling toxicology work and initial clinical studies. If a mode of presentation or formulation of a chemical form is changed, some care is required to assure that the strategy and rationale for the change can be supported. For example, if an in situ HCl salt were used (as a solution) in toxicology and subsequently a crystalline HCl salt (presented as a solid) is proposed for the clinical supplies, bridging data would be needed to argue suitability. Crafting such an argument is the joint responsibility of CMC, regulatory, and toxicology professionals, generally led by the responsible toxicological representative working through a regulatory liaison.

Toxicology Formulations In parallel with scale-up of the compound, a toxicology formulation should be defined and selected with an aim for simplicity: A clear preference should be given to a minimum formulation approach to focus the evaluation on the new compound rather than formulation per se. Consideration of the drug product is also a key step to (1) deliver the compound in a suitable dosage form to volunteers in the FIH studies, and (2) launch formulation design and development for later stages of testing should a compound continue past its initial testing in humans. These points should be kept in mind as a toxicology formulation is being developed. To reiterate a point, GLP toxicology formulations have two main purposes: convenient delivery to animals with minimal ancillary effects of vehicle, and provision of high and dose-related plasma/serum exposures to facilitate determination of toxicological profiles.

Regulations such as 21 CFR Part 58 [7] do not speak specifically to vehicles for toxicology studies. Acceptable vehicles and carriers are discussed in Chapters 3, 7, and 8. The ideal toxicology vehicle for an oral compound is water or an aqueous solution of a polymer with a long-standing track record of safety in animals. Examples of such polymers are hydroxypropyl cellulose (HPC) and hydroxypropyl methylcellulose (HPMC). If the compound dissolves readily in water across the dose range anticipated, pure water may be preferable, whereas if a compound due to lack of solubility needs to be in suspension, the presence of the polymer is often preferred to ensure homogeneity of the suspension for dosing. Properties of the drug substance, such as chemical form, particle size, and shape, become especially important for suspension dosing, and hence it is important to develop and document an understanding of the form of the compound before starting the GLP toxicology program.

Given the objective of high plasma/serum exposures in animals relative to anticipated human exposures, the challenge of delivery in animal studies is often greater than that encountered in the phase I clinical program. If exposures from aqueous suspensions are limited in animals, which can occur at the high doses proposed for toxicology, some remedies can be considered. For example, from the CMC perspective, an alternative vehicle can be suggested to help overcome a dissolution limitation of absorption in an oral program. Various lists of acceptable vehicles for toxicology programs exist, and certain company preferences are known to exist. Chapters 3, 7, and 8 refer to some sources for vehicle information. Additional references are provided in the resource section at the end of this chapter.

As the integrity of toxicology data is critical, appropriate stability must be provided to support the use of the vehicle and the goals of the study. If the drug substance is placed in the chosen vehicle on a schedule during a GLP study (say, e.g., that a weekly preparation of suspension is required), a quantitative study of the stability of the material under the same conditions needs to be documented to provide coverage for the use period. To make conclusions regarding the effect of exposure to the therapeutic drug, it may suffice to control and record the level of the API alone. However, at little to no cost to the development time line, the purity-indicating analytical method developed for the drug substance can be used to record the purity profile over the intended period of use in the toxicological formulation. This quantitation and control of impurities in the GLP toxicological studies can serve to qualify these chemicals for subsequent clinical administration. Ideally, the cycle of formulation preparation should be selected to minimize any changes over the time frame of use.

For unstable compounds, which may be anticipated to exhibit increases in degradates over the course of preparation, shipping, and storage of clinical materials, it may be necessary to introduce stress to the toxicology supplies to induce the formation of degradates proactively. The choice to invoke process steps to induce degradate formation in GLP toxicology studies is dependent on careful consultation with expert toxicologists and good data to support the viability of such an approach. A drug development organization must balance the need for qualification of components with artificial introduction of variables that may complicate interpretation of toxicology findings.

5.4.2 Bridging to Formulations for FIH Studies

The types of formulations one might consider for FIH studies range from simple (e.g., a toxicology formulation) to complex, such as an oral tablet dosage form or a lyophilized powder for reconstitution into an injectable solution. The range of options for dosage forms for the FIH evaluation is illustrated in Table 5.6. The choice is dependent on many factors, including feasibility, cost, risk profile, and confidence in the particular molecule and/or mechanism of action. The route of administration for initial studies is determined by the toxicology program, which will seek to define the organ toxicity and dose limits to be placed on the first study in humans.

A proposed dosage form for humans should satisfy the stated criteria of maintaining the qualitative and quantitative impurity profile covered by the toxicity studies that enables the human study while utilizing inert components that meet safety and cGMP standards. Introduction of a new excipient or component will raise regulatory questions, and in the case of a previously untested component, a toxicological program will probably be required to "qualify" any new excipient. Given that the cost to develop a toxicology package to qualify a new component is on the same order of magnitude as the toxicology program for the API itself, there would need to be significant strategic benefits to taking the option of using the previously untested component. Examples of excipients that were specifically qualified to support ultimate use in marketed dosage forms include the solubilizing agents sulfabutyl-β-cyclodextrin (Cydex Inc.; licensed by Pfizer for use in two injectable products) and hydroxypropyl-β-cyclodextrin (Janssen Pharmaceutica; used in itraconazole oral solution and intravenous injection).

Technologies to support intranasal, ocular, transdermal, buccal, rectal, inhalation, and other routes were not included in Table 5.6, for the following reasons:

- These routes are less common than injection or the oral route for FIH evaluation of a compound.
- Formulation requirements for some routes overlap with those for other routes (e.g., intranasal and ocular dosage forms require similar treatment to sterile injections, with some additional irritation evaluations).

By using preferred routes of delivery and simple formulation prototypes, the focus in ADME and initial clinical evaluation of an NCE is placed appropriately on understanding molecular properties (e.g., attributes that are independent of formulation). Essentially, the assumption is that any influence of formulation has been disconnected at the site and time of metabolism, and distribution and excretion are also assumed to be independent of how the formulation was delivered to the body. There are clear exceptions to this assumption, such as long-circulating injectable liposomes and polymer-based subcutaneous or intramuscular injections. To avoid stacking excessive risk onto a program by adding technology risk to the compound's inherent risk, formulation elaborations are generally introduced at a later stage of human testing rather than being the leading approach when a new compound is being tested.

When aiming for high oral bioavailability and the aqueous solubility is low or a molecule's permeability through membranes is limited, the "A" part of

TABLE 5.6 Possible Prototypes for FIH Dosage Forms

Type, Route	Image, Example(s)	Main Variables	Advantages	Disadvantages
Aqueous solution, oral	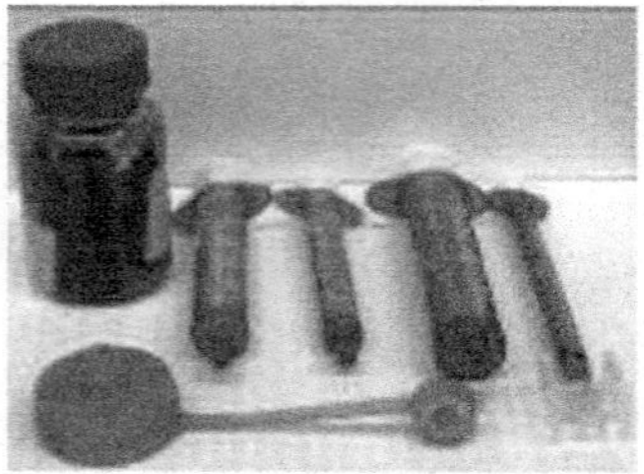	Ready to use or powder for reconstitution Preserved if for long-term storage in reconstituted form	Dosing flexibility Automated filling possible Uniformity of dose strength assured	Not appropriate for compounds susceptible to hydrolysis, other instability Defers development effort: support not applicable to ultimate dosage forms Clinical site restrictions/qualification requirements Taste/smell? Preservative?
Aqueous suspension, oral	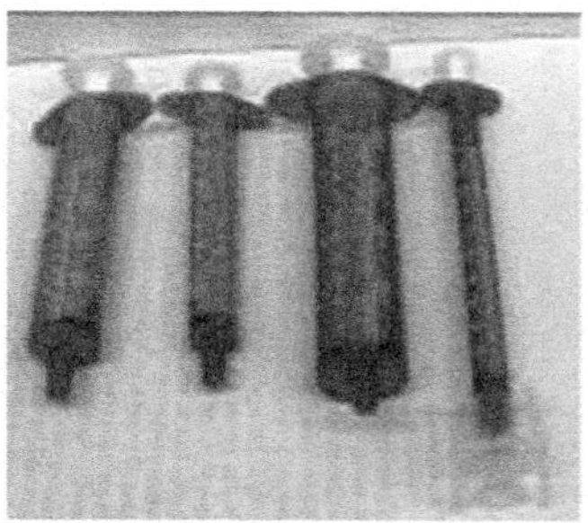	Same as above, plus: particle size control and characterization recommended	Same as above, plus: usually comparable to tox formulation Limited development	Same as above, plus: settling of drug, redispersibility/dose uniformity Significant CMC component of clinical protocols required

Aqueous solution, injection: i.v. (intravenous), i.m. (intramuscular), or s.c. (subcutaneous).	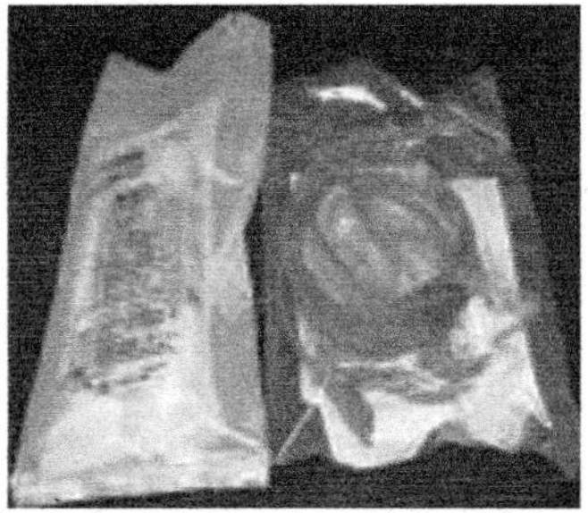	Ready to use or powder for reconstitution Buffer and tonicity agent Method of solution sterilization	Dosing flexibility Automated filling possible Uniformity of dose strength assured	Need compatibility with packaging (e.g., glass, plastic) Particle-formation risk in ready-to-use formulations Lyophilization or spray-drying cost
Aqueous suspension, injection: i.m. or s.c.	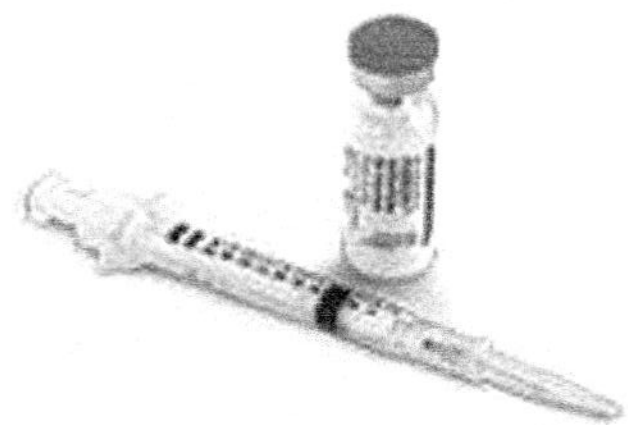	Same as above, plus: use of polymers or oils for rate control	Often prolonged release from a depot (i.m. > s.c.) compared with i.v. injection	Risk of pain on injection and site irritation Volume constraint: <1 mL s.c., ~ 3 mL i.m.
Dispersion of compound in a nonaqueous vehicle in capsule, oral	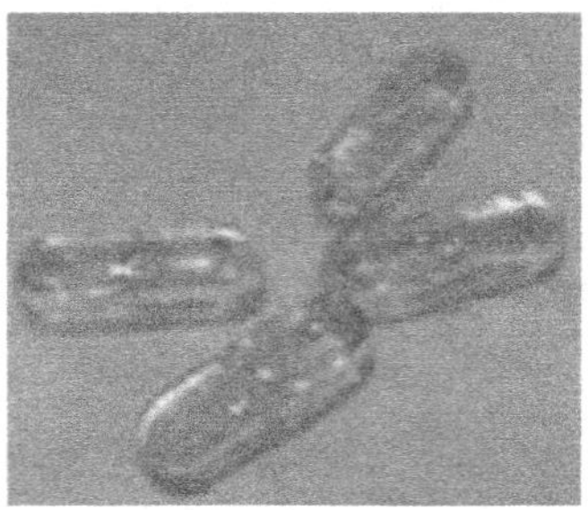	Gelatin or HPMC capsules Semisolid filled at elevated temp. Beads coated with drug solution, spray-dried material, softgel	Can enable high bioavailability of poorly soluble and first-pass metabolized Access to GMP-qualified technology	Complexity of compositions Acceptability of components Risk of physical instability Cost and market acceptability

(*Continued overleaf*)

TABLE 5.6 *(Continued)*

Type, Route	Image, Example(s)	Main Variables	Advantages	Disadvantages
Neat or blend of compound in capsule, oral	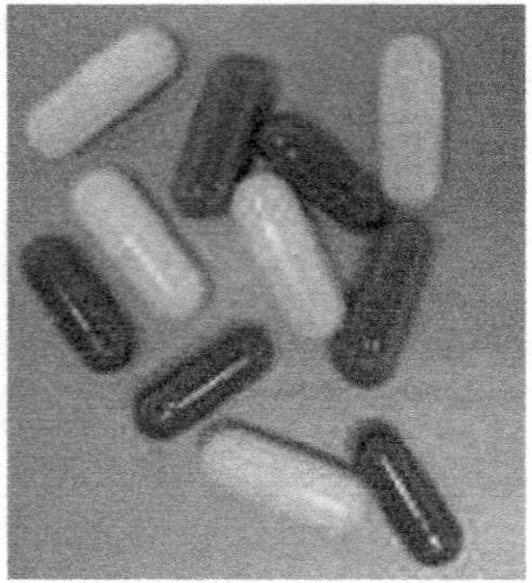	Gelatin or HPMC capsules; pure compound (if water-soluble), formulated blend	Simpler than dispersions to make and store Can be automated effectively	Cost and market acceptability post-phase I
Tablets	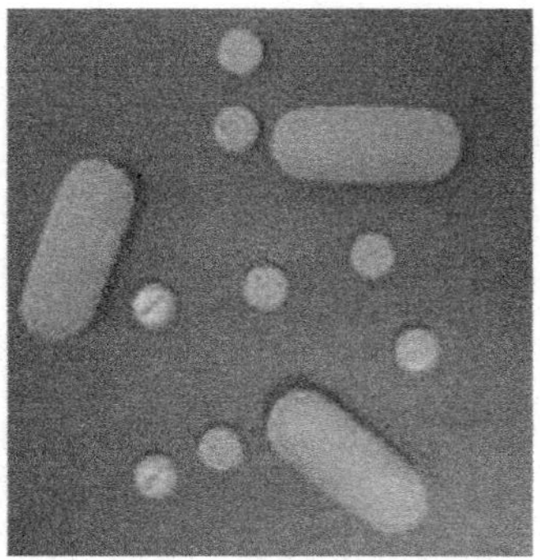	Dry processing (granulation, direct compression or roller compaction) Wet granulation, fluid-bed drying and compression *Materials-sparing approaches*	Elegant prototypes Reflective of future dosages Stability (physical and chemical) often assured High-speed, scalable operations	Requires discipline in dose selection May require more compound than other types to develop

ADME can become a significant variable in the pharmacokinetic and pharmacology assessment. For an oral compound, the elements of material properties and formulation composition thus can become a point of possible elaboration at an early stage. A strategic choice needs to be made as to whether or not salt selection, micronization of drug substance, or a special formulation effort is warranted for the FIH study. Also, if chemical stability is a challenge (e.g., if a prodrug approach is being employed or if chemical functional groups that are known to be labile are included), it is useful to get a quantitative evaluation of stability under conditions of storage and use at an early stage to examine future liabilities in toxicology and the clinic.

References dealing with the evaluation of routes other than oral and injections are suggested at the end of the chapter. Additionally, evaluation of controlled release is generally secondary to an FIH evaluation of pharmacokinetices and tolerability, and hence we only suggest resources to study the controlled-release aspect rather than devoting further discussion to such special cases.

5.5 CMCs TO MEET CLINICAL TRIAL MATERIAL REQUIREMENTS

Clinical trial material (CTM) is the fuel that supports a clinical study, whether it is a safety evaluation in volunteers or a study of efficacy and safety in patients. In this section, the requirements for suitable clinical formulations, ingredients, GMP manufacturing, packaging, and labeling will be highlighted, and the subject of placebos and blinding will receive a short description. Finally, a short section on strategic considerations is included to help raise awareness of interdependencies in early drug development.

5.5.1 Drug Substance Comparability with Material Used in Pre-FIH GLP Studies

In parallel with the GLP toxicological and safety testing executed with pre-GMP drug substances (above, and Chapters 7, 8, and 9), process chemistry efforts continue to refine the GLP synthetic process with a goal of producing a batch of cGMP drug substance of a specified quantity and purity. While GLP drug substance can be qualified for its targeted studies by moderate characterization (as discussed in Section 5.4.1), the qualification of GMP drug substance starts with control of the manufacturing process and environment, with associated increased testing and characterization. The quantity required is a strategic decision based on intended use of this first cGMP batch, perceived probability of success of the candidate in clinical evaluations, maturity of the clinical concept (first-time test of target validity or backup compound to a probe NCE), cost of goods, chemical yield, time line strategy, and availability of technical and capital resources.

A significant technical aspect of the chemical development includes designing the latter steps of the process with the goal of rejecting impurities from inclusion in the finished material to produce a crystalline drug compound of high purity. As discussed above, the crystalline form of the drug substance has a number of advantages compared to amorphous powders, including higher purity due to geometric and energetic selectivity during precipitation from the mother liquor, as well as a desired resistance to degradation during drug substance storage due to the lower energy state of the crystalline form relative to a less crystalline or amorphous state.

The goal of drug substance batch manufacture is to achieve acceptable yields while controlling the purity (fraction of the drug substance mass comprised by the stoichiometric drug compound) as well as the impurity profile of the drug substance. A typical target of drug substance purity is on the order of greater than 98.0%. Certain classes of drugs that are difficult to purify, such as some antibiotics, may have lower purity expectations. Biopharmaceutical compounds are also in this latter category, where purity in the range of 95% may be considered acceptable for use.

5.5.2 Good Manufacturing Practices

In the United States, development, manufacture, packaging, testing, and storage of drug substances and drug products for clinical testing or marketing is accomplished under 21 CFR Parts 210 and 211 [9]. Together, Parts 210 and 211 comprise the current good manufacturing practices (cGMPs) applicable to drugs and finished pharmaceuticals intended for human use. GMPs or cGMPs are accepted and instituted in other regulatory regions as well. It is critical for clinical sponsors to incorporate a contemporary and sophisticated quality assurance (QA) group, a required element of an organization that aims to test compounds in humans. As cGMP regulations are necessarily broad to ensure wide coverage of drug development activities, science-focused QA personnel can add significant value to clinical efforts by ensuring focus on the critical quality attributes of the CTM rather than procedure-driven checklists.

5.5.3 Analytical Development for Assay of Drug Substance and Drug Product

Methods Development and Validation Analytical methods development is a critical qualification aspect of materials used for GLP toxicology and human studies. It should be noted that the term *analytical* applies to analyte measurement in dosage forms and chemical mixtures, while *bioanalytical* is used for analyte(s) measurement in biological matrices (Chapter 4). Assay, the measured potency of the dosage form via comparison with a suitable reference standard, establishes the dose of the administered compound(s) for study. Quantification of the number and level of each undesirable material is required both to ensure safety of the material and to demonstrate control of the production and storage processes. Undesirable material may include *extraneous matter* such as fiber or dust, which is inadvertently incorporated into the stored material, *impurities*, which are technically only chemicals that do not increase with storage time, such as a residual solvent, unreacted reagent, or a quenched (side) reaction product, and *degradates*. Degradates (sometimes referred to as *degradants* or *degradation products*) are conversion products that increase with storage time as a result of a continuing slow reaction in the drug substance or drug product. Although it is true that genuine impurities can be quantified solely through drug substance purity methods, and drug product purity methods need only be selective for degradation products in the early stages of program development, the driver of value for methods development is to achieve a level quantification and control sufficient to enable a single ascending dose and a multiple ascending dose for safety evaluation. This is achieved most efficiently by a drug substance purity method that is selective for both constant level and degradate species, and a very similar or identical drug product purity method. The resources necessary to identify the source and kinetics of a given undesirable chemical unequivocally are probably best reserved for later-stage activities. In this chapter addressing FIH activities, then, the term *impurity* is used to denote any material outside the API subject to quantification and control.

The quantification and control requirements for impurities are driven by their anticipated risk. Prior to regulatory submission, the possibility of genotoxin or carcinogen presence can be evaluated via analysis of the drug substance synthetic pathway using a knowledge-based expert system for the qualitative prediction of toxicity such as DEREK (see the resources section at the end of the chapter). Impurities that are suspected or established genotoxins or carcinogens may require strict control and therefore quantitation from less than 10 to about 100 parts per million. For suspected genotoxins or carcinogens, as with all impurities, the control limit is a strong function of both the acute exposure (i.e., total daily intake) and the chronic exposure (i.e., the duration of the clinical evaluation or therapeutic administration) [10].

Due to the need to quantify impurities to trace levels in pharmaceutical systems, chemical separation techniques are ubiquitous in the quantitative analysis of both drug substances and drug products. Since the 1980s, HPLC has become the indispensible technique for such separation and quantification. Impurities retained by a stationary phase, either normal-phase silica gel or the more common reversed-phase functionalized silica, are invariably organic impurities which may share functional groups with the API. Impurities that are likely not to be retained, and therefore require additional methodology, include residual solvents (limited to levels of 0.05 to 0.5%) and inorganic impurities.

For ordinary organic impurities (i.e., those not known to be genotoxic or carcinogenic), three generic thresholds are of interest to development scientists. The guideline discussion below is based on the International Conference on Harmonization (ICH) Tripartite Guideline, Impurities in New Drug Products Q3B(R2) [11]:

1. Organic impurities at or above the *reporting* threshold must be tabulated and reported in all regulatory communications. The reporting threshold

for drug substances and drug products is on the order of 0.05 to 0.1%, depending on total daily intake.

2. Organic impurities at or above the *identification* threshold of about 0.2% must be identified via a proposed chemical structure consistent with acquired mass spectrometry and/or nuclear magnetic resonance (NMR) data.
3. Organic impurities present at the 0.20 to 1% level and above typically need to be *qualified* via laboratory tests for biological safety (Chapters 6 to 9).

Specifications of a drug substance or drug product are designed to ensure safety as well as assure the quality of clinical material. Development of specifications throughout the program cycle is a significant component of product development, which can be used to develop understanding of the material's critical quality attributes and focus effort on controlling these attributes in clinical manufacture. In early development, the specifications for drug substances and drug products may be somewhat generic, as there is an insufficient lot history to establish specific control targets. Also, there is a need to obtain clinical data to establish correlations between laboratory test results and clinical performance of early drug products. Typically, impurity and potency specifications for early phase drug substances and drug products may be assigned using guidelines from an applicable ICH monograph. Note, however, that these monographs are intended for product registration, and the published guidelines may require adaptation for early phase material intended for short-term evaluation. Although regulatory agencies accept reference and comparisons to ICH in early development, the ICH guidelines are considered significantly more relevant for phase III product candidates than for phase I drug substance and clinical trial materials.

Setting Specifications Specifications consist of a quality parameter (e.g., assay), a method for testing the parameter [e.g., purity analysis by high-performance liquid chromatography (HPLC)], and an acceptance criterion (98.0 to 102.0%). Once specifications are established by the relevant standard operating procedures (SOPs) as required by cGMP regulations 21 CFR Parts 210 and 211 [9], the finished drug substance or drug product can be tested using the appropriate analytical methods. Pharmaceutical compendia such as the *United States Pharmacopeia*, the *European Pharmacopeia*, and the *Japanese Pharmacopeia* comprise a significant repertoire of methodology for use in testing compendial drug substances and products. Although compendial methods can be used for generic impurities (e.g., heavy metals, or refractory material via residue on ignition), new chemical or biological entity testing will require specific methods developed as part of the specification and testing process. The analytical method that typically requires the most development effort is a stability-indicating method capable of quantitating drug-related organic impurities and degradates. The stability-indicating qualifier simply means that the method has been shown to be specific for the degradation products of the drug substance. The degradation products are typically explored by directed and purposeful degradation studies in which the drug substance is exposed to such stresses as excess acid, base, chemical oxidants, and thermal and photonic energy.

Once a specific group of analytes has been targeted, analytical methods are developed to quantify these components to support drug product prototype development. An analytical test method is an experimental protocol targeted to achieve a certain level of accuracy, sensitivity, reproducibility, and associated measurement characteristics by prescribing the sample preparation, chemical separation, data acquisition, and quantification methodology of the test. Not all methods contain all these components; for example, chemical separation may only be required for accurate quantitation of compounds present at relatively low levels. Analytical methods may be shown to be applicable for their intended use over a specified range of results through method validation, a series of experiments in which the method components are subject to a series of challenges. This external body of data validates the results obtained via execution of the analytical test procedure as written.

Upon completion of the drug substance manufacture, the lot is tested to determine if the material meets specifications. The execution of these tests, and reporting of the test results on a drug substance certificate of analysis (CofA), are critical quality activities that need to be executed under the review of the appropriate quality assurance personnel. The drug substance for a phase I clinical trial will probably be the first cGMP batch of the program and the first batch manufactured above a scale of hundreds of grams. With no prior clinical data or lot history to set drug substance targets addressing desired processability or clinical performance, the specifications at this stage are driven largely by safety and efficacy: for example, appearance, assay, related substances (which are typically either process impurities or degradates of the API), residual solvents, heavy metals, residue on ignition to address inorganic impurities, microbial testing, and perhaps moisture. Acquisition of results within specifications, and documentation of results via the drug substance CofA, enables use of the qualified drug substance lot in the CTM drug product. Ancillary data such as drug substance particle size may be collected to begin characterization of the campaign and allow examinations of process parameters, but would typically not appear on the CofA until a point in the program where a meaningful set of acceptance criteria can be established. The components of the FIH drug product CofA are also focused on safety and efficacy, and typically include appearance, assay, and related substances. If the FIH CTM is a solid dosage form, disintegration or dissolution data should be collected to ensure reasonable drug release in the clinic and to begin drug product lot history characterization. As critical acceptance criteria have not yet been established for this parameter, dissolution or disintegration may not be included on the early phase drug product CofA.

Stability Testing The purpose of drug substance and drug product stability testing for regulatory submissions is determination of the principal degradation rates in the drug substance, in prototype formulations, and in the clinical trial material in relevant packaging to ensure that the material is safe and within specifications for all administrations. A stability protocol with prescribed time points and tests at each point is useful; nonetheless, given the dynamic nature of the exploration of early drug substance and formulation concepts, a need for flexibility is emphasized. As before, the potency of the compound is a key metric, as are impurities. In principle, only impurities expected to increase (i.e., degradates) are monitored in clinical drug product stability testing. In practice, a single test procedure may be selective for the API, the drug substance organic impurities, as well as the drug substance organic degradates, so all impurities are monitored during stability testing. The API and its degradates, as reactants and products of chemical processes occurring during storage of the clinical material, require quantitative test procedures, which are test methods capable of determining an amount present within known accuracy and precision. Impurities that either remain constant or decrease with storage, such as residual solvents or heavy metals, are tested at release but need not be monitored on stability. For these impurities, the safety of the clinical trial material can be assured with a *limit* test procedure. A limit test is not designed to quantify the level of the chemical within a stated uncertainty but rather, is intended to show that the level of the analyte is less than the standard level used in the test.

Shelf Life and Expiration Dating As indicated earlier, the FIH dosage form may be a solution, a suspension, a neat drug substance contained in a capsule, or a tablet designed for the specific drug substance's physicochemical properties. Regardless of the vehicle, the CTM intended must be shown to be safe at the time of administration. This is achieved by development of prototype formulation(s), which are chemically and physically representative of the intended clinical dose with respect to level of chemical excipients, storage conditions, and packaging, then measuring the expiration time, that is, the time required for the material to fail specifications. To decrease the CTM development time, such excipient compatibility and prototype stability testing can cautiously be accelerated by increasing the severity of the storage conditions to substitute for time (i.e., based on careful extrapolation of Arrhenius kinetics). For example, four weeks at 40°C/75% relative humidity may be considered to be roughly equivalent to four months at 25°C/60% relative humidity. These types of probe stability data support development of the CTM formulation and process and provide the initial expiration dating of the CTM. With respect to science-driven pharmaceutical development and regulatory submissions, it is important to realize that ICH stability conditions (25°C/60% relative humidity, 30°C/65% relative humidity, and 40°C/75% relative humidity) are designed for phase III registration studies to determine required market packaging in specific global climate zones. Opportunistic and flexible testing conditions such as open dish or temperatures greater than 40°C, however, may be appropriate for acquisition of the CTM stability profile for phase I submissions [8,12]. As always, for development of high-value experimental protocols and standard practices, it is imperative to understand the intended use and scope of the stability data acquired.

A typical single ascending dose phase I clinical protocol can generally be supported by a six- to eight-month use-by period, whereas a marketed product probably requires a two-year shelf life for commercial viability. The most common threats to drug product stability are moisture (degradation via hydrolysis, increase in solid-state kinetics via mobility increases, or plasticization of drug product components via water) and/or oxygen (oxidation). Packaging protecting the drug product from moisture, such as desiccant inserts, or from oxygen, such as oxygen scavengers, can have a profound impact on the expiry date of the CTM. During FIH development, it is critical to probe the degradation mechanism that can affect the CTM, to enable the phase I dosing, but also to evaluate the longer-term viability of the NCE, including the packaging and storage conditions.

As indicated in the preceding sections, sponsor CMC personnel are well advised to stay current regarding developments in CTM quality guidelines from governmental agencies with jurisdiction applicable to the company's efforts in drug development and administration. Changes in guidances comprising the tripartite ICH: the FDA, the Ministry of Health, Labor, and Welfare of Japan, and the European Medicines Agency (EMEA)/Committee for Medicinal Products for Human Use (CHMP) are generally of greatest relevance. The globalization of both early phase CTM development and subsequent market authorization has been accompanied by a recognition that worldwide patient need is best served by a convergence of quality guidelines and test procedures. A current example of this effort is quality guideline Q4B, which is a series of evaluations and recommendations of pharmacopoeial texts for use in ICH regions [13]. At this time, the Q4B Expert Working Group is proceeding through a series of quality parameters and tests (e.g., disintegration, uniformity of dosage units, sterility), examining the associated tests in the pharmacopoeial text (the *United States Pharmacopoeia*, the *Japanese Pharmacopoeia*, and the *European Pharmacopoeia*), and submitting recommendations to regulatory authorities regarding test interchangeability in ICH jurisdictions. A recent (2009) example of this effort is publication in the U.S. *Federal Register* of a Q4B Guidance for Industry addressing microbial examination of nonsterile products [14]. In sum, it is advisable, to ensure safety, quality, and successful continuity of programs, for clinical trial sponsors to remain up to date with international CTM quality guidelines.

5.5.4 Placebos and Blinding

An important but often underappreciated area of CMC development is the provision of placebo and assurance of blinding. Placebo-controlled studies are the norm in nonclinical and clinical drug development, and pharmaceutical and analytical groups are usually tasked with providing the placebo article(s). A placebo for the purposes of early human studies is defined (source: *Stedman's Medical Dictionary*) as "An inactive substance or preparation used as a control in an experiment or test to determine the effectiveness of a medicinal drug." Table 5.7 gives some examples of possible placebos for early clinical trials.

TABLE 5.7 Examples of Placebos for Early Stage Clinical Trials

Dosage Form Type	Placebo Option(s)	Comments
Tablet	Compressed avicel or lactose, etc.	Same tools used as for the active tablets to minimize visual differences; match each unit's size, shape, etc.
Capsule	Gelatin or HPMC capsule bodies	Fill with lactose or other excipient for similar weight and handling as active-containing capsules
Injection, colorless	Dextrose, saline	Commercially available sterile injections
Injection, slight yellowish hue	Multivitamin concentrate, diluted with saline	Dilute to match visually to active solution; may need to use masking foil or other obscuring method (Note: MVI solution has a slight "vitamin B odor")
Oral suspension or solution	Bitrex (denatonium benzoate) in water, quinine	Bitrex is a potently bitter substance; the taste may be "differently unpleasant" from that of the active

General points about placebos and blinding are:

1. Best efforts should be put forth to provide a placebo that matches the active to the extent possible without compromising inertness. This can be reasonably simple in the case of tablets, for example, but blinding becomes more challenging in other cases (Table 5.7).
2. Labeling considerations include whether an unblinded investigator at a clinical study site can handle and dispense the drug product and placebos, or if elaborate kits that are blinded to participants in the field are needed to support double-blind studies.
3. Careful discussions of options with clinical groups are essential to ensure that appropriate expectations are set for the placebo effort; it is important to recognize and accept technical, practical, and safety limitations as to how well blinding can reasonably be done.

5.6 CMC STRATEGIC CONSIDERATIONS

5.6.1 Interactions Across Disciplines

It is critical to align CMC with the initial pharmacokinetic and safety objectives of the pre-FIH toxicity and the first clinical studies. Strategic alignment should be created early on items such as "what type of application to file, where," dose selection and projected range in phase I, the format(s) of dosing, and dose escalation schemes for advancing the clinical program (Chapters 10, 11, 13, and 14). Pharmaceutical development, with its deliverable of a dosage form to help meet clinical objectives, needs to be linked with clinical and regulatory planning. For example, selection of processes and technologies to prepare the drug product can influence both regulatory acceptance and the long-term prospects for delivering dosage form to pivotal studies, as well as ultimate registration and launch. Forward thinking is useful as always but need not constrain early efforts by introducing artificial requirements that are not aligned with the goal of initial safety evaluation in human volunteers. Analytical development, shelf life, and specifications need to be regarded as evolving and some flexibility is required, i.e., achieved through negotiation between analytical development, regulatory/CMC and quality assurance (QA) functions due to lack of batch experience at early stages. Finally, the relationship between the proposed dosage forms and the clinical protocol requires careful attention. In addition to understanding material requirements, labeling of the product and blinding, a sponsor needs to take care to answer questions whether the dosage form is suitable for use as provided or whether GCP-trained staff is required to modify the materials in any way at the clinical site, as this aspect may drive selection of countries and sites (Chapter 13).

Part of the innovation opportunity in any program lies in the integration of CMC aspects with discovery, nonclinical, and clinical insights. An evolving, scientifically driven co-optimization approach can lead to both elegant and innovative ways to deliver a compound and bring about pharmacokinetic or pharmacodynamic effects that are derived from a combination of molecular and material properties. Attention to possible synergies can provide a strategic advantage, especially where existing compounds are being studied for new uses. It is not the intent of this chapter to discuss patents and intellectual property. Suffice it to state that formulation and crystal form efforts have provided patentable inventions on a plethora of compounds in clinical use. Ongoing interactions between scientists and experienced patent attorneys are indicated in the event that a sponsor's strategy includes seeking protection by way of patents.

5.6.2 Outsourcing (and Insourcing) CMC Work

Sponsor companies, expanding business boundaries as have other industries in the mobile economy, are broadening the means by which pharmaceutical development and other components of drug development are achieved. Although a detailed discussion is beyond the scope of this chapter, the outsourcing topic deserves some comment, due to frequent application in contemporary development efforts. Outsourcing to CROs or other institutions implies the transfer of defined work to a vendor company, which is typically off-site, sometimes many time zones removed from the sponsor, and is independent of the compound sponsor company. Some considerations regarding outsourcing to CROs are described in Chapter 1. Insourcing is the hiring of a dedicated "resource" that is aligned with the internal operation on an ongoing and usually exclusive basis. For example, a dedicated full-time person is assigned to a sponsor's process chemistry effort across a number of compounds and over time. The desired outcome is the same: on-time delivery of a task or material to meet the requirements of a given study or program. The sponsor's major imperative is often to avoid fixed costs such as overhead or long-term headcount commitment, and to create a variable cost that acknowledges the business risk inherent in the endeavor of initiating a clinical program.

Main advantages of outsourcing are tighter management of fixed and variable resources, leading to optimization of cost. The disadvantages are generally increased time required to respond to unexpected or emerging data, a greater incidence of making decisions without all available information or observations, innovation risk, and quality management logistics. The risks can be mitigated, but generally only to a degree that still carries greater risk than keeping activities internal. If a compound is being evaluated as a component of a larger portfolio of projects, strategic outsourcing decisions can be made based on relative priority, tolerance for time line risk, capability gaps, and so on. Minimizing time line risk can depend on technical complexity as well as the priority in the vendor's schedule. Innovation risk is more difficult to quantify, but it relates to concern over the vendor's intentions as well as the sponsor being absent when "interesting," unusual, but relevant observations are made regarding the materials. It can be especially important to be able to tie together seemingly disparate aspects related to complex synthetic or formulation problems.

Quality management is ultimately the gatekeeper to the use of a material slated for human studies. Significant quality systems need to be in place at the vendor and sponsor to accomplish the ultimate goal of getting a compound into a study that meets regulatory requirements. As a general matter for CMC outsourcing, a sponsor is well advised to have access to two strong and accountable persons to counsel on the outsourcing subject: a CMC sciences expert (with API and formulation experience) and a quality assurance professional experienced in CMC and current with respect to cGMPs.

5.7 CASE STUDIES

Examples often inform thinking and approach for future projects as much as general information. Two case studies are presented in this section to illustrate (1) interconnections and synergy of CMC support with discovery, nonclinical, and early clinical efforts; (2) the value of solid-state form selection to ultimate product definition, and (3) opportunities to build in quality through good science at the early development stage.

5.7.1 Indinavir

The HIV protease inhibitor indinavir (Figure 5.3) was approved in 1996 and remains a mainstay of HIV therapy, as part of combination regimens. Merck markets the drug under the tradename Crixivan. The history of the discovery and early development of this compound was published by Lin et al. [15]. First, their paper is an excellent account of the iterations and interactions that are frequently

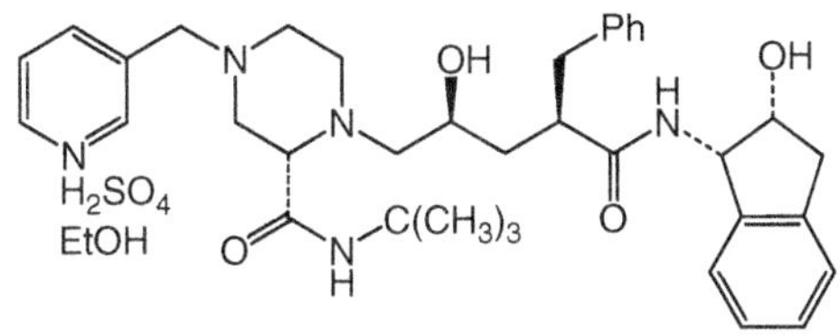

FIGURE 5.3 Chemical structure of indinavir sulfate ethanolate solvate, the HIV protease inhibitor active agent in Crixivan.

needed to solve the challenge of NCE selection. Second, the CMC aspect is integrated into the discussion of the lead generation process and early clinical evaluation of indinavir. Although the physical properties of the compound are not ideal, the benefits achieved by making this crystalline salt form proved vital to the success of formulation development and ultimate commercialization of Crixivan.

The key issues for early clinical evaluation were (1) significant first-pass metabolism of candidates and (2) low aqueous solubility and lack of oral bioavailability in animals, which led to limited availability of appropriate formulation options. Both the poor absorption and extensive metabolism properties can be related to the structure of the leads and the target itself, which is an aspartyl protease. Earliest leads were peptides (e.g., Boc-protected Phe-Phe linked to a hydrophobic γ-amino acid core capped with an N-terminal Leu-Phe-NH_2; L-365,505). Iteration to produce L-689,502, a less-peptidelike compound with a morpholine base appendage, gave the first instance of a compound that elicited some bioavailability in dogs and thus was an important milestone in the program. The quest for a candidate suitable for a GLP toxicology program eventually led to L-735,524 (MK-869; indinavir), which showed pharmacokinetic properties in dogs that exceeded the closest contenders by an order of magnitude or more. However, methyl cellulose suspensions of the crystalline free base gave low and variable oral bioavailability in animals. Nonetheless, the balanced hydrophobic/hydrophilic properties (log P of 2.92), adequate solubility at pH 7.4 (0.02 mg/mL at room temperature) and opportunities to create high-solubility salts due to the presence of a pair of basic functions in the molecule provided the optimal overall profile for a clinical candidate. In fact, acidic solutions of indinavir (in situ salt solutions) gave high exposures in animals and thus allowed the candidate to proceed to further evaluation.

The toxicology program for indinavir was facilitated by the use of acidic solutions using a pharmaceutically acceptable acid. The solutions were sufficiently stable to chemical degradation to allow the GLP program to proceed, but instability and bitter taste were factors that eliminated the option of an oral solution product for long-term clinical study and marketed formulation. A critical event for the program was the discovery of the crystalline sulfate salt (chemical composition in Figure 5.3). This breakthrough came as the culmination of significant joint effort of medicinal chemistry and the CMC chemist. Some key properties of indinavir sulfate ethanolate are listed in Table 5.8.

TABLE 5.8 Properties of Indinavir Sulfate Ethanolate, the Crystalline Drug Substance in Crixivan

Property	Observations	Comments
Form	Monosulfate, ethanolate	>99% purity; ethanol is part of the structure; if removed or exchanged for water, crystallinity is lost
Solubility	>500 mg/mL (pH < 3); 0.02 mg/mL (pH > 7; base compound)	Strong pH dependence of solubility translates to pH-dependent absorption; important to ensure acidic gastrointestinal environment to achieve highest possible exposures
Pharmacokinetics	Same as for other acidic solutions	Oral bioavailability of acidic solutions significantly better in dogs and humans than with free base
Moisture sorption	Hygroscopic above 40% relative humidity at room temperature; chemical instability at high % relative humidity	Challenge for handling, manufacture, storage; pharmacokinetics outweighs this consideration, so the production of Crixivan takes into account the requirement for low % relative humidity during all handling of the compound
Processability	Incompatible with water, due to instability	Absolute requirement for dry processing of the salt to maintain chemical and physical stability
Long-term stability	Room-temperature storage achieved	Desiccated powder (drug substance) and gelatin capsules in bottles (drug product) provided

The pH-dependent oral absorption of indinavir was well characterized and the understanding proved vital to the toxicology program as well as the clinical evaluation and ultimate labeling. Dogs were chosen as the nonrodent toxicology species, and it is well known that dogs that are fasted—as is generally the case in chronic dosing—have very limited acid output and thus have high stomach pH. For indinavir, this condition led to low and variable oral bioavailability of a solid form, except when the intrinsically acidic sulfate salt was used. In humans, the HIV condition is known to be associated with high stomach pH (achlorhydria is thought to affect about a third of the patient population). Once again, the acidic sulfate salt obviates a concern over lack of performance of a solid dosage form in such patients. As for the impact on labeling, an interaction with gastric acid–reducing drugs is required.

The Crixivan story provides a remarkable example of the power of strong interactions of discovery with ADME and CMC experts. Although early studies with the compound were made possible by the short-term formulation option of an acidified aqueous solution, the advent of the crystalline sulfate salt unlocked the option of extensive efficacy studies and ultimately, development of a marketable solid dosage form. For a decade after its introduction, Crixivan capsule was the simplest and arguably most elegant dosage form in the HIV protease inhibitor class. The value or early interdisciplinary collaboration to enable this product is evident.

5.7.2 Doxorubicin Peptide Conjugate

A published example of an injectable compound designed to treat prostate cancer illustrates further the impact of CMC expertise on compound selection. The choice of the injection route places a greater emphasis on solubility and formulation than do most oral drug candidate programs. Although the compound is not approved and there is not yet an integrated review of the type that was written for indinavir, the case study of the doxorubicin peptide conjugates can be constructed from three literature references [16–18]. Doxorubicin is a known cytotoxic agent, and is also known as adriamycin. The structure of the compound evaluated in patients is shown schematically in Figure 5.4.

The discovery effort focused on the consensus sequence on the peptide that would allow the targeting of PSA (prostate-specific antigen) [16]. The essential requirement for this approach to succeed is that PSA is active principally at the target site (tumor) and is not significantly active in the systemic circulation. In this way, cleavage of the doxorubicin (Dox) peptide conjugate would be essentially restricted to the diseased tissue. The potent cytotoxics in the molecule were assigned as Dox (see the left-hand box in Figure 5.4 and Leu-Dox (representing one C-terminal amino acid remaining linked to the amine of doxorubicin). Residual concern over distribution of cleaved material out of the tumor and into the circulation cannot be allayed, but full evaluation of the dose-limiting toxicity in patients would shed light on the impact of the proposed targeting on the tolerability profile.

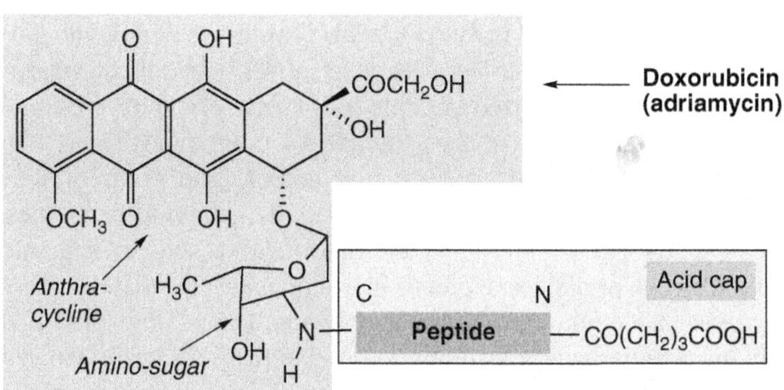

FIGURE 5.4 Structures of doxorubicin peptide conjugates discovered at Merck Research Laboratories.

Garsky et al. [16] outline the general design principles. The amine function of Dox was acylated with a series of peptides and key properties of cytotoxicity in PSA-expressing and nonexpressing cell lines were characterized. Initial compounds contained long peptides (>8 residues) based on consensus sequences from semenogelin I, a key seminal fluid protein that served as a design guide for medicinal chemistry. The amine terminus of the peptides was generally amidated ($-CONH_2$) or acetylated ($-COCH_3$). In either case, the basic function of Dox and the overall peptide conjugate was eliminated. The impact of this lack of ionizable function became important when the team approached the NCE stage.

Doxorubicin HCl is a well-behaved material from the pharmaceutical perspective: It has high aqueous solubility, good stability, and is suitable for injection formulations. The compound is, however, toxic to the heart, and injection-site adverse events are also quite serious, as the compound is necrotic. Due to its cytotoxic nature, doxorubicin is a PBOEL class 4 agent and must be handled with great care and containment in the laboratory as well as in manufacturing [19]. In the absence of data, the peptide conjugates had to be assumed to possess similar toxicity.

Given the prodrug targeting strategy in this case, the medicinal chemistry effort required significant metabolism input; hence, Garsky et al. [16] describe the comparison of metabolic $t_{1/2}$ and EC_{50} potency and selectivity (vs. a non-PSA-secreting cell type). Additionally, some preliminary estimates of maximum tolerated dose (MTD) were generated in rats. Pharmaceutical chemistry input was provided regarding chemical stability in solution, but material limitations hampered the assessment of material properties of solid-state compounds. Once tens of milligrams became available, it was clear that the preparation of a non-ionizable conjugate (e.g., with acetyl groups capping the peptide N-termini) led to very water-insoluble aggregates. Although these solid materials were poorly crystalline by physical techniques, they were nevertheless stable and difficult to solubilize in pharmaceutically acceptable vehicles. Lack of an ionizing group meant that pH dependence of solubility was negligible and that no salt form could be made to attempt a solubility enhancement for an intravenous formulation.

The successful drug candidate from this program is a compound represented by the structure in Figure 5.4. In Garsky et al. [16] this is compound 27: glutaryl-Hyp-Ala-Ser-Chg-Gln-Ser-Leu-Dox. Karki et al. [17] detail the pharmaceutical properties, which are summarized in Table 5.9. The key benefit of using the diacid capping agent (glutaric acid, in the example of compound 27) is the aqueous solubility gained for the ionized form, the sodium salt form of the prodrug, without a negative impact on the biological and metabolic properties. Having the option to deliver a simple aqueous solution of a sodium salt instead of a complex mixture of organic excipients in water made the conduct of all safety studies (human and nonhuman) considerably more appealing than if a number of solubilizing agents had been required. A contrast can be drawn with Taxol, which uses a complex vehicle and reconstitution process at the time of use (see the product label insert for this important cancer drug). Risk and benefit evaluation is essential in any case, and for the situation where an NCE was to be selected based

TABLE 5.9 Properties of Doxorubicin Peptide Conjugate 27

Property	Observations	Comments
Form	Sodium salt, weak crystallinity	Anhydrous material, chemically distinct and >95% pure
Solubility	>150 mg/mL (pH 5.6); 3 mg/mL (pH < 4; free acid compound)	Strong pH dependence of solubility, with sodium salt being sufficiently soluble for formulation development
Pharmacokinetics	Linear PK with intravenous formulation	Sterile formulation: aseptically filtered solution at 40 mg/mL drug; citrate and sucrose inactive ingredients
Moisture sorption	Hygroscopic above 70% relative humidity at room temperature; instability at high % relative humidity	Minor challenge for handling, manufacture, storage; No specific requirement for control of % relative humidity during handling of the compound as a drug substance
Processability	Salt conversion to lyophilizate viable	Karki et al. [17] describe the development of a lyophilized formulation for phase II and beyond
Long-term stability	Room-temperature storage achieved	Desiccated powder (drug substance) and lyophilized powder (drug product) developed

Source: Adapted from [16].

on a problematic anthracycline such as doxorubicin, it was ultimately beneficial to incorporate water solubility as a criterion and thus simplify the formulation approach.

Clinical evaluation of the compound proceeded with a lyophilized version of the solution that was provided for GLP toxicology. The composition and process design is described by Karki et al. [17]. As an example of anticipatory design, the intravenous formulation for toxicology evaluation included sucrose, as this ingredient was shown early to be useful for a putative lyophilized formulation. Citrate was also used as a buffer in both cases, as it was important to maintain good pH control in the injection regardless of concentration, handling, storage etc. (Inclusion of buffer in injectable products is highly recommended in any situation). In summary, the composition for GLP and GMP manufacture was the same, and hence no bridging GLP work was required to gain approval to test the compound in refractory patients. Important conclusions drawn in DiPaola et al. [18] were that (1) pharmacokinetics is linear up to an MTD of 315 mg/m^2, (2) metabolites included Dox and Leu-Dox as expected, (3) neutropenia was the dose-limiting toxicity, and (4) a clinical response was seen below the MTD, supporting further evaluation of the compound.

The case studies here are but two examples where the investigators had ready access to the information and insights required to put the story together with the inclusion of CMC considerations, which often are obscure in these examples. It is our hope that future publications will succeed in describing amalgams of effort from nonclinical and clinical groups that include the CMC component, especially when the input has affected the design and development of a drug candidate.

5.8 EVOLUTION OF DRUG DEVELOPMENT: IMPLICATIONS FOR CMCs IN THE FUTURE

At the beginning of the twenty-first century, the pharmaceutical research and development enterprise worldwide is suffering a productivity crisis. Approximate doubling of drug research and development expenditure over the last decade has not led to anticipated gains in innovation and associated value in terms of novel compounds and treatments. A recent review and projection was published by PricewaterhouseCoopers in 2007 [20]. An adaptation of one of the figures presented is shown in Figure 5.5. The prognosis for the next decade is for an

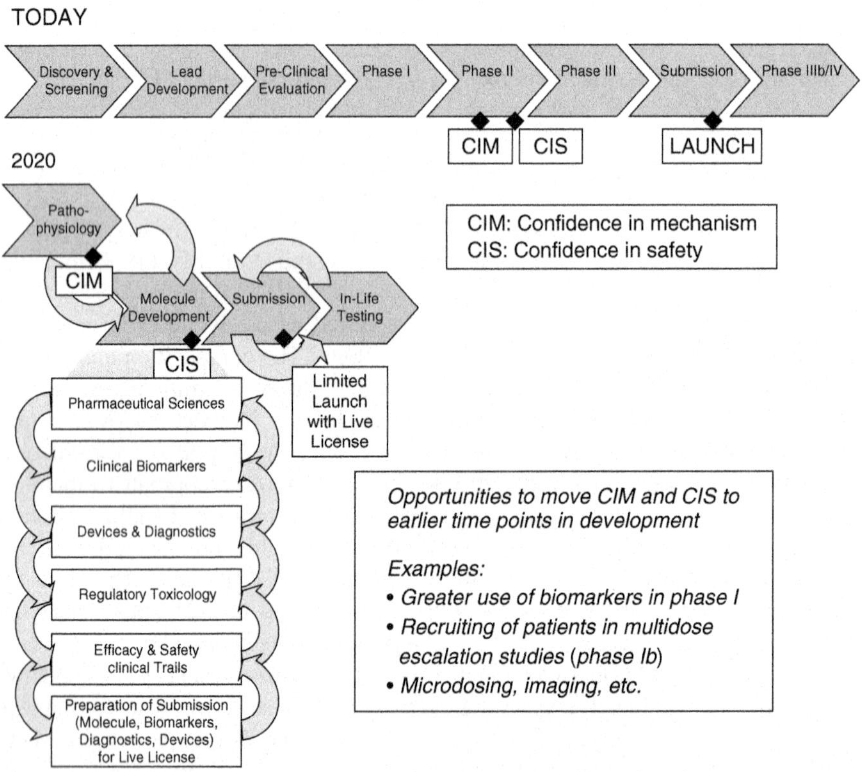

FIGURE 5.5 Drug development scenarios at the beginning of the twenty-first century. (Adapted from the PricewaterhouseCoopers 2007 report: "Pharma 2020: The Vision. Which Path Will You Take?")

evolution toward sharper focus on the key milestones of confidence in mechanism (CIM) and subsequently confidence in safety (CIS), in favor of sharp regulatory specification of the process. For example, such traditional mileposts of development as phase IIa may in some cases be moved earlier and into phase I, to intersect or overlap with initial safety testing in volunteers. Put another way, volunteer studies may have more frequent inclusion of disease populations. Such shifting and overlap of studies is highly target specific, but one can see the strategic implications of narrowing or eliminating gaps between studies, to the point of creating significant acceleration. The impact will be felt in nonclinical work, where GLP toxicology and other mechanistic work needs to keep pace with the duration of human testing of the compound, and in the CMC process, where in providing supplies for various uses and planning for critical registration studies, the dosage form must be locked in to allow regulatory review and discussion of the CMC aspects.

An alternative, more specific viewpoint on early development was provided by the Chorus initiative, which was built within Eli Lilly with the goal to rapidly advance non-core assets (e.g. discovery compounds with uncertain pathways of development) to proof-of-principle in humans [21]. The general idea of Chorus is to identify and answer the key question on a given project. In this way, when an experiment is successful, the risk reduction per unit of cost is maximized. If the experiment fails or otherwise proves that a project is not viable, cost has been minimized to get to this answer. On occasion, CMC is a limiting issue, but most frequently the burning question relates to performance and pharmacological validity in humans—hence, the drive must be to get data in humans as fast as possible with a minimal formulation in most cases. The "truth-seeking" approach of Chorus to managing early development has merit, but the main caveat is that there must at all times be clear understanding and communication of risks that are being absorbed—be the risks in CMC, nonclinical, regulatory, or clinical.

CMC is invariably and increasingly a parallel development activity, which in the early development corridor is focused on gaining scientific insight and developing batch history. Process capabilities are largely unknown at the time of initiation of the first GMP batch of drug substance, and the challenge for the nonclinical research and development groups is to integrate information in real time to begin creating the physical image, for both drug substance and drug product. In later stages of development, post CIM or at CIS in the vernacular of PricewaterhouseCoopers, the focus shifts to locking in the attributes of the product and executing on the delivery of supplies and the documentation that will be required for ultimate market authorization applications.

RESOURCES

- FDA Web site: www.fda.gov; includes list of excipients in drug products (identity only), and provides links to the CFRs.

- cGMP and GLP regulations: part of 21 CFR and accessible through the FDA Web site.
- ICH guidelines (list and Web sources): www.ich.org.
- Pharmacopeias: *United States Pharmacopeia, National Formulary* (U.S.), *European Pharmacopeia*, and *Japanese Pharmacopeia*; available in hard copy and some electronically. Contents include monographs of drug substances and excipients for use in drug products, as well as test methods and references.
- *Merck Index*, 14th edition (2006) and electronic version (CD). Essential information on a large number of compounds: www.merckbooks.com/mindex/index.html.
- *Analytical Profiles of Drug Substances and Excipients*. Founding editor Klaus Florey, current editor Harry G. Brittain. Academic Press, San Diego, CA, Vol. 26, 1999. Includes the monographs for citric acid and indinavir sulfate, for example.
- *Handbook of Pharmaceutical Excipients*, 3rd ed. Ed. H. Kibbe. Pharmaceutical Press, London, 2000.
- *Handbook of Injectable Drugs*, 14th ed. Ed. L. A. Trissel. American Society for Hospital Pharmacists, Bethesda, MD, 2007.
- *Excipient Toxicity and Safety*. Ed. M. L. Weiner and L. A. Kotkoskie. Marcel Dekker, New York, 2000.
- *Handbook of Pharmaceutical Additives*. Compiled by M. Ash and I. Ash. Gower, VT, 1997.
- *Rational Design of Stable Protein Formulations: Theory and Practice*. J. F. Carpenter and M. C. Manning. Vol. 13 in *Pharmaceutical Biotechnology*, series ed. R. Borchardt. Kluwer Academic/Plenum Publishers, New York, 2002.
- *Integration of Pharmaceutical Discovery and Development: Case Histories*. R. T. Borchardt, R. M. Freidinger, T. K. Sawyer, P. L. Smith. Series ed. R. Borchardt. Kluwer Academic/Plenum Publishers, New York, 1998. This volume contains an integrated review of indinavir discovery and early development.
- *Ansel's Pharmaceutical Dosage Forms and Drug Delivery Systems*, 8th ed. L.V. Allen, Jr., N. G. Popovich, H. C. Ansel. Lippincott, Williams & Wilkins, Chicago, 2005.
- *Oral Drug Absorption: Prediction and Assessment*. J. B. Dressman and H. Lennernas. Marcel Dekker, New York, 2000.
- *Gastrointestinal Physiology*, 6th ed. L. R. Johnson, Mosby (an affiliate of Elsevier), St. Louis, MO, 2001.
- DEREK program: Genotoxicity ranking based on chemical structures: www.lhasalimited.org.

REFERENCES

1. Gardner CR, Walsh CT, Almarsson Ö. Drugs as materials: valuing physical form in drug discovery. *Nat Rev Drug Discov*. 2004;3(11):926–934.
2. Liu R, ed. *Water-Insoluble Drug Formulation*, 2nd ed. Boca Raton, FL: CRC Press; 2008.
3. Clas S-D, Faizer R, O'Connor RE, Vadas EB. Assessment of the physical stability of lyophilized MK-0591 by differential scanning calorimetry. *Thermochim Acta*. 1996;288(1–2):83–96.
4. European patent EP0658103. Beads having a core coated with an antifungal and a polymer. Assigned to Janssen Pharmaceutica N.V., Nov. 20, 1996.
5. Bernstein J. *Polymorphism of Molecular Crystals*. New York: Oxford University Press; 2002.
6. Stahl PH, Wermuth CG, Eds. *Handbook of Pharmaceutical Salts: Properties, Selection, and Use*. Weimar, TX: C.H.I.P.S. Books; 2008.
7. FDA regulation 21 CFR Part 58, Section 105 (test and control article characterization).
8. Guidance for Industry: Current Good Manufacturing Practice for Phase 1 Investigational Drugs. U.S. Department of Health and Human Services, Food and Drug Administration; 2008.
9. 21 CFR Parts 210 and 211.
10. Genotoxicity Task Force White Paper on Establishment of Allowable Concentrations of Genotoxic Impurities in Drug Substance and Product. PhRMA; 2005 (*Regul Toxicol Pharmacol*. 2006). Guidance for Industry and Review Staff: Recommended Approaches to Integration of Genotoxic Study Data. U.S. Department of Health and Human Services, Food and Drug Administration; Jan. 2006.
11. ICH Quality Guideline: Impurities in New Drug Products. ICH Q3B (R2). International Conference on Harmonization; 2006. Available at: www.ich.org.
12. 2.2.1.P.8 of Guideline on the Requirements to the Chemical and Pharmaceutical Quality Documentation Concerning Investigational Medicinal Products in Clinical Trials. Committee for Medicinal Products for Human Use; 2006.
13. ICH Quality Guideline: Evaluation and Recommendation of Pharmacopoeial Texts for Use in the ICH Regions. ICH Q4B. International Conference on Harmonization; 2007. Available at: www.ich.org.
14. *Federal Register*. 2009; 74(66):15992–15993. Available at: www.fda.gov/cder/Guidance/8669fnl.pdf, and www.fda.gov/cder/guidance/7386dft.htm.
15. Lin JH, Ostovic D, Vacca JP. The integration of medicinal chemistry, drug metabolism, and pharmaceutical research and development in drug discovery and development: the story of Crixivan, an HIV protease inhibitor. *Pharm Biotechnol*. 1998;11:233–255.
16. Garsky VM et al. The synthesis of a prodrug of doxorubicin designed to provide reduced systemic toxicity and greater target efficacy. *J Med Chem*. 2001;44(24):4216–4224.

17. Karki SB et al. Design of an IV formulation of an unstable prodrug candidate for prostate cancer treatment: solution chemistry of *N*-(glutaryl-hyp-ala-ser-cyclohexylglycyl-gln-ser-leu)-doxorubicin. *Drug Dev Ind Pharm*. 2006;32(3):327–334.
18. DiPaola RS et al. Characterization of a novel prostate-specific antigen-activated peptide–doxorubicin conjugate in patients with prostate cancer. *J Clin Oncol*. 2002;20(7):1874–1879.
19. The PB-OEL classification system is outlined in: Naumann BD, Sargent EV, Starkman BS, Fraser WJ, Becker GT, Kirk GD. Performance-based exposure control limits for pharmaceutical active ingredients. *Am Ind Hyg Assoc J*. 1996;57(1):33–42.
20. Pharma 2020: The Vision. Which Path Will You Take? PricewaterhouseCoopers report. 2007.
21. Bonabeau E, Bodick N, Armstrong RW. A more rational approach to new-product development. *Harvard Bus Rev*. Mar. 2008.
22. Connors K, Amidon G, Stella V. *Chemical Stability of Pharmaceuticals: A Handbook for Pharmacists*, 2nd ed. New York: Wiley; 1986.
23. Florey K, ed. *Analytical Profiles of Drug Substances*, Vol. 9. New York: Academic Press; 1980:87–106.
24. Brittain HG, ed. *Analytical Profiles of Drug Substances*, Vol. 26. New York: Academic Press; 1999:319–357.

6

NONCLINICAL SAFETY PHARMACOLOGY STUDIES RECOMMENDED FOR SUPPORT OF FIRST-IN-HUMAN CLINICAL TRIALS

DUANE B. LAKINGS

6.1 INTRODUCTION AND OVERVIEW

Nonclinical studies conducted to investigate and characterize the pharmacological profile of new chemical entities (NCEs), either small organic molecules or macromolecules, are frequently classified as follows:

1. Primary pharmacodynamics or pharmacology studies within in vitro systems or animal models that are designed to investigate the mechanism or mode of action of an NCE and to define the pharmacological profile of various doses of an NCE administered to animals using the projected clinical route of administration. *Mechanism of action* is defined as the specific biochemical interaction through which an NCE produces a pharmacological effect and usually includes mention of the specific molecular target, such as an enzyme or receptor, to which the NCE binds. *Mode of action* is defined as the means by which an NCE achieves an intended therapeutic effect or action.
2. Secondary pharmacodynamics or pharmacology studies designed to explore and evaluate the broader pharmacological activity of an NCE that may arise from additional actions of an NCE unrelated to its primary mode or mechanism of action.

Early Drug Development: Strategies and Routes to First-in-Human Trials, Edited by Mitchell N. Cayen

3. Safety pharmacology or studies designed to investigate and evaluate potential undesirable pharmacodynamic effects of an NCE on physiological functions in various organ systems at exposures within and higher than the expected therapeutic range (defined during primary pharmacodynamic studies on an NCE).

During drug discovery and early drug development, most sponsors will conduct pharmacology studies on an NCE in each of these areas. The results should be documented in study reports and summaries of the results prepared for inclusion in a regulatory agency submission for the first-in-human (FIH) clinical trial on an NCE. Primary and secondary pharmacodynamic studies do not need to be conducted in compliance with good laboratory practice (GLP) regulations. The safety pharmacology core battery (discussed later) should ordinarily be conducted in compliance with GLP regulations. Supplemental (discussed below) and follow-up safety pharmacology studies on an NCE (which are usually conducted after clinical trials have been initiated) should also be conducted in compliance with GLP regulations to the greatest extent feasible. Safety pharmacology assessments that are part of toxicology studies on an NCE would also be conducted in compliance with GLP regulations.

The results from safety pharmacology studies on an NCE are used to guide and define the starting dose for the FIH clinical trial and to establish possible stopping criteria for the initial clinical studies. These safety pharmacology studies also provide possible guidance on potential adverse events for which monitoring in clinical trials is appropriate and warranted. Results from safety pharmacology studies can also assist in the understanding of toxicological findings identified during nonclinical toxicology studies and in humans during clinical trials.

The design and conduct of nonclinical safety pharmacology studies are defined in the International Conference on Harmonisation (ICH) S7a guideline [1] entitled "Safety Pharmacology Studies for Human Pharmaceuticals" that was introduced in 2001. Additional information, including timing in relationship to clinical trials, on safety pharmacology studies for small organic molecules is available in the ICH M3 guideline [2] entitled "Nonclinical Safety Studies for the Conduct of Human Clinical Trials for Pharmaceuticals" and for many macromolecules, in the ICH S6 guideline [3] entitled "Preclinical Safety Evaluation of Biotechnology-Derived Pharmaceuticals." Thus, prior to an FIH trial, the sponsor of an NCE is expected to complete the ICH S7a recommended core battery (central nervous, cardiovascular, and respiratory system assessments) and possibly some of the supplemental battery (renal/urinary, autonomic nervous, gastrointestinal, and other system) studies to investigate and characterize the safety pharmacology profile of an NCE. For each of the three primary ICH regions (United States, European Union, and Japan) and for most other countries throughout the world, these safety pharmacology assessments are expected to have been completed prior to the initiation of clinical trials on an NCE, and the results are to be summarized and the study reports included in submissions to the regulatory authority in the country where the FIH trial is to be conducted.

An additional nonclinical ICH guideline [4] entitled "Safety Pharmacology Studies for Assessing the Potential for Delayed Ventricular Repolarization (QT Interval Prolongation) by Human Pharmaceuticals" (ICH S7b guideline) was finalized in 2005. Unless other results indicate a substantial potential for adverse effects to the cardiovascular system, the safety pharmacology studies recommended in ICH S7b are not conducted prior to the FIH clinical trial on an NCE but are performed concurrently with clinical testing. Copies of these guidelines can be obtained at the ICH Web site (www.ich.org).

The specific program of safety pharmacology studies considered necessary to support an FIH trial on an NCE depends on a number of factors, which include, but are not limited to, the disease indication, the route of administration, and the pharmacokinetic profile of the NCE. In general and as noted above, most sponsors will need to have completed the standard battery of safety pharmacology studies to support an FIH clinical trial conducted in any ICH region or other country. However, and is the case for many drug development programs, exceptions are common. For some life-threatening diseases for which no therapeutic agents are available, fast track development of an NCE is the norm, and safety pharmacology assessments can often be delayed (but not eliminated) until after the clinical development program on the NCE has been initiated. For some routes of administration, such as dermal or ocular, where absorption into systemic circulation is not necessary, desirable, or observed for treatment of the disease, safety pharmacology assessments are not warranted since the target organ systems will not be exposed to the NCE or its metabolites. On the other hand, some supplemental safety pharmacology evaluations may be necessary for an NCE administered orally where adverse gastrointestinal effects may occur or for an NCE cleared from the body primarily by the kidney, which may lead to adverse effects on the renal system. The sponsor of an NCE should design the safety pharmacology study package to effectively characterize the safety profile of the drug candidate in each organ system that potentially might be affected adversely when exposed to the NCE and/or its metabolites.

Understanding the safety pharmacology associated with a new or existing disease target has significant potential for reducing failure during later nonclinical and clinical development of an NCE. Furthermore, the design of the pre-FIH safety pharmacology program should be influenced by an understanding of the disease target [both distribution (where the target is located in body and the extent of expression in those locations) and function in the body] and not simply through fulfillment of safety pharmacology studies recommended in ICH S7a. Mechanistic understanding of the entire pharmacological profile of an NCE will probably provide a better understanding of risk–benefit in humans. For example, the target for an NCE designed to treat a central nervous system (CNS) disease or disorder will be expressed in a particular region of the CNS system. However, the target may also be expressed in other CNS regions where interactions with the NCE could lead to undesirable CNS effects. Thus, CNS safety pharmacology studies are necessary to evaluate these potential undesirable interactions. In addition, the CNS target could also be expressed in other organ systems, such as the cardiovascular system or the renal system, and interaction with the target in these organ systems could also lead to undesirable effects, which can be discovered and characterized by appropriately designed safety pharmacology assessments. Thus, understanding how an NCE interacts with its target and where in the body that target is expressed are important aspects to be considered when designing the safety pharmacology package necessary for supporting an FIH trial and later clinical development of the candidate drug.

The history of these types (i.e., safety pharmacology evaluations) of pre-FIH studies is not discussed in this chapter. This history has been documented in at least one book [5] and summarized in a number of book chapters, including two by this author [6,7]. In general, the need for safety pharmacology assessments was recognized during the 1970s, when toxicological evaluations of NCEs (mostly small organic molecules, since macromolecules, with the exception of insulin, were not being developed as therapeutic agents at that time) were insensitive for detecting many of the severe pharmacodynamic properties that were ultimately detected during clinical development. During the 1980s, many sponsors initiated safety pharmacology evaluations on NCEs, but the study protocols and the selection of organ systems to be evaluated did not follow a systematic approach. In the early 1990s, regulatory agencies throughout the world recognized the need for specific guidelines for evaluating the safety pharmacology profiles of drug candidates. Thus, both the sponsors of NCEs and regulatory agencies were involved in the design and development of the ICH S7a guideline that was implemented in 2001. An important topic that was not fully addressed in the ICH S7a guideline was the effect of an NCE on cardiac ventricular repolarization, which is considered as a surrogate biomarker for *torsades de pointes* proarrhythmic risk. To address this topic, ICH S7b was designed and implemented in 2005.

This chapter describes various study designs that the sponsor of an NCE may adapt for evaluating the pre-FIH safety pharmacology profile of a drug candidate. Since the development of an NCE may require unique and specific assessments to fully define and provide understanding of the potentially adverse effects of an NCE on the various organ systems, the study designs outlined in this chapter should be used only as templates and not as final designs.

6.2 TIMING OF SAFETY PHARMACOLOGY STUDIES

The following statement is contained in the ICH M3 guideline with regard to a small organic molecule NCE.

> Safety pharmacology includes the assessment of effects on vital functions, such as cardiovascular, central nervous and respiratory systems, and these should be evaluated prior to human exposure. These evaluations may be conducted as addition to toxicity studies or as separate studies.

The ICH S6 guideline contains the following statement with regard to safety pharmacology studies on biopharmaceuticals or macromolecules.

> It is important to investigate the potential for undesirable pharmacological activity in appropriate animal models and, where necessary, to incorporate particular monitoring for these activities in the toxicity studies and/or clinical studies. Safety pharmacology studies measure functional indices of potential toxicity. These functional indices may be investigated in separate studies or incorporated in the design of toxicity studies. The aim of the safety pharmacology studies should be to reveal any functional effects on the major physiological systems (e.g., cardiovascular, respiratory, renal, and central nervous systems). Investigations may also include the use of isolated organs or other test systems not involving intact animals. All of these studies may allow for a mechanistically-based explanation of specific organ toxicities, which should be considered carefully with respect to human use and indication(s).

The ICH S7a guideline contains the following statement with regards to the timing of safety pharmacology studies on an NCE.

> The effects of a test substance on the functions listed in the safety pharmacology core battery should be investigated prior to first administration in humans. Any follow-up or supplemental studies identified as appropriate, based on a cause for concern, should also be conducted. Information from toxicology studies adequately designed and conducted to address safety pharmacology endpoints can result in reduction or elimination of separate safety pharmacology studies.

Thus, each of these guidelines recommends that safety pharmacology be conducted early in the drug development process so that the results can be available to assist in the design and interpretation of results from toxicity studies and in the design of the FIH trial.

Although most safety pharmacology studies do not include an assessment of plasma exposure (or toxicokinetics) to an NCE, the pharmacokinetic profile of an NCE in the animal species to be employed for a given safety pharmacology study can be highly beneficial in the design of the study. Thus, sponsors should consider conducting preliminary pharmacokinetic studies in each animal species to be used in safety pharmacology studies (and in toxicology studies) and over the proposed dose range to be evaluated in those studies. The route of administration for these preliminary pharmacokinetic studies should be the proposed clinical route of administration and be intravenous, if feasible (which may not be possible for some NCEs, particularly those with limited aqueous solubility where intravenous administration of the NCE may result in precipitation in the blood). The results provide important information on the rate and extent of absorption (for a nonintravenous route of administration), which when compared to the extent of exposure after intravenous dosing determines the absolute bioavailability of the NCE, and the plasma disposition profile, which determines how long the NCE stays in the body (Chapter 2). These pharmacokinetic profiles on an NCE can be used to determine the optimal assessment times for safety pharmacology studies. For an NCE with a relatively short terminal disposition half-life, assessments shortly after dosing (i.e., 1 to 2 h) would be important.

However, for an NCE with a relatively prolonged terminal disposition phase, assessments should be made shortly after dosing and at later times (i.e., 6, 8, 12, or even 24 h after dosing), when the NCE has had a chance to distribute into various organ systems and is now slowly being cleared from the body. To obtain these pharmacokinetic profiles, a developed and appropriately validated bioanalytical chemistry (BAC) method is necessary (Chapter 4). For most small organic molecules, the development of such a BAC method for the quantification of an NCE in plasma is usually relatively uncomplicated. However for biopharmaceutics, a BAC method commonly requires the generation of antibodies, and the development time is long, which usually prevents the generation of preliminary pharmacokinetic results on these NCEs. Sponsors of biopharmaceuticals need to take this into consideration when designing safety pharmacology (and toxicity) studies with these drug candidates.

Some sponsors include toxicokinetic assessments as a part of safety pharmacology evaluations. As noted earlier, safety pharmacology studies are expected to be conducted in compliance with GLP regulations. Thus, assessments of exposure for these studies should also be conducting in compliance with GLP regulations, which requires that the BAC methods be validated appropriately (Chapter 4).

6.3 CNS SAFETY PHARMACOLOGY

Parameters commonly evaluated during CNS safety pharmacology studies include motor activity, behavioral changes, coordination, sensory/motor reflex responses, and body temperature. Following single-dose administration to rats, the Irwin's test is commonly used to identify any possible gross effects of an NCE on a battery of behavioral and physiological parameters, covering the main central and peripheral nervous system functions. Table 6.1 presents a standard study design for the Irwin's test in rats [8]. During the Irwin's test, a number of clinical signs are evaluated to determine if an NCE has a potential adverse effect on various CNS functions or profiles, such as the behavior profile (awareness, mood, motor activity, motor incoordination), neurological profile (central excitation, muscle tone, body posture, refluxes), and autonomic profile. Table 6.2 summarizes the various clinical signs and the observation conditions.

6.4 CARDIOVASCULAR SAFETY PHARMACOLOGY

6.4.1 Study Designs

Prior to conducting in vivo cardiovascular safety pharmacology studies, many sponsors conduct an in vitro study to evaluate the potential of an NCE to inhibit hERG (human ether-a-go-go related gene) [9–11]. The hERG gene encodes a potassium (K^+) ion channel responsible for the repolarizing current in the cardiac action potential. Abnormalities in this channel may lead to either long- or short-QT syndrome, both of which are potentially fatal cardiac arrhythmias

TABLE 6.1 Standard Study Design for CNS Safety Pharmacology (Irwin's Test) in Rats

Parameter	Specification
Species, strain, gender	Rats, Sprague–Dawley or Wistar; commonly, only males used, but males and females should be evaluated if gender differences have been noted for an NCE. The choice of rat strain should be based on the proposed strain to be used in toxicology studies, which in turn can depend on geographical area and the availability of animals. When gender differences for an NCE are observed in pharmacological response, pharmacokinetic profile, or other parameters, both males and females should be evaluated.
Age at initiation of treatment	Approximately 8 to 9 weeks.
Approximate body weight range at initiation of treatment	About 250 to 380 g for males and about 200 to 250 g for females.
Dose groups and number of animals per group	Commonly, five dose groups with $n = 6$ or 8/group or $n = 3$–4/gender/group: Group A: naive or with no treatment Group B: vehicle control Group C: X mg/kg (low dose) Group D: $2X$ to $4X$ mg/kg (middle dose) Group E: $4X$ to $10X$ mg/kg (high dose) where X is the pharmacologically active dose in the test species.
Rationale for dose selection	The low dose or pharmacological active dose is commonly selected based on the primary pharmacological action in other rat studies. The pharmacological active dose is the minimal dose level that produces the desired biological effect in an animal model of the disease indication or disorder to be evaluated during clinical trials. If the animal species to be evaluated during safety pharmacology studies is different from that used in primary pharmacodynamic studies, the pharmacological active dose should be converted to mass per body surface area (i.e., mg/m^2) for the pharmacology animal species and the dose for the safety pharmacology animal species determined. The higher doses are commonly selected to establish a dose–response relationship while avoiding doses that may produce frank or substantial dose-related toxicities (observed during toxicology studies in rats) that may interfere with result interpretation.
Dose formulation	Solution or suspension in the vehicle proposed for or used during toxicity studies in rats.
Route of administration	Clinical route proposed.

(*Continued overleaf*)

TABLE 6.1 (*Continued*)

Parameter	Specification
Fasting	Animals are not fasted prior to the test.
Testing conditions	The test is conducted in a quiet room. On the test day, the animals are first observed before dosing, using the standardized battery of tests listed in Table 6.2. After the baseline measurements have been recorded, the animals are dosed with an NCE and then evaluated at various times after dosing.
Observation times	A commonly used time series is 0.5, 1, 2, 6, and 24 h after dosing, but the times should be selected based on the pharmacokinetic and pharmacological profiles of the NCE and should include observations when the plasma concentration of an NCE is at or near maximum and when the maximum pharmacological effect is observed. When the maximum plasma concentration time and maximum pharmacodynamic effect time are different, both times should be included.
Testing procedure	Measurements are first carried out in the home cage, which is where the animal is maintained before and between assessments. The posture of the animal, tremors, convulsions, stereotypes (e.g., licking, gnawing, biting, head movements, sniffing, circling, writhing), vocalizations, and palpebral closure are recorded. The ease of removal and the reactivity of an animal to handling during removal from the home cage and transfer to the open field are then rated. The observer notes and/or ranks body tone, palpebral closure, exophthalmus, lacrimation, the presence of crusts around the eyes, salivation, piloerection, fur appearance, and bite marks on the tail or paws (in relation to stereotypes). In a third step, the animal is placed in an open field (commonly 58.5 × 68.5 cm with a 6-cm rim) and observed for 3 min. The presence of tremors, convulsions, or stereotypes is again noted. The number of rearing occasions (supported and nonsupported) and grooming episodes are counted. The arousal level and gait characteristics are ranked. At the end of the 3-min observation period, the number of fecal boluses and pools of urine is counted. The reflex testing is conducted, which consists of recording the animal's response to the approach of a vertical rod, a touch to the rump, a finger snap, or a tail pinch. Righting reflex and catalepsy are rated. The grip strength is measured with a grip strength test that determines the maximal force developed by a rat on the front paws when the operator tries to pull the rat out of a designed grid. The measure (in newtons) is performed three times.
Temperature	Rectal temperature (°C) variation throughout the test period is calculated for each rat. The temperature variation is the difference of temperature (delta temperature) between predose (time 0) and the different subsequent observation times.

TABLE 6.1 ***(Continued)***

Parameter	Specification
Other observations	Any other clinical and/or behavioral abnormalities observed are also noted.
Results	Results of clinical examination are expressed as frequency of occurrence of the various clinical signs within each dose group at each observation time.
	Data are frequently reported on a score grid derived from a spreadsheet. Results are expressed, where applicable, as averages ± SEM of scores (rank order data, count data, and quantal data) or as descriptive data. These results, and individual animal data, are presented in an appendix to the study report.
Data evaluation	The effects of an NCE or method control (if used) on the frequency of occurrence of the various clinical signs at each measurement time are compared with those of the vehicle control using an appropriate statistical test such as Fisher's test, or using nonparametric procedures such as the Kruskal–Wallis test, followed, if statistically significant, by Wilcoxon's rank sum test.
	Delta body temperatures (average ± SD) are compared to values of naive and vehicle-treated animals at each observation time using parametric procedures (analysis of variance followed, if statistically significant, by Dunnett's test).

TABLE 6.2 CNS Safety Pharmacology: List of Clinical Signs Observed During the Irwin's Test in Rats

Clinical Sign	Correspondence or Observation Conditions
	Behavior Profile
Awareness	
Hyperalertness	Active freezing or rapid head or body exploratory movements (observation while in cage)
Decrease in visual placing	Visual placing only after vibrissae contact after lowering the rat handled by the tail at a height of 15 cm
Passivity to finger approach	No motor response to finger approach toward the head
Passivity when touched	No motor response to touching the head with a finger
Absence of reactivity	No motor response to flank approach (no touch)

(Continued overleaf)

TABLE 6.2 ***(Continued)***

Clinical Sign	Correspondence or Observation Conditions
Stereotyped movements	Repeated jumpy movements (observation while in cage)
Catalepsy	Homolateral paw-crossing test
Mood	
Vocalization	Observation in cage and during handling
Restlessness	Sudden movements of rat, agitation or inability to remain long in a given position (observation while in cage)
Aggressiveness/irritability	Biting reflex when touched or when near other rats
Increase in fear	Exaggerated withdrawal when rapid finger approach toward the head
Decrease in fear	Slowed withdrawal when rapid finger approach toward the head
Grooming	Observation while in cage
Motor activity	
Absence of spontaneous locomotor activity	Observation of locomotor activity while in cage
Slowed spontaneous locomotor activity	Observation of locomotor activity while in cage
Increased spontaneous locomotor activity	Observation of locomotor activity while in cage
Motor incoordination	
Staggering gait	Observation of gait while in cage
Abnormal gait	Observation of gait while in cage
Loss of righting reflex	Inability to land squarely on all fours when somersaulted 30 cm above the floor
	Neurological Profile
Central excitation	
Absence of startle response	No motor response to a finger snap
Increase in startle response	Exaggerated response to a finger snap
Insensitivity to pinching of tail	No motor response to pinching tail with a forceps at about 2.5 cm above the base of the tail
Hyperreactivity to pinching of tail	Exaggerated fleeing or biting to pinching tail with a forceps at about 2.5 cm above the base of the tail
Tremors	Observation while in cage
Twitches	Observation while in cage
Clonic seizures	Observation while in cage
Tonic seizures	Observation while in cage

TABLE 6.2 ***(Continued)***

Clinical Sign	Correspondence or Observation Conditions
Muscle tone	
Body sag	Observation while in cage
Decrease in limb tone	Decrease in resistance to passive flexion of hind paw
Increase in limb tone	Increase in resistance to passive flexion of hind paw
Decrease in grip strength	Decrease in grid-gripping performance
Decrease in body tone	Decrease in body tone by gently compressing the sides of the rat with the index finger
Decrease in abdominal tone	Decrease in abdominal tone by gently compressing the abdomen of the rat with the index finger
Body posture	
Flattened position	Observation (while in cage) of body position
Lying on side	Observation (while in cage) of body position
Sitting up	Observation (while in cage) of body position
Rearing	Observation (while in cage) of body position
Virtually permanent reared position	Observation (while in cage) of body position
Reflexes	
Loss of pinna reflex	No response to tactile stimulation of pinna
Loss of corneal reflex	No response to tactile stimulation of cornea
Hind limb reflex	No response to tactile stimulation of hind limb
	Autonomic Profile
Skin color (cyanosis)	Observation of the plantar surface and digits of fore limbs
Tachycardia	Estimated by pressing the chest
Bradycardia	Estimated by pressing the chest
Dyspnea	Observation while in cage
Bradypnea	Observation while in cage
Polynea	Observation while in cage
Myosis	Pupil contracted (observation during handling)
Mydriasis	Pupil dilated (observation during handling)
Ptosis	Eyes half closed or closed (observation while in cage and immediately after handling)
Exophthalmos	Prominent eyes (observation while in cage and immediately after handling)
Writhing symptom	Ondulatory wavelike movement over the abdomen (observation while in cage)
Caudal catatonia	Observation while in cage
Piloerection	Observation while in cage
Salivation	Observation during handling

(*Continued overleaf*)

TABLE 6.2 ***(Continued)***

Clinical Sign	Correspondence or Observation Conditions
Lacrimation	Observation during handling
Diarrhea	Observation while in cage and during handling
Soft feces	Observation while in cage and during handling
Straub	Observation while in cage
	Toxicity
Acute death	Observation of death between 0 and 2 h after dosing
Delayed death	Observation of death between 2 and 24 h after dosing

caused by repolarization disturbances of the cardiac action potential. As mentioned earlier, cardiac ventricular repolarization is considered as a surrogate biomarker for *torsades de pointes* proarrhythmic risk in humans. This risk was first identified in drugs approved for marketing, which required changes in the package inserts for some drugs. Regulatory agencies now expect this potential risk to be evaluated during in vitro and in vivo cardiovascular safety pharmacology studies on an NCE that are conducted prior to the FIH trial. Table 6.3 presents a possible study design for evaluating the potential of an NCE to inhibit hERG.

Commonly, experiments are conducted using CHO-K1/hERG cells because hERG-transfected cells allow the electrophysiological properties of an NCE on K^+ currents implicated in cardiac repolarization to be determined during a single study. Another commonly used system for evaluating the ability of an NCE to inhibit hERG uses rubidium flux and is described in Table 6.4.

Another objective of cardiovascular safety pharmacology studies is the determination of potential hemodynamic [heart rate (HR) and blood pressure (BP)] adverse effects of an NCE. Table 6.5 provides a standard study design for evaluating potential hemodynamic effects caused by an NCE in rats.

To be in compliance with the ICH S7b guideline, information on the hemodynamic effects and potential changes in electrocardiograms (ECGs) are necessary for an NCE. The study design in Table 6.6 describes a determination of potential effects on BP, HR, and ECG following administration of an NCE to monkeys or dogs. The species of choice depends on the pharmacological profile of the NCE and the projected nonrodent toxicology animal species. For many small organic molecules, the nonrodent species is commonly the dog, whereas for most biopharmaceuticals the nonrodent species is frequently a nonhuman primate such as the cynomolgus monkey (Chapters 7 and 12).

Thus, a sponsor of an NCE should carefully select (using available data, such as in vitro protein binding and drug metabolism results where plasma and hepatocytes from humans can be employed and the human results generated can be compared to those from various animal species to determine if some animal

TABLE 6.3 Cardiovascular Safety Pharmacology: Study Design for Evaluation of hERG Inhibition

Parameter	Specification
Culture system	CHO-K1/hERG cells are cultured in Dulbecco's modified Eagle's medium–F12 and grown onto sterile tissue culture plate at 37°C in a humidified atmosphere containing 5% CO_2.
NCE concentrations	The effects of the NCE in 1% dimethyl sulfoxide (DMSO) on hERG K^+ current parameters are commonly evaluated at five concentrations (e.g., 0.01, 0.1, 1, 10, and 100 μM), with each concentration evaluated five times.
Experimental procedure	Cells plated on coverslips are placed in a thermally conductive perfusion chamber mounted on the stage of an inverted phase contrast microscope. Cells are superfused with buffer (superfusate solution) containing 150 mM NaCl, 4 mM KCl, 1.2 mM $CaCl_2$, 1 mM $MgCl_2$, and 10 mM HEPES adjusted to pH 7.4 ± 0.05 using NaOH. An electronically controlled, constant-flow perfusion system is used to deliver solutions at a flow rate of 1 mL/min. Cells are maintained at a constant temperature (30 ± 1°C) by a thermistor feedback loop. Bath temperature is recorded together with the electrophysiological signals, by an analog output connected to an analog input channel of the digitizer.
Recording procedures	After recordings with the vehicle have been made, at least five cells are exposed to increasing concentrations of an NCE. After control recordings with the superfusate solution, three cells are exposed to the positive control. *Note:* If all the concentrations of an NCE cannot be tested on the same cell, the remaining concentrations are tested using another cell.
Cell stabilization	During the control period, the cell is allowed to stabilize for a minimum of 10 sweeps before switching to the first concentration of an NCE or to the reference item. Thereafter, the cell is allowed to equilibrate for 25 sweeps before recording and switching to the next concentration.
Recordings	Recordings are performed in a whole-cell voltage-clamp configuration of a patch-clamp method, using a fire-polished micropipette positioned with a micromanipulator. The micropipette filling solution contains 140 mM KCl, 5 mM EGTA, 5 mM Na_2-ATP, and 10 mM HEPES adjusted to pH 7.2 ± 0.05 using KOH. Once whole-cell configuration is obtained, the resting membrane potential is maintained at −80 mV (holding potential). To induce K^+ currents through hERG channels, the protocol described below is used. Currents are recorded using an amplifier in combination with an analog-to-digital converter.

(*Continued overleaf*)

TABLE 6.3 (*Continued*)

Parameter	Specification
Voltage protocol	Steady-state and fully activated tail currents are obtained by using: 1. Depolarizing pre-pulse at +20 mV for 1250 ms (steady-state current), 2. Hyperpolarizing pulse at −120 mV for 1150 ms (tail current), 3. Intersweep interval for 10 s.
Results	Currents are expressed as pA/pF (to correct for variation in cell size) of hERG specific currents after subtraction of leak current using a subtraction technique and corrected for the time-dependent rundown. Vehicle control tail currents are measured immediately before the superfusion of the first concentration of an NCE. The results for each concentration of an NCE are expressed as a percentage inhibition of the vehicle tail current. The results for the reference item are expressed as a percentage inhibition of the control tail current.
Calculations	The amplitude of the tail current (I_{tail}) is calculated as the difference between the baseline current (average current recorded before the depolarizing pre-pulse) and the maximum inward current recorded at the beginning of the hyperpolarizing pulse. For each test item concentration, data are expressed as averages of a minimum of five pulse-induced currents of one experiment, then as averages ± SEMs for five experimental values. The data for the reference item is expressed as the average ± SEM for three experimental values. If the results so indicate, the IC_{50} (inhibitory concentration at 50%) value of an NCE is determined.
Statistical evaluations	NCE values (averages ± SEMs) are compared to vehicle control values and analyzed using one-way ANOVA, followed by Dunnett's *t*-test. Statistical analyses are performed using appropriate software and significance is considered at $p < 0.05$ versus vehicle controls.

species have profiles different from those of humans) the nonrodent species for toxicology assessments and that same species should be utilized for cardiovascular safety pharmacology studies. If the sponsor selects the dog as the nonrodent toxicology species and later determines that the dog is not a relevant animal species for the NCE and switches to the nonhuman primate, the cardiovascular safety pharmacology evaluations should be repeated in this species. Many sponsors do not conduct the study recommended in the ICH S7b guideline prior to the

TABLE 6.4 Cardiovascular Safety Pharmacology: Study Design for Evaluation of hERG Inhibition Using Rubidium

Parameter	Specification
Culture	A CHO cell line expressing hERG is grown in Ham's F12 supplemented with 10% FCS (fetal calf serum), 100 μg/mL streptomycin/100,000 U/L penicillin at 37°C and in 5% CO_2. The cells are plated at a density of 50,000 cells/well in 96-well microtiter plates and incubated at 37°C with 5% CO_2 until 60 to 90% confluency is attained (approximately 24 h).
Rubidium (Rb^+) loading	Cells are washed with 200 μL of Rb^+ load buffer (5.4 mM of RbCl at pH 7.4). The cells are then loaded with 200 μl of Rb^+ load buffer/well and incubated for 1 h at 37°C with 5% CO_2.
Positive control	E-4031, which can be obtained from Sigma Chemical Co. and is a known blocker of hERG channels, or other suitable agent.
Wash	Excess Rb^+ is removed by two successive washes using 200 μL of Rb^+ wash buffer (5 mM KCl at pH 7.4).
NCE application	Aliquots (2 μL) of the NCE stock solutions over the concentration range to be tested are added to individual wells and incubated for 30 min at 37°C with 5% CO_2. The primary NCE stock solutions (at 100 times of the NCE stock solutions to be tested) are prepared in 100% DMSO and then diluted with the Rb^+ wash buffer so that the final DMSO concentration in each of the stock solutions is 1%.
Channel activation and NCE application	The Rb^+ wash buffer is replaced with 198 μL of channel open buffer (60 mM KCl at pH 7.4) and 2 μL of the NCE stock solution in 100% DMSO. Channel activation is performed for 6 min.
Cell lysis	A 200-μL extracellular sample is collected from the supernatant and stored in 96-well microtiter plates. Intracellular samples are then obtained by whole-cell lysis with the application of 200 μL of lysis buffer (0.1% sodium dodecyl sulfate).
Analysis	The level of Rb^+ in both the intracellular and extracellular samples (100-μL samples) are measured. The percentage efflux of Rb^+ (Rb^+ concentration out divided by Rb^+ concentration total) is used as an indicator of hERG channel blockage.

FIH trial. If the NCE has been shown to have potential adverse cardiovascular effects in other safety pharmacology studies or in acute and subchronic toxicity studies conducted prior to the FIH trial, the sponsor should consider conducting more detailed cardiovascular safety pharmacology studies to further characterize and extend the earlier findings. For most drug candidates (with the possible exception of an NCE being developed to treat a life-threatening disorder for which no therapeutic treatment is available), the potential of adverse cardiovascular effects needs to be evaluated carefully to determine if an FIH trial is justified and warranted.

TABLE 6.5 Cardiovascular Safety Pharmacology: Study Design for Evaluating Hemodynamic Effects in Rats

Parameter	Specification
Species, strain, gender	Rats, Sprague–Dawley; commonly, only males used, but males and females should be evaluated if an NCE has a known or potential gender effect in pharmacological response or pharmacokinetic profile.
Dose groups	Commonly, five dose groups: Group A: naive or with no treatment Group B: vehicle control Group C: X mg/kg (low dose) Group D: $2X$ to $4X$ mg/kg (middle dose) Group E: $10X$ to $20X$ mg/kg (high dose) where X is the pharmacologically active dose in the test species.
Number	$n = 6$ or 8: 6 or 8 males/group or 3 or 4/gender/group.
Dose formulation	Solution or suspension using the same vehicle proposed for or used during toxicology studies in rats.
Route of administration	Proposed clinical route. (*Note:* Other acceptable route is intravenous to evaluate potential cardiovascular adverse effects when the NCE is 100% available, as with an intravenous bolus injection or short infusion.)
Dosing frequency	Once. (*Note:* Dosing to steady state may be appropriate for some NCEs, particularly those that may accumulate after multiple-dose administration and thus have a different exposure profile than that after a single dose.)
Volume administered	Listed in mL/kg, with 2 mL/kg common for oral dosing and 1 mL/kg common for other routes.
Fasting	Not necessary.
Measurements	Rats dosed with vehicle, positive control, or NCE are monitored for mortality and adverse clinical observations after dosing. At various times after dosing, BP is determined using an indwelling carotid arterial cannula, and HR is determined from the peak-to-peak time of the arterial pressure trace.
Duration of measurements	This depends on the pharmacological and pharmacokinetic profiles of an NCE. Measurements should be made at or near the time of maximum pharmacological response and at or near the maximum plasma concentration (at T_{max}) of an NCE and should continue until an NCE is cleared from systemic circulation almost completely. Typical measurement times are 0 (predose), 0.5, 1, 2, 4, 8, and 24 h after dosing.
Date evaluation	Graphs of the systolic BP, arterial pressure, diastolic BP, and HR for the rats in each dose group are used to determine if changes in various hemodynamic parameters occurred over the dose range evaluated.

TABLE 6.5 (*Continued*)

Parameter	Specification
Statistical comparisons	Homogeneity between groups before any treatment is tested by ANOVA. Effects of an NCE or positive control are compared with those of the vehicle using appropriate statistical tests, such as a two-way ANOVA with treatment as a factor at each measurement time in case of significant interaction, followed by a Dunnett's test if significant ($p \leq 0.05$). Pre- and posttreatment values are compared for each group using one-way ANOVA with time as a factor and with repeated measures at each time, followed by a Dunnett's test in case of a significant time effect ($p \leq 0.05$).

TABLE 6.6 Study Design for Evaluating Cardiovascular Profiles in Monkeys or Dogs

Parameter	Specification
Species, strain, gender	Monkey, cynomolgus, or dog, beagle; commonly, only males used, but males and females should be evaluated if an NCE has a known or potential gender effect in pharmacological response or pharmacokinetic profile.
Dose groups	Commonly, five dose groups: Group A: naive or with no treatment Group B: vehicle control Group C: *X* mg/kg (low dose) Group D: 2*X* to 4*X* mg/kg (middle dose) Group E: 10*X* to 20*X* mg/kg (high dose) where *X* is the pharmacologically active dose in the test species.
Number	8 males for four dose groups or 2/gender/group and 10 males for five dose groups or 2/gender/group.
Design	Either a parallel group design or crossover design can be employed. For a balanced crossover design, the number of animals can be reduced to 5 [all the same gender or 3 males and 2 females or 3 females and 2 males (depending on which gender is more sensitive)] so that each monkey or dog receives each treatment after an appropriate wash-out period. Alternatively, an unbalanced crossover design could be employed.
Dose formulation	Solution or suspension using the same vehicle proposed for or used during toxicology studies in the nonrodent species for an NCE.

(*Continued overleaf*)

TABLE 6.6 ***(Continued)***

Parameter	Specification
Route of administration	Proposed clinical route or intravenous if the NCE has limited systemic exposure after the proposed clinical route (such as dermal), and the safety pharmacology profile of the NCE may not be assessed appropriately by that route.
Dosing frequency	Once for each dose level and route of administration. (*Note:* Dosing to steady state may be appropriate for some NCEs. If dosing to steady state is considered necessary in order to obtain the desired exposure profile of an NCE, a crossover study design would not be feasible. For this case, a parallel dose group design should be considered.)
Washout period	For a crossover design, commonly 1 or 2 days between doses, but the period should be determined from the pharmacokinetic profile of an NCE in the test species.
Volume administered	Listed in mL/kg, with 5 mL/kg common for oral dosing and 1 mL/kg for other routes.
Fasting	If desired, test species can be fasted overnight. Fasting may be necessary, particularly if results have shown that food adversely affects the rate and extent of NCE absorption.
Measurements	Monkeys or dogs are monitored for mortality and adverse clinical observations after each treatment. A telemetric system (surgically implanted under aseptic conditions into the abdominal cavity) is used for measurement of BP [systolic (SBP), diastolic (DBP), and mean arterial (MBP)], HR, ECG, and temperature.
Duration of measurements	Measurements are usually begun 2 h before dosing and then continued for 24 h after dosing. The ECG is examined for QRS complex duration, PR interval, RR interval, and QT interval duration. A corrected QT interval (QTc) is calculated using Bazett's and Fridericia's formulas: Bazett's formula: $QTc = QT/RR^{1/2}$ Fridericia's formula: $QTc = QT/RR^{1/3}$
Date evaluation	The SBP, MBP, DSP, and HR for each animal for each treatment are evaluated to determine if an NCE compared to the vehicle caused a meaningful effect on any of the parameters and if any change was related to the dose level. The ECG parameters for each animal for each treatment are also compared to determine if an NCE adversely affected any of these parameters. The results from the positive control are used to certify that the study was performing as desired.

6.4.2 Additional Information on QT-Interval Prolongation or Delayed Ventricular Repolarization

As discussed in the ICH S7b guideline, one component of the ECG, the QT interval, is of particular importance for assessing cardiovascular system safety in drug development. If other results, such as hERG channel inhibition, other cardiovascular safety pharmacology results, and/or initial toxicology study results, indicate that the heart may be affected adversely after administration of an NCE, the sponsor should consider conducting detailed studies to evaluate the potential of the NCE to cause prolongation of the QT interval prior to the FIH trial. Prolongation of the QT interval is currently considered to be the "best" surrogate biomarker available for very serious cardiac events, including sudden cardiac death. The ECG comprises several segments, including the P-wave, the QRS complex, and the T-wave, and each of these segments is associated with certain cardiac electrical activity that occurs during each heartbeat. The time interval between the onset of the QRS complex and the offset of the T-wave is defined as the QT interval. For a test species with a steady heart rate of 60 beats per minute (bpm), the total length (in the time domain) of all ECG segments during one beat adds up to 1 s or 1000 ms. Each component of the ECG can therefore be assigned a length, or duration, in milliseconds. The length of the QT interval is obtained by inspecting the ECG and identifying the QRS onset and the T-wave offset.

As the heart beats faster, the time duration of each cardiac cycle decreases. Since the QT interval should be evaluated at various heart rates, the interval can be "corrected" for HR. This correction leads to the term QTc, which is calculated (by one of several methods, such as Bazett's formula or Fridericia's formula; Table 6.6) by taking into account the actual QT and the HR (the duration of the entire cardiac cycle, sometimes referred to as the RR interval) at that point. The title of the ICH E14 guidance [12] uses the term *QT/QTc interval* to indicate that both QT and QTc are of interest to regulatory agencies.

Thus, during early drug development (including nonclinical studies and early clinical trials), a sponsor needs to ascertain whether or not the NCE causes prolongation of the QT interval. Such a finding, which represents delayed cardiac repolarization of the myocardial cells, is regarded as the best surrogate marker currently available for certain dangerous cardiac arrhythmias: namely, polymorphic ventricular tachycardia, *torsade de pointes*, and sudden cardiac death.

6.5 RESPIRATORY SYSTEM SAFETY PHARMACOLOGY

As one of the core battery of safety pharmacology studies, the effects of an NCE on the respiratory system are to be assessed before the FIH trial. Respiratory parameters commonly studied include respiratory rate, tidal volume, and hemoglobin saturation. As noted earlier, respiratory system safety pharmacology evaluations are frequently conducted in beagle dogs as a combination cardiovascular and respiratory safety pharmacology assessment. Tables 6.7 to 6.9 are

TABLE 6.7 Study Design for Respiratory System Safety Pharmacology Study in Rats

Parameter	Specification
Species, strain, gender	Rat, Sprague–Dawley; commonly, only males used, but both males and females should be evaluated if gender effects in pharmacological activity or pharmacokinetic profile are known.
Dose groups	Commonly, five dose groups: Group A: vehicle control Group B: positive control (e.g., sodium pentobarbital) Group C: *X* mg/kg (low dose) Group D: 2*X* to 4*X* mg/kg (middle dose) Group E: 10*X* to 20*X* mg/kg (high dose) where *X* is the pharmacologically active dose in the test species.
Number	8 males/group or 4/gender/group, for a total of 40 rats.
Dose formulation	Solution or suspension using the same vehicle as proposed for or used during toxicology studies in the rat.
Route of administration	Proposed clinical route. (*Note:* Other acceptable route is intravenous if considered necessary to evaluate potential respiratory system adverse effects when the NCE is 100% bioavailable, as with an intravenous bolus injection or short infusion.)
Dosing frequency	Once. (*Note:* Dosing to steady state may be appropriate for some NCEs, particularly those that may accumulate after multiple-dose administration and thus have a different exposure profile than that after a single dose.)
Volume administered	Listed in mL/kg, with 2 mL/kg common for oral dosing and 1 mL/kg common for other routes.
Fasting	Overnight (approximately 17 to 22 h).
Animal preparation	Rats are anesthetized (1.4 to 1.6 g/kg of urethane or other acceptable agent) prior to dosing with supplemental anesthesia administered as needed. Catheters are placed in the esophagus to measure esophageal pressure, in the trachea to facilitate spontaneous breathing, and in the jugular vein for treatment administration (if an NCE is to be administered intravenously). Animals are allowed to stabilize for a minimum of 5 min prior to dosing.
Measurements	Changes in airway resistance (R_f) (cm H_2O/ mL/s). Dynamic lung compliance (C_{dyn}) (mL/cm H_2O). Respiratory rate (f) (breaths/min). Tidal volume (TV) (mL). Minute volume (MV) (mL/min).
Measurement techniques	TV, MV, and f are obtained from integration of the respiratory flow signal passing through a pneumotachograph milled directly into a plethysmograph and connected to a differential pressure transducer. Intrapleural pressure (cm H_2O) is estimated from esophageal pressure measured with a pressure transducer. Changes in R_f and C_{dyn} are calculated on a breath-by-breath basis from intrapeural pressure, TV, and airflow rate measurements.

TABLE 6.7 ***(Continued)***

Parameter	Specification
Measurement frequency	Using an acceptable recording device, results are recorded and summarized every minute for the first 5 min and then every 5 min thereafter for a duration of 30 min.
Method of analysis	Individual values of R_f, C_{dyn}, f, TV, and MV at each time point for animals in each dose group are averaged and then compared to average values at each time point for animals administered vehicle as well as to the average baseline values (predose or time 0 values) for each dose group using appropriate statistical tests (e.g., ANOVA followed by Tukey HSD multiple comparison test or Bonferroni multiple comparison test).
Results evaluation and reporting	The various measurements per rat at each time point per dose group are averaged and the average values are compared to predose values for that dose group and to the average values for rats in the control group at each time point. Average values that have statistically significant ($p < 0.05$) changes from time 0 for a dose group or changes from the average time point value for the rats in the control group are noted to determine if changes in any of the respiratory parameters are drug related and dose dependent.

TABLE 6.8 Study Design for Respiratory Safety Pharmacology Study in Rats Using Whole-Body Plethysmograph Chambers

Parameter	Specification
Species, gender	Rats, commonly both males and females.
Dose groups	Commonly, five dose groups: Group A: vehicle control Group B: positive control Group C: X mg/kg (low dose) Group D: $2X$ to $4X$ mg/kg (middle dose) Group E: $10X$ to $20X$ mg/kg (high dose) where X is the pharmacologically active dose in the test species.
Number	3/gender/group.
Dose formulation	Solution or suspension in the same vehicle as proposed for or used during toxicology studies in rats.
Route of administration	Clinical route proposed.
Acclimatization	Rats are placed in plethysmography chambers for at least 60 min prior to test initiation for acclimation.

(*Continued overleaf*)

TABLE 6.8 (*Continued*)

Parameter	Specification
Testing conditions	Once the rats are acclimatized, baseline respiratory signals are recorded and measured for at least 30 min. The chambers are then opened and the rats are dosed as defined in a randomization plan. After dosing, rats are maintained for 240 min under the plethysmography environment.
Recovery test conditions	After a 2-week recovery period, the rats are again acclimatized to the chambers, and baseline respiratory signals are measured for at least 30 min.
Measurements	A respiratory signal is created by the sum of the nasal flow and flow due to changing thoracic volume. Under normal conditions, these flows are out of phase and largely cancel each other out. When a rat inspires, air is removed from the chamber and enters the lungs, driving the chamber pressure down. At the same time, however, the lungs expand, increasing the chamber pressure. Air is taken from the WBP at box temperature and humidity and placed in the lungs where the air is warmed to body temperature and saturated with water vapor at body temperature. The increased volume of that air, due to the temperature and humidity increase, expands the thorax beyond the volume of air inspired. The difference between these two processes creates the respiratory signal, which is recorded via a transducer connected to a preamplifier module.
Date evaluation	After the acclimatization period, respiratory parameters are continuously recorded electronically at 100 Hz and analyzed as follows: Baseline: Values are collected continuously over the 30-min baseline period and averaged over 5 min for every 5-min interval. After dose administration: Values are collected continuously and averaged over 15-min intervals from 30 to 240 min. After 14-day recovery period: For vehicle control and NCE dose groups, values are collected over a 30-min period and averaged over 5 min for every 5-min interval. The results are expressed as average ± SEM.
Statistical comparisons	Homogeneity between groups before any treatment is tested by ANOVA. Effects of an NCE or positive control are compared with those of the vehicle using a two-way ANOVA with treatment as a factor at each time in case of significant interaction, followed by a Dunnett's test if significant ($p \leq 0.05$). Pre- and posttreatment values are compared for each group, using one-way ANOVA with time as factor and with repeated measures at each time, followed by a Dunnett's test in case of a significant time effect ($p \leq 0.05$).

TABLE 6.9 Study Design for Combination Cardiovascular and Respiratory Safety Pharmacology Study in Beagle Dogs

Parameter	Specification
Species, strain, gender	Dogs, beagle; commonly, both males and females.
Dose groups	Commonly, rising doses starting with control (vehicle) and followed by at least three dose levels of the NCE, with the low dose at or twice the pharmacologically active dose and the high dose usually 10 to 20 times the low dose.
Number	4/gender.
Dose formulation	Solution or suspension using the same vehicle as proposed for or used during toxicology studies.
Route of administration	Proposed clinical route. (*Note:* For oral dosing, intraduodenal administration is commonly used so that the NCE is placed at the site of absorption and does not have to pass through the stomach, which may have a prolonged emptying time for an anesthetized animal.)
Anesthetization	The dogs are anesthetized, typically with pentobarbital sodium (30 mg/kg intravenons (i.v.) bolus injection at a volume of 1 mL/kg followed by continuous i.v. infusion of 5 mg/kg administered at 2.5 mL/h throughout the experiment).
Testing conditions	After a dog is anesthetized, testing begins with the administration of the control vehicle to obtain baseline cardiovascular and respiratory measurements. The dog is then administered the low dose and after an appropriate washout period (which depends on the pharmacokinetic and pharmacological profiles, but is usually 30 to 60 min), the next-higher dose is given. This process is continued until the NCE has been administered all dose levels.
Cardiovascular measurements	Lead II ECG can be obtained using subdermal needle electrodes and an ECG signal conditioner. HR can be measured with a pulse rate tachometer. The right femoral artery can be cannulated with a catheter connected to a pressure transducer and pressure processor for recording mean, systolic, and diastolic BP. The left femoral artery can be exposed by a flank incision and a probe connected to an electromagnetic flowmeter (placed around the artery) for measurement of blood flow (BF). These parameters (ECG, HR, BP, BF) can be recorded and displayed on a thermal writing oscillograph.
Respiratory measurements	A 5.0-mm endotracheal tube (connected to a pneumotachograph) can be used to record flow integrated to obtain a continuous recording of respiratory rate (RR). Intrapleural pressure can be obtained from an esophageal balloon placed in the lower third of the esophagus. Transpulmonary pressure [the difference between thoracic (i.e., external end of the endotracheal tube) and pleural pressure] can be measured with a differential

(*Continued overleaf*)

TABLE 6.9 (*Continued*)

Parameter	Specification
	pressure transducer. Measurements from respiratory flow and transpulmonary pressure are used to compute total lung resistance (R_L) and C_{dyn}.
Results	All of the recorded parameters (ECG, HR, BP, RR, TV, R_L, and C_{dyn}) are monitored for 30 or 60 min following each dose. The average readouts over a 1-min period are calculated at preset intervals, commonly pre-dose and 5, 15, 30, 45, and 60 min after administration, but the intervals should be selected based on the pharmacokinetic and pharmacological profiles of the NCE.
Data evaluation	The results for each dog at each dose level of an NCE are compared to the baseline values (vehicle control) to determine if changes are present in any of the parameters and at what dose any changes occurred.

possible study designs for evaluating respiratory system safety pharmacology. The first and second designs are for rat studies, with the second using plethysmography chambers. The third design is for a cardiovascular and respiratory combination safety pharmacology evaluation in beagle dogs, which could also be used for such a study in the nonhuman primate.

Table 6.8 is a study design for respiratory function evaluations in rats using whole-body plethysmography (WBP) chambers. For a study with eight available chambers (a common number for most testing laboratories) and five dose groups (common for most studies with a positive control group), a matrix design can be used where some rats in each dose group are evaluated on five consecutive days. After a 14-day recovery period, the animals (except for the rats in the positive control group) are retested using the same matrix design. Use of the WBP method fully meets the ICH S7a guideline for in vivo safety pharmacology studies using conscious animals under the preferred condition of nonrestraint. However, respiratory data cannot be analyzed when airflow is disrupted by sniffing activity. Respiratory values are not calculated when sniffing behavior occurs for at least 50% of the time interval to be analyzed. When sniffing occurs for less than 50% of this time interval, analysis is performed using the WBP trace "cleaned up" for sniffing activity.

From the computerized respiratory box flow, the following parameters are obtained:

1. Inspiratory time (T_I, milliseconds), defined as the time from the start of inspiration to the end of inspiration.
2. Expiratory time (T_E, milliseconds), defined as the time from the end of inspiration to the start of the next inspiration.

3. Relaxation time (RT, milliseconds), defined as the elapsed time between the beginning of the expiration and the moment when the remaining 30% of the tidal volume has been reached.
4. Peak inspiratory flow (PIF, mL/s).
5. Peak expiratory flow (PEF, mL/s).
6. Penh = $[(T_E/\text{RT})-1](\text{PEF/PIF})$. Penh, which stands for "enhanced pause," is a dimensionless value that characterizes the expiratory shape change. Penh consists of two ratios: one compares the level of box flow during early expiration to the level of box flow during late expiration, and the other compares the level of the peak expiratory box flow to the peak inspiratory box flow. Penh is considered by some researchers [13] to be an indicator of bronchoconstriction and has been demonstrated to correlate with resistance in histamine response in guinea pig. Others [14] have questioned the interpretation of the quantitative changes in Penh and thus the validity of this parameter to measure lung function.
7. Respiration rate (f, breaths/min), by using PEF for counting the number of breath cycles.
8. Tidal volume (V_T, mL). Computing the effects of the temperature and vapor pressure of water change on box flow according to the Drobaugh and Fenn equation [15], the relation of the tidal volume of the animal (volume of air displaced during a breath cycle) to the flow changes recorded within the plethysmograph can be calculated.

$$V_T = (\text{respiratory box flow})(\text{calibration factor})\frac{T_b(P_a - P_c)}{T_b(P_a - P_c) - T_c(P_a - P_r)}$$

where

T_b = body temperature of the animal (assumed to be 310.5 K)
T_c = animal chamber temperature (assumed to be stable at 298 K after acclimatization period)
P_a = barometric pressure (assumed to be constant at 730 mmHg)
P_c = vapor pressure (mmHg) of water at T_c (considered to be a constant parameter of 29.3 mmHg.
P_r = vapor pressure (mmHg) of water at T_b (considered to be a constant parameter of 64.6 mmHg)

9. Minute volume (V_E, mL/min); $V_E = fV_T$.

As mentioned earlier, many sponsors conduct a combination cardiovascular and respiratory safety pharmacology study. This combination study is commonly conducted in beagle dogs but can also be conducted in cynomolgus monkeys. Table 6.9 presents a standard study design for such a combination study in beagle dogs.

6.6 RENAL/URINARY SAFETY PHARMACOLOGY

As with all supplemental safety pharmacology studies, the sponsor of an NCE should evaluate the route of drug elimination and the organs of toxicity to determine if renal/urinary system safety pharmacology studies are warranted. Frequently, information on the rate and route of elimination for an NCE is not available prior to the FIH trial. When that information becomes available (commonly concurrently with the clinical data) and the kidney has been shown to be a primary organ of elimination, renal/urinary safety pharmacology assessments should be conducted. If the kidney has been shown to a primary clearing organ for an NCE and/or any of its known metabolites prior to the FIH trial and toxicology results indicate the kidney may be a primary organ of toxicity, sponsors should consider conducting a renal/urinary safety pharmacology study prior to the FIH trial so that appropriate evaluations in humans can be conducted to determine if adverse effects are being observed in the renal/urinary system. For an NCE not cleared from the body by the kidney and where the renal/urinary system is not affected adversely after administration of an NCE, renal/urinary system safety pharmacology studies are usually not necessary. If considered necessary, these studies are commonly conducted in rats and parameters usually evaluated include urinary volume, urine pH, specific gravity, osmolality, various electrolytes, proteins, and cytology. These parameters can also be assessed from urine samples collected during toxicology studies in a rodent (usually, the rat) and a nonrodent (commonly, the dog or monkey) species. If the conduct of a renal safety pharmacology study is deemed advisable pre-FIH, a recommended study design in rats is outlined in Table 6.10.

6.7 GASTROINTESTINAL SYSTEM SAFETY PHARMACOLOGY

The potential adverse effects on the gastrointestinal (GI) system are to be assessed for an NCE to be administered orally to humans, and the results should be available to support the FIH trial. For an NCE to be administered by another route (e.g., intravenous, nasal, pulmonary, dermal. ocular), GI safety pharmacology studies are usually not necessary.

Possible parameters that may be evaluated include gastric secretion, GI injury potential, bile secretion, in vitro ilead contraction, gastric pH measurements, and in vivo transit time. The most common safety pharmacology study on the GI system is GI motility or in vivo transit time. The mouse is the most common animal species used for this study, but other animal species, such as the rat, can also be used. If the rat is the animal species for primary pharmacodynamic studies and is the rodent species employed for toxicological evaluations, GI safety pharmacology studies in the rat would be beneficial, so that results across studies can be compared. As with other supplemental safety pharmacology studies, GI safety pharmacology should be conducted prior to the FIH trial when other results indicate a potential concern for adverse effects in the GI system. Generally, for

TABLE 6.10 Study Design for a Renal Safety Pharmacology Study in Rats

Parameter	Specification
Species, strain, gender	Rats, Sprague-Dawley or Wistar; commonly, only males used, but both males and females should be evaluated if gender differences in pharmacological activity or pharmacokinetic profile have been noted.
Dose groups	Commonly, five dose groups: Group A: vehicle control Group B: positive control Group C: X mg/kg (low dose) Group D: $2X$ to $4X$ mg/kg (middle dose) Group E: $10X$ to $20X$ mg/kg (high dose) where X is the pharmacologically active dose in the test species.
Number	$n = 6$/group: 6 males or 3/gender.
Dose formulation	Solution or suspension using the same vehicle as proposed for or used during toxicology studies.
Route of administration	Clinical route proposed.
Hydration	Saline (15 mL/kg) is commonly administered to hydrate the animals.
Testing conditions	Animals are placed in individual metabolism cages and urine is collected over various intervals after dosing. Intervals commonly used are 0–6 h, 6–12 h, and 12–24 h, but are dependent on the pharmacokinetic profile of the NCE.
Measurements	Urine volume for each interval is measured and the pH determined. After centrifugation, aliquots are assayed for specific gravity, osmolality, various electrolytes, proteins, and cytology.
Results evaluation	The average ± SEM values of the various parameters (except pH) are calculated. Dunnett's test (or other acceptable statistical technique) is applied for comparison between vehicle and treated groups. Differences are considered significant at $p < 0.05$.

any NCE to be administered orally, GI safety pharmacology assessments are warranted prior to the FIH study. Table 6.11 presents a possible study design for evaluating GI motility in mice.

6.8 AUTONOMIC NERVOUS SYSTEM SAFETY PHARMACOLOGY

Safety pharmacology studies on the autonomic nervous system are not commonly conducted with most NCEs or are conducted as part of the CNS safety pharmacology study (discussed above). These studies are usually not conducted before the FIH trial unless other results are suggestive of a potential adverse effect

TABLE 6.11 Study Design for Gastrointestinal Motility Study in Mice

Parameter	Specification
Species	Mice; commonly, only males used, but both males and females may be used. Rats or other species may also be used.
Dose groups	Commonly, five dose groups: Group A: vehicle control Group B: positive control Group C: *X* mg/kg (low dose) Group D: 2*X* to 4*X* mg/kg (middle dose) Group E: 10*X* to 20*X* mg/kg (high dose) where *X* is the pharmacologically active dose in the test species.
Number	$n = 10$/group: 10 males or 5/gender for mice. Fewer animals may be used for other species.
Dose formulation	Solution or suspension in a vehicle proposed for or used during rodent toxicology studies.
Route of administration	Oral gavage, commonly at 0.2 mL/kg.
Testing conditions	At 1 h after dosing, animals are given a 5% charcoal in 10% gum arabic suspension by oral gavage (0.3 mL/animal) and are sacrificed at 15 min after dose administration.
Sample collection and measurements	The intestine of each animal is removed and the length of the gut [gut length (GL) in mm] as well as the extent of the charcoal movement from the pylorus to the ending of the charcoal column (CP in mm) is measured.
Intestinal transit (IT)	IT for each animal is calculated as IT = (CP/GL) × 100%.
Results evaluation and reporting	The IT average ± SD or SEM value for each treatment group is calculated and Dunnett's test (or other appropriate statistical text) is applied for comparison between control and treated groups. Differences are considered significant at $p < 0.05$.

to the autonomic nervous system. When conducted (based on other results which suggest that the autonomic nervous system may be at risk or for an NCE that is in a class of compounds, such as some chemotherapeutic agents, that are known to cause adverse effects in this system), parameters evaluated include binding to receptors in the autonomic system, functional responses to agonists or antagonists in vitro and in vivo, direct stimulation of autonomic nerves, and measurements of cardiovascular responses, baroreflex testing, and heart rate variability.

6.9 OTHER SYSTEMS

The results from other studies on an NCE should be used to determine if safety pharmacology studies on other organ systems are justified and warranted and when these studies should be conducted. If toxicology results indicate that a particular organ system is at risk, a sponsor should consider designing and conducting safety pharmacology studies on that organ system. In this case, these studies should be conducted prior to the FIH trial so that the clinical study can be designed appropriately to evaluate potential adverse effects in this organ system. If the results from this (or other) safety pharmacology study suggest possible unacceptable risk to humans, the FIH trial should be delayed until the concern has been evaluated and characterized more fully. For most NCEs, especially those being developed to treat a life-threatening disease or disorder and for which no therapy is presently available, both risk and benefit need to be considered. If an NCE has a potential human benefit that is considered to outweigh the risk of adverse effects to a particular organ system, sponsors need to be aware of the potential risk and design the FIH trial to ensure that the risk is acceptable in relation to the benefit. One such organ system is the eye. A number of NCEs have been shown to cause adverse effects (such as retinal detachment) in the eye, and in such situations, ocular safety pharmacology assessments should be considered. Other possible organ systems include skeletal muscle, the immune system, and organs involved in endocrine functions. Since a sponsor is commonly not aware of the potential adverse effect on an other organ system until after the FIH trial has been conducted, these safety pharmacology evaluations cannot be conducted prior to the FIH trial. Once information on potential adverse effects to a given organ system become available, the sponsor of the drug candidate needs to more fully evaluate and characterize that adverse effect, and these assessments can usually be made in animals with appropriately designed experiments that should be considered as safety pharmacology evaluations in other organ systems.

6.10 DISCUSSION AND CONCLUSIONS

Nonclinical safety aspects, which include safety pharmacology assessments, have become a very important component in the discovery and development of an NCE. Until 15 to 20 years ago, discovery was a sequential process starting with the selection of the most active compound (determined using special pharmacological assays for a given human disease or disorder) from a series of newly synthesized compounds. Nonclinical safety aspects were addressed, at least in part, by additional pharmacological testing at high doses of the NCE selected in tests directed at disease indications or disorders other than the intended indication to be evaluated during clinical trials. These secondary pharmacodynamic studies on an NCE were followed by animal pharmacokinetic and metabolism studies. Safety profiles were obtained from acute and subchronic rodent and nonrodent toxicity studies. However, the results from these toxicity studies gave information primarily on changes in organ structure rather than organ function. The results of these nonclinical pharmacology, pharmacokinetic, and toxicity studies were used to support a regulatory agency submission for an FIH trial. This strategy has been abandoned for several reasons, which include:

1. Some negative effects on organ function (e.g., ventricular tachycardia) were not detected until after clinical trials had been initiated, putting humans at unacceptable risk.
2. Many findings from animal toxicology studies were found not to be relevant in humans.
3. New scientific approaches offered new possibilities for assessing safety profiles.
4. The "druggability," having acceptable druglike properties, of discovery leads was underestimated considerably by many sponsors when the probability of success for an NCE was assessed.

The strategy described above was employed mostly for small organic molecules and not for biopharmaceuticals since the recommendations for characterizing biopharmaceuticals had not yet been fully defined either by the sponsor or by regulatory authorities. During this time, sponsors and regulatory agency scientists worked together to define the nonclinical studies, including safety pharmacology assessments, considered necessary to support an FIH trial on a macromolecule NCE.

As the success rate and introduction of new drugs to the market each year began to decline and the overall development time and cost of drug development increased (Chapter 1), a change in development strategy included the following:

1. Parallel instead of sequential involvement of the various scientific disciplines was started first for the assessment and selection of discovery leads and then for the nonclinical development of an NCE.
2. The inclusion of safety pharmacology assessments on various organ systems during the pre-FIH stage of development was implemented.
3. The results of ICH-recommended safety pharmacology studies were to be included in a submission to a regulatory agency for the FIH trial.

Most regulatory agencies expect sponsors to be in compliance with the various ICH guidelines, including the ICH S7a and S7b safety pharmacology guidelines. Since these guidelines recommend that safety pharmacology studies be completed prior to an FIH trial, sponsors generally attempt to meet these recommendations. However, not all NCEs or regulatory agencies are the same. Thus, safety pharmacology assessments on some NCEs, such as those for life-threatening disorders for which no medical therapy is available or for routes of administration, such as dermal, where no systemic exposure is expected or has been observed, can be delayed until after clinical testing has been initiated or may even be waived by regulatory authorities,. However, if other nonclinical results indicate a potential adverse effect to a particular tissue or organ system, sponsors should conduct the necessary safety pharmacology studies to more fully define and characterize this effect prior to the FIH study. Also, regulatory authorities in some countries (usually those not in a primary ICH region) allow the initiation of clinical testing, particularly for less than pharmacologically active doses, so that the pharmacokinetic profiles of an NCE in humans can be determined, before a complete nonclinical safety package has been generated. However, most regulatory authorities still expect sponsors to submit sufficient nonclinical safety data, which includes safety pharmacology assessments, to ensure that humans are not being subjected to unnecessary risk. Prior to initiating an FIH trial, a sponsor should meet with the regulatory agency to determine if the nonclinical safety package available is sufficient to support the clinical trial proposed. If considered to be insufficient by the regulatory agency, the additional nonclinical safety studies, including any safety pharmacology evaluations, would need to be completed before the FIH trial was initiated.

Although this new strategy has been used for the past 15 years or so, the number of drugs reaching the marketplace has not increased. However, the safety profiles of those drug candidates that are entering clinical trials have been characterized in much more detail than previously, and thus the risks to humans during clinical trials have been reduced substantially, since many, but not all, compounds with unacceptable safety profiles, including unacceptable safety pharmacology in various organ systems, are eliminated from the drug development process prior to the FIH trial.

REFERENCES

1. ICH Safety Guideline: Safety Pharmacology Studies for Human Pharmaceuticals. ICH S7A. International Conference on Harmonisation; 2001. Available at: www.ich.org.
2. ICH Multidisciplinary Guideline: Nonclinical Safety Studies for the Conduct of Human Clinical Trials for Pharmaceuticals. ICH M3. International Conference on Harmonisation; 1997. Available at: www.ich.org.
3. ICH Safety Guideline: Preclinical Safety Evaluation of Biotechnology-Derived Pharmaceuticals. ICH S6. International Conference on Harmonisation; 1997. Available at: www.ich.org.
4. ICH Safety Guideline: Safety Pharmacology Studies for Assessing the Potential for Delayed Ventricular Repolarization (QT Interval Prolongation) by Human Pharmaceuticals. ICH S7B. International Conference on Harmonisation; 2002. Available at: www.ich.org.
5. Gad SC. *Safety Pharmacology in Pharmaceutical Development and Approval*. London: CRC Press, Taylor & Francis; 2003.
6. Lakings DB. Nonclinical drug development: pharmacology, drug metabolism, and toxicology. In: Guarino RA, ed. *New Drug Approval Process: Accelerating Global Registrations*, 4th ed. Drugs and the Pharmaceutical Sciences, Vol. 139. New York: Marcel Dekker; 2004.
7. Siegel EB, Lakings DB. In: Gad SC, ed., *Preclinical Drug Development Handbook: Regulatory Considerations*. Pharmaceutical Development Handbook Series. Weinheim, Germany: Wiley-VCH; 2006.

8. Irwin S. Comprehensive behavioral assessment: a systematic quantitative procedure for assessing the behavioral and physiologic state of the mouse. *Psychopharmacologia*. 1968;13:222–257.
9. Sanguinetti MC, Jiang C, Curran ME, Keating MT. A mechanistic link between an inherited and an acquired cardiac arrhythmia: HERG encodes the IKr potassium channel. *Cell*. 1995;81(2):299–307.
10. Moss AJ, Zareba W, Kaufman ES, et al. Increased risk of arrhythmic events in long-QT syndrome with mutations in the pore region of the human ether-a-go-go-related gene potassium channel. *Circulation*. 2002;105(7):794–799.
11. Sanguinetti MC, Tristani-Firouzi M. hERG potassium channels and cardiac arrhythmia. *Nature*. 2006;440(7083):463–469.
12. ICH Efficacy Guideline: Clinical Evaluation of QT/QTc Interval Prolongation and Proarrhythmic Potential for Non-antiarrhythmic Drugs. ICH E14. International Conference on Harmonisation; 2005. Available at: www.ich.org.
13. Chong BT, Agrawal DK, Romero FA, Townley RG. Measurement of bronchoconstriction using whole-body plethysmograph: comparison of freely moving versus restrained guinea pigs. *J Pharmacol Toxicol Methods*. 1998;39(3):163–168.
14. Petak F, Habre W, Donati YR, Hantos Z, Barazzone-Argiroffo C. Hyperoxia-induced changes in mouse lung mechanics: forced oscillations vs. barometric plethysmography. *J Appl Physiol*. 2001;90(6):2221–2230.
15. Drobaugh JE, Fenn WO. A barometric method for measuring ventilation in newborn infants. *Pediatrics*. 1955; 16(1):81–87.

PART IV

PRE-IND DRUG DEVELOPMENT

7

TOXICOLOGY PROGRAM TO SUPPORT INITIATION OF A CLINICAL PHASE I PROGRAM FOR A NEW MEDICINE

HUGH E. BLACK, STEPHEN B. MONTGOMERY, AND RONALD W. MOCH

7.1 INTRODUCTION

In the United States, it is a regulatory requirement that an investigational new drug (IND) application be filed and approved by the U.S. Food and Drug Administration (FDA) before any clinical study can be initiated in human subjects with a new medicine. There are now similar requirements in most developed countries. The IND is submitted to obtain regulatory permission to evaluate a potential new drug candidate in human subjects to determine its safety, tolerability, and pharmacokinetics. The initial two clinical studies are a single rising dose safety and tolerance study and a multiple rising dose safety and tolerance study. Among the key goals of these two clinical studies are (1) to relate dose administered to systemic exposure achieved, (2) to determine the maximum tolerated dose or dose-limiting toxicity, (3) to determine the systemic exposure associated with onset and duration of any adverse event, and (4) to establish the relationship between nonclinical and clinical systemic exposures to parent drug (and possibly metabolites).

The principal objective of this chapter is to present the steps that lead to the orderly development of a toxicology program that supports the IND submission to initiate these first-in-human (FIH) studies. The discussion excludes consideration

Early Drug Development: Strategies and Routes to First-in-Human Trials, Edited by Mitchell N. Cayen

of exploratory INDs (described in Chapter 11). In this chapter we also include a perspective on the very early role of toxicologists in the drug discovery/drug development continuum. Most of the pre-FIH toxicity program discussed herein may not apply equally to biotherapeutics (typically, administered parenterally), although the safety endpoints are the same as with small-molecule drugs. Toxicology testing with these large biologically derived molecules is typically focused on immunological or adverse primary pharmacological effects [1,2]. The regulatory requirements for nonclinical safety assessment of biopharmaceuticals [3] are different from those of small-molecule NCEs, and the specific toxicology program is designed on a case-by-case basis.

7.2 TOXICOLOGY SUPPORT OF DISCOVERY

It is important to point out that the role of the toxicologist should not begin at the stage of the pre-FIH good laboratory practice (GLP)–supported toxicology program, but that the discipline needs to participate in the nomination of a new chemical entity (NCE) as a candidate drug targeted for development [4]. The principal reason for this early involvement is that adverse clinical responses remain the leading cause of NCE attrition at all stages of development, and about 70% of safety-related toxicity is identified nonclinically [4]. As a result, many pharmaceutical companies are applying innovative approaches to help minimize attrition and to deliver safer drug leads from discovery into development. Some of these emerging approaches include expanded in vitro receptor/enzyme drug screening, toxicogenomics, proteomics, and metabolomics, although if used independent of more traditional toxicological principles, such technologies may do little to advance compounds into development. To be of value, newer technologies must be shown to be predictive of the human response, as it is those traditional approaches that have been shown to have at least some counterpart in humans and affect more profoundly the cost and time leading to FIH and ultimate compound attrition [5,6].

Appropriately targeted investigative toxicology and pathology should be part of the drug discovery armamentarium during the hit-to-lead and lead optimization stages [4]. For example, quantitative microscopy (morphometry, stereology) and molecular pathology techniques (immunohistochemistry; in situ hybridization) can be very useful in the validation of nonclinical models for pharmacological effects and of the potential druggability of novel targets. Prospective in vitro screens can be used to identify toxicities for which there may be no histopathological counterpart in short-term in vivo studies, such as safety pharmacology or mutagenicity. Many of these toxicity tests can be carried out in high-throughput assay format during the hit-to-lead stage of drug discovery and can help identify potential liabilities associated with a chemical template. Such studies are not conducted under the GLP umbrella. Subsequent interactions with medicinal chemistry and pharmacology disciplines can then enable synthesis of potentially more viable NCEs. Although it is beyond the scope of this chapter to list and describe these tests, the ultimate goal is to allow the application of target organ–specific or other in vitro assays to generate structure–toxicity relationships, to screen out compounds with predictable toxicities as early as possible, thereby delivering superior lead candidates from discovery into development.

7.3 GOALS OF THE PRE-FIH TOXICOLOGY PROGRAM

It is the primary tenet of toxicology that all xenobiotics are toxic at some dose or exposure level, and a key goal in the design and interpretation of a toxicology program is whether dose-limiting toxicity is a potential handicap to further development. Development-limiting toxicity is more elusive and involves the totality of drug properties in laboratory animals and humans, such as safety margin ("therapeutic index" in humans), reversibility of the toxicity, treatment duration, therapeutic indication, and overall risk/benefit ratio.

The pre-FIH toxicity studies are designed to determine in a rodent and a nonrodent species the target organs of toxicity, the maximum tolerated dose (MTD), the no observed adverse effect level (NOAEL), and the exposures associated with the doses administered. The NOAEL is defined as the highest dose tested in an animal species that does not produce a significant increase in adverse effects compared to the control group [1], and the MTD is defined as the highest dose that does not produce unacceptable toxicity. The commonly used definition of the nonclinical safety margin used by the pharmaceutical industry and regulatory agencies is the ratio of the total exposure [i.e., the area under the plasma or serum concentration–time curve ($AUC_{0-24\ h}$)] at the NOAEL divided by the total exposure ($AUC_{0-24\ h}$) predicted at the human efficacious dose or at the maximum anticipated human therapeutic dose. As the human efficacious dose or plasma exposure to drug-derived material is difficult to predict prior to the conduct of the FIH trial or with relevant pharmacokinetic/pharmacodynamic modeling, the exposure at pharmacological (efficacious) doses in animal models of disease can be used as the temporary default denominator until human plasma exposures are obtained. An acceptable therapeutic/safety margin (>10) to enable proceeding to human trials will depend on many factors, such as type of toxicity and disease target.

The toxicity studies that support an FIH trial are conducted using the same route of administration as planned for the clinical studies and using a dose regimen similar to that proposed for human subjects. The duration of the repeat dose toxicity study should be at least as long as that of the clinical rising multiple dose safety and tolerability study. Thus, the number of days that the laboratory animals are dosed will support up to the same number of dosing days in the clinic. It should be noted that a different paradigm is used if the initial submission is an exploratory IND (Chapter 11).

7.4 IMPORTANCE OF A CLINICAL REVIEW OF THE NONCLINICAL PHARMACOLOGY DATA

A thorough review and discussion of the nonclinical pharmacology data should be held with the physician(s) [expert(s)], who will then develop the clinical study plan. The clinical study plan includes the proposed therapeutic indication, the route of administration, dose levels proposed, and the duration of dosing. Having this information prior to establishing the toxicology program is important since it is the purpose of the toxicology program to support the clinical development plan proposed. To be avoided is the situation in which the toxicology studies are planned and conducted without consideration of the clinical development plan. This approach may lead to unexpected problems and can prove to be a waste of time and resources. For example, the route of administration may have been wrong, the dosing regimen was not followed, or the duration of the toxicology studies was insufficient to cover the dosing interval planned for the clinic. Under these circumstances the toxicity studies may put constraints on the route, doses, or duration of dosing in the clinic. As a result, some or all of the toxicity studies may have to be redesigned and repeated to correct such problems.

7.5 TAKE THE TIME TO PLAN APPROPRIATELY

Taking the time to plan the toxicology program carefully based on the clinical program proposed is essential. In addition to making sure that the toxicology program supports the clinical plans, it helps avoid the situation where unrealistic time lines are projected that will ultimately lead to failure and frustration on the part of everyone within the organization and frustration by the investors who are supporting the company financially. Therefore, before the IND submission date is made public, it is important that management have a clear understanding of when the test compound will be available to initiate the toxicity studies, and appreciates the time, cost, and staff resources required to complete the studies and assemble the submission document. Attempting to take shortcuts to meet a publically announced unrealistic IND submission deadline almost always leads to unexpected difficulties.

7.6 THE ACTIVE PHARMACEUTICAL INGREDIENT

7.6.1 Availability Issues

The availability of an active pharmaceutical ingredient (API) is a critical component of a toxicology program. The API is used not only for dosing of the test species but is also utilized for assay development in verifying dose formulations and for estimating systemic exposures (toxicokinetics), both of which are essential components of GLP toxicity studies. A realistic understanding is needed of any difficulties associated with the synthesis and release of the API in the quantities and quality needed to develop and validate analytical assays for the drug product (Chapter 5) and bioanalytical assays (Chapter 4) for the drug in plasma or serum, and then to initiate and complete the toxicology program. It is futile to plan the initiation of the toxicity studies if the API has not been made available for assay development and validation well before the assays are needed. The approximate compound requirements for such assay development are low-gram amounts.

Providing an API of the quality required and the amount needed well in advance of the initiation date proposed for the toxicity studies is important. In contrast to the low-gram quantities for analytical and bioanalytical assay development, the quantities required for the toxicology program may reach a kilogram, depending on the doses to be administered, study duration, and whether the non-rodent animal model will be a dog (8 to 10 kg) or a cynomolgus monkey (3.5 to 4.5 kg). Supplying the compound well in advance of the study start date provides the time needed by the laboratory staff to identify and resolve problems such as preparation of the compound in a formulation suitable for the proposed route of delivery, or achieving the required concentrations for the route of administration proposed. Thus, delivery of the drug to a toxicology laboratory only one or two days prior to the planned start of a study increases the risk of encountering difficulties and potentially stressful delays. These delays, if significant, can lead to penalties against the company for holding unused laboratory space for periods of time beyond those agreed to when the contracts were signed originally. These delays can create significant issues for the sponsor if not managed carefully.

7.6.2 Impurity Considerations

It is also important to consider whether the API for toxicology testing will be qualified as GMP (good manufacturing practice) or non-GMP. GMP material offers the opportunity to test material that can be or will be utilized in the clinical investigations. If GMP material is used in the toxicology program, the impurity profile will have been qualified for clinical investigations. Using GLP (non-GMP) material in the toxicology program always raises the specter of whether the GMP impurity profile will be fully qualified.

The qualification and quantification of impurities in an API is discussed fully in the International Conference on Harmonisation (ICH) Q3 guidance [7]. Needless to say, the qualification of impurities has become quite complex and may be subject to additional in silico (computer) structure–activity investigations pre-FIH to identify possible genotoxic and carcinogenic alerts [8]. It should also be noted that a certificate of analysis (CofA) for the test material covering the dates of the toxicology testing for each study in which a particular lot (or batch) was used is required by GLP as evidence of API stability during the course of investigation.

7.6.3 Inactive Ingredients

Often overlooked, inactive ingredients that will be used in the FIH clinical formulation should be considered prior to adoption. The FDA database on inactive ingredients in approved drug products provides a starting point to assess whether the inactive ingredients proposed for inclusion in the pharmaceutical formulation are appropriate for their intended use. The toxicology program should encompass the inactive ingredients in the vehicle and test article formulations intended for testing. This becomes of particular concern for novel pharmaceutical excipients or inactive ingredients intended to be used at higher doses or by a different route than approved previously.

7.7 TIMELY CONDUCT OF IN VITRO ASSAYS

From the toxicologist viewpoint, two initial questions asked in developing a candidate drug are: What species should be selected for the pre-FIH GLP toxicology program? Does the chemical structure possess any genotoxicity properties that would otherwise preclude it from further development? These can be answered from the timely conduct of in vitro studies.

Of critical importance to the initiation of the pre-FIH toxicology program is species selection. The decision on the appropriate rodent and nonrodent species for the toxicology program utilizes information obtained from the pharmacological (efficacy) response in animal models, background (historical control) data available on the species, and most important, on comparable in vitro metabolic profiles. Justification for the species selected for a toxicology study is a GLP requirement. Comparative in vitro metabolic profiles are accepted by regulatory authorities as part of that justification.

7.7.1 Comparative In Vitro Metabolism

Species comparison of the in vitro metabolic profile of the candidate drug is usually investigated in liver microsomes and/or hepatocytes. As discussed in Chapter 2, the goal of early evaluation of the metabolic profile of an NCE is to select the appropriate rodent and nonrodent species for the toxicity studies which metabolize the candidate drug in a manner similar to that in humans. Typically, microsomes are studied initially to evaluate phase I metabolism, but the totality of the biotransformation of the drug candidate is best achieved by using hepatocytes, so as to capture both phase I and phase II metabolites across species.

At this early pre-FIH phase of the development program, exact identification and quantification of the metabolites are not necessary for selection of appropriate toxicology species. This can be quite expensive and time consuming in early development of a drug candidate and is not required for regulatory submission of an IND for initiation of an FIH clinical trial. Rather, a species comparison can be achieved from the chromatographic peaks assayed using appropriate analytical methods following incubation of the candidate drug with hepatocytes from human (donors) and laboratory species (e.g., mouse, rat, dog, monkey, minipig). The chromatographic peaks in the culture medium after a defined period of time are interpreted to represent metabolites of the parent compound. Such metabolite profiling may be supported by preliminary liquid chromatograph (LC)-mass spectrometry (MS)/MS analyses. Thus, the rodent and nonrodent species whose peaks most closely resemble those produced by the human hepatocytes should be selected for the pre-FIH toxicology program. These in vitro results are accepted by regulatory authorities as justification for selection of the laboratory species used in IND enabling studies.

During a clinical phase I/II program, the identification and quantification of metabolites in vitro and in vivo will be completed for the toxicology species selected as well as for humans. It should be recognized that subsequent post-IND in vivo metabolism studies in human subjects or patients may result in the identification of circulating metabolites that were not uncovered in the initial in vitro studies. This may necessitate a change in the laboratory species that will be used in chronic toxicity studies, or a separate evaluation of such a human metabolite (Chapters 4 and 8). The safety assessment strategies for qualifying human metabolites are discussed further in an FDA guidance [10].

7.7.2 Genetic Toxicology

Genetic toxicity assays are used to screen a candidate drug (and its metabolites) for possible mutagenic (DNA damage) and clastogenic (chromosomal aberrations) effects. These arrays provide an early means to identify whether a candidate drug (and metabolites) has carcinogenic potential. It is therefore recommended that the most commonly used test for mutagenicity—the bacterial reverse mutation assay (Ames test) [11,12], conducted as a GLP study—be one of the first studies completed in the toxicology program. Although some 35 years old, this reverse-mutation assay remains the gold standard test for early detection of potential genotoxicity. The purpose is to determine early in the development program if the compound is genotoxic. This is particularly important if the compound will be used clinically in a broad patient population where there will be chronic or frequent intermittent administration, such as with antihistamines. Compounds for such clinical use will require carcinogenicity assays. The results of the carcinogenicity studies usually become available during or near the completion of phase III studies because of the 90-day studies required to justify the doses selected for the carcinogenicity studies as well as the approximately three years needed to complete and finalize the report. If there is an indication of a tumor finding in the carcinogenicity studies and the compound has already been shown to be genotoxic in the Ames assay, it may be exceedingly difficult, after the expenditure of all these resources and time, to get approval to complete the clinical program or to get the product approved. Because of these potentially costly consequences, if the compound is positive in the Ames assay very early in the development program, it is prudent to review any analogs of the compound to determine if any have similar pharmacologic activity and are negative in the Ames assay.

With that information, an informed decision can be made as to which compound to advance into development. Accordingly, many drug sponsors will conduct preliminary (non-GLP) bacterial reverse mutation assays in selective tester strains as part of the discovery paradigm well before the drug candidate enters into formal pre-FIH development. An exception to abandoning further development of a candidate drug with a positive result in the in vitro bacterial reverse mutation assays is for an anticancer chemotherapeutic agent because the mechanism of action is directed at modulating DNA. The completion of a GLP bacterial reverse mutation assay is required for regulatory submission of an IND for initiation of an FIH clinical trial.

7.8 DEVELOPMENT OF VALIDATED BIOANALYTICAL AND ANALYTICAL ASSAYS

7.8.1 Validated Bioanalytical Assay for Determining Plasma Concentrations of the NCE

It is important to have in place a validated plasma or serum assay for each of the laboratory species to be used in the toxicology program, prior to beginning the in vivo GLP toxicology studies (Chapters 4 and 10). Plasma exposure data and their relationship to dose and observed toxicity are important in interpreting the significance of the findings. The ultimate purpose is to compare the exposure of the animals at the maximum tolerated dose and at the NOAEL in the toxicity studies to the human exposure at the maximum recommended clinical dose.

The quantities of compound required for assay development (typically, an LC-MS/MS assay) are relatively small. Some plasma assays are very difficult and time consuming to develop and validate. Not having validated bioanalytical assays in place before initiating the toxicology studies can complicate the interpretation of the toxicity data and can significantly delay the issuance of the final report for a study. An important reason for not proceeding with the toxicity studies prior to having the assays in place is the issue of possible instability of the compound in the plasma of the test species. If the compound is not sufficiently stable in plasma for the length of storage time prior to the bioanalyses, the levels measured may be an underestimate of the actual exposure that occurred. Those data then belong to the study permanently and cannot be corrected or used to develop safety factors. Further, the results must be explained in a regulatory submission when they are shown to be inconsistent with results from later studies.

7.8.2 Validated Analytical Assays for Dosing Solutions or Suspensions

In addition to validated bioanalytical methods for determining plasma drug concentrations, a validated analytical assay is needed to demonstrate the accuracy of the concentrations of compound in the dosing solutions and suspensions used in the GLP toxicology studies (Chapter 5). If the assay is not available at the time the study is conducted, there is no way of proving that the animals received the nominal doses called for by the protocol. If dosing solutions are not assayed until well after the actual dosing of the animals has occurred and the results show that there has been a major miscalculation in the preparation of one or more of the dosing solutions, there is no way of taking corrective action to save the study. Therefore, it is critical to have this assay in place before the GLP studies are initiated. Unfortunately, history teaches that miscalculations in the preparation of dosing solutions are not rare.

7.8.3 Validated Assays for Dosing Solution Stability

As well as validated assays to demonstrate the concentration of the NCE in the dosing solutions, data are required to affirm that the dosing solutions are stable over time under the conditions of storage recommended. This is to assure that the concentrations in the dosing solutions on the day the solutions are administered are the same as those on the day the solutions were prepared (i.e., if prepared once every 14 days, they should be stable over that period).

7.9 PLANNING FOR THE CONDUCT OF TOXICITY STUDIES

Planning for the conduct of the toxicity studies requires development of the appropriate protocols, as well as making arrangements to have the studies conducted either within the corporate laboratories or in an appropriate contract research organization (CRO). To arrive at an initiation date, the animals must be available for acclimation purposes prior to the study start date, and the activities of the personnel and equipment in the formulation, analytical, clinical pathology, necropsy, and histology laboratories, in addition to quality assurance, must all be available to work on the study. Thus, if the studies are to be conducted by a CRO, the time should not be underestimated to bid the study, establish meaningful start dates, and conclude equitable contracts between the sponsor and the laboratory. A general rule of thumb is to add at least one month to these planning activities prior to arrival of the animals for initiation of the study.

7.9.1 Timing of the IND/CTA

There are a number of items to be considered in calculating the time required to complete the studies necessary to submit an IND/or clinical trial application (CTA). As a rough estimate, it takes approximately 12 to 18 months to file an IND from the time the API is available in quantities sufficient to conduct the in vivo toxicity studies. This includes the time required to conduct the in vitro assays and develop the pilot study data for selection of doses for the GLP studies. Complicating factors such as difficulties in assay development or formulation development or lack of available laboratory space can delay start dates and lead to the longer times required.

7.9.2 The Danger of Shortcuts

One of the most expensive ways to consume time and money is to design shortcuts into protocols for the toxicity studies. Shortcuts can cause delays in study completion by requiring additional work to assist in interpretation of equivocal findings and may even lead to additional studies to resolve the questions or issues created by the shortcuts. Potentially, expensive shortcuts include reducing the numbers of animals per dose group, not including a recovery phase in the study, not processing all tissues to slides, using one gender only, reading the slides of high-dose and control animals only, or using two pathologists to read the slides (one for each gender). At this early stage of drug development, the sponsor has minimal or no information about the toxicity of the compound, and obvious gaps or shortcuts in the study design will almost certainly lead to regulatory questions or challenges that have the potential to lead to the IND being put on hold. Having the IND put on hold can be expensive for drug sponsors and sometimes disastrous for a small company.

7.9.3 Pilot In Vivo Studies for Dose Selection and Bleeding Time Determinations

Prior to initiating pre-FIH toxicity studies, it is important to conduct pilot (non-GLP) studies to help select the appropriate doses and determine correct bleeding times for the collection of plasma for drug concentration analysis. To provide the most useful data, the pilot studies should determine the maximum doses that each species will tolerate as a single dose and then as repeated doses given for a period of from 7 to 14 days. The objective is to develop sufficient information to permit an appropriate dose selection regimen. It is very costly to start a GLP study and then find that it has to be terminated because the animals will not tolerate the compound at one or more of the doses selected for the study.

It is recommended that that the word *pilot* be included in the protocol titles for pilot toxicity studies that are not conducted according to GLP. This signals that the protocol probably was not conducted according to GLPs and was not conducted for the purpose of supporting a clinical study. This may seem trivial, but it will preclude pressing to shortcut the development process by using these studies to support the planned clinical development program.

An additional early benefit from pilot studies is the identification of toxicities which may indicate that further development of an NCE should be terminated. Examples include unexpected adverse ocular effects, central nervous system (CNS) effects such as convulsions, adverse effects on the heart at doses near the clinical dose proposed, and finding a steep dose response in the pilot studies where the difference is narrow between a dose that has no apparent adverse effect (NOAEL) and a dose that produces deaths. Any of these types of findings in the pilot studies indicate that thoughtful consideration should be given before additional resources are expended on development of a compound.

Because the results of pilot toxicity studies are related to the safety of a compound, the results from these studies, even though non-GLP, must be written up and submitted with the IND. A sponsor cannot decide to file the information in its archives and not include the data in its submission to a regulatory agency if the sponsor decides to progress with development of the NCE as a candidate drug.

7.10 GLP TOXICOLOGY PROGRAM

The in vivo toxicology program to support the IND application is conducted in a rodent and a nonrodent species, the selection of which is justified predominantly based on the results of the in vitro metabolite profiles in hepatocytes as compared to humans. Most toxicity studies are conducted in one of the common laboratory species because of the importance of having access to historical control data for interpretative purposes. Such data may show that any values in question, although different from the concurrent controls, are still within the range of values for the historical controls from the laboratory in which the study was conducted. This information is very valuable in assessing and justifying the interpretation of a finding. It is important that the historical control database use species or strains from the same supplier covering a two- to three-year time span from the date of initiation of the study. If historical control information is cited in the study report, these data must be included in the final report as an appendix.

The repeated-dose studies supporting an IND are most often of 28 days' duration, are conducted by the dose route and dose regimen proposed for the clinical program, and utilize doses selected from the pilot toxicity studies. Studies of shorter duration may be appropriate if the period of dosing in the phase I and II clinical studies will be of short duration. The number of days that a compound is studied in the GLP in vivo toxicology studies is the maximum duration of dosing that can occur in the human studies. Thus, two weeks of dosing in toxicology limits dosing in humans to two weeks.

The idea that two weeks of dosing in the toxicology studies will shorten considerably the time to submission of the IND is a mistake. The only time savings will be the two weeks required for dosing the animals, as the time required to complete all other aspects of the study is the same as for a 28-day study. The only financial savings are the costs associated with requiring less compound for dosing the animals and lower housing, feeding, and animal handling activities. Thus, justification for shortening the repeated-dose toxicity studies from 28 days to 14 days based on cost is somewhat limited.

If the new medicine is being developed as an anticancer agent, use in the toxicity studies of the dose regimen proposed for the clinic is important. Some anticancer agents are not well tolerated. If administered daily, the toxicity profile that is developed may indicate that the compound is significantly more toxic than it would have been had the proposed clinical dosing regimen been followed. Most clinical treatments with these drug candidates are intermittent, allowing for a recovery period between dose regimens. A study design that includes a recovery period before an animal is exposed to another dose regimen will provide a more accurate assessment of the toxicity profile of the compound.

The ultimate purpose of conducting GLP repeated-dose toxicity studies is to protect the patient or volunteer from the potentially adverse effects of the NCE as well as to inform the physician of changes in clinical signs, hematology, serum chemistry, or urinalysis that may indicate that a compound-related toxicity is developing.

7.10.1 Toxicology Requirements for Initiating an FIH Trial

The conduct of nonclinical safety studies has been described in ICH guideline M3 [13] and its two revisions of 1997 (R1) [14] and 2008 (R2) [15] entitled "Nonclinical Safety Studies for the Conduct of Human Clinical Trials for Pharmaceuticals." The M3 guideline was intended to harmonize the nonclinical toxicity studies to support the various stages of clinical development among the regions of Europe, the United States, and Japan. This supersedes other guidances that had been used or issued by the various regulatory authorities in these countries. All clinical trials in the United Kingdom and the EU now proceed via a clinical trial application (CTA) similar to that of the U.S. IND through the FDA. The supposed advantage once considered for initiating the first clinical trials in the UK under a CTX (exemption), essentially an investigator's IND but without the IND filing, is no longer accepted.

As excerpted from the ICH M3(R2) guideline [15], Table 7.1 provides information on the duration of rodent and nonrodent toxicity studies required to support clinical investigations. Thus, "repeated dose toxicity studies in two species (one nonrodent) for a minimum duration of 2 weeks [Table 8.1] would generally support any clinical development trials of up to 2 weeks in duration" [15]. Clinical trials of longer duration should be supported by repeated-dose toxicology studies of at least equivalent duration. Six-month rodent and nine-month nonrodent studies would generally support dosing for longer than six months in clinical trials. There are additional notes and special (regional) exceptions detailed in the ICH M3(R2) guidance, but for general purposes this table reflects the industry standard when considering early clinical development of an NCE.

TABLE 7.1 Duration of Repeated Dose Toxicity Studies to Support the Conduct of Worldwide Clinical Trials in All Regions

	Minimum Duration of Repeated Dose Toxicity Studies to Support Clinical Trials	
Maximum Duration of Clinical Trial	Rodents	Nonrodents
Up to 2 weeks	2 weeks	2 weeks
Between 2 weeks and 6 months	Same as clinical trial	Same as clinical trial
>6 months	6 months	9 months

Source: Adapted from [15].

From a practical drug development standpoint, we recommend that the following toxicity studies be considered to support the approval of an FDA IND application to initiate an FIH study with an orally administered NCE:

1. A study to compare in vitro the metabolism across species (species justification)
2. Single (acute)-dose toxicity studies (GLP) in a rodent species by the oral and intravenous routes of administration and orally to the nonrodent species
3. Repeated-dose range-finding studies (non-GLP) by the oral route of administration once daily in a rodent and a nonrodent species of five to seven days in duration (with toxicokinetics)
4. Repeated-dose toxicity studies in a rodent and a nonrodent species (GLP) by the oral route of administration once daily for 28 days (with toxicokinetics) with a two-week recovery phase
5. In vitro genotoxicity studies [bacterial reverse mutation assay (Ames test) and a chromosomal aberration assay using human peripheral blood lymphocytes] in accordance with ICH S2(R1)[20] [A study to assess in vivo clastogenic activity (e.g., mouse micronucleus test) should be completed during the clinical phase I program.]

As noted previously, the total cost and time of conducting a 14-day versus a 28-day study are not that different, with the 28-day study allowing further clinical exploration in early phase II clinical trials while toxicity studies of longer duration are being conducted.

Pilot studies to assess potential effects of the NCE on reproduction and fertility and on embryo–fetal development may be appropriate to ascertain risks associated with the inclusion of women of childbearing age into the FIH trial. For trials conducted in the United States, legal requirements are such that women cannot be excluded from participating in the clinical trials (including FIH) unless there is sufficient scientific justification based on the toxicology results.

Additional studies needed to complete the general toxicity profile of the NCE during clinical phase II/III are beyond the scope of this chapter; these include chronic studies (ICH S4) [16], reproductive and developmental toxicity studies [ICH S5(2R)] [17], carcinogenicity studies [ICH S1A, ICH S1B, ICH S2(R1)] [18–20], and if necessary, special studies to assess phototoxicity, sensitization, and/or immunotoxicity (ICH S8) [21]. [Teratology studies in rats and rabbits should be completed prior to initiation of phase II clinical trials if women of childbearing age are not part of exclusion criteria.]

7.10.2 Toxicology Protocols

Study Director As described in the GLP regulations (Chapter 9), the study director has the responsibility for the technical conduct of the study as well as for interpretation, analysis, documentation, and reporting of results. The study director is the single point of study control. There is only one study director identified for a toxicity study. Other participants who play special roles in supporting bioanalytical or toxicokinetic efforts of the study are referred to as *principal investigators* and should be so listed in the study protocol. A principal investigator is obligated to provide a final signed audited report to the study director for that particular aspect of the work product.

Study directors who are familiar with the therapeutic area and have the opportunity to review the pharmacology of an NCE prior to initiation of the toxicity study offer better insight on study observations and data interpretation than do those who without such familiarity. Also, to provide a desired level of attention to a GLP toxicity study, it is advisable that a study director be responsible for a single study at a time rather than overseeing multiple studies concurrently. It is of utmost importance that a study director be in constant communication with the development team or study sponsor.

Study Protocol Considerations A study protocol is a written document that immortalizes the objective of the study and the specific means taken in the study to reach that objective. Once it is signed by the study director, it becomes the guidance for the tasks that must be followed during the study. Detailed protocols may also provide a description on what is to be included in the final study report. The signed protocol also provides a summary that allows a reader or regulatory reviewer to understand what should have taken place during the study. If the study is to be conducted under contract by a CRO, the protocol will be the basis for guiding the CRO for what they have been contracted to perform. The various portions of the protocol are discussed in the following paragraphs.

A statement should be included as to whether or not the study will be conducted in accordance with GLP regulations (Chapter 9). Pivotal studies submitted to regulatory agencies in support of drug submissions are, in general, expected to be GLP compliant. Pilot studies are often not GLP compliant but meet the scientific objectives of the protocol. A decision not to conduct a study under GLP should be made with careful consideration to potential problems that may arise due to a lack of acceptable documentation and results.

The study objective states the purpose of the study. It also forms the basis for what is included in the conclusion section of the study report. Most objectives are stated in one to four sentences. An example of a study objective follows.

> *Objective:* The purpose of this study is to evaluate the responses in rats to once-daily oral administration of XXXX-XXX [code or drug candidate name] for 13 weeks and to determine the reversibility, persistence, or delayed occurrence of effects after four weeks of recovery. Any adverse findings associated with XXXX-XXX will be correlated to peak (C_{max}) and total ($AUC_{0-24\ h}$) plasma exposures of the parent compound [and, if appropriate, metabolites]. Any differences in sensitivity between genders will be evaluated. The NOAEL and MTD will be determined and potential target organs for toxicity identified.

The study design section begins by explaining how many vehicle and test article groups will comprise the study, provides a justification for the dose levels that will be tested, states the species of animal that will be used, how long the animals will be acclimated before dosing begins, and how the animals will be housed. It should indicate whether or not there will be any interim sacrifice as well as whether there will be a terminal sacrifice and, if so, when the sacrifice will take place. This section should give any specific instructions as to how the vehicle and test article should be prepared, and once prepared, the route by which it is to be administered and how frequently it is to be administered. If there are specific instructions as to the time of day that dosing should occur, these should also be listed.

Guidance specific to the study regarding mortality observations, clinical observations, and physical examinations of the animals should be provided. Major areas of data collection, such as body weights and food consumption, need to indicate when these data will begin to be collected and how frequently they will be collected. Whether or not there will be clinical pathology analyses (e.g., hematology, coagulation, serum chemistry, urinalysis) and/or toxicokinetic sampling should be stated clearly as well as what tests will be run, when samples will be collected, and how the samples will be collected and handled. If there are specific areas to be addressed in a study report or a special manner in which they are to be presented, these should be specified in detail in the study protocol.

If there is to be an interim or terminal sacrifice of animals, this should be specified. Guidance as to when animals may be sacrificed outside of these time points and what samples (blood, tissue) will be taken should be stated clearly. Instructions as to what will be observed (gross pathology), what organ weights and tissues will be taken for microscopic examination, and how they will be prepared (tissue fixation, processing, staining) should also be included. If a board-certified veterinary pathologist is to supervise the gross necropsies or perform a microscopic examination of tissues, this should also be included in the protocol.

Detailed protocols will include similar sections on how data will be collected, whether or not there will be statistical analysis of the data collected, and what statistical methods will be employed. Often overlooked in a study protocol is the composition of the final narrative report: that is, will text tables be included, will there be signed separate reports for the toxicokinetic report or reports by the pathologist and/or clinical pathologist, and how will study deviations be handled or included in the report? A complete protocol will indicate how study results will be communicated to the study sponsor, consultant, or monitor and how study-related materials will be archived once the study is completed.

When developing a protocol, it should be remembered that if a specific procedure or process is not covered in a study protocol, it does not have to be done in any particular manner or at all. If a specific method or procedure is desired in a given study, it must be described in the protocol. Some CROs have simplified study protocols that may work to the benefit of the CRO rather than the sponsor of the study. These simplified protocols are often provided when a CRO is asked to develop a study protocol for a client. Time spent in developing, expanding, editing, and assuring that all important points are covered in the study protocol is time well spent, as the protocol drives the study conduct. Study protocols should be completed and approved by both the sponsor's representative (sponsor's consultant and/or monitor as appropriate) and the study director before the animals are ordered. Modification of the protocol is accomplished by an amendment and is covered in the following section.

Sample Protocol Outline Often, a protocol outline is developed to capture the essential design elements for developing the complete protocol. This protocol outline can be used for internal discussions within an organization before a complete detailed protocol is developed and/or to obtain bids from CROs on an equable design if a CRO is to be used. An example of a protocol outline that may be used to begin development of a detailed study-specific protocol is provided below.

Pilot Oral Gavage 7-Day Toxicity Study of XXXX in Sprague–Dawley Rats

GLP Status: *This study will be conducted according to good laboratory practices.*

Objective: The purpose of this study is to evaluate the responses in rats to once-daily oral administration of XXXX-XXX [code or drug candidate name] for four weeks. Any adverse findings associated with XXXX-XXX will be correlated to peak (C_{max}) and total ($AUC_{0-24\ h}$) plasma exposures of the parent compound [and if appropriate, metabolite(s)]. Any differences in sensitivity between genders will be evaluated. The NOAEL and MTD will be determined and potential target organs for toxicity identified.

Organization of the Study Test Groups

Group	Group Number	Treatment Group	Dose Level	Concentration	Dose Volume (mL)	Number of Rats/Dose
Main	1	Control	0	TBD	TBD	3M-3F
	2	Low	TBD	TBD	TBD	3M-3F
	3	Middle	TBD	TBD	TBD	3M-3F
	4	High	TBD	TBD	TBD	3M-3F
TK	1	Control	0	TBD	TBD	9M-9F
	2	Low	TBD	TBD	TBD	9M-9F
	3	Middle	TBD	TBD	TBD	9M-9F
	4	High	TBD	TBD	TBD	9M-9F

TBD, to be determined.

Study Design:

Dose groups: Four groups—one control group, three test article groups

Dose justification: Doses will be based on the results of the acute oral (gavage) single-dose toxicity study in rats with a 14-day recovery period.

Animals: Young adult Sprague–Dawley rats (total of 96 rats on study)

Main study: 3 rats/gender/group (total of 12 males and 12 females)

Toxicokinetic study: 9 rats/gender/group (total of 36 males and 36 females)

Acclimation period: Approximately seven days of acclimation

Housing: One rat/cage

Interim sacrifice: None

Terminal sacrifice: All surviving rats on day 7

Test article preparation for dosing: Formulation methods will be discussed with the sponsor. Stability and storage information on the bulk test material is available. Duplicate samples of the control and the dosing formulations of each test article will be collected for possible verification of the concentration of the dosing solution using a validated assay. Any analysis of the test article in the dosing solutions will be performed at a sponsor-designated analytical laboratory.

Test article administration: Oral (gavage) on days 0 through 6.

Time of dosing: The time of dosing will be documented in the records. Dosing will occur within ±30 minutes of the preceding day.

Viability/mortality observations: Twice daily—as early in the morning and as late in the afternoon as possible. The two observations will be separated by at least 6 hours.

Clinical observations: All rats, immediately prior to dosing and approximately 2 and 6 hours (±15 minutes) postdose.

Detailed physical examinations: All rats prior to dosing and weekly thereafter.

Body weights: Weekly during pretest and on days 0, 2, and 6.

Food consumption: Weekly during pretest and on days 0, 2, and 6.

Ophthalmology: None

Toxicokinetics: At dosing day 6, blood samples will be collected from three rats/gender/group/time point at 0, 5, 15, 30 minutes and 1, 3, and 6 hours postdosing. [One group of 3 rats/gender will be sampled at 0 minutes, 30 minutes, and 6 hours after dosing; a second group of 3 rats/gender will be sampled at 5 and 60 minutes after dosing; and a third group of 3 rats/gender will be sampled at 15 minutes and 3 hours after dosing.] A total of 168 blood or plasma samples will be collected. After final sampling, all rats used for toxicokinetics will be euthanized humanely without further examination. [Analysis of plasma for parent drug will be performed at an independent sponsor-designated bioanalytical laboratory.]

Clinical pathology: All main study rats at time of necropsy will have samples taken for hematology (24 samples), serum chemistry (24 samples), and coagulation (24 samples) parameters (total: 72 samples).

Necropsy: On main study rats, complete necropsy with collection and fixation of tissues from the STP standard list of tissues on all rats that die on study or are terminally sacrificed. Tissues will be fixed for microscopic examination (see "Histopathology").

Organ weights: A standard list of organ weights will be taken from main study rats at the time of terminal necropsy.

Histopathology: On main study rats, all tissues will be processed to glass microslides. The control and high-dose groups will be examined microscopically. All gross lesions from all dose groups will be examined microscopically.

Reporting: An audited draft report and final report are to be provided as a searchable PDF file that can be integrated seamlessly into an electronic submission.

Protocol Amendments At any time after the protocol is signed, during the course of a study, modification of existing protocol requirements may be desired. A protocol amendment is the means by which any change in a study protocol is documented. It is preferred that a protocol amendment be discussed by all contributing parties [the study sponsor, study consultant (if one is involved) and the CRO] prior to affecting any change to the study. Putting the proposed change into writing assures that all specifics of the change to be made are stated clearly for all parties concerned and documented for those reading the study report subsequent to study completion.

Communication of the need for change is the responsibility of whoever is requesting the modification. A draft of the proposed change should be developed that shows (1) the current protocol wording, (2) the new protocol wording, and (3) the justification for the change. This amendment should be approved/signed by the study director and if conducted at an CRO, it should also be signed by the sponsor's representative (the sponsor's consultant if there is one), and the CRO study director. Subsequent protocol amendments should be numbered sequentially.

An example of a protocol amendment to change the name of the study pathologist is provided below.

Protocol Amendment No. 1

Section VII. Designation of Study Pathologist

Current version: The study pathologist will be

Don Small, D.V.M, Ph.D., ACVP

Amended version: The study pathologist will be

~~Don Small, D.V.M., Ph.D., ACVP~~

Sarah Little, D.V.M., ACVP

Justification: To indicate a change in the study pathologist.
Approved by:

XXXXXXXX ________, ________
Study Director Date

XXXXXXXX________, ________
Sponsor's Representative Date

XXXXXXXX________, ________
Study Consultant Date

Protocol Deviations Whenever an action is taken in the study that is not in accordance with the study protocol or when an action required in the study protocol is not taken, a protocol deviation has occurred. Protocol deviations need to be summarized in such a way that any person reading the study report can understand what took place and how this affected the overall study outcome. Each deviation should be addressed separately as to the significance of the deviation, and reasoning should be provided for that determination.

A summary of protocol deviations should be provided by the study director in the overall final study report. Some study directors prefer to include deviations in the narrative text to the study. We prefer to include all summary deviations in an appendix to the study report. Including deviations in a separate appendix allows all deviations to be summarized in one location and does not interfere with the reader's ease in reading the overall study report.

An example of a suggested format for the recording of deviations is provided below.

Study Deviation No. 1

Protocol: Give the section of the protocol (page, paragraph, and specific wording) from which the deviation occurred.

Deviation period: Give the date and time of the deviation.

Deviation: State what occurred to make it a deviation.

Evaluation: Provide an evaluation of the deviation and state specifically whether or not the deviation had an effect on carrying out the objectives of the study or interpretation of the results; if so, why; if not, why not.

Study Deviation No. 2 (Continue with similar format/information.)

7.10.3 Study Monitoring

When a drug sponsor is a large pharmaceutical company or other institution that has its own toxicology department(s), typically the infrastructure is in place whereby the corporate sponsor, study director, toxicology laboratory, and other disciplines, such as quality assurance, are contained within a single facility. In such instances, study monitoring is part of the institutional procedures and is often described with in-house standard operating procedures (SOPs). However, many sponsor organizations require the use of outside laboratories such as CROs, in which case it is critical that procedures are in place to assure that the studies are conducted according to the sponsor's goals and approved protocol. Studies left to run themselves are prone to disaster. When a CRO is involved, study monitoring begins before the laboratory is selected and continues after the study protocol is signed through to the generation and approval of the final report.

Prior to placing a study at a CRO, the laboratory should be inspected by someone qualified to evaluate the ability of the laboratory to run the study. In the interest of getting a study placed at a laboratory, CRO business representatives may claim that all the work required can be done within the facility. Unfortunately, this has not always proved to be the case. A facility inspection by a person trained in such a review may save considerable time and money in the long run by identifying potential problems in running the study at any facility (Chapter 1).

If a study is placed in a CRO, some degree of monitoring will be done by the CRO's quality assurance unit. Additional monitoring may be performed by the study supervisor and study director. When considering a CRO to perform a study, one of the items that should be discussed with the CRO is how they are going to monitor the study: by whom, how frequently, how the monitoring activities will be documented, and whether such documentation will be available for review by the sponsor. Similarly, if a CRO is going to subcontract a portion of the study, how will the subcontractor be monitored?

Either the sponsor or a representative of the sponsor familiar with CROs and their carrying out of study procedures should monitor the study as it is being performed. In general, the longer and more detailed the study, the more monitoring will be required. Having a sponsor-provided study monitor present to observe the formulation of test articles and the first day of dosing indicates to a CRO more than a passing interest in the conduct of the study. Trained monitors will observe all aspects of the start of the study and provide the sponsor with a written report of their observations. This report may serve as a basis for indicating areas of the CRO's performance that need improvement or other areas that were performed adequately or in an exemplary manner. If there is an area that needs improvement, monitoring will identify the problem early in the study and allow for needed adjustment on behalf of the people performing the study.

Major or unique study events should be monitored. If animals are to undergo interim or terminal necropsy, having a study monitor familiar with necropsy procedures is particularly helpful. Potential treatment-related lesions may be identified at the time of the necropsy and the sponsor made aware of them within hours/days rather than waiting for a report from the laboratory, which may not occur until months later.

7.10.4 Microscopic Examination of Tissues

On main study animals (i.e., the non-toxicokinetic group), all tissues normally collected [22] should be processed to glass microslides. The FDA guidance [13–15] states that control and high-dose groups should be examined microscopically and that all gross lesions from all dose groups should be examined microscopically. If tissues are processed and examined microscopically in the control and high-dose groups, according to the FDA's recommendation, the need to read tissues from the additional groups may arise. In a CRO, a major bottleneck to study completion is frequently the time to process the additional tissues and to reschedule the pathologist's time to read them. Some CROs will offer to expedite reading of the additional tissues; however, this may be quite expensive compared to the original reading. Therefore, to optimize time and cost effectiveness, it is advisable to stain and read all tissues in all groups at the end of the study, and then, if needed, to process and read additional tissues at a later date.

7.10.5 Considerations of the NOAEL and MTD in Protocol Design

The endpoints of the general toxicology protocol are designed to determine the NOAEL and the MTD along with identification of potential target organs for toxicity as a function of systemic exposure. As discussed previously, these should be included as distinct study objectives to ensure that these essential endpoints are captured in the study outcome. In our experience, not all study directors readily address the NOAEL or MTD in the discussion or conclusion sections of the study report. Some study reports do not address the NOAEL. In the absence of identifying the NOAEL, the identification and interpretation of the NOAEL is left to the reader/reviewer, and this can have regulatory consequences.

Interpretation of the NOAEL In the design of a toxicity study, the selection of the lowest dose is anticipated to be the NOAEL. This dose should be five- to 10-fold higher relative to the clinical therapeutic dose (or dose range) estimated and based on a body surface area using an average body weight of 65 kg. The NOAEL is used principally to estimate the maximum safe starting dose in the FIH trial [9] and to provide assurance on relative margins of safety during clinical development. The NOAEL also provides guidance on the relative merits of the early acute nonclinical efforts to define therapeutic index (ED_{50}/LD_{50}) and relative margins of safety (LD_1/ED_{99}) [23].

The NOAEL is not necessarily equivalent to the no observable effect level (NOEL). The key difference is in the term *adverse*. An extension of the pharmacological or biological activity of an NCE is not necessarily considered adverse. The NOEL may represent a dose where pharmacological activity may be present (e.g., local bruising associated with anticoagulant therapy) in the absence of clinical or anatomic pathological findings.

There are situations where the NOAEL cannot be determined from the results of a completed toxicity study. This can occur when the NOAEL cannot be estimated because of adverse effects encountered at the lowest dose that was tested. For shorter-term (subchronic) toxicity studies, the solution is typically to repeat the study but at lower doses, keeping in mind that the decision on dose-level selection still needs consideration of safety margins relative to the clinical therapeutic dose anticipated. For longer-term (chronic) studies, the solution usually resides in the adverse finding(s) and relevance to the existing clinical safety database. However, repeating a chronic toxicity study is usually an exception.

Interpretation of the MTD Determination of the MTD is important for two reasons: (1) decisions on the high-dose levels in subchronic and chronic toxicity studies are dependent on the MTD as an estimate of threshold response for adverse effects; and (2) the MTD or highest not significantly toxic dose serves as a means to determine the starting dose in patients for special therapeutic categories (e.g., anticancer chemotherapeutics). The selection of doses for the toxicology protocol should span the anticipated maximum tolerated dose and toxic dose levels. Initially, this is based on preliminary dose-range-finding studies and subsequently on definitive toxicity studies. Justification for selection of the MTD is defined in each toxicology study protocol. The selection of the MTD is usually based on the toxicity profile but can also be defined by the toxicokinetic profile (Chapter 9), where saturation of absorption (or plateau) limits further systemic exposure with higher dose administration or where limits in the elimination or metabolism of an NCE results in continuous systemic accumulation of the active moiety. For anticancer cytotoxic drug development, the MTD is identified as the highest nonsevere toxic dose (HNSTD) [24]. This HNSTD is used for estimating the maximum safe starting dose in initial clinical trials of chemotherapeutics in patients.

In summary, determination of both the NOAEL and the MTD plays a critical role in the drug development process and requires careful consideration when selecting the doses to be used in a toxicology protocol.

7.11 PRE-IND MEETING

The pre-IND meeting (Chapters 13 and 14) is a tool whereby a sponsor can present to the FDA its available nonclinical data and proposed nonclinical/clinical development plan in a written document and seek FDA concurrence or guidance. Data presented may include chemistry, manufacturing, and controls, pharmacology data (in vitro and in vivo), pharmacokinetic data, available toxicology data, the proposed toxicology program and toxicology protocols, and an outline of the proposed clinical development plan. The plan must include the clinical indication, dose route, and regimen, and the phase I clinical protocol outline and preliminary phase II plans.

The sponsor may be granted a meeting with the regulators to discuss specifically the questions that have been raised. Often, the reviewing group provides written responses to each question and in addition may follow these with a conference call. For those proposed plans with which the reviewers do not agree, there is a written discussion as to why the agency does not agree with the proposal and a suggestion of what the agency expects to receive in the IND package. How the sponsor develops the specific data that are requested is left to the creativity of the sponsor.

These pre-IND contacts are as effective as the sponsor chooses to make them. If the data package prepared by the sponsor is very complete and the data, plans, and questions are prepared carefully and thoughtfully, this contact is most constructive. If the sponsor intends to present minimal data and then attempts to convince the agency that further studies are not needed, the sponsor usually comes away frustrated and sometimes angry. These contacts are designed to provide the sponsor with an opportunity to present their data and plans and to receive constructive feedback, which indicates what information, in addition to that which is proposed, will be adequate to support an approvable IND.

7.12 CONCLUSIONS

It is a regulatory requirement that an IND application be filed with and approved by the FDA before *any* clinical study can be conducted in the United States by a drug sponsor using human subjects. There are guidelines to be followed in developing the information package that supports the FIH trial. A principal concern associated with approval of the resulting IND is the presentation of data that supports the safety of the test article in human subjects. In the submission the sponsor must demonstrate that the drug candidate has been synthesized under controlled conditions and has the same structure, level of purity, and stability as the compound evaluated in the nonclinical toxicity studies. The pre-FIH toxicity studies must have been conducted using doses, dose route, dose regimen, and study durations that support the specific clinical studies proposed in the IND, and thus provide a basis for selection of the initial dose in the FIH trial. This starting dose is usually one-tenth the NOAEL obtained from the repeated-dose toxicity study conducted in the most sensitive animal species. For a cancer indication this dose may be one-sixth of the NOAEL in the nonrodent species to allow higher starting doses in patients in order to provide a possible benefit from the drug should their cancer be responsive to the activity of the compound.

The most important conclusion in the IND is the statement that the data support safe evaluation of the compound in humans. The time taken to develop an approvable IND is time well spent. Efforts to develop an IND package based on a management-imposed inappropriately short deadline can lead to an IND package that is inadequate and is ultimately put on hold because of deficiencies or questions that will most certainly arise. The time, effort, and resources to get an IND off hold more than justifies the effort to do it right the first time. Shortcuts in this process can be very costly.

REFERENCES

1. Serabian MA, Pilaro AM. Safety assessment of biotechnology-derived pharmaceuticals. ICH and beyond. *Toxicol Pathol*. 1999;27:27–31.
2. Medjitna TD, Stadler C, Bruckner L, Griot C, Ottiger HP. DNA vaccines: safety aspect assessment and regulation. *Dev Biol*. 2006;126:261–207.
3. ICH Safety Guidelines: Preclinical Safety Evaluation of Biotechnology-Derived Pharmaceuticals. ICH S6 (1997); ICH S6(R1) (2008). International Conference on Harmonization. Available at: www.ich.org.
4. Kramer JA, Sagartz JE, Morris DL. The application of discovery toxicology and pathology towards the design of safer pharmaceutical lead candidates. *Nat Rev/Drug Discov*. 2007;6:636–648.
5. Olson H, Betton G, Robinson D, Thomas K, Monro A, Kolaja G. Concordance of the toxicity of pharmaceuticals in humans and in animals. *Regul Toxicol Pharmacol*. 2000;32:56–67.
6. Greaves P, Williams A, Eve M. First dose of potential new medicines to humans: how animals help. *Nat Rev/Drug Discov*. 2004;3:226–236.
7. ICH Quality Guideline: Impurities in New Drug Products. ICH Q3B(R2). International Conference on Harmonization; 2006. Available at: www.ich.org.
8. Guidance for Industry: Genotoxic and Carcinogenic Impurities in Drug Substances and Products: Recommended Approaches. U.S. Department of Health and Human Services, Food and Drug Administration; 2008.
9. Guidance for Industry: Estimating the Maximum Safe Starting Dose in Initial Clinical Trials for Therapeutics in Adult Healthy Volunteers. U.S. Department of Health and Human Services, Food and Drug Administration, Center for Drug Evaluation and Research; 2005.
10. Guidance for Industry: Safety Testing of Drug Metabolites. U.S. Department of Health and Human Services, Food and Drug Administration, Center for Drug Evaluation and Research; 2008.
11. Ames BN, McCann J, Yamasaki E. Methods for detecting carcinogens and mutagens with the *Salmonella*/mammalian-microsome mutagenicity test. *Mutat Res*. 1975;31:347–364.
12. Maron DM, Ames BN. Revised methods for the *Salmonella* mutagenicity test. *Mutat Res*. 1983;113:173–215.

13. ICH Multidisciplinary Guideline: Nonclinical Safety Studies for the Conduct of Human Clinical Trials for Pharmaceuticals. ICH M3. International Conference on Harmonization; 1997. Available at: www.ich.org.
14. ICH Multidisciplinary Guideline: Nonclinical Safety Studies for the Conduct of Human Clinical Trials for Pharmaceuticals. International Conference on Harmonization; ICH M3(R1). 1997. Available at: www.ich.org.
15. ICH Multidisciplinary Guideline: Nonclinical Safety Studies for the Conduct of Human Clinical Trials and Marketing Authorization for Pharmaceuticals. ICH M3(R2). International Conference on Harmonization; 2008. Available at: www.ich.org.
16. ICH Safety Guideline: Duration of Chronic Toxicity Testing in Animals (Rodent and Non-rodent Toxicity Testing). ICH S4. International Conference on Harmonization; 1999. Available at: www.ich.org.
17. ICH Safety Guideline: Detection of Toxicity to Reproduction for Medicinal Products and Toxicity to Male Fertility. ICH S5(R2). International Conference on Harmonization; 1994. Available at: www.ich.org.
18. ICH Safety Guideline: Guideline on the Need for Carcinogenicity Studies of Pharmaceuticals. ICH S1A. International Conference on Harmonization; 1996. Available at: www.ich.org.
19. ICH Safety Guideline: Testing for Carcinogenicity of Pharmaceuticals. ICH S1B. International Conference on Harmonization; 1998. Available at: www.ich.org.
20. ICH Safety Guideline: Guidance on Genotoxicity Testing and Data Interpretation for Pharmaceuticals Intended for Human Use. ICH S2(R1). International Conference on Harmonization; 2008. Available at: www.ich.org.
21. ICH Safety Guideline: Immunotoxicity Studies for Human Pharmaceuticals. ICH S8. International Conference on Harmonization; 2006. Available at: www.ich.org.
22. Center for Food Safety and Applied Nutrition's Redbook. U.S. Food and Drug Administration. Available at: www.cfsan.fda.gov/~redbook/red-ivb1.html.
23. Eaton DL, Klaassen CD. Principles of toxicology. In: Klaasen CD, ed. *Casarett and Doull's Toxicology: The Basic Science of Poisons*, 5th ed. New York: McGraw-Hill, Chap. 24.
24. DeGeorge JJ, et al. Regulatory considerations for preclinical development of anticancer drugs. *Cancer Chemother Pharmacol*. 1998;41:173–185.

8

TOXICOKINETICS IN SUPPORT OF DRUG DEVELOPMENT

GARY EICHENBAUM, VANGALA SUBRAHMANYAM, AND
ALFRED P. TONELLI

8.1 INTRODUCTION

In its simplest terms, toxicokinetics is the evaluation of the pharmacokinetics of a compound at doses used in toxicity studies. Its primary purpose is to correlate the dose administered to the systemic exposure and toxic effects that are observed in all subtypes of nonclinical toxicity studies [1,2]. Toxicokinetic data are typically obtained by analysis of plasma, serum, and occasionally, blood or urine samples taken from main toxicology or satellite test animals. The studies are generally designed to enable estimates of the maximum plasma concentration (C_{max}) and area under the plasma (or serum) concentration versus time curve (AUC). Although the original objective for toxicokinetics was simple (i.e., validation of drug exposure in toxicity studies), it has evolved into a critical enabling methodology, which helps to rationalize species and dose selection, dosing vehicles and frequency, and animal/human safety margin assessments.

Throughout the course of drug development, toxicokinetics plays an important role in clinical dose selection and escalation, but perhaps one of the most critical roles is to support the initial single and multiple ascending dose studies in healthy volunteers. At this stage there are no human safety data and the critical questions are [3]: What is the starting human dose and exposure in the first-in-human (FIH) study? What should be the "stopping" dose and corresponding plasma drug concentration?

Starting and stopping criteria for an FIH study are very much driven by the nature of the toxicities, the doses, and the exposure at which those toxicities

Early Drug Development: Strategies and Routes to First-in-Human Trials, Edited by Mitchell N. Cayen

were observed in the pre-FIH studies. Although toxicity study designs can vary considerably depending on the type of study, most investigators seek to define no observed adverse effect level (NOAEL) as well as toxic doses and associated plasma analyte concentrations. Establishing safety margins is one of the first steps in estimating the safe human starting doses. These may be calculated by dividing either the toxicology dose corrected for body surface area, or the toxicokinetic exposure, at the NOEL (no effect level)/NOAEL by the dose, or exposure, desired in the clinic. Additional factors influencing toxicokinetics include species differences in pharmacokinetics, metabolism, and protein binding. Assessing safety margins relative to the toxicity profile and the pharmacological target desired forms the basis for setting clinical starting doses and criteria for stopping dose escalation.

Toxicokinetics generally does not include traditional characterization of the absorption, distribution, metabolism, and elimination (ADME). However, these dispositional parameters play an important role in species and dose selection for the initial toxicity studies and help complement the toxicokinetic data [4] (Chapter 7). In contrast to ADME studies, the purpose of toxicokinetic studies is to observe and react to, but not to determine mechanistically, the underlying rationale for differences in exposure that may occur across species, genders, intradose group, or following single versus multiple dosing [1].

In the first part of this chapter we provide a brief history, a regulatory perspective, and factors to consider in the design of toxicokinetic studies. In the second part we address the role of toxicokinetics in the various types of toxicology and safety pharmacology studies and approaches to interpret toxicokinetic results. Examples to help illustrate the concepts are presented in both sections. Although the focus of this book is on drug development to support FIH studies, nonclinical drug development is a continuum, and toxicity studies to support phase II are generally under way prior to completing the phase I safety and pharmacokinetic studies. Therefore, additional information has been included to provide guidance for those nonclinical studies that are ongoing during phases I and II.

8.2 HISTORICAL PERSPECTIVES

Prior to the 1980s, the nonclinical safety of many xenobiotics was often evaluated in toxicity studies by noting their effects on the behavior and survival of test animals and by observing changes in organ function and morphology but without measuring corresponding systemic exposure levels [5]. In the absence of exposure data, estimates of safety margins relied solely on extrapolation of the dose administered in a nonclinical model to the dose in humans based on body surface area or mass. Although estimates of safety margins by this approach are still employed [2] and can provide important insights for setting clinical doses, they do not account for potential differences in exposure that can occur across species, genders, intradose group, or following single versus multiple dosing. However, such data can be misleading because after oral drug administration, the toxic effects can be dependent on the ADME behavior of the compound and may not relate directly to the dose administered. Toxicokinetics started to evolve into its modern form in the early 1980s, when quantitative pharmacokinetic principles were developed to validate drug exposure in animals [6,7].

The more widespread use of toxicokinetics was enabled by two major changes in bioanalytical technologies [4]. Advances in high-performance liquid chromatography (HPLC) as a sensitive and robust analytical tool, amenable to automation, allowed simpler method development and lower costs for plasma analysis. The second major breakthrough was the advent of LC-mass spectrometry (MS) as a routine bioanalytical tool (Chapter 4). Recent advances in mass spectrometric instrumentation revolutionized the sensitivity of quantitative analysis of drugs and their metabolites in biological fluids. Currently, drug concentrations in the picogram to nanogram/mL range can be detected in as little as ≤ 10 μL of blood plasma or other biological matrix. These advances also had some impact in minimizing animal use in pharmacokinetic evaluations, by allowing multiple samplings from the smaller species.

8.3 REGULATORY CONSIDERATIONS

In June 1995, the International Conference on Harmonization (ICH) issued the ICH S3 guidance, entitled: "Toxicokinetics: A Guidance for Assessing Systemic Exposure in Toxicity Studies" [2], wherein toxicokinetics is defined as "the generation of pharmacokinetic data, either as an integral component in the conduct of nonclinical toxicity studies or in specially designed supportive studies, in order to assess systemic exposure." The guidance states that "the primary objective of toxicokinetics is to describe the systemic exposure achieved in animals and its relationship to dose level and the time course of the toxicity study"; secondary objectives are to "relate the exposure achieved in toxicity studies to toxicological findings and contribute to the assessment of the relevance of these findings to clinical safety, to support the choice of species and treatment regimen in nonclinical toxicity studies, to provide information which, in conjunction with the toxicity findings, contributes to the design of subsequent nonclinical toxicity studies" [2]. Although bioanalytical considerations were addressed only partially in ICH S3, they have evolved through joint regulatory and industry meetings known as the Crystal City bioanalytical meetings as probably the best defined and internationally understood supportive guidelines in use today (Chapter 4).

The toxicokinetics guidance intentionally leaves significant room for interpretation on how to properly conduct the toxicokinetic portion of a toxicity study. It states that the objectives described above may be achieved by the derivation of one or more pharmacokinetic parameters from measurements made at appropriate time points during the course of the individual studies. These measurements usually consist of plasma (or whole blood or serum) concentrations for the parent compound and/or metabolite(s) and should be selected on a case-by-case basis. Plasma (or whole blood or serum) AUC, C_{max}, and t_{max} are the parameters commonly used in assessing exposure in toxicokinetics studies. Importantly, the toxicokinetic guidance states that due to its integration into toxicity testing and its bridging character between nonclinical and clinical studies, the focus is primarily on the interpretation of toxicity tests and not on characterizing the basic pharmacokinetic parameters of the substance studied. The guidance also states that "for some compounds it will be more appropriate to calculate exposure based on the [plasma protein] unbound concentration" [2]. In practice, many drug sponsors have found that regulatory authorities will consider animal or human exposure multiples for unbound drug only when the free fraction is greater in human plasma than in plasma of the toxicity species. These data may be obtained from all animals on a toxicity study, in representative subgroups, in satellite groups, or in separate studies.

Toxicokinetic analyses that support good laboratory practices (GLP) toxicity studies must also be conducted in accordance with GLPs (Chapter 9) using fully validated bioanalytical methods (Chapter 4). However, it is important to note that pharmacokinetic studies in support of formulation assessments, general ADME–pharmacokinetics characterization, and non-GLP pilot toxicity studies are not required to be conducted under GLPs. GLP toxicokinetic work requires documented training records for involved staff, dosing, bleeding, and sample storage/shipping records and validated bioanalytical methods [8,9]. The validation report should include information on the analyte stability, a calibration curve with a definition of the lower limit of quantification (LLOQ), and the specificity, precision, accuracy, and sensitivity of the method. The bioanalysis and toxicokinetic assessment may be performed by the same investigator and combined in a single report or conducted by separate groups and included in separate reports. An independent quality assurance unit must also review all reports generated to support the toxicokinetic analysis.

Although not formally accepted in non-ICH countries, these principles should be considered to be applicable for non-ICH affiliated regions (e.g., India and China), as modern drug development is generally a global process.

8.4 FACTORS TO CONSIDER IN THE DESIGN OF TOXICOKINETIC STUDIES

Although the recommendations contained in the ICH S3A guideline [2] provide a basis for designing toxicokinetic studies, as discussed above, there are multiple factors to consider regarding the study design that are left up to the investigator. These considerations can vary with the type of study and stage of development and are discussed in the sections that follow.

8.4.1 Drug Supply Requirements

The ability to conduct adequate toxicokinetic assessments may be limited by the availability of drug supply. Depending on the species, dose levels, and duration

TABLE 8.1 Study Design Example for a One-Month Rat Toxicity Study[a]

Group	Dose Level (mg/kg)	Dose Volume (mL/kg)	Dose Concentration (mg/mL)	Number of Animals: Tox Males	Tox Females	Recovery Males	Recovery Females	TK Males	TK Females	Drug Substance Required (g)[b]
1	0	10	0	10	10	0	0	0	0	0.00
2	200	10	20	10	10	0	0	0	0	42.00
3	600	10	60	10	10	0	0	0	0	126.00
4	1750	10	175	10	10	0	0	0	0	367.50
5	0	10	0	0	0	0	0	3	3	0.00
6	200	10	20	0	0	0	0	4	4	16.80
7	600	10	60	0	0	0	0	4	4	50.40
8	1750	10	175	0	0	0	0	4	4	147.00

[a]The drug substance requirements for the toxicokinetic portion relative to the toxicology portion of the study.
[b]The total drug substance calculations assume an average weight per rat of 0.5 kg, resulting in an estimated amount of drug required for the toxicokinetic portion of the study (groups 5 to 8) of 214.2 g and 535.5 g for the toxicology portion (groups 1 to 4).

of the toxicity study, the drug supply requirements can be significant, especially in the early stages of development, prior to optimizing synthesis processes. In the example shown for a drug with low toxicity (from our laboratories) in Table 8.1, more than 200 g of additional drug substance may be required to support toxicokinetic evaluation in the satellite animals (companion study animals used for plasma sampling and toxicokinetics only; see Section 8.4.13) of a rat one-month toxicity study. Therefore, it is important to provide estimates of the drug requirements for the toxicology and toxicokinetic portions early in the planning process so that an adequate drug supply can be synthesized and made available in a timely manner. For GLP toxicity studies, an overage factor of 20% is generally applied to ensure that there is sufficient drug for bioanalytical characterization. Generally, for toxicokinetic characterization in nonrodents the same animals are used for blood collection as in the toxicity study, and no additional drug supply is needed.

In cases where drug supply is limited, it may be necessary to consider performing sparse or limited sampling (see Section 8.4.2) from the main toxicology animals to support the toxicokinetic assessment. Another alternative to consider when the drug supply is limited is to file an exploratory investigational new drug (IND) application (Chapter 11) or clinical trial application (CTA), which generally requires an abbreviated toxicology program and much less drug supply for the toxicology enabling studies [10].

8.4.2 Species Selection

Selection of the appropriate species is a critical consideration in toxicity studies that support an FIH trial. With rare exceptions, the pre-FIH rodent species is the rat (Sprague–Dawley or Wistar), and the nonrodent species is usually a choice between the dog and a nonhuman primate. It is highly desirable to select species that are similar to humans with respect to activity at the biological target, metabolism, and pharmacokinetics (Chapter 7). From the toxicokinetic perspective, if there are much lower plasma concentrations of metabolites in the nonclinical species compared to humans, it can be difficult to evaluate safety at sufficient multiples of the clinical target. Exposures to a metabolite that is not present, or is present at much lower levels, in humans could confound the toxicologic assessment and necessitate further evaluation in a more relevant species. Selection of a nonrepresentative species can result in increased cost and time for development. Nevertheless, since prior to FIH dosing, no data are available on the in vivo metabolism in humans, if there are no obvious species differences based on in vitro metabolism in liver microsomes and/or hepatocytes, the rat and dog are typically the default species used. Toxicokinetics and metabolism are important parameters in species selection but must also be weighed with the appropriate species from a pharmacological target and activity perspective.

8.4.3 API Properties: Salt/Crystal Form, Particle Size, and Impurities

The salt/crystal form, particle size, and impurity profile can have a significant impact on the kinetic solubility and absorption as well as the chemical and physical stability of the NCE, which can in turn have a significant impact on plasma drug exposure. These properties may not be fully characterized in the batches used in the early stage non-GLP dose-range-finding toxicity studies, and as a result, when the compound is scaled up for GLP studies, the exposure and resulting toxicity profile in the new batch may change substantially. Therefore, when a new batch is synthesized using different processes resulting in different dissolution profiles, or other changes in the physicochemical characteristics, single-dose bridging pharmacokinetic escalation studies, at a toxicologically relevant dose, are often conducted to support dose selection for the toxicity studies instead of relying on data from previous batches. This is more important for compounds that have low solubility such that major changes in absorption may occur with a change in dosage form or formulation. This is shown in Figure 8.1, which illustrates how the change in dosage form of a low-solubility drug can markedly affect the plasma exposure. Form 1 attained much higher exposures than form 2 at similar doses. Form 1 shows a dose proportional increase in exposure up to a dose of approximately 550 mg/kg and a saturation of absorption at doses above 750 mg/kg. Form 2 shows a saturation of absorption at doses greater than 375 mg/kg.

8.4.4 Dose-Related Exposure

One of the goals in the selection of dose levels for toxicity studies is that plasma exposure to parent drug and/or relevant metabolites should be dose related.

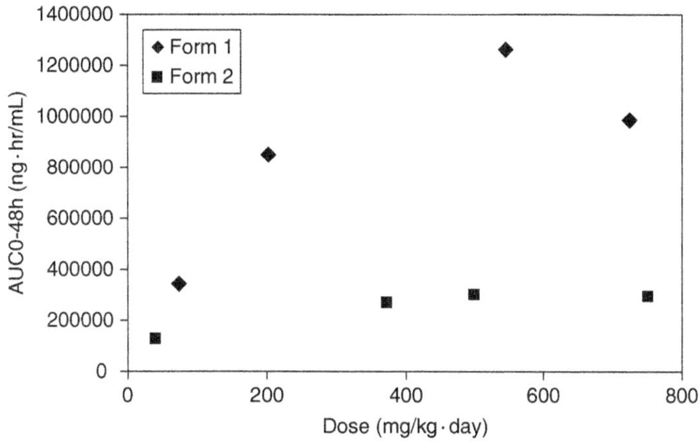

FIGURE 8.1 AUC versus dose for two forms of a low-solubility drug.

Thus, drugs that have limited exposure due to poor aqueous solubility, absorption, efflux, emesis, extensive first-pass metabolism (gut or liver) [11], or that are subject to rapid elimination may not achieve sufficient exposure to support a comprehensive toxicology assessment. For compounds with these properties, exploratory single escalating dose pharmacokinetic studies may be useful prior to initiating toxicity studies to evaluate if these limitations can be overcome. For example, in the case of compounds that undergo extensive first-pass metabolism or efflux, by evaluating the pharmacokinetics at higher doses it may be possible to identify doses at which these processes are saturated. In the case of low-solubility compounds, it may be helpful to try alternative vehicles (see Section 8.4.6) with improved dissolution to identify a suitable formulation that can deliver higher circulating drug levels. For compounds with high first-pass clearance, alternate dosing regimens may be tested to identify one that has sustained exposure to the test article over the dosing interval (e.g., twice or three-times daily dosing for orally administered and longer-duration infusions for compounds administered intravenously). For compounds that cause emesis in nonrodents, it may be possible to mitigate the frequency or extent of emesis by changing the time of feeding relative to dosing, the dosing regimen, or the formulation type (e.g., suspension to capsules). Unfortunately, for many compounds with dose-limited absorption, it is very difficult to find methods that generate significant increases in absorption.

8.4.5 Changes in Pharmacokinetics Following Multiple Dosing

Following multiple dosing, the drug metabolism and transport systems can become inhibited or induced based on the chemical nature of the new chemical entity (NCE), or less frequently on the effects of the compound's toxicity on the metabolic or clearance mechanism in the test animals [12]. To evaluate the potential for inhibition or induction, or animal toxicity, toxicokinetic measurements are usually made on the first and last days of dosing in the toxicity study. Autoinduction or inhibition in animals is usually observed within two weeks of dosing. The interpretation of differences in exposure on day 1 versus at steady state are discussed in Section 8.6.4. The most appropriate comparisons to human exposure for safety window estimates are conducted using multiple-dose data from the toxicity studies compared to steady-state human exposure.

8.4.6 Selection of Dosing Vehicles

It is highly desirable to select a vehicle for toxicity studies that is nontoxic, inert (i.e., does not enhance or mask the toxicologic effects), and delivers the dose in a form that has adequate stability and absorption. Preferred vehicles for oral toxicity studies are aqueous solutions or suspensions consisting of 0.5% methylcellulose or carboxymethylcellulose. Preferred vehicles for intravenous toxicity studies are aqueous sterile saline solutions. However, alternative vehicles [13,14] may be required to deliver low-solubility compounds, for which exposure is dissolution limited in standard vehicles. The need to use alternative vehicles is being driven in large part by the increasing numbers of low-solubility compounds that have entered drug development in recent years [15].

Potential challenges with nonstandard excipients or cosolvents include confounding effects on pharmacokinetics [16,17] and/or interference with the assessment of the pharmacologic or toxic effects [18,19] of the NCE. In addition, there may not be sufficient historical control data to differentiate excipient versus drug-related effects. For example, it has been shown that certain excipients can interact with uptake or efflux transporters and thereby affect the exposure of the test article [20,21]. Although it is desirable to use the same vehicle for all toxicology studies on a particular test agent, formulations may change depending on compound or project needs. In those cases, formulation comparison studies should be completed prior to re-initiating the toxicology program.

8.4.7 Bioanalytical Method

Development of a fully validated bioanalytical method is a critical component of the GLP toxicokinetic analyses and can be on the critical path for completing a toxicity study. The ICH S3A toxicokinetics guidance recommends that:

> The analytical methods to be used in toxicokinetic studies should be specific for the entity to be measured and of an adequate accuracy and precision. The limit of quantification should be adequate for the measurement of the range of concentrations anticipated to occur in the generation of the toxicokinetic data. The choice of analyte and the matrix to be assayed (biological fluids or tissue) should be stated and possible interference by endogenous components in each type of sample (from each species) should be investigated. Plasma, serum or whole blood are normally the matrices of choice for toxicokinetic studies. The analyte and matrix assayed in non-clinical studies should ideally be the same as in clinical studies. If different assay methods are used in non-clinical and clinical studies they should all be

suitably validated. An outline of the analytical method should be reported or referenced. In addition, a rationale for the choice of the matrix analyzed and the analyte measured should be given.

Bioanalytical methods are generally modified or improved during the course of drug development as study objectives and sensitivity requirements change. The most significant driver for the change is the requirement to support GLP-based studies using a validated bioanalytical method with well-characterized assay performance. Some other factors that need to be considered in bioanalytical method development include red blood cell (RBC) partitioning, matrix effects [22–24], and plasma stability. Whole blood/plasma ratios are typically evaluated in vitro as part of the bioanalytical method development. If significant partitioning into RBCs [or white blood cells: (WBCs)] is present, more complete work on capacity and saturability of blood cells is required, as well as characterization of in vivo blood partitioning. For those compounds where whole blood will be the compartment compared across clinical and toxicity studies (e.g., for evaluating exposure margins for efficacy or safety), plasma concentrations are also typically measured.

Depending on the nature of the drug, several factors may influence the partition of drugs into RBCs or WBCs from the plasma compartment. These include organic, cationic, anionic transporters, lipophilicity, ion trapping, and drugs binding to carbonic anhydrase. Drugs that penetrate RBCs are also subject to metabolism by RBC enzymes and binding to hemoglobin. Drugs that preferentially distribute to white blood cells are relatively rare; however, due to the low volume of white cells, this compartment may saturate early, spilling drug into RBCs and plasma proteins for secondary binding. Bioanalysis and sampling of drugs in the white cells or the buffy-coat interface between RBCs and plasma is very difficult, due to potential plasma or RBC contamination, and analysis usually defaults to measuring whole-blood drug concentrations. The reader is referred to Section 8.7.3 for a discussion of the impact of RBC partitioning on estimation of exposure margins and to the review on RBC partitioning by Hinderling [25] for details on RBC partitioning of drugs and its impact on bioanalytical method development. More detailed information on matrix effects, plasma stability, and bioanalytical method validation is discussed in detail in Chapter 4 and relevant guidance documents and publications [26].

8.4.8 Evaluation of Metabolites

The role of metabolites in safety testing during drug development is currently an evolving area with significant progress made in recent years [26–29]. It is accepted that drug toxicity can be due to the parent compound and/or its metabolites. Therefore, metabolism data in the nonclinical species and humans are required to evaluate if the toxicity profile is due to the parent drug or metabolites and its relevance to humans. Under debate are when the data need to be generated, what metabolite levels must be achieved in nonclinical testing, and the impact on the clinical development program.

Toxicokinetic support for metabolites starts with assisting in the selection of the most appropriate species for toxicity studies. Ideally, both toxicology species selected should have exposure to the parent compound and its metabolites preferably greater than, or at least equal to, their exposure in humans. In practice, this is often not the case, since quantitative species differences in metabolism are common. Accordingly, it is acceptable if all of the major human metabolites are covered in at least one of the toxicology species. In recent years, experts from both the pharmaceutical industry [27,28,30,31] and the regulatory agencies [29,32] have attempted to develop some basic guidelines in metabolite evaluations and quantification.

The current ICH S3A toxicokinetic guideline does not identify specific thresholds for qualifying metabolites but recommends evaluating metabolites in the following circumstances:

- When the administered compound acts as a "pro-drug" and the delivered metabolite is acknowledged to be the primary active entity.
- When the compound is metabolized to one or more pharmacologically or toxicologically active metabolites, which could make a significant contribution to tissue/organ responses.
- When the administered compound is very extensively metabolized and the measurement of plasma or tissue concentrations of a major metabolite is the only practical means of estimating exposure following administration of the compound in toxicity studies.

In February 2008, the U.S. Food and Drug Administration (FDA) issued a guidance describing specific requirements for metabolite exposure in toxicity studies [32]. Strict interpretation of the document implies that any metabolite present in humans to greater than 10% of the parent drug's AUC in humans must be measured in toxicity studies to demonstrate exposure, with the target exposure at least equivalent to that in humans. Ongoing discussions with the FDA and industry scientists have shown that in the case of highly metabolized drugs, or very potent, low dose drugs, this goal is not possible and it appears there will be a more flexible, and a case-by-case interpretation of the "10% rule." A major quandary encountered in early nonclinical studies is to decide which metabolite(s) are relevant to humans, since no in vivo human data are available. Often, some in vitro data in human hepatocytes or subcellular fractions are generated as an initial guide to potential in vivo human metabolism (Chapters 2 and 7), but interpretation of these data is often problematic.

The following are some factors to consider in evaluating the safety, impact, and toxicokinetics of metabolites:

1. Known species differences in the properties of cytochrome P450 enzymes and other metabolizing systems can generate quantitative and qualitative differences across species. In general, the metabolites of interest that should be measured in later stage toxicity studies are only those that are considered

significant in humans. The sponsor should develop a proposal as to what specific metabolites are considered significant and/or major, based on the totality of data on the specific drug candidate. Major metabolites in animals that are not relevant to humans should not be measured unless there are other factors that support analysis (active metabolite, toxic metabolite).

2. The liver is the principal site of xenobiotic metabolism and elimination; therefore, a minor circulating metabolite may be a major metabolite that is cleared directly from the liver. This also sometimes explains why in vitro metabolism data often do not correlate with in vivo plasma or serum exposure to metabolites.
3. The cytochrome P450 enzymes are subject to species-specific autoinduction or autoinhibition, depending on the nature of the NCE. The higher doses used in toxicity studies result in more frequent induction in animals, which often does not translate to therapeutic doses in humans.
4. The nature of metabolites produced (e.g., stable or reactive) should be considered in data interpretation. Reactive metabolites do not generally circulate in the body and thus are not amenable to bioanalytical quantification methods. Stable metabolites, often but not always, have high clearance rates and are excreted rapidly. In such cases, a small amount (<1%) of a reactive metabolite can theoretically pose safety problems, whereas 200% (compared to plasma exposure of the parent drug) of a stable metabolite may not have any safety concerns.
5. The uptake, distribution, and excretion of an NCE and its metabolites in animals and humans are also dependent on species- and organ-specific transporters.
6. Biliary versus renal excretion of parent drug and metabolites often demonstrate species differences in the elimination route. Biliary excretion of NCEs and their metabolites is often more predominant in rodents than in nonrodents, with efficient drug elimination often occurring without systemic exposure through plasma. Although the metabolite guidance places the emphasis on the measurable plasma compartment for exposure assessments, demonstrating high "local" tissue exposure but low plasma exposure can be used to support the position that the test animal has been exposed to high concentrations of a metabolite in at least one critical organ (i.e., liver) and therefore the metabolite should not be considered unique to humans or underexposed in the toxicology species.
7. Phase II (conjugated) metabolites usually have less extensive distribution and lower pharmacological activities than those of parent drug and phase I metabolites. They are also generally cleared more rapidly and have lower distribution to tissues. Therefore, conjugated metabolites are not analyzed routinely in toxicology or clinical studies. However, potentially reactive metabolites, such as unstable acylglucuronides or active conjugates, will require further evaluation. Bioanalysis of conjugates can be complicated by difficult synthesis and analyte instability. For those compounds, hydrolysis

of the conjugate and measurement of the unconjugated product is often used, although many variables make this difficult and better for estimation than full quantification.

With these considerations, it is difficult to prescribe a "one size fits all" path for metabolite analysis, particularly at the pre-FIH phase of development. However, the metabolite guidance is likely to encourage the pharmaceutical industry to accelerate metabolite identification programs (both reactive and stable) during late drug discovery and early development, so that potential metabolite-related safety issues are addressed in the earlier stages of a clinical program rather than later.

A generic approach has evolved for early metabolite analysis integrated into the safety assessment program. To support selection of an appropriate species from a metabolism perspective, the initial assessment typically involves qualitative determination of the metabolites formed both in vitro in nonclinical species and humans following incubation of the unlabeled NCE in microsomes and/or hepatocytes, and in vivo after administration to the nonclinical species. These studies enable identification of potential "unique" metabolites and provide some information on potential differences in the levels of metabolites between species. A quantitative assessment of metabolite levels can be obtained through the use of radiolabeled compound, but this requires the investment of resources to synthesize the radiolabeled compound (typically ^{14}C or ^{3}H) prior to the toxicology evaluation. Comparisons of in vitro profiles with actual circulating metabolites are then made with in vivo samples from pharmacokinetic or toxicokinetic studies. Ideally, this is done with radiolabel material for absolute quantification, but nonlabeled methods are used routinely at the early stages of development. The first in vivo comparisons in humans usually occur with samples from the highest doses used in the FIH study. This is generally a semiquantitative assessment, whose purpose is to identify major human metabolites for qualitative or semiquantitative comparison to the toxicology species. LC-MS/MS is the standard instrument for quantification and early metabolite identification. It is extremely sensitive and can detect even trace levels of metabolites. However, due to the inherent potential differences in ionization response that can occur with even minor structural changes, metabolite quantification is difficult without standards or alternative means to compare response. Initial metabolite evaluations are almost never performed under GLP. However, for those metabolites designated as major, which need to be followed in toxicity studies, fully validated bioanalytical methods with sufficient sensitivity will ultimately be required. Although individual concentrations of parent and metabolite are clearly preferred by regulators for safety assessment purposes, total drug load should also be considered, especially when there is toxicity in animals and the ratio of parent drug to metabolite is much smaller than that observed in humans.

From a toxicokinetics perspective, if there are human metabolites that circulate at levels that are greater than 10% of the parent and are considered major, based on the current FDA guidance, it may be necessary to develop a bioanalytical method to evaluate the toxicokinetic profile of the metabolite as part of the toxicokinetic assessment for the pivotal toxicity studies. However, this must be evaluated in light of the ICH S3A recommendation of using the threshold of 10% of total drug as the cutoff point. These may include some of the key genetic toxicology, general toxicology, safety pharmacology, reproductive toxicology, and carcinogenicity studies. However, in support of the pre-FIH toxicity studies, the measurement of parent compound only (with the exception of prodrugs) is acceptable for toxicokinetic assessments, the primary goal being the demonstration that different dose levels of the NCE generate discrete circulating concentrations of the drug administered. Technical difficulties often preclude or delay development of validated methods for early metabolite assessments in support of toxicity studies. Therefore, initially the toxicokinetic support often relies on semiquantitative assessments, with quantitative confirmation following thereafter.

8.4.9 Evaluation of Enantiomers

If a drug candidate is a racemic mixture, the component enantiomers may exhibit different pharmacological and possibly toxicologic effects, as well as different pharmacokinetic properties from the perspective of absorption, metabolism, and excretion [33,34]. As a result, it is necessary to develop a stereoselective bioanalytical method for measurement of the individual enantiomers (Chapter 4) to support evaluation of the toxicokinetic profiles of these components. Characterization of enantiomer pharmacokinetics and potential interconversion generally builds with the development program. Pre-FIH, in the absence of data on activity differences between enantiomers, a nonchiral assay may be acceptable to support pre-FIH toxicity studies. The ICH S3A toxicokinetic guidance states: "If the drug substance is a racemate or some other mixture of enantiomers, additional justification should be made for the choice of the analyte [racemate or enantiomer(s)]." Generally, as a program advances past phase I, activity differences between enantiomers are characterized and a chiral bioanalytical method is developed to measure the levels of the enantiomers. It should be noted, however, that sponsors currently prefer to select individual stereoisomers rather than racemic mixtures, as drug candidates due to the resource intensive need to evaluate the properties of the component enantiomers of a racemate during nonclinical and clinical development.

8.4.10 Matrix Considerations

The most common matrix for toxicokinetic analysis is plasma (or serum), as it is readily accessible, easily analyzed, and generally representative of the kinetic changes in concentration in other body compartments. Most important, it provides a direct link to human plasma concentrations. However, in some unusual cases, there may be accumulation in specific organs or tissues not evident by plasma analysis. Separate tissue distribution studies using radiolabeled compound may be used to determine the extent to which compounds distribute to other organs or tissues following single or, preferably, multiple doses. Partitioning of drug into specific tissue compartments rarely requires analysis of that tissue compartment as a routine event. However, depending on the target site of action and target organs for toxicity, an evaluation of the concentrations in other fluids or tissues may be appropriate (e.g., if the target site of action is the colon, sampling in plasma may not be sufficient) [12]. One potential challenge in measuring tissue concentrations (e.g., brain) as part of a GLP toxicity study is the difficulty in developing a validated method for extracting and measuring concentrations. One way to address this is to perform the assessment using a qualified method in a separate mechanistic pharmacokinetic study. Alternatively, the toxicity study protocol must specify that tissue concentrations and exposures will be evaluated by nonvalidated methods. A major limitation in measuring tissue concentrations is that unlike plasma, it is not possible to bridge exposure in most tissues from nonclinical to clinical studies. Therefore, the value of measuring tissue concentrations is limited to evaluating toxicology findings in that species. Drug in urine is filtered from plasma and therefore is an indirect measurement of systemic exposure. Urine is a compartment that can be sampled in animals and humans, but it is rarely used for toxicokinetic purposes, as it is difficult to relate urine concentrations directly to plasma concentrations. However, in assessing if a metabolite is truly unique to humans, its presence in urine should be considered as part of the weight of evidence for animal exposure in the toxicity studies.

8.4.11 Number of Animals

In cases where the toxicokinetic assessment is performed on the main toxicology animals, the number of animals per dose group is determined by the main toxicity study design (generally, 10 animals/gender/group for rodents and 3 to 5 animals/gender/group for nonrodents). In rodent toxicity studies in which the toxicokinetic assessment is performed on separate satellite animals, there are generally 3 or 4 animals/gender/group to support serial sampling and 3 or 4 animals/gender/group/time point to support sparse sampling.

8.4.12 Gender

As both genders are usually included in toxicity studies, the toxicokinetic assessment of the exposure in both genders is also included. It is not uncommon for gender differences in exposure to be observed due to differences in metabolism [35] and active transport [36–39], particularly in rodents, which can result in differences in toxicity. An example of gender differences in the exposure (C_{max} and AUC) and pharmacokinetics of an NCE in rats is shown in Table 8.2. When there are substantial gender differences in exposure, it may be necessary to use different dose levels for each gender to achieve sufficient exposure multiples or to account for differences in toxicity. Furthermore, in cases where significant gender differences in exposure are due to a similar mechanism (e.g., a common

TABLE 8.2 Compound for Which There Is a Substantial Gender Difference in Clearance and Bioavailability Due to More Extensive Metabolism in Female Than in Male Rats

Route	Dose (mg/kg)	Gender	C_{max} (ng/mL)	t_{max} (h)	$AUC_{0-\infty}$ (ng•h/mL)	$t_{1/2}$ (h)	CL/F (mL/h ·kg)	Vd_{ss} (mL/kg)	F (%)
Intravenous	2	Male	788	NA	592	0.86	3,400	3,400	NA
			(31)	NA	(54)	(0.08)	(294)	(217)	NA
	2	Female	810	NA	411	0.49	4,870	2,780	NA
			(63)	NA	(22)	(0.02)	(263)	(109)	NA
Oral	10	Male	405	0.50	767	1.35	13,200	NA	25.91
			(81)	(0.00)	(93)	(0.15)	(1,540)	NA	(3.14)
	10	Female	57	0.50	83	0.96	121,000	NA	4.03
			(3)	(0.00)	NA	NA	NA	NA	NA

NA, not available.

metabolic pathway) in animals and humans, it may be appropriate to calculate gender-specific animal/human exposure multiples. Although toxicokinetic (TK) reports list values by gender, in those instances where pharmacokinetics-based gender differences are similar, male and female TK data can be pooled for summary assessments.

8.4.13 Dose Selection

Toxicity study dose levels are selected to enable evaluation of toxicity at exposure comparable or higher than the target exposure for efficacy. In all studies, dose selection should be such that plasma exposure to drug and/or relevant metabolite(s) is dose related. Target exposure for human efficacy is generally estimated from nonclinical pharmacology models. The degree of confidence in the extrapolation of PK and/or pharmacodynamics (PD) targets from animal species to humans depends on the therapeutic class and the clinical experience with a given target. For example, in the case of antibiotics, nonclinical models have been shown to be predictive of the target exposure [40]. In contrast, for novel biological targets, predictive confidence in the pharmacodynamic models and therefore target exposure is more limited. As the NCE progresses into clinical studies, the target exposures for efficacy are refined based on evaluation of clinical biomarkers. Therefore, the target TK exposures that are evaluated in early toxicity studies should cover broad ranges of anticipated exposures [5], especially for those conditions where no dose-limiting animal toxicity was observed.

There is debate among toxicologists regarding the extent to which the high dose levels in toxicity studies should be governed by the toxicology findings (the current practice) and the pharmacodynamic responses of the test species compared to consideration of the toxicokinetic exposure data and safety margins [5].

Some toxicologists argue that a dose level that saturates absorption, metabolism, or excretion is inappropriate because it results in atypical exposure of the test species, with little relevance to exposure to human patients. However, the strong regulatory preference is that target organ toxicity must be observed to have a valid study. This places toxicokinetics as a valuable tool to evaluate the relevance of observed toxicity and less frequently as a direct mechanism to limit dose escalation.

8.4.14 Dose Volume

Dose volumes (mL/kg) used in toxicity studies are covered in Chapter 7. From a toxicokinetics perspective, it is important to recognize that changes in the dose volume can affect pharmacokinetic parameters such as the AUC, C_{max}, and t_{max}, particularly for low-solubility compounds.

8.4.15 Blood Sampling Variables

Blood Volume Toxicokinetic study designs need to consider the maximum blood volume that can be withdrawn without adversely affecting the health of the animal. Guidelines have been proposed for volumes of blood and recovery periods, which take into account the stress of single versus multiple sampling (Table 8.3). Additional recovery time is proposed for animals in the dose groups that are part of the main toxicity studies since a critical evaluation of hematological parameters is required in these animals. The institutional animal care and use committee at the site where the study is being performed should be consulted regarding specific guidelines, as they may differ from those shown in Table 8.3. To facilitate serial sampling for toxico- or pharmacokinetic purposes, a higher volume (20%) is presented in the multiple-sampling scenario. However, it should be remembered that there could be an impact on the half-life or clearance of the drug as a result of withdrawal of such large volumes. Since the half-life is generally not a critical parameter in toxicokinetic evaluation, this is generally

TABLE 8.3 Limit Volumes for Blood Sampling and Recovery Periods

Single Sampling (e.g., Toxicity Study)		Multiple Sampling (e.g., Toxicokinetic Study)	
Circulatory Blood Volume Removed (%)	Approximate Recovery Period (weeks)	Circulatory Blood Volume Removed in 24 h (%)	Approximate Recovery Period (weeks)
7.5	1	7.5	1
10	2	10–15	2
15	4	20	3

Source: Adapted from [41].

TABLE 8.4 Total Blood Volume and Maximum Blood Sample Volume Recommended for Various Species

Species (Average Weight)	Total Circulating Blood Volume) (mL)	Sample Volume Recommended 7.5% (mL)	10% (mL)	15% (mL)	20% (mL)
Mouse (25 g)	1.8	0.1	0.2	0.3	0.4
Rat (250 g)	16	1.2	1.6	2.4	3.2
Rabbit (4 kg)	224	17	22	34	45
Dog (10 kg)	850	64	85	127	170
Macaque (rhesus) (5 kg)	280	21	28	42	56
Macaque (cynomolgus) (5 kg)	325	24	32	49	65
Marmoset monkey (350 g)	25	2.0	2.5	3.5	5
Minipig (15 kg)	975	73	98	146	195

Source: Adapted from [41].

not a consideration. Blood or fluid replacement has not been considered since the volumes proposed do not warrant such intervention. Table 8.4 is a helpful reference guide to the blood volumes that can be removed without significant disturbance to an animal's normal physiology [41].

Blood Sampling Sites A summary of the sites for blood sampling for toxicokinetic assessment and the advantages and disadvantages for each species are summarized in Table 8.5. The sites recommended for repeated blood sampling in each species are as follows [41]:

- *Mouse:* saphenous, lateral tail
- *Rat:* saphenous, lateral tail, sublingual
- *Rabbit:* marginal ear, central ear artery, jugular
- *Dog:* cephalic, jugular, saphenous
- *Macaque:* cephalic, saphenous, femoral
- *Marmoset:* femoral, saphenous
- *Minipig:* cranial vena cava

It is important to minimize the number of needle punctures at the blood sampling site; the same puncture site along the vein should not be reused. Surgical implantation of a indwelling catheter can be a useful technique for repeated blood sampling that minimizes distress and discomfort of the animal. However, cannulation requires proper surgical technique to avoid clotting and infection, may require that the animals be restrained or separated from their peers to prevent removal or biting, and may not be suitable for long-term studies, in which penetration of the vessel can occur or the animal outgrows the cannula. For more

TABLE 8.5 Toxicokinetics: Summary of the Advantages and Disadvantages of Various Methods of Blood Sampling from Laboratory Animals

Sampling Site/Vein	General Anesthesia	Tissue Damage[a]	Repeat Bleeds	Species
Jugular	No	Low	Yes	Rat, dog, rabbit
Cephalic	No	Low	Yes	Macaque, dog
Saphenous/lateral tarsal	No	Low	Yes	Mouse/rat, marmoset/macaque, dog
Marginal ear	No (local)	Low	Yes	Rabbit, minipig
Femoral	No	Low	Yes	Marmoset/macaque
Sublingual	Yes	Low	Yes	Rat
Lateral tail	No	Low	Yes	Rat, mouse/marmoset
Central ear artery	No (local)	Low	Yes	Rabbit
Cranial vena cava	No	Low	Yes	Minipig
Tail tip amputation (<1–3 mm)	Yes	Moderate	Limited	Mouse/rat
Retrobulbar plexus	Yes	Moderate to high	Yes	Mouse/rat
Cardiac[b]	Yes	Moderate	No	Mouse/rat/rabbit

Source: Adapted from [41].

[a]The potential for tissue damage is based on the likelihood of incidence and the severity of any sequelae (e.g., inflammatory reaction or histological damage).

[b]Only carried out as a terminal procedure under general anesthesia.

information on the advantages and disadvantages of blood sampling sites and proper sampling techniques, the reader is referred to Diehl et al. [41].

Serial Sampling Generally, because of the higher blood volumes in nonrodent species compared to rodents, there is sufficient circulating blood to support serial collection for clinical chemistry, hematology, and toxicokinetic assessment without having a significant impact on the toxicology evaluation. However, in rodent toxicity studies, serial blood sampling from the main study animals is not generally used for toxicokinetic assessment because the stress and trauma associated with frequent venipuncture and blood loss could cause adverse changes in physiology, thus jeopardizing the integrity of the toxicity study [42]. Conversely, standard pharmacokinetic or formulation support studies will often use cannulated rats with serial blood sampling and blood replacement after scheduled sampling times.

In the design of rodent toxicity studies, a satellite group of animals is housed with the main study animals but are used solely for toxicokinetic sampling. The drawbacks of using satellite animals for toxicokinetic sampling are the greater number of animals required, increased drug substance requirements, and increased labor for dosing and veterinary care. Another approach is to use sparse sampling from the main study animals, which is described in more detail in the next section

TABLE 8.6 Toxicokinetics: Study Design of Serial Blood Sampling from the Main Toxicology Animals on Days 1 and 28 of a 28-Day Study of an Orally Administered NCE

Group Number Identification	Dose Level (mg/kg · day)	Number of Animals	
		Males	Females
1: Vehicle control	0	101–103	151–153
2: NCE-001	25	201–203	251–253
3: NCE-001	75	301–303	351–353
4: NCE-001	150	401–403	451–453

[42–44]. An example of a study design consisting of serial sampling from the main toxicology animals is shown in Table 8.6.

According to the ICH S3A toxicokinetic guideline, it is not mandatory to assay samples from control groups [2]. However, currently, most toxicity studies routinely sample and analyze control animals based on European regulatory agency requests to provide confirmatory information that these animals have not been exposed to test article. Additionally, this sampling ensures that control and main toxicology animals are treated identically throughout the study. Sampling from control animals can also confirm that the bioanalytical method is free of matrix effects; although a predose sample from the treatment groups on day 1 can also be used to show that there is no matrix interference with the bioanalytical assay. When satellite animals are used for toxicokinetic assessment, blood collections in the control group are generally limited to a maximum of two or three time points and serve only as a confirmation that there is no exposure to test article.

Sparse Sampling As a result of limitations on blood sampling volume, it may be necessary or desirable, particularly in the case of rodents, to use sparse sampling on satellite toxicokinetic animals or on the main study animals. For example, if the bioanalytical method requires a blood sample volume of 0.5 mL/time point and a total of seven time points are needed for toxicokinetic assessment, sparse sampling can reduce the volume per rat from 3.5 mL, which exceeds the limit for a four-week study (see Table 8.7) to 1.5 to 2 mL. Using sparse sampling on satellite animals can help to minimize stress to the animals [42,44]. An example of a study design consisting of sparse sampling from the satellite toxicokinetics animals is shown in Table 8.7.

Approaches have been proposed for applying sparse sampling directly from the main study animals to help minimize the number of animals required and number of samples collected [42,44,45]. Sparse sampling of main toxicology animals typically involves the collection of a single blood sample on a given study day from each animal in a treatment group. Samples are collected at predesignated time points to provide for replicates, and sufficient time is scheduled between sample days to allow for recovery. Selection of appropriate time points based on detailed pharmacokinetic studies conducted previously is critical for the approach

TABLE 8.7 Study Design of Sparse Sampling from Satellite (for Toxicokinetics) Animals on Days 1 and 28 of a 28-Day Rat Toxicity Study

Group	Number of Animals		Dose Level	Time Points
	Male	Female	(mg/kg·day)	(hours postdose)
		Toxicity Groups		
1 (Control)[a]	10	10	0	No samples collected
2 (Low)	10	10	20	No samples collected
3 (Middle)	10	10	40	No samples collected
4 (High)	10	10	80	No samples collected
		Toxicokinetic Groups[b]		
5 (Control)[a]	4	4	0	0 (predose) and 4
6 (Low)				
Subgroup A	4	4	20	0 (predose), 2, and 8
Subgroup B	4	4	20	1, 4, and 24
7 (Middle)				
Subgroup A	4	4	40	0 (predose), 2, and 8
Subgroup B	4	4	40	1, 4, and 24
8 (High)				
Subgroup A	4	4	80	0 (predose), 2, 8, and 24
Subgroup B	4	4	80	1, 4, and 24

[a]Group 1 will receive vehicle/control article only.
[b]Toxicokinetic animals included solely for the purpose of blood sample collections. One additional animal per gender from group 5 and two animals per gender from groups 6 to 8 will be included as replacement toxicokinetic animals, if needed.

to work properly. An appropriate statistical procedure is employed to assess the population mean exposure to the compound, with some indication of the variance of the data [42].

The risks in using a sparse toxicokinetic sampling approach on main toxicity study animals include the possibility that reduced blood sampling volumes can still have an adverse impact on the toxicological outcomes and cause variability in terms of the toxicity. In addition, use of limited time points selected based on preliminary pharmacokinetic studies may not be sufficient because they do not account for time-dependent changes that can occur. Due to these concerns, although the application of sparse sampling on main toxicology animals received attention in the mid- to late 1990s [42,44,45], it does not appear to have gained widespread adoption in the industry.

Limited Sampling There are a number of toxicity study types wherein full toxicokinetic profiles are not required:

- In vivo micronucleus
- In vivo single-cell gel electrophoresis assay for DNA damage (e.g., COMET)
- In vivo unscheduled DNA synthesis

- Safety pharmacology
- In vivo phototoxicity
- Bridging formulation studies

The toxicokinetic goal in these studies is to confirm exposure by measuring plasma concentrations at a limited number of time points and, relying on the full toxicokinetic assessment in the same species from previous studies, to determine parameters such as the AUC. As a result, these studies may not require a separate toxicokinetic report and the individual and mean plasma concentrations can be included in the main toxicology or bioanalytical report. In these studies the protocol will generally state something to the effect that "Individual and mean (e.g., $n = 3 \pm \text{SD}$) plasma concentrations will be reported at each sampling time at each dose level. The relationship between exposure and dose will be evaluated by comparison of the plasma concentrations at each dose level." Comparisons for gender differences in exposure should not be made with this type of toxicokinetic sampling design and should only be made when full toxicokinetic analysis is conducted.

8.4.16 Sampling Times

Sample collection and analysis may be limited to one to two time points when the only toxicokinetic goal is to confirm that there are detectable circulating levels of drug, but not to evaluate any other kinetic parameters. This minimal sampling approach may be used when the kinetic profile after single and multiple dosing has been well characterized in previous studies (see the discussion of limited sampling above). One risk in relying on the full kinetic data from previous studies to support longer-duration toxicity studies is that there could be changes in kinetics that do not become apparent until later in a study. If only one or two time points are being analyzed, it is preferable to choose time points that are close to $t_{\max}$ to maximize the likelihood that there are detectable concentrations of drug. In the case of intravenous bolus administration, this time point should be almost immediately after dosing, and in the case of intravenous infusion it should be right before discontinuing the infusion. Although comparisons can be made between dose groups and genders using samples from one or two time points, it may be difficult to determine whether these differences are real or are due to animal-to-animal variability in kinetics.

When the toxicokinetic goals are to determine the exposure (AUC and $C_{\max}$) and also to evaluate the relationships among dose, exposure, and gender, previous pharmacokinetic data can be used to select the appropriate plasma sampling time points. It should be noted that with the limited sampling schedules inherent in toxicokinetic studies, it is difficult to "capture" $t_{\max}$ after oral administration, and thus $C_{\max}$ values observed are considered less precise than would be obtained with more extensive sampling in formal pharmacokinetic evaluations. The sampling schemes presented below address both extra- and intravenous routes of administration. In addition, practical considerations such as the scheduling of plasma collections within the constraints of an 8- to 12-hour workday can also limit to 8 to 10 hours the range of time points that may be selected after dose administration and would require overtime to support collection at times between 10 and 24 hours. It should be noted that it is usually important to include a 24-hour sample in any scheme, as the dosing regimen in toxicity studies is typically once a day, and thus a full 24-hour AUC within the dosing interval is very valuable. It is emphasized that the goal of toxicokinetics is to evaluate plasma exposure, and thus limited sampling generally does not enable calculation of pharmacokinetic parameters such as clearance or elimination half-life with sufficient accuracy for interpretation.

Extravascular (Including Oral) Administration Following extravenous dosing, a minimum of five to six time points is recommended, consisting of two time points during the absorption phase, one at the t_{max} estimated, and two to three time points during the elimination phase. If there is sufficient plasma volume, additional information may be obtained by taking a predose sample (see the discussion below) and a sample at the end of the dosing interval (e.g., 24 hours after a single dose), at which time concentrations are above the lower limit of quantification (LLOQ). If there are no previous pharmacokinetic data, the following time points can be used as a default: predose, 0.5, 1, 2, 4, 8, and 24 hours; at steady state, the predose concentration can be used as an estimate of the 24-hour value, and an additional time point (e.g., 12 hours) can be inserted into the collection scheme.

Intravenous Bolus Administration Following intravenous bolus administration, a minimum of five or six time points is also recommended, consisting of two or three samples during the distribution phase, a sample immediately after injection, and two or three time points during the elimination phase. If there are no previous pharmacokinetic data, the following time points after dosing can be used as a default: predose, 0.083, 0.25, 1, 2, 4, 8, and 24 hours.

Intravenous Infusion Following intravenous infusion administration, a minimum of five or six time points is also recommended, consisting of one time point during the infusion, one sample at the end of the infusion, and two or three time points during the elimination phase. Although a predose sample is not required, collection of predose samples provides confirmation that there is no compound in the systemic circulation prior to dosing on the first day of dosing and provides information about the extent of accumulation for predose samples collected at steady state. The collection of a predose sample is not essential but can provide useful control information when there is drug detected in control samples or there are questions regarding the potential for accumulation.

Frequency of Sampling In toxicity studies of three months' duration or less, toxicokinetic samples are generally collected only on the first and last days of dosing. In toxicity studies that are longer than three months, an additional sampling day may be added midway through the study. The benefit of evaluating the exposure over different time intervals is that it provides an ability to determine whether there is evidence of time-dependent changes in pharmacokinetics over the course of the study, which could be due to enzyme induction, inhibition, changes in clearance due to target organ toxicity, or other effects.

8.4.17 Considerations with Biopharmaceutics

The various types of biopharmaceutics include proteins, peptides, cytokines, plasminogen activators, recombinant plasma factors, growth factors, fusion proteins, enzymes, receptors, hormones, monoclonal antibodies, recombinant DNA protein vaccines, chemically synthesized peptides, plasma-derived products, endogenous proteins extracted from human tissue, and oligonucleotide drugs. Unlike small-molecule pharmaceuticals, a majority of biologics are not orally absorbable and are therefore administered either by an intravenous, subcutaneous, intraperitoneal, intramuscular, or intranasal route. In contrast to small molecules, which are more likely to have adverse effects that are off-target, the adverse effects of biopharmaceutics are almost always a direct consequence of primary pharmacologic action or a consequence of an immune mediated hypersensitivity response [46]. Therefore, translation of pharmacological and toxicological effects to humans based on nonclinical toxicity studies depends on extrapolating species specificity and exposure at the biological target. Consideration should be given to the minimum anticipated biologic effect level (MABEL). The application of MABEL and considerations for safety margins as it relates to biopharmaceutics is discussed in more detail in Chapters 10 and 12.

The importance of toxicokinetic evaluation in the development of biopharmaceutics is debatable. One primary reason for this is that safety issues related to biologics are often associated with their extended pharmacology or to their immunogenicity profile. The S6 guidance document for biologics [47] considered these points and provided some useful guidance points in the design of pharmacokinetic and toxicokinetic studies for biologics:

> It is difficult to establish uniform guidances for pharmacokinetic studies for biotechnology derived pharmaceuticals. Single and multiple dose pharmacokinetics, toxicokinetics, and tissue distribution studies in relevant species are useful; however, routine studies that attempt to assess mass balance are not useful. Differences in pharmacokinetics among animal species may have a significant impact on the predictiveness of animal studies or on the assessment of dose–response relationships in toxicity studies. Alterations in the pharmacokinetic profile due to immune-mediated clearance mechanisms may affect the kinetic profiles and the interpretation of the toxicity data. For some products, there may also be inherent, significant delays in the expression of pharmacodynamic effects relative to the pharmacokinetic profile (e.g., cytokines) or there may be prolonged expression of pharmacodynamic effects relative to plasma levels.
>
> Pharmacokinetic studies should, whenever possible, utilize preparations that are representative of those intended for toxicity testing and clinical use and employ a

route of administration that is relevant to the anticipated clinical studies. Patterns of absorption may be influenced by formulation, concentration, site, and/or volume. Whenever possible, systemic exposure should be monitored during the toxicity studies.

When using radiolabeled proteins, it is important to show that the radiolabeled test material maintains activity and biological properties equivalent to that of the unlabeled material. Tissue concentrations of radioactivity and/or autoradiography data using radiolabeled proteins may be difficult to interpret due to rapid in vivo metabolism or unstable radiolabeled linkage. Care should be taken in the interpretation of studies using radioactive tracers incorporated into specific amino acids because of recycling of amino acids into non-drug related proteins/peptides.

Some information on absorption, disposition, and clearance in relevant animal models should be available prior to clinical studies in order to predict margins of safety based upon exposure and dose.

8.4.18 Practical Considerations in Planning a Toxicokinetic Program

As regulators and drug sponsors continue to understand the value added from toxicokinetic studies, the demand, complexity, and costs can spiral upward. For example, a one-month GLP toxicity study may cost $200,000 to 250,000 at a high-quality contract research organization (CRO). GLP bioanalysis at study start and conclusion, may add another $40,000–60,000 to the study. Bioanalytical and toxicokinetic protocol writing, data analysis, report writing, quality control/quality assurance (QC/QA) analysis, and integrating results into reports and investigator brochures adds several more workdays to the program. Although toxicokinetic assessment generally represents less than 20% of the total toxicity study costs, as these costs are applied across the 10 to 20 toxicity studies that need toxicokinetic support, the resource and drug supply requirements can become substantial. Adding multiple metabolites, more frequent sampling times, or full toxicokinetic characterization for all toxicity studies can drive up cost with little actual benefit to the safety aspect toxicokinetics provides. Therefore, as with all aspects of drug development, a toxicokinetics program should be efficiently planned and goal oriented. For example, the value of bridging studies or sparse sampling to evaluate exposure should always be considered before moving to full-size studies or incorporating metabolite analysis into routine toxicity studies.

8.5 TOXICOKINETIC PARAMETER ESTIMATES AND CALCULATIONS

8.5.1 Data Analysis (Noncompartmental Versus Compartmental)

Although there is flexibility in the type of pharmacokinetic model that can be applied to toxicokinetic data, generally noncompartmental analysis is applied because it does not require the investigator to make any assumptions about the number of compartments that best describes the data; the approach also provides

AUC and C_{max}, the two major descriptive pharmacokinetic parameters required. The only decision that may be desirable in using a noncompartmental model to estimate the basic pharmacokinetic parameters is the time points that should be used to estimate the terminal elimination rate constant, if indeed it was determined that $t_{1/2}$ was a parameter necessary for the study goal. Several validated commercial software packages are available for evaluating toxicokinetic data (e.g., WinNonlin, www.pharsight.com). A discussion of compartmental modeling is beyond the scope of this chapter; the reader is referred to Roland and Tozer for more detail on this approach [48].

8.5.2 Noncompartmental Kinetic Parameters

Figure 8.2 is a plot of the plasma concentration versus time following single oral administration of an NCE, and Figure 8.3 is a plot of the plasma concentration versus time following intravenous bolus administration of another NCE. The plots demonstrate the key toxicokinetic parameters (C_{max}, t_{max}, and AUC) that may be estimated by noncompartmental analysis. Additional parameters that may be estimated but are not necessary, can be misleading, and are not required in toxicokinetic assessment are the terminal phase half-life ($t_{1/2}$), clearance, and volume of distribution. Definitions of each of these parameters, as well as those employed in standard pharmacokinetics studies and approaches for estimating them, are presented in the sections that follow.

Time to Peak Concentration Peak time (t_{max}) is the time at which the highest concentration is measured after administration of an extravascular dose, obtained by visual inspection of the data. Its precision is dependent on the number of time points used for sample analysis.

Maximum Concentration Maximum concentration (C_{max}) is the highest concentration observed after administration of an extravascular dose, obtained by visual inspection of the data. As with t_{max}, its precision is dependent on the number of time points used for sample analysis. This is one of the two primary variables (with AUC) included in toxicokinetic evaluations.

Area Under the Concentration Versus Time Curve The area under the concentration versus time curve (AUC) is one of the two primary variables (along with C_{max}) included in toxicokinetic evaluations, and may be determined by a *linear* or *linear up/log down trapezoidal method*. In both cases the linear trapezoidal method is used for each part of the curve for which $C_{i+1} \geq C_i$, and for the linear method it is used for the entire curve. The advantage of the linear trapezoidal method is that it is simple and easy to calculate by hand; the disadvantages are that it assumes a straight line between points; if the curve is steep, the error may be large and can result in under- or overestimates, depending on whether the curve is ascending or descending. The advantages of the linear up/log down

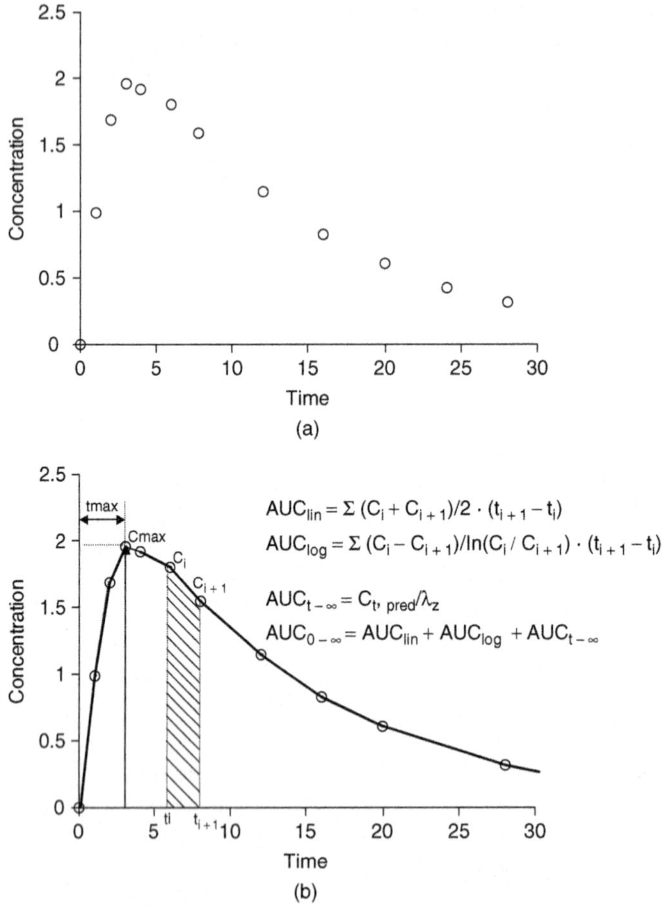

FIGURE 8.2 Plasma concentration–time curve of an NCE following an oral dose: (a) individual raw data; (b) calculations for t_{max}, C_{max}, and AUC. Note that generally the number of time points in a toxicokinetic assessment will be 5 to 7, not the 10 time points shown

method are that it is very accurate for monoexponential curves and more accurate at later time points, where the interval between time points is increased; the disadvantage is that it may not be as accurate for a steeply declining polyexponential curve, and in these situations a compartmental model may be more appropriate.

The sum of these areas (AUC_{lin}) by the linear method is given by

$$AUC_{lin} = \frac{\Sigma(C_i + C_{i+1})}{2}\Delta t$$

with $\Delta t = t_{i+1} - t_i$ and $AUC_{0-t} = AUC_{lin}$. In the linear up/log down method, the log trapezoidal method is used for every part of the curve for which $C_{i+1} < C_i$.

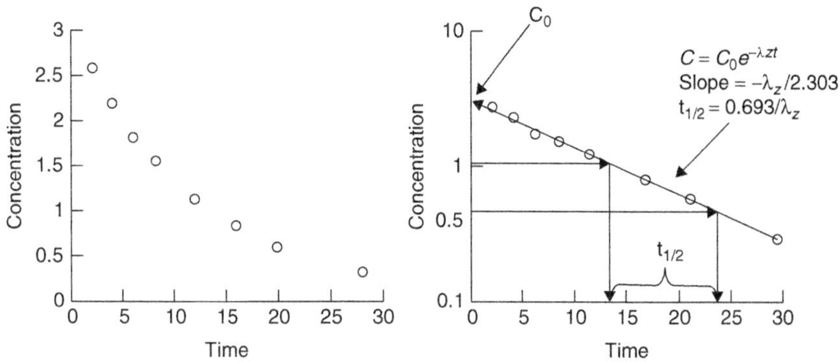

FIGURE 8.3 Plasma concentration–time curve of an NCE following an intravenous bolus dose to illustrate determination of C_0 (theoretical drug concentration at time zero) and $t_{1/2}$

The sum of these areas (AUC_{log}) is then given by

$$AUC_{log} = \frac{\Sigma(C_i - C_{i+1})}{\ln(C_i/C_{i+1})} \quad \Delta t$$

where $AUC_{0-t} = AUC_{lin} + AUC_{log}$. However, the linear trapezoidal method is always used for area segments before and after a zero concentration value.

t, the time of a quantifiable concentration for the determination of AUC_{last}, is the last time sampled in the dosing interval (τ) for $AUC_{0-\tau}$. AUC_{last} is defined as the area under the curve from the time of dosing to the last measurable concentration. $AUC_{0-\tau}$, where τ is the dosing interval, is defined as the area under the curve from the time of dosing to the time of the last time point sampled in the dosing interval. If the last concentration is nonzero, $AUC_{last} = AUC_{0-\tau}$. Otherwise, $AUC_{0-\tau}$ will be greater than AUC_{last}, as it includes the additional area from the last measurable concentration down to zero. Based on the data available, the investigator can decide to use another method for AUC calculation (e.g., the linear trapezoidal method), which should be documented in the raw data of the study.

After *single administration*, extrapolation is done from t (the time of the last measured concentration > LLOQ) to infinity (∞):

$$AUC_{t-\infty} = \frac{C_{t,\text{pred}}}{\lambda z} \rightarrow AUC_{0-\infty} = AUC_{lin} + AUC_{log} + AUC_{t-\infty}$$

After *multiple dosing*, extrapolation is done from t to τ (the dosing interval) when $t < \tau$:

$$AUC_{t-\tau} = \frac{C_{t,\text{pred}}}{\lambda}(1 - e^{-\lambda(\tau - t)}) \rightarrow AUC_{\tau} = AUC_{lin} + AUC_{log} + AUC_{t-\tau}$$

If the percentage extrapolated area, $\text{AUC}_{\text{ex}} = \text{AUC}_{t-\infty}/\text{AUC}_{0-\infty} \cdot 100\%$ or $\text{AUC}_{\text{ex}} = \text{AUC}_{t-\tau}/\text{AUC}_{0-\tau} \cot 100\%$, exceeds 20–25%, the investigator may want to note this in the report.

After steady state has been reached by applying *constant infusion*, AUC_τ is calculated as

$$\text{AUC}_\tau = C_{\text{ss}}\tau$$

with C_{ss} as the steady-state concentration and τ as the dosing interval.

Rate Constant The rate constant (λ_z or λ) is the absolute value of the slope calculated by log-linear regression on the data points determined during a well-defined phase on the log(plasma concentration) versus time plot. If this phase is the terminal phase, this is the terminal rate constant λ_z. The terminal phase is the phase in which the drug is eliminated from the body and is characterized by the terminal decrease in the concentrations. The terminal phase is determined by visual inspection of the data. Selection of time points requires scientific judgment on the suitability of the data to support estimation of a *terminal half-life* (sometimes called the *terminal-phase half life*) and the selection of which time points should be included.

Half-Life The terminal half-life ($t_{1/2}$) is the time required for the plasma concentration to decrease to one-half of its value during any portion of the terminal phase. The $t_{1/2}$ value is calculated as $t_{1/2} = \ln(2)/\lambda_z = 0.693/\lambda_z$. The (terminal or terminal-phase) half-life can only be calculated using the quantifiable concentrations determined during a well-defined (terminal) phase in which the plasma concentrations are decreasing over time.

Estimated Concentration at the Time of Intravascular Administration The estimated plasma drug concentration at the time of intravascular dosing (C_0) is calculated by log-linear regression on the first two data points after dosing, if these data show a trend to decrease. This is a calculated value, as it is impossible to collect a plasma sample for analyses at the precise time when a dose is administered intravascularly.

Clearance Although the single parameter typically used to describe the rate of elimination of a drug from the body is the half-life ($t_{1/2}$), this variable is in reality a hybrid of two pharmacokinetic parameters: clearance and volume of distribution. It can be argued that clearance provides a better description of drug elimination, as it represents the totality of all elimination processes from the body. Thus, a strict definition of plasma clearance is the volume of plasma cleared of drug per unit time as a result of all elimination processes. Clearance is basically dose (in mg/kg) divided by the AUC, but it should be noted that if a truncated AUC is used, which may be all that is available from the data, an overestimation of plasma clearance will result. Thus, clearance after both intravenous and nonintravenous routes of administration involves the calculation of $AUC_{0-\infty}$.

The total plasma clearance of the drug in plasma after a single intravenous administration (CL) is calculated as

$$CL = \frac{D_{iv}}{AUC_{0-\infty}}$$

After multiple intravenous administrations or a constant intravenous infusion, the AUC_{τ} at steady state is used instead of $AUC_{0-\infty}$.

After a single oral or other nonintravenous route of administration, the total plasma clearance is expressed as CL/F [i.e., CL divided by the bioavailability (F)] and is calculated as

$$\frac{CL}{F} = \frac{\text{dose}}{AUC_{0-\infty}}$$

In case of multiple nonintravenous administration, AUC_{τ} at steady state is used instead of $AUC_{0-\infty}$.

Volume of Distribution The volume of distribution is a theoretical concept that represents the overall distribution of the drug after administration and is utilized as an estimate of the extent of distribution outside the central compartment (plasma or serum). The higher the value, the greater the theoretical extent of drug uptake to the periphery. There are several means of expressing this parameter:

1. The apparent volume of the central (= initial distribution) compartment (V_c) is calculated after intravenous (i.v.) administration as

$$V_c = \frac{D_{iv}}{C_0}$$

2. The apparent volume of distribution at steady state ($V_{d_{ss}}$) after i.v. administration is calculated as

$$V_{d_{ss}} = CL \cdot MRT$$

where MRT is the mean residence time (ratio AUMC/AUC).

3. The apparent volume of distribution during the elimination phase (V_{d_β}) after i.v. administration is calculated as the total plasma clearance (CL)/terminal rate constant:

$$V_{d_\beta} = \frac{CL}{\lambda_z}$$

8.5.3 Statistics and Outliers

The ICH S3A toxicokinetics guidance states that "consideration should be given to the calculation of mean or median values and estimates of variability, but in some cases the data of individual animals may be more important than a refined statistical analysis of group data" [2]. Therefore, individual concentrations as well as mean and standard deviations at each time point should be presented in a tabular format in the toxicokinetics report. When serial sampling is performed on individual animals, individual means and standard deviations for the pharmacokinetic parameters are also presented. Statistical comparisons using t-tests or F-tests on raw data are not usually performed, due to the small number of samples and animals and the large intra- and interanimal variation; such properties do not conform to required statistical distributions.

Mean values ($\pm$ standard deviation if $n \geq 3$) may be calculated if all of the data to be averaged are quantifiable. As stated above, since it is difficult to determine statistically whether the mean plasma exposure is gender independent, if a combined mean is calculated, it is still recommended to present mean values for male and female animals separately.

There are several approaches to calculating a mean when one or more of the samples is below the lower limit of quantification (BLOQ). One technique is to assign a value of zero to concentrations below the limit of quantification and use this for the mean calculation, irrespective of this value being higher or lower than the LLOQ. Accordingly, the mean can actually be less than the LLOQ, and it is acceptable to report this value as long as a footnote describes how the mean was calculated. An alternative approach is not to report any discrete mean concentration if it is BLOQ and simply report it as BLOQ. Irrespective of which strategy is used, the approach should be defined as part of a standard operating procedure and/or in the protocol. Case studies on the statistical analysis of toxicokinetic data have been presented by Igarashi et al. [43,49].

8.5.4 Physiologically Based Toxicokinetic Modeling

In recent years there has been increasing interest in physiologically based pharmacokinetic modeling in the pharmaceutical industry [50–56]. The aim of physiologically based toxicokinetic modeling is to accurately predict the tissue concentrations and associated risks for toxicity. Although concentrations and exposures may be obtained by sampling individual tissues in animals, this is much more difficult or often not possible in humans; thus, the extrapolation of tissue distribution across species is difficult to assess. Furthermore, the measurement of tissue drug concentrations in toxicity studies to verify model predictions can be laborious and time consuming. Physiologically based toxicokinetic models involve tissue compartments connected by blood circulation. Since drug uptake into tissues is a function of both thermodynamic and membrane transport properties, and tissue partitioning, such models are interpreted with mass balance equations designed to predict drug concentrations in each organ and compartment.

The adoption and application of physiologically based toxicokinetics have faced several challenges, which include difficulty in obtaining reliable estimates for the numerous model inputs without the benefit of experimental data and challenges in knowing how to extrapolate model results from nonclinical species to humans. Although physiologically based pharmacokinetics and toxicokinetics have applications in other areas, the requirements for tissue concentration assessment and difficulty in linking to clinical concentrations have limited its application in pharmaceutical development [57].

8.6 INTERPRETATION OF TOXICOKINETIC DATA

8.6.1 Review of In-life Results

Prior to determining the individual and mean toxicokinetic parameters, it is important to review carefully the in-life portion of the study, including the dosing sheets, the clinical observations, the toxicology findings, the blood and plasma sample collection sheets, and the bioanalytical data sheets to identify any issues that may have affected the quality or integrity of the toxicokinetic results. Examples of issues that could affect the toxicokinetic study results and should be noted in the data tables of the report include dose analysis errors, incomplete dosing, emesis, mortality (provides an explanation for missing toxicokinetic time points postmortem), insufficient plasma sample volumes collected, or bioanalytical sample analysis failures. The relationship of toxicokinetic data to toxicological findings is discussed later in this chapter. The occurrence of missing values must be documented appropriately (e.g., as "NS" or "no sample"). The reason for "no sample" should be specified where applicable. The investigator should be sure to highlight these issues in the text to the extent that they affect interpretation of the data.

8.6.2 Protocol Deviations

In some cases there are protocol deviations that occur during the in-life portion of the study or during the subsequent analysis. When a deviation occurs, it is required under GLPs to notify the study director and is generally a best practice to document the deviation as part of the toxicokinetic report. If the deviation is more than a one-time event (e.g., a change to the dose level for the duration of a study due to toxicity), it should be documented in a protocol amendment and would no longer be considered a deviation.

8.6.3 Confirmation of Exposure and Evaluation of Dose Proportionality

In the summary and conclusion sections of a toxicokinetics report, statements are generally included, confirming that there was exposure as measured by detectable concentrations of the test article in the groups treated and that no test article was found in the vehicle control group (provides evidence that there was no cross-contamination during the in-life or bioanalytical phases of the study).

True dose proportionality requires that appropriate statistics be used to demonstrate that the increases in doses are correlated directly to increases in exposure (C_{max} and/or AUC). With the high dose levels required to generate toxicity along with the low solubility of many drugs, statistically supported dose proportionality is often not achieved in toxicity studies. Also, even if mean exposure values may appear to be dose proportional, toxicokinetic study designs are such that there are too few animals and high interanimal variability to demonstrate statistical proportionality. However, this is not a problematic finding, as one of the goals of toxicokinetic measurements is to demonstrate that increases in exposure levels were at least dose related, even though true dose proportionality may not be attained. Saturation of absorption, not proportionality, is really the toxicokinetic information the toxicologists will use in selecting top doses for future studies. In addition to saturation of exposure, supraproportional increases in exposure can be observed, but less frequently. This generally implies saturation of some clearance mechanism but may also be a partial bioanalytical artifact if seen at lower doses and due in part to poor assay sensitivity, where terminal time points cannot be captured accurately. When there are fewer than three animals per dose group, caution should be used in drawing conclusions about dose proportionality.

Several scenarios for the evaluation of dose proportionality of exposure when concentrations at only one or two time points (limited sampling for confirmation of exposure where kinetics have been characterized in previous studies) are presented in Table 8.8, and the conclusions that can be drawn are as follows:

- *Scenario 1.* The plasma concentrations in group $1 < 2 < 3 < 4$ and the conclusion could be written as follows: "Exposure to the test article based on mean plasma concentrations was observed in all of the treated groups and increased with dose."
- *Scenario 2.* The plasma concentrations in group $1 < 2 < 3 < 4$ at only one or both of the two time points and the conclusion could be written as follows: "Exposure to the test article, based on mean plasma concentrations, was observed in all of the treated groups and generally increased with dose."
- *Scenario 3.* The plasma concentrations in group $1 < 2 < 3 \cong 4$ and the conclusion could be written as follows: "Exposure to the test article based on mean plasma concentrations was observed in all of the treated groups. The exposure increased with dose when the dose was increased from 200 to 600 mg/kg but did not increase when the dose was increased from 600 mg/kg to 1250 mg/kg."
- *Scenario 4.* The plasma concentrations in group $1 < 2 \geq 3 \geq 4$ and the conclusion could be written as follows: "Exposure to the test article, based on mean plasma concentrations, was observed in all of the treated groups; however, exposure did not increase with dose."
- *Scenario 5.* The plasma concentrations in group $1 < 2$ with variability precluding evaluating differences in exposure between groups 2, 3, and 4 and

TABLE 8.8 Plasma Drug Concentrations in Individual Plasma Samples After Oral Administration of a Single Dose of an NCE (Illustrative)

	Mean Drug Concentration (ng/mL) (± SD)					
Group: Dose (mg/kg)	Scenario 1: Dose-Related Increase in Exposure; Sample Collection at 1 h Postdose	Scenario 2: Dose-Related Increase in Exposure; Sample Collection 0.5 h Postdose	Scenario 2: Dose-Related Increase in Exposure; Sample Collection 4 h Postdose	Scenario 3: Partially Dose-Related Increase in Exposure; Sample Collection at 1 h Postdose	Scenario 4: No Increase in Exposure with Dose; Sample Collection at 1 h Postdose	Scenario 5: Dose Relationship Inconclusive; Sample Collection at 1 h Postdose
Group 1: 0	0	0	0	0	0	0
Group 2: 200	872 ± 220	200 ± 20	872 ± 220	872 ± 220	1000 ± 500	1000 ± 1000
Group 3: 600	1500 ± 500	250 ± 93	1500 ± 500	1000 ± 500	872 ± 220	1100 ± 1253
Group 4: 1250	3500 ± 1228	125 ± 20	3500 ± 1228	1110 ± 433	789 ± 150	1200 ± 890

the conclusion could be written as follows: "Exposure to the test article, based on mean plasma concentrations, was observed in all of the treated groups; due to variability in the data it is not possible to determine the relationship between exposure and dose."

It is important to note that if there is only one outlier in a dose group and yet there is a general increase in exposure with dose, the following conclusion should be used: "Exposures based on mean plasma concentrations generally increased with dose." In addition, if a predose sample is being used to serve in lieu of vehicle control, following multiple dosing (e.g., cardiovascular studies that involve escalating doses with a washout) there may be measurable levels of test article in predose samples, and this may be expected based on the compound's half-life and should not be viewed as evidence of cross-contamination.

Similar principles apply when evaluating dose proportionality using AUC values. AUC values are generally more reliable in evaluating dose proportionality since they incorporate multiple time points that can account for delayed absorption, which can occur upon dose escalation.

8.6.4 Exposure after Single and Multiple Dosing: Accumulation Perspectives

Generally, toxicokinetic sampling in a multiple-dose toxicity study is conducted on the first day of dosing and on the last day of the study, which depending on the half-life and duration of the study will generally represent steady-state

TABLE 8.9 Number of Half-Lives Required to Reach Steady State

Number of Half-Lives	Dose (mg)	Amount in Body (mg)	Amount Eliminated (mg)	% of Steady State
1	100	100	50	50
2	100	150	75	75
3	100	175	87.5	87.5
4	100	187.5	93.75	93.75
5	100	197.5	98.75	98.75

exposure. Table 8.9 shows the number of half-lives that it takes to reach steady state following a 100-mg dose. Steady state is reached when the amount of drug entering the body equals the amount eliminated from the body. As a rule of thumb, it takes 4 half-lives to reach about 93.75% and 5 half-lives to reach 98.75% of the steady-state concentration. In practice, it is generally acceptable to assume that steady state has been reached after 4 or 5 half-lives. Therefore, if possible, to ensure that the second toxicokinetic sampling day represents steady-state exposure, toxicokinetic sampling should be conducted at least 4 half-lives after the start of dosing.

Exposure following multiple dosing may increase based on the duration of the dosing interval relative to the half-life. For a compound that follows linear kinetics, the expected accumulation index (r), which is the ratio between the highest initial concentration at steady state, $C_{p,\max\text{-ss}}$, and the highest concentration after the first dose, $C_{p,\max\text{-1stdose}}$, can be expressed as the ratio

$$r = 1/1 - R \qquad \text{where} \quad R = e^{-\tau/t_{1/2}}$$

R is the fraction of the initial plasma concentration remaining at the end of the dosing interval, τ is the dosing interval, and $t_{1/2}$ is the elimination half-life. This accumulation ratio also describes the relative $\text{AUC}_{0-\tau}$ at steady state as compared to a single dose. Table 8.10 presents the expected accumulation index as a function of the ratio of the dosing interval relative to the half-life. In cases where the dosing interval is equal to the half-life, an accumulation index of 2 is expected.

Unexpected accumulation following multiple dosing can occur for two primary reasons. First, following multiple dosing, drug metabolism and transport systems can be either inhibited or induced, based on the chemical nature of the test drug, which can result in either higher or lower exposures at steady state compared with exposures following a single dose. Second, toxicity can affect drug clearance directly or indirectly. Liver and kidney are two common target organs, and drug-induced toxicity can result in changes in clearance from these organs. Changes in protein binding, body mass, and general health status can affect drug distribution and clearance. Understanding tissue effects and clearance mechanisms is required to help interpret toxicokinetic differences associated with toxicity.

There are several approaches to evaluating whether there is unexpected accumulation (i.e., exposure exceeds that predicted based on the relationship of the

TABLE 8.10 Accumulation Index (r) as a Function of the Ratio of the Dosing Interval (τ) Relative to the Half-Life ($t_{1/2}$)

Dosing Interval τ (h)	$t_{1/2}$ (h)	Ratio $\tau/t_{1/2}$	R^a	r
24	6	0.25	0.06	1.1
24	12	0.5	0.25	1.3
24	24	1	0.50	2.0
24	36	1.5	0.63	2.7
24	48	2	0.71	3.4
24	96	4	0.84	6.3

[a] R is the fraction of the initial plasma concentration remaining at the end of the dosing interval.

dosing interval and the half-life). One approach is to compare the $AUC_{0-\infty}$ value on day 1 to the $AUC_{0-\tau}$ (or AUC_{last}) value at steady state. Assuming linear kinetics as shown below, these exposures should be equal.

$$AUC_0^{\infty} = \frac{FD}{CL}$$

$$C_{SS,av} = \frac{FD}{CL \cdot \tau}$$

$$AUC_{ss} = C_{SS,av}\tau = \frac{FD}{CL} = AUC_0^{\infty}$$

If these values are significantly different, this suggests a time-dependent change in pharmacokinetics. However, in some cases it may not be possible to estimate $AUC_{0-\infty}$ accurately if the terminal half-life is greater than half the dosing interval and/or there are insufficient time points to estimate the terminal phase accurately. Implicit in the estimation of the $AUC_{0-\infty}$ is the determination of a terminal half-life, which provides information about the expected accumulation for a given dosing interval. Other approaches to evaluating if there is a time-dependent change in pharmacokinetics causing unexpected accumulation are to evaluate if the ratio of maximum concentration in plasma at steady state ($C_{p,\text{max - ss}}$) and the highest concentration after the first dose ($C_{p,\text{(max -1)st dose}}$) are greater or less than the accumulation index or to compare the minimum plasma concentration at 24 hours postdose on the first day of dosing to the predose concentration at steady state.

Given the small sample sizes and inherent variability in toxicokinetic data from nonclinical toxicity studies, generally the potential for accumulation due to induction or inhibition is reported only if it is a factor of 2 above or below the accumulation index expected.

8.6.5 Gender Effects

Quantitative gender differences in metabolism [35] and active transport [36–39] are fairly common in rodents, and thus gender differences in drug exposure are often observed. These are especially well known in rats where gender-based metabolism differences driven by growth hormone effects on hepatic expression of gender-dependent forms of CYP450 manifest as severalfold-higher parent exposure in female versus male rats. However, the reverse can occur (i.e., exposure in males> females), as shown in a previous example [35]. The mouse model, in which the gender differences (F > M) in drug-metabolizing enzyme activities vary by only 40 to 100% versus 300 to 500% in rats, are also regulated by gender-dependent plasma growth hormone profiles [35]. When extrapolated to other species, such as humans, the magnitude of the gender differences is much smaller or nonexistent [58–61]. Therefore, caution should be used in extrapolating nonclinical gender differences in exposure to humans or across species. When there is substantially greater metabolism in one gender of a nonclinical toxicology species (e.g., absolute oral bioavailability of 3% in male rodent versus 90% in humans), it can be challenging to reach sufficient exposure multiples to evaluate the toxicological effects on the reproductive organs. To overcome the extensive metabolism in one gender and reach target clinical exposures can require very high drug loads (e.g., 1000 mg/kg in rat versus 8 mg/kg in humans) and result in exposures to multiple metabolites, due to the extensive metabolism unique to the rat and that therefore may not be relevant to humans. In these situations alternative routes (e.g., intravenous infusion or subcutaneous administration) may be considered to reach higher exposures.

Similar to assessment of dose proportionality, statistical analysis to evaluate gender differences can be utilized but in actuality provides little benefit over observational analyses. In general, mean AUC and C_{max} observations which are less than twofold are not considered meaningful. The benefit in understanding gender differences is in assisting with dose selection, evaluating gender-specific effects on the reproductive system, or understanding different toxicity thresholds across genders. Qualitative gender differences in metabolism are much less frequent than quantitative differences and, if present, should be evaluated relative to any differences in the toxicity profile. When there are fewer than three animals per dose group, caution should be exercised when drawing conclusions about gender differences due to considerable intersubject variability.

8.6.6 Relationship to Toxicology Findings

It is important to understand whether observed toxicological effects can be mitigated or avoided by reducing the C_{max} or whether the effects are AUC mediated. Comparing once versus twice daily dosing for oral administration, or bolus versus infusion dosing in the case of intravenous administration and the corresponding toxicokinetics can facilitate this comparison. In cases where a toxicological finding is C_{max} related, it may be possible to apply controlled-release drug delivery methods to minimize C_{max} levels [62–65].

Another important question to consider is whether the toxicological effects are pharmacologically mediated or are due to an off-target event. An evaluation of the in vitro and in vivo pharmacodynamic activity of a compound in the toxicological model compared to humans coupled with the determination of the relative concentrations or exposures achieved in toxicity studies can provide insights as to whether the effects are due to exaggerated pharmacology or are an off-target effect [5]. This question is discussed in more detail in Section 8.8.1.

Correlation of toxic effects to plasma drug or metabolite concentrations in practice is usually made at the group mean level. Unlike nonrodent species, wherein the toxicokinetic sampling may be conducted with main study animals, with pooled samples in rats and the use of satellite animals for the toxicokinetic portion of the study, it is very difficult to assign toxicities to specific rodents. Time-dependent changes in the exposure to a compound within a dose group can be indicative of toxicity to the organs responsible for clearance of the compound (e.g., liver or kidney [7]).

8.6.7 Midstudy Changes in Dosing Duration or Dose Level

When severe toxicity resulting in mortality is observed in a main toxicity study, the study director may choose to stop dosing and euthanize the remaining animals prior to the scheduled study termination date to ensure that a thorough toxicological assessment can be made. In these situations the toxicokinetic assessment is also performed in parallel prior to the scheduled termination date. Alternatively, the study director may choose to continue the study but lower the dose level. In these situations, the plasma drug concentrations in the toxicokinetic satellite animals are also lowered. From a toxicokinetic perspective, when the dose level is lowered midstudy, it can be difficult to evaluate if there are time-dependent changes in pharmacokinetics between the beginning and end of the dosing period and also to interpret the relationship between exposure and observed toxicity (i.e., exposure at the initial dose or reduced dose). A separate multiple-dose study can be conducted at the reduced-dose level to evaluate the time-dependent changes in pharmacokinetics; however, relating the exposure to the toxicities observed may not be possible without conducting another toxicity study at the reduced dose level.

8.7 ROLE OF TOXICOKINETICS IN DIFFERENT TYPES OF TOXICITY STUDIES

In this section the role of toxicokinetics in acute, dose-range finding, repeat dose, subchronic and chronic, genetic, and reproductive toxicity studies as well as in safety pharmacology, carcinogenicity, and bridging studies is described. Although the focus of this chapter is generally on the pre-FIH program, toxicokinetic strategies in support of all standard toxicity studies are discussed. The ICH guidelines for toxicity studies, in which toxicokinetics may be applied, are listed in Table 8.11. Not all of these guidelines explicitly mention toxicokinetics, and therefore ICH S3A [2] is generally the most appropriate guideline to refer to with respect to the role of toxicokinetics in these different study types.

TABLE 8.11 Toxicity Studies in Which Toxicokinetics Is Applied by Drug Development Sponsors and the Appropriate ICH Guidelines[a]

Toxicity Study	Relevant ICH Guideline
Single dose	S4
Repeat dose	S4A and M3
Safety pharmacology	S7A and S7B
Genotoxicity	S2A and S2B
Reproductive toxicity	S5A and S5B
Carcinogenicity	S1A, S1B, and S1C

[a]ICH S3A is the most appropriate reference for guidelines on the application of toxicokinetics to these different study types.

8.7.1 Acute Studies

The ICH S3A guideline on toxicokinetics states that: "Single dose studies are often performed in a very early phase of development before a bioanalytical method has been developed and toxicokinetic monitoring of these studies is therefore not normally possible. Plasma samples may be taken in such studies and stored for later analysis, if necessary; appropriate stability data for the analyte in the matrix sampled would then be required" [2]. The guideline does not require toxicokinetics for single-dose studies and since single-dose toxicokinetics are generally evaluated as part of the multiple-dose toxicity studies, most drug sponsors do not perform toxicokinetic sampling in acute studies.

8.7.2 Dose-Range-Finding and Tolerability Studies

When discovery stage compounds have shown promise in nonclinical pharmacology models, they are generally first tested in tolerability studies that consist of a single-dose escalation phase followed by a short-duration (<10-day) repeat dose phase in a rodent and a nonrodent species (Chapter 7). These studies are non-GLP and generally utilize a bioanalytical method that is only partially validated (Chapter 4). Unless data exist which suggest that rats or dogs have very different pharmacokinetic, metabolism, or pharmacological response and receptor profiles from those of humans, at this stage most companies default to these species. In some cases single-dose pharmacokinetic escalation studies are conducted prior to the tolerability studies to determine whether sufficient multiples of the target exposure can be achieved. Doses start at pharmacologic levels and are increased to supra-pharmacologic levels in the escalation phase based on clinical observations, pathological endpoints, or limitations of formulation, and in some cases no toxicokinetic data are collected. Toxicokinetic evaluation of system exposures can be particularly helpful in cases where emesis is observed (e.g., in dogs or monkeys) to confirm that there is systemic exposure to the compound and that the clinical observations are not due only to local gastrointestinal effects.

Dose-range-finding and tolerability studies are generally conducted using discovery material to support species or dose selection, and toxicokinetic exposure data may be collected on the first and last days of dosing. Often, the tolerability studies represent the first opportunity to evaluate the effects of single versus multiple dosing regimens, and fewer animals are used. Additionally, some sponsors will save the livers from the toxicokinetic animals to evaluate whether there is evidence for CYP450 induction *in vivo*.

8.7.3 Subchronic Studies (Two Weeks to Three Months)

The ICH guideline on any GLP repeated dose study states:

> Toxicokinetics should be incorporated appropriately into the design of the studies. It may consist of exposure profiling or monitoring at appropriate dose levels at the start and towards the end of the treatment period of the first repeat dose study. The procedure adopted for later studies will depend on the results from the first study and on any changes in the proposed treatment regimen. Monitoring or profiling may be extended, reduced or modified for specific compounds where problems have arisen in the interpretation of earlier toxicity studies.

Subchronic toxicity studies are generally used as the pivotal FIH-enabling toxicity studies and are conducted in a rodent and a nonrodent species. Doses in the subchronic studies are set based on the toxicology and toxicokinetic results, especially as a function of the saturation of drug absorption of the tolerability studies. Toxicokinetic sampling is usually conducted in satellite animals for rodents and in the main study animals for nonrodents, due to limitations on blood sample volume in rodents.

8.7.4 Chronic Studies (Six to 12 Months)

Chronic studies of six months duration in rodents and nine to 12 months in nonrodents are generally conducted to support phase II and III clinical development and registration. They are not required for initial IND submissions and are generally scheduled in time to support phase II programs, so may actually start prior to completion of the FIH study. Toxicokinetic sampling is usually conducted at the beginning, middle, and end of the study to evaluate the potential for time-dependent changes in exposure. Given the low cost of toxicokinetic analysis relative to the overall cost of the chronic studies, full toxicokinetic sampling that supports determination of AUC, C_{max}, and t_{max} values is recommended.

8.7.5 Safety Pharmacology and Specialty Studies

Safety pharmacology studies (Chapter 6) are required for FIH-enabling programs. Although the ICH S3A guideline does not specifically discuss toxicokinetic evaluations in these studies, ICH S7A states:

> Generally, any parent compound and its major metabolites that achieve, or are expected to achieve, systemic exposure in humans should be evaluated in safety pharmacology studies. Evaluation of major metabolites is often accomplished through studies of the parent compound in animals. If the major human metabolites are found to be absent or present only at relatively low concentrations in animals, assessment of the effects of such metabolites on safety pharmacology endpoints should be considered. Additionally, if metabolites from humans are known to substantially contribute to the pharmacological actions of the therapeutic agent, it could be important to test such active metabolites. When the in vivo studies on the parent compound have not adequately assessed metabolites, as discussed above, the tests of metabolites can use in vitro systems based on practical considerations.

Therefore, it is a standard practice in most pharmaceutical companies to obtain the GLP quality toxicokinetic data for these studies. So as not to affect the sensitive measurements in these studies, generally sparse or limited plasma sampling is used. Studies such as in vivo phototoxicity assessments or mechanistic studies generally include the ability to characterize exposure either directly or through the use of bridging studies discussed below.

8.7.6 Genetic Toxicology

In Vitro genetic toxicity studies are also core studies required for the initial IND/CTA filing. The ICH S2A and S2B guidances, which cover the in vitro and in vivo GLP–genotoxicity studies, state: "For negative results of in vivo genotoxicity studies, it may be appropriate to have demonstrated systemic exposure in the species used or to have characterized exposure in the indicator tissue." In tests such as the bacterial reverse mutation assay, concentrations of the test article in the dosing solutions may be determined, but generally no toxicokinetics assessment is performed. In the in vivo chromosomal aberration or micronucleus assays in bone marrow cells of rats or mice, typically three or four dose levels up to an MTD with five animals per dose and males only is sufficient unless there are qualitative gender differences in metabolism. Blood sampling for toxicokinetic assessment is recommended up to 24 hours (all doses) and 48 hours (top dose only). In the in vivo rodent studies a confirmation of exposure by sampling at a single time point may be sufficient if toxicokinetic data are available from other studies at the doses used.

8.7.7 Reproductive Toxicology

Reproductive toxicity studies are generally initiated after initial phase I safety and tolerability studies and are not typically included in FIH packages. However, many drug targets are expressed more frequently in women, and therefore rapid enrollment of women of childbearing potential are critical in phase I to early phase II testing. On those occasions, reproductive toxicity studies are advisable pre-FIH, both to test for safety in the target population and to enable rapid recruitment for the phase II program. The ICH guidelines provide the following recommendations with regard to the application of toxicokinetic evaluations in reproductive toxicity studies (e.g., fertility studies as well as studies in pregnant and lactating animals):

- Maternal toxicity is typically dose limiting for these studies, but plasma concentrations are important for assessing the NOAEL, safety margins, and next steps forward.
- Consideration should be given to the possibility that the kinetics will often differ in pregnant and nonpregnant animals and therefore must be characterized for both conditions.
- Plasma is the standard matrix. It is also appropriate to study embryo/fetal transfer and secretion in milk as specific study objectives related to developmental toxicology but as separate programs.

Typically, reproductive toxicity studies are conducted in rats and/or rabbits. Since toxicokinetic data have already been generated in repeat dose rat studies, it is not essential but is generally most efficient to include toxicokinetics in the fertility and peri- and postnatal studies, to confirm that there are no differences in exposure in pregnant and nonpregnant animals. In practice, many sponsors include toxicokinetics, either as part of the range-finding study or part of the main study, due to observed pharmacokinetic profile differences for some compounds in pregnant animals. Recent regulatory requirements mandate that human metabolites are also present in plasma in at least one reproductive toxicology species to have a valid program for human safety assessment. A more detailed review on toxicokinetic support for reproductive toxicity studies has been published by Schwartz [66].

8.7.8 Carcinogenicity Studies

Two-year carcinogenicity studies in rodents (typically, mice and rats) are not conducted prior to the FIH trial but are required at later stages of development of drug candidates target for chronic use. Thirteen-week dose-range-finding studies are generally used in the strain of interest to determine the MTD before conducting the definitive carcinogenicity bioassays. The toxicokinetic evaluations in these dose-ranging studies are crucial in dose selection for the carcinogenicity studies. In the definitive bioassays, the ICH guidance suggests monitoring toxicokinetics at several occasions up to six months. Toxicokinetic data beyond six months are not required unless other confounding data are obtained from dose-ranging studies and definitive bioassays. The top dose in these studies is required to reach an MTD, a 25-fold AUC ratio (rodent to human) or a maximum feasible dose (e.g., due to saturation of absorption) [67]. Since most drugs cause toxicity in rodents at AUC values that are 5 to 10 times higher than the human therapeutic exposure, it is often not possible to reach a 25-fold exposure ratio, and thus doses are usually set at an MTD.

Drug is often formulated in the animal feed to reduce the labor and chances for gavage error during the two-year carcinogenicity studies. To determine the appropriate doses in a diet–drug mixture that provide sufficient exposure, it is helpful to conduct pilot pharmacokinetic studies with the drug in animal feed prior to the start of the definitive studies. Toxicokinetic evaluation immediately following dosing on the first day can also be used to confirm that appropriate doses are being administered.

8.7.9 Bridging Toxicity Studies

In the context of this discussion, bridging studies are toxicity studies that are usually conducted to qualify a new formulation, salt form, or a batch containing various impurity levels. These studies are generally 2 to 4 weeks in duration but can be as short as a single dose with 14-day sacrifice, depending on the duration of clinical use and stage of development. The toxicity profile of the new formulation, salt form, or batch is generally evaluated side by side with the previous batch, formulation, or form at the NOAEL dose level to confirm that no new toxicities are observed. In cases where the previous batch is not available, it may be acceptable to compare results between the bridging study on the new formulation and the results from the previous study but run the risk of leading to confounding toxicity results that require follow-up investigation. Toxicokinetic sampling in these studies can be quite important because differences in exposure with a new formulation could cause new and unexpected toxicities. For compounds with dissolution-limited exposure, it is prudent to conduct single- or multiple-dose pharmacokinetic studies prior to conducting the toxicity study to determine if there are likely to be substantial differences in exposure. If there are substantial differences in exposure, it may be necessary to conduct additional standard toxicity studies.

8.8 ROLE OF TOXICOKINETICS IN INTEGRATED SAFETY ASSESSMENT

8.8.1 Safety Margins: Role in Setting Clinical Doses for FIH Studies

Considerations for the estimation of a safe starting dose in the FIH trial are discussed in Chapter 10. Toxicokinetics can provide helpful information in selecting a safe starting dose and maximum acceptable exposure in a FIH single ascending dose study. Generally, a safe human starting dose must be determined based solely on nonclinical toxicology and pharmacokinetic studies and without any information about the pharmacokinetics in humans. Interestingly, in the FDA guidance on approaches for determining the maximum recommended starting dose [68], the primary approach emphasizes scaling the dose at the NOAEL in the most sensitive nonclinical toxicology species to humans based on body surface area. Pharmacokinetic differences between species are cited as providing supportive

TABLE 8.12 Relationship Between Key Findings and Exposures in Studies with an NCE and the Estimated Exposure in Humans Based on Allometric Scaling

C_{max} (ng/mL)	AUC (ng·h/mL)	Key Pharmacology and Toxicology Findings Across Studies
4,060	57,700	Convulsion in one male dog in 2-week study at 10 mg/kg
3,940	43,900	Convulsion in two female dogs in 2-week study at 10 mg/kg
5,976	25,078	Substantial pharmacologic effect in 28-day rat pharmacology study (30 mg/kg)
1,000	17,000	NOAEL (10 mg/kg) in 14-day dose-range finding study in male and female monkeys
891	11,200	NOAEL (2 mg/kg) in male dogs in 14-day GLP toxicity study
904	11,100	NOAEL (2 mg/kg) in female dogs in 14-day GLP toxicity study
901	6,070	NOAEL (10 mg/kg) in female rats in 14-day GLP toxicity study
568	3,400	NOAEL (10 mg/kg) in male rats in 14-day GLP toxicity study
100–300	18,000	High-target human efficacy concentrations based on nonclinical PK/PD
570	3,082	Significant pharmacologic effect in 28-day rat study (2 mg/kg)
415	1,756	Moderate pharmacologic effect in 28-day rat pharmacology study (1 mg/kg)
5.79	659	2-mg single oral dose in humans ($F = 100\%$); 70 kg (scaling estimate)
2.32	264	2-mg single oral dose in humans ($F = 40\%$); 70 kg (scaling estimate)

information but are not the drivers in this guidance. However, in practice, worldwide regulators place a higher emphasis on the toxicokinetic exposures than on absolute dose for initiating and stopping human dose escalation.

Toxicokinetics has evolved to be a major factor in projecting safe working margins of exposure in human volunteers, based on animal data. Table 8.12 shows an example of an integrated way to present the relationship between key findings and exposures in nonclinical studies and the proposed starting dose in humans (exposure estimated based on allometry [69,70]). Table 8.12 contains the target efficacious range for C_{max} and AUC in humans based on the nonclinical PK/PD model (row shown in boldface type). In the rows above the target exposure in humans, the exposures at the NOAEL doses in the nonclinical toxicity studies as well as the levels and types of adverse effects that were observed are presented; in the rows below, the pharmacologic effects expected at lower exposures based on the nonclinical PK/PD model as well as the projected exposure at the recommended starting dose of 2 mg based on estimated bioavailability values in humans of 40% and 100% are presented. Presentation of the information in this tabular format is particularly useful for evaluating the relationship of the projected exposure at the recommended starting dose relative to the exposures at which pharmacological or adverse effects have been observed for the drug candidate in the nonclinical studies. For subsequent doses, projections of exposure are more dependent on the pharmacokinetic and safety data obtained in humans.

In establishing a safety window for single and multiple ascending dose studies, both for selection of the first dose and also for limiting dose escalation, toxicokinetics are evaluated with the NOAEL dose. Key considerations in setting a maximum exposure for dose escalation in humans that is above the NOAEL is whether the toxicity observed at that exposure may be readily monitored in a clinical setting and if the toxicological effect observed nonclinically is reversible.

8.8.2 Role of Protein Binding and Blood Partitioning

Protein binding, or free drug fraction in plasma, is an area where guidelines and practices are open to interpretation. The ICH S3A guideline states that protein-binding differences should be "considered" as factors for interpreting exposure differences, citing that it may be most appropriate to consider for highly bound drugs. In practice, most toxicokinetic comparisons use total drug concentrations unless there are significant binding differences across species, which in turn can significantly alter safety window assessments for free "available" drug. Species with the highest plasma free fraction theoretically have more drug available to tissue sites of toxicity or activity. Experimentally, binding is characterized initially in separate in vitro studies encompassing clinical and nonclinical concentrations. If there are significant binding differences across species, especially if there is saturable binding at higher concentrations, more detailed studies are usually conducted. These can include protein-binding assessments directly on toxicology samples or using in vitro binding estimates to adjust total concentrations. For drugs that are very highly protein bound (>99%), smaller differences in bound fraction result in larger differences in free fraction, as illustrated in Table 8.13. A 1% difference in protein binding for a highly protein-bound drug (e.g., 99.8% in human versus 98.8% in rat) can result in a 500% difference in the free fraction. When presenting exposures based on free fractions in regulatory support documents, it is important to include uncorrected (total) exposures. It should be noted that, in practice, regulatory agencies often do not accept animal or human exposure multiples based on the free fraction when the binding is greater in humans than in animals; therefore, if it is important for the program, this approach should be discussed proactively with the appropriate regulatory agencies.

Partitioning into red blood cells can also have an impact on drug toxicokinetics and should be considered in the estimation of safety margins and in correlating exposures to toxicity [25]. Although plasma (or serum) is typically the main compartment of interest for toxicokinetic assessments, and is generally used without issue, whole blood is also an accessible compartment for evaluation of

TABLE 8.13 Changes in Protein Binding for Highly Bound Drugs Compared to Moderately Bound Drugs

Total Concentration (μg/mL)	Fraction Bound	Fraction Free	Free Concentration μg/mL	Free Fraction Difference
		Drug with Moderate Protein Binding		
100	45%	55%	55	Baseline (e.g., rat)
100	40%	60%	60	110% (e.g., human)
		Drug with High Protein Binding		
100	99.8%	0.2	0.2	Baseline (e.g., rat)
100	98.8%	1.2	1.2	600% (e.g., human)

drug exposure in animals and humans. Partitioning into whole blood should be understood and under certain conditions considered for interpreting toxicokinetic data. For example, in the case of the neuroleptic drugs butaperazine, haloperidol, and thioridazine, the RBC concentrations have been reported to correlate better with therapeutic effects or dose than plasma concentrations [25]. Similarly, the measurement of RBC concentrations has been recommended for lithium in evaluating adverse reactions and toxicity of the drug; with digoxin, RBC concentrations were found to better distinguish between toxic and nontoxic drug levels than were plasma concentrations [71]. Extrapolation of toxicokinetic data across species may be complicated by interspecies differences in RBC distribution, as was shown for trimetrexate [72].

8.8.3 Toxicokinetics: Caution about Safety Margins

Initially, toxicokinetics was designed simply to document dose-related exposure and was more of an interpretive tool to include with the overall data package for toxicity studies. However, the concept of animal to human safety margins and safe versus toxic doses is now a fundamental part of the safety evaluation package, and often becomes the primary consideration for the human starting and stopping doses. The safety margin concept has moved into almost all types of toxicity studies, at all stages of development, and into many regulatory guidelines. Although there is strong rationale for this as an acceptable general rule, when applied blindly it is often overly conservative and can result in inadequate testing of drug candidates or stopping clinical development prematurely.

Without exception, industry scientists and regulators must always protect study subjects while trying to move from an NCE to a viable drug with patient benefits. Factors such as therapeutic area, onset, monitorability, and reversibility of toxicity, along with patient population, phase of development, risk/benefit ratio of the clinical study, and eventual indication, must all be factored in to set the most appropriate safe margins for drug testing. Setting an acceptable safety margin should be an integrated effort by the toxicologists, clinicians, and other scientists on the development team.

One of the dangers in applying exposure-based safety margins is that this approach ignores the substantial differences in total drug burden often present between toxicology animals and humans. Many animals metabolize drugs faster than humans do, and through multiple pathways; elimination rates are often higher in laboratory animals. Therefore, to generate target organ toxicity, large doses are administered (up to 2000 mg/kg) and the total drug burden (drug and metabolites) is often at levels that will never be attained in humans. For example, a clinically effective plasma concentration of 2 μg/mL could be achieved with a 100-mg dose (2 mg/kg) in humans, whereas in animals, due to more rapid metabolism and clearance, it could require more than 400 mg/kg. Although parent concentrations are the same, the overall drug burden is much larger (>80-fold on a mg/kg basis) in the toxicology animals. These perspectives should be considered in the interpretation of safety windows.

Another important consideration is whether pharmacologically mediated toxicity can be monitored or evaluated in the nonclinical species due to differences in the in vitro and in vivo pharmacodynamic activity of a compound compared to humans. In situations where a drug has much lower potency in the nonclinical toxicology species, the safety margins may be misleading [5]. Conversely, if the drug is more potent against the receptors in the nonclinical species, it can be difficult to evaluate off-target toxicity at sufficient multiples of the clinical target because pharmacologically mediated toxicity at supratherapeutic doses may arise. As discussed above, the impact of differences in biological effect is embodied in the concept of the minimum anticipated biological effect level (MABEL) and is of particular concern in the case of biologics that have the potential to illicit a much larger immune response [46].

As the toxicokinetic approach is attractive in simplicity and rationale, its application to metabolites is also expanding. Requirements for metabolite exposure comparisons to "validate" the toxicology species have moved from a more qualitative and staged approach targeted to support the larger enrollment of phase III trials to generating quantitative information as early as possible in the drug development program. Although this is attractive on the surface, common sense must be applied regarding the decision as to which human metabolites, which may represent only a relatively small percentage of parent drug in plasma, should be evaluated for "coverage" in the toxicology species.

8.8.4 Safety Margins for Different Toxicity Profiles

Although it is tempting to select a number that feels comforting as an acceptable safety margin (e.g., a human therapeutic AUC of 5 or 10 times greater than that at the animal NOAEL), this is not practical. Toxicokinetics provides C_{max} and AUC values that can be compared to clinical target exposure. However, setting acceptable safety margins depends on the type and severity of toxicity, if it is a monitorable or a reversible toxicity, if the drug is first in class versus one where there is significant clinical experience with the class, and even the target indication or medical need for the product. Many marketed drugs have safety margins below 1 for serious toxicities in the toxicology species, which were not observed in humans. For example, many central nervous system (CNS) drugs have dose-limiting CNS side effects in animals that are at, or lower than, the target concentrations in humans. The exposure-based safety margin for these type compounds is often at, or below, unity. Generally, cautious dose escalation in the clinical program, with dose-limiting toxicity of human CNS effects, has helped establish safer and more appropriate exposures in humans than if safety margins were applied without considering relevant drug and patient characteristic cofactors.

8.9 CONCLUSIONS

Toxicokinetics has become fully integrated into all phases of drug safety evaluation programs. The discipline directly influences toxicity study design, interpretation of results, and how those results are evaluated by regulatory agencies. As such, the more basic aspects of toxicokinetics (i.e., how and when it is applied) have evolved through regulatory guidelines, workshops, and GLP requirements. Although these more mechanical factors are becoming standardized and are generally very helpful, when considered in isolation they can sometimes lead to missed opportunities in optimizing toxicity study design and data interpretation. The many factors described in this chapter should be evaluated in the context of the individual toxicity study, the entire nonclinical program, and the clinical results, as they can significantly influence how the toxicokinetic data are generated, how they are interpreted, and what follow-up actions may be required.

REFERENCES

1. DeGeorge JJ. Food and Drug Administration viewpoints on toxicokinetics: the view from review. *Toxicol Pathol*. 1995;23(2):220–225.
2. Toxicokinetics: A Guidance for Assessing Systemic Exposure in Toxicity Studies. ICH-S3A. International Conference on Harmonization; 1995. Available at: www.fda.gov/cder/guidance/index.htm.
3. Nonclinical Safety Studies for the Conduct of Human Clinical Trials for Pharmaceuticals. ICH-M3. International Conference on Harmonization; 1997. Available at: www.fda.gov/cder/guidance/index.htm.
4. Baldrick P. Toxicokinetics in preclinical evaluation. *Drug Discov Today*. 2003;8(3):127–133.
5. Morgan DG, Kelvin AS, Kinter LB, Fish CJ, Kerns WD, Rhodes G. The application of toxicokinetic data to dosage selection in toxicology studies. *Toxicol Pathol*. 1994;22(2):112–123.
6. Yacobi A, Barry H. In: Yacobi A, Barry HIII, eds. *Experimental and Clinical Toxicokinetics*. Washington, DC: American Pharmaceutical Association; 1984. *J Clin Pharmacol*. 1985;25(4):313.

7. Welling P, Iglesia F. *Drug Toxicokinetics*, Vol. 9. New York: Marcel Dekker; 1984.
8. Shah V, Midha K, Dighe S. Analytical method validation: bioavailability, bioequivalence, and pharmacokinetic studies (Conference Report). *Pharm Res*. 1992;9:588–592.
9. Shah VP, Midha KK, Findlay JW, et al. Bioanalytical method validation: a revisit with a decade of progress. *Pharm Res*. 2000;17(12):1551–1557.
10. Robinson WT. Innovative early development regulatory approaches: expIND, expCTA, microdosing. *Clin Pharmacol Ther*. 2008;83:358–360.
11. Zhang L, Strong JM, Qiu W, Lesko LJ, Huang SM. Scientific perspectives on drug transporters and their role in drug interactions. *Mol Pharm*. 2006;3(1):62–69.
12. Frantz SW, Beatty PW, English JC, Hundley SG, Wilson AG. The use of pharmacokinetics as an interpretive and predictive tool in chemical toxicology testing and risk assessment: a position paper on the appropriate use of pharmacokinetics in chemical toxicology. *Regul Toxicol Pharmacol*. 1994;19(3):317–337.
13. Brewster M, Mackie C, Noppe M, Lampo A, Loftsson T. *Solvent Systems and Their Selection in Pharmaceutics and Biopharmaceutics*, Vol. VI. New York: Springer; 2007.
14. Strickley RG. Solubilizing excipients in oral and injectable formulations. *Pharm Res*. 2004;21(2):201–230.
15. Lipinski CA. Drug-like properties and the causes of poor solubility and poor permeability. *J Pharmacol Toxicol Methods*. 2000;44(1):235–249.
16. Bittner B, Mountfield RJ. Intravenous administration of poorly soluble new drug entities in early drug discovery: the potential impact of formulation on pharmacokinetic parameters. *Curr Opin Drug Discov Dev*. 2002;5(1):59–71.
17. Buggins TR, Dickinson PA, Taylor G. The effects of pharmaceutical excipients on drug disposition. *Adv Drug Deliv Rev*. 2007;59(15):1482–1503.
18. Himmel HM. Suitability of commonly used excipients for electrophysiological in-vitro safety pharmacology assessment of effects on hERG potassium current and on rabbit Purkinje fiber action potential. *J Pharmacol Toxicol Methods*. 2007;56(2): 145–158.
19. Pifferi G, Restani P. The safety of pharmaceutical excipients. *Farmaco*. 2003; 58(8):541–550.
20. Cornaire G, Woodley J, Hermann P, Cloarec A, Arellano C, Houin G. Impact of excipients on the absorption of P-glycoprotein substrates in vitro and in vivo. *Int J Pharm*. 2004;278(1):119–131.
21. Subrahmanyam VV, Tonelli AP. Chapter 4, Pharmacokinetics/ADME of small molecules. In: *Preclinical Drug Development*. New York: Informa Healthcare; 2005: 99–158.
22. Little JL, Wempe MF, Buchanan CM. Liquid chromatography–mass spectrometry/mass spectrometry method development for drug metabolism studies: examining lipid matrix ionization effects in plasma. *J Chromatogr B*. 2006;833(2): 219–230.
23. Matuszewski BK, Constanzer ML, Chavez-Eng CM. Matrix effect in quantitative LC/MS/MS analyses of biological fluids: a method for determination of finasteride in human plasma at picogram per milliliter concentrations. *Anal Chem*. 1998;70(5):882–889.

24. Hong Mei YH. Investigation of matrix effects in bioanalytical high-performance liquid chromatography/tandem mass spectrometric assays: application to drug discovery. *Rapid Commun Mass Spectrom*. 2003;17(1):97–103.

25. Hinderling PH. Red blood cells: a neglected compartment in pharmacokinetics and pharmacodynamics. *Pharmacol Rev*. 1997;49(3):279–295.

26. Viswanathan CT, Bansal S, Booth B, et al. Quantitative bioanalytical methods validation and implementation: best practices for chromatographic and ligand binding assays. *Pharm Res*. 2007;24(10):1962–1973.

27. Baillie TA, Cayen MN, Fouda H, et al. Drug metabolites in safety testing. *Toxicol Appl Pharmacol*. 2002;182(3):188–196.

28. Baillie TA, Cayen MN, Fouda H, et al. Reply. *Toxicol Appl Pharmacol*. 2003; 190(1):93–94.

29. Hastings KL, El-Hage J, Jacobs A, Leighton J, Morse D, Osterberg RE. Drug metabolites in safety testing. *Toxicol Appl Pharmacol*. 2003;190(1):91–92; author reply 93–94.

30. Prueksaritanont T, Lin JH, Baillie TA. Complicating factors in safety testing of drug metabolites: kinetic differences between generated and preformed metabolites. *Toxicol Appl Pharmacol*. 2006;217(2):143–152.

31. Smith DA, Obach RS. Seeing through the mist: abundance versus percentage—commentary on metabolites in safety testing. *Drug Metab Dispos*. 2005;33(10): 1409–1417.

32. Guidance for Industry: Safety Testing of Drug Metabolites. U.S. Food and Drug Administration; 2008. Available at: www.fda.gov/cder/guidance/index.htm.

33. Rippley RK, Yan KX, Matthews ND, Greenberg HE, Herman GA, Wagner JA. Human pharmacokinetics and interconversion of enantiomers of MK-0767, a dual PPAR{alpha}/{gamma} agonist. *J Clin Pharmacol*. 2007;47(3):323–333.

34. Zhongzhou Shen RB. Enantiomer ratio of MK-0767 in humans and nonclinical species. *Rapid Commun Mass Spectrom*. 2005;19(9):1125–1129.

35. Shapiro BH, Agrawal AK, Pampori NA. Gender differences in drug metabolism regulated by growth hormone. *Int J Biochem Cell Biol*. 1995;27(1):9–20.

36. Buist SC, Klaassen CD. Rat and mouse differences in gender-predominant expression of organic anion transporter (Oat1–3; Slc22a6–8) mRNA levels. *Drug Metab Dispos*. 32(6):620–625.

37. Maher JM, Slitt AL, Cherrington NJ, Cheng X, Klaassen CD. Tissue distribution and hepatic and renal ontogeny of the multidrug resistance-associated protein (Mrp) family in mice. *Drug Metab Dispos*. 2005;33(7):947–955.

38. Urakami Y, Nakamura N, Takahashi K, et al. Gender differences in expression of organic cation transporter OCT2 in rat kidney. *FEBS Lett*. 1999;461(3):339–342.

39. Buist SC, Cherrington NJ, Choudhuri S, Hartley DP, Klaassen CD. Gender-specific and developmental influences on the expression of rat organic anion transporters. *J Pharmacol Exp Ther*. 2002;301(1):145–151.

40. Craig WA. Pharmacokinetic/pharmacodynamic parameters: rationale for antibacterial dosing of mice and men. *Clin Infect Dis*. 1998;26(1):1–10; quiz 11–12.

41. Diehl KH, Hull R, Morton D, et al. A good practice guide to the administration of substances and removal of blood, including routes and volumes. *J Appl Toxicol*. 2001;21(1):15–23.

42. Tse FL, Nedelman JR. Serial versus sparse sampling in toxicokinetic studies. *Pharm Res*. 1996;13(7):1105–1108.
43. Igarashi T, Sekido T. Case studies for statistical analysis of toxicokinetic data. *Regul Toxicol Pharmacol*. 1996;23(3):193–208.
44. Pai SM, Fettner SH, Hajian G, Cayen MN, Batra VK. Characterization of AUCs from sparsely sampled populations in toxicology studies. *Pharm Res*. 1996;13(9):1283–1290.
45. Burtin P, Mentre F, van Bree J, Steimer JL. Sparse sampling for assessment of drug exposure in toxicological studies. *Eur J Drug Metab Pharmacokinet*. 1996;21(2):105–111.
46. Tabrizi MA, Roskos LK. Preclinical and clinical safety of monoclonal antibodies. *Drug Discov Today*. 2007;12(13–14):540–547.
47. Preclinical Safety Evaluation of Biotechnology-Derived Pharmaceuticals. ICH-S6. International Conference on Harmonization; 1998. Available at: www.fda.gov/cder/guidance/index.htm.
48. Roland M, Tozer T. *Clinical Pharmacokinetics: Concepts and Applications*, 3rd ed. Philadelphia: Williams & Wilkins; 1995.
49. Igarashi T, Yabe T, Noda K. Study design and statistical analysis of toxicokinetics: a report of JPMA investigation of case studies. *J Toxicol Sci*. 1996;21(5):497–504.
50. Bjorkan. Prediction of the disposition of midazolam in surgical patients by a physiologically based pharmacokinetic model. *J Pharm Sci*. 2001;90(9):1226–1241.
51. Liao KH, Dobrev ID, Dennison JE Jr et al,. Application of biologically based computer modeling to simple or complex mixtures. *Environ Health Perspect*. 2002;110 (suppl 6):957–963.
52. Moghadamnia AA, Rostami-Hodjegan A, Abdul-Manap R, Wright CE, Morice AH, Tucker GT. Physiologically based modelling of inhibition of metabolism and assessment of the relative potency of drug and metabolite: dextromethorphan vs. dextrorphan using quinidine inhibition. *Br J Clin Pharmacol*. 2003;56(1):57–67.
53. Poulin P, Theil FP. A priori prediction of tissue:plasma partition coefficients of drugs to facilitate the use of physiologically-based pharmacokinetic models in drug discovery. *J Pharm Sci*. 2000;89(1):16–35.
54. Poulin P, Theil FP. Prediction of pharmacokinetics prior to in vivo studies: II. Generic physiologically based pharmacokinetic models of drug disposition. *J Pharm Sci*. 2002;91(5):1358–1370.
55. Price K, Haddad S, Krishnan K. Physiological modeling of age-specific changes in the pharmacokinetics of organic chemicals in children. *J Toxicol Environ Health A*. 2003;66(5):417–433.
56. Theil FP, Guentert T, Haddad S, Poulin P. Utility of physiologically based pharmacokinetic models to drug development and rational drug delivery candidate selection. *Toxicol Lett*. 2003;138:29–49.
57. Nestorov I. Whole-body physiologically based pharmacokinetic models. *Expert Opin Drug Metab Toxicol*. 2007;3(2):235–249.
58. Harris RZ, Benet LZ, Schwartz JB. Gender effects in pharmacokinetics and pharmacodynamics. *Drugs*. 1995;50(2):222–239.

59. Tanaka E. Gender-related differences in pharmacokinetics and their clinical significance. *J Clin Pharm Ther*. 1999;24(5):339–346.

60. Meibohm B, Beierle I, Derendorf H. How important are gender differences in pharmacokinetics? *Clin Pharmacokinet*. 2002;41(5):329–342.

61. Salphati L, Benet LZ. Modulation of P-glycoprotein expression by cytochrome P450 3A inducers in male and female rat livers. *Biochem Pharmacol*. 1998;55(4):387–395.

62. Sathyan G, Chancellor MB, Gupta SK. Effect of OROS controlled-release delivery on the pharmacokinetics and pharmacodynamics of oxybutynin chloride. *Br J Clin Pharmacol*. 2001;52(4):409–417.

63. Sood A, Panchagnula R. Design of controlled release delivery systems using a modified pharmacokinetic approach: a case study for drugs having a short elimination half-life and a narrow therapeutic index. *Int J Pharm*. 2003;261(1–2):27–41.

64. Vetrovec GW, Parker VE, Cole S, Procacci PM, Tabatznik B, Terry R. Nifedipine gastrointestinal therapeutic system in stable angina pectoris: results of a multicenter open-label crossover comparison with standard nifedipine. *Am J Med*. 1987;83(6B):24–29.

65. Wong PSL, Gupta SK, Stewart BE. Osmotically controlled tablets. *Drugs Pharm Sci*. 2003;126(Modified-Release Drug Delivery Technology):101–114.

66. Schwartz S. Providing toxicokinetic support for reproductive toxicology studies in pharmaceutical development. *Arch Toxicol*. 2001;75(7):381–387.

67. Dose Selection for Carcinogenicity Studies of Pharmaceuticals. ICH-S1C. International Conference on Harmonization; 1995. Available at: www.fda.gov/cder/guidance/index.htm.

68. Guidance for Industry: Estimating the Maximum Safe Starting Dose in Initial Clinical Trials for Therapeutics in Adult Healthy Volunteers. U.S. Food and Drug Administration; 2005. Available at: www.fda.gov/cder/guidance/index.htm.

69. Tang H, Mayersohn M. Accuracy of allometrically predicted pharmacokinetic parameters in humans: role of species selection. *Drug Metab Dispos*. 2005;33(9):1288–1293.

70. Mahmood I. Allometric issues in drug development. *J Pharm Sci*. 1999;88(11):1101–1106.

71. Kawai S, Ogawa K, Satake T. Erythrocyte digoxin concentration. *Clin Pharmacol Ther*. 1982;31(5):541–547.

72. Whittfield L, Pegg D. Drug toxicokinetics. In: Welling P, Iglesia F, eds. *Drug and Chemical Toxicology*, Vol. 9. New York: Marcel Dekker; 1984: 267–303.

9

GOOD LABORATORY PRACTICE

ANTHONY B. JONES, KATHRYN HACKETT-FIELDS, AND SHARI L. PERLSTEIN

9.1 INTRODUCTION*

Good laboratory practice (GLP): three letters that have caused more than their fair share of debate, controversy, and angst in the research and development community; three letters that have been the root of much misunderstanding at all organizational levels, up to and including senior management. In this chapter we simplify and demystify GLP, give practical advice and encouragement to those embarking on the GLP journey, and show that GLP really does rhyme with R&D; applying a rational, well-designed GLP system should result in a harmonious ensemble, not a discordant cacophony. To achieve such harmony, as with any orchestra, everyone involved has to understand the fundamental principles which, once identified, can produce successful results through constant practice and repetition. For the musician, these components are easily discerned—the melody, rhythm, and dynamics of the composition—however, in GLP we must first study the *raison d'être* for the regulations in order to appreciate the underlying principles. In the United States, the Food and Drug Administration's (FDA's) GLPs were developed to prevent recurrences of questionable practices uncovered during investigation of nonclinical safety testing in the pharmaceutical industry. Valuable information on their genesis and purpose is contained in the final report of the FDA investigation of the G.D. Searle Company [2], in charges brought against personnel associated with the Industrial Bio-Test Laboratories [3], and

*Parts of Section 9.1 have been adapted from [1], with permission. Copyright © 2003 John Wiley & Sons, Ltd.

Early Drug Development: Strategies and Routes to First-in-Human Trials, Edited by Mitchell N. Cayen

in the preambles to the GLP and electronic records regulations [4,5]. Further information on the preambles to the FDA regulations is included in Appendix 9.1.

The FDA investigation of Searle in the 1970s was the starting point for the GLP regulations, uncovering so many problems that the findings of the FDA task force were "too voluminous" to include them all in their final report. It is worth recapping these findings here (paraphrased from [2]); as an illustration of what lies at the heart of GLP:

- Technical personnel had a disregard for important aspects of their work, including the significance of the studies, the need to adhere to protocols, the need to record and verify data accurately, and the need to sign and date their records. Particular problems were the inaccurate transcription of results from original documents to reports and the absence or noncompliance with proper procedures in key areas.
- Management did not adequately evaluate and control the performance and analysis of research. Insufficient assurance of personnel qualifications and training, and the (lack of) verification of the accuracy and completeness of data are cited as examples of this deficiency.
- Decisions were made seemingly to minimize the chance of discovering toxicity in the products tested and to allay FDA concern.
- Other decisions, perhaps unintentional or inadvertent, resulted in too few data being collected, or in data being lost. Clerical or arithmetic errors resulted in underreporting of observations: for example, four malignant mammary tumors were omitted from a particular statistical analysis. These tumors were reported in the data sheets submitted with the report, however, allowing the FDA to find the inconsistency. The reason for this omission was the employment of a clerk typist to enter the data into the statistical analysis program. This typist had "15 to 20 minutes" of training, and used her own handwritten list (which did not contain the category "mammary tumors") to make decisions on the tumor classification.
- It was concluded that the lack of quality assurance was a common factor in many of the problems observed.
- In one study it was "impossible to determine who made observations," referring to the inconsistency and absence of identification of those who made data entries.
- Overall, the findings made it impossible, in some cases, to draw any conclusions regarding the toxic potential of the products being tested.

The principles embodied in the current GLP regulations are thus easily perceived from reviewing such "historical" documents:

1. *Accuracy.* Accurate data recording is an essential element in performing GLP studies. Accuracy also implies that the data have been verified and have been recorded indelibly in a direct, prompt, and legible fashion.

2. *Completeness and consistency.* Together with accuracy, completeness and consistency are components of data integrity [6]. It is of note that the entire investigation into practices at Searle was triggered by a question related to consistency. The company was asked to clarify "discrepancies" seen by the FDA in a histopathology report. The "corrected" report was subsequently returned to the FDA, with data corrected in the *original data sheet* for the animal involved but not in the summary of the report. The inconsistency between raw data and summary caused sufficient suspicion for the FDA to justify a scaled-up inspection.
3. *Reconstruction.* The need to be able to reconstruct a study from the original observations and the associated prescriptive [e.g., standard operating procedures (SOP)] and descriptive documentation (e.g., the study report) is a central precept of GLP. On a practical level this means that all data must have an associated audit trail, ranging from a handwritten reason, signature, and date to a validated, secure electronic audit trail for electronic records.
4. *Training: sufficient and documented.* Personnel are required to have sufficient education, training, and experience to perform their roles.
5. *Personnel responsibilities.* All personnel, including management, must understand and assume their responsibilities.
6. *Security.* Both paper and electronic records must be kept securely.
7. *Need for checks and controls.* Procedures must be established to ensure that critical operations are controlled and that documentation is maintained. A system of controlling documents (including SOPs and protocols) should be designed to allow control of study activities. As applied to electronic records, checks and controls on devices, operators (users), and system validation documentation are all needed to ensure integrity of the resulting records.

All the quality principles noted above are listed in Table 9.1 together with a reference to the relevant section of the U.S. *Code of Federal Regulations* (CFR). Although the principle of confidentiality is not mentioned in the GLP regulations, the requirement to maintain confidentiality of records is included in 21 CFR Part 11 (electronic records) [5] and is included in the table as a good principle to keep in mind. This is a key business consideration for any organization that works for multiple clients, such as a contract research organization (CRO).

9.2 HAZARD AND RISK

In designing and implementing an effective GLP system, other basic concepts to keep in mind are those of hazard and risk. There are comprehensive systems available to assess and mitigate risk (see, e.g., [7]), but for the purposes of this chapter a very simple, intuitive scheme is described. Analogous to evaluation

TABLE 9.1 GLP Principles

Principle	21 CFR Reference and Excerpts	Notes
Accuracy	58.1(a): "Compliance with this part is intended to assure the quality and *integrity* of ... data" 11.10: "Persons who use closed systems to create, modify, maintain, or transmit electronic records shall employ procedures and controls designed to ensure the authenticity, *integrity*, and, when appropriate, the confidentiality of electronic records"	• This refers to accuracy of recorded data as well as intrinsic data accuracy • Data integrity = accuracy, completeness, consistency • Accuracy implies: Verification [58.33(b)] Direct, prompt, and legible data recording [58.130(e)]
Completeness	As above for Accuracy	Especially important related to electronic records
Consistency	As above for Accuracy	
Reconstruction	58.3(k): "Raw data ... are necessary for the *reconstruction* and evaluation of the report of that study"	Similarly, 21 CFR Part 11 requires audit trails for reconstruction purposes
Training: sufficient and documented	58.29(a): "Each individual ... shall have [the] education, *training* and experience to perform the assigned functions" 11.10(i): "Determination that persons who develop, maintain, or use electronic record/electronic signature systems have the education, *training*, and experience to perform their assigned tasks"	Also 58.29(b): Each testing facility shall maintain a current *summary of training*...
Personnel responsibilities	58 Subpart B	
Security	58.190: Storage and retrieval of records and data. 11.10(c): "Protection of records to enable their accurate and ready retrieval throughout the records retention period"	

TABLE 9.1 **(*Continued*)**

Principle	21 CFR Reference and Excerpts	Notes
Need for checks and controls	11.10: "Persons who use closed systems to create, modify, maintain, or transmit electronic records shall employ *procedures and controls* designed to ensure the authenticity, integrity, and, when appropriate, the confidentiality of electronic records" 11.10(k): "Use of appropriate *controls* over systems documentation"	Also applies to controls introduced by SOPs, protocols, systems for authorization and review
Confidentiality	11.10: "Persons who use closed systems to create, modify, maintain, or transmit electronic records shall employ procedures and controls designed to ensure the authenticity, integrity, and, when appropriate, the *confidentiality* of electronic records"	

of laboratory safety, *hazard* is the potential to cause harm, whereas *risk* is the likelihood of that hazard occurring. To illustrate this related to laboratory safety, an example of a high hazard would be a large waste solvent container containing flammable solvent residues. If ignition of this container occurred, the resulting explosion could be catastrophic, causing significant harm to facilities and personnel. Hopefully, the *risk* of remote ignition of the solvent container is negligible, minimized by procedures, staff training, adequate ventilation, and exclusion of sources of ignition. An example of a low hazard would be that posed by a trailing power cord, where potential harm is limited to a minor trip injury to an individual member of the staff. In the latter case, although the hazard represented by the trailing cord may be low, the risk of the hazard occurring could be high if the cord is raised from the ground and trails across a busy laboratory thoroughfare. In GLP terms, hazard categories as they apply to study data integrity are defined in Table 9.2. A very high potential hazard would be one that could affect an entire study or series of studies: for example, key equipment unknowingly being out of calibration. Minor hazards would be those that would affect only an isolated portion of data in a relatively insignificant fashion: for example, a missing date on one data entry within a series.

TABLE 9.2 Hazard

High Hazard	Medium Hazard	Low Hazard
Potential major effect on data integrity for entire study(ies)	Potential major effect on data integrity for *part* of a study Potential multiple minor data integrity problems for entire study(ies)	Potential minor isolated data integrity problems

TABLE 9.3 Risk[a]

Function	High Risk	Medium Risk	Low Risk
Process	No process	Insufficient process	Established process
Visibility	Low visibility	Insufficient or incomplete visibility	High visibility
QC	No QC review	Insufficient QC review	Extensive QC review
QA	No QA review	Insufficient QA review	Extensive QA review

[a]Absence of process, low visibility of records, absence of quality control, and quality assurance review all raise the risk of a potential hazard occurring, and vice versa.

In conceiving a quality system, the aim is to minimize hazard occurrence through process, quality control (QC), and quality assurance (QA) systems. As shown in Table 9.3, risk is reduced by having a robust process using validated systems, maintaining high visibility (e.g., easy access through a computerized system, data review steps), and quality control review. An effective quality assurance program can be instituted by considering these factors and overlaying a system of inspection and audit that meets the intent of the regulations while not simply re-reviewing data or expending disproportionate amounts of resource on low-hazard records or processes. Although consideration of hazard and risk is not mentioned explicitly in the GLP regulations, it is embodied in current FDA guidance [8], and together with an appreciation of the underlying principles of GLP, this will help the adoption of an effective GLP quality system.

9.3 U.S. GLP REGULATIONS

Having reviewed these basic themes, we can now turn our attention back to the regulations to see how these concepts are integrated into a comprehensive GLP rule. In this chapter we focus on the U.S. FDA GLP regulations and provide a basic overview of their content, subpart by subpart, referring to them interchangeably as "GLPs" or "the regulations." Where other regulations are discussed, they are referenced specifically, and a brief review of international GLP regulations is given in Appendix 9.2. As discussed earlier, the FDA GLP regulations were finalized in 1978 [9] in response to practices that undermined FDA's confidence in the quality of data provided in support of drug safety. Revised FDA GLP regulations became effective in 1987 [10], and current FDA GLPs contain nine subparts:

- *Subpart A:* General Provisions
- *Subpart B:* Organization and Personnel
- *Subpart C:* Facilities
- *Subpart D:* Equipment
- *Subpart E:* Testing Facilities Operation
- *Subpart F:* Test and Control Articles
- *Subpart G:* Protocol for and Conduct of a Nonclinical Laboratory Study
- *Subpart J:* Records and Reports
- *Subpart K:* Disqualification of Testing Facilities

9.3.1 Subpart A: General Provisions

Scope of GLP The GLP regulations begin with a statement of scope, which is sufficiently important to merit citation in full here (italic added for emphasis):

> This part prescribes good laboratory practices for conducting *nonclinical laboratory studies* that support or are intended to support applications for research or marketing permits for products regulated by the Food and Drug Administration, including food and color additives, animal food additives, human and animal drugs, medical devices for human use, biological products, and electronic products. Compliance with this part is intended to assure the quality and integrity of the safety data filed pursuant to . . . the Federal Food, Drug, and Cosmetic Act and . . . the Public Health Service Act. Animal studies to determine *safety* intended to be submitted for an IND have to be conducted in accordance with GLP [10].

This scope statement makes it very clear that the regulations apply only to *nonclinical safety* studies. The word *intended* is included to make it clear that tests that are never intended to be submitted to the FDA as the basis for the approval of a research or marketing permit do not need to be performed under GLP, even though they may eventually be submitted to the agency. The associated preambles [4,10] give further details on the study types that fall outside the scope of GLP, including:

- Pharmacological and effectiveness studies
- Studies to develop new methodologies for toxicology experimentation
- Basic research, preliminary exploratory studies
- All studies done on medical devices that do not come into contact with or are not implanted in humans

In deciding which studies do need to be performed under GLP, it should be remembered that if a nonclinical study is submitted to provide justification for the safety of a drug, the FDA will expect this to be conducted to GLP standards. However, as shown in the list above, research studies and preliminary exploratory studies are excluded from the scope of the regulations. As such, in vitro–in vivo ADME studies or in vitro metabolism studies performed to select the species prior to toxicity studies would not fall within the scope of the regulations. The extent to which quality systems such as GLP are incorporated into discovery and preliminary research activities is a business decision; there are very good reasons to adopt a robust quality system in early research, and additional information on this topic has been provided by the World Health Organization [11] and the British Association of Research Quality Assurance [12]. For studies that do fall within the scope of GLP, the FDA will assess any compliance deficiencies to determine if they are significant and, if they are, whether they invalidate the entire study or necessitate further validation of the study.

Definitions and Roles Subpart A goes on to provide a basic structure for GLP through definition of its principal components, including: test article, control article, test system, nonclinical laboratory study (with dates of study initiation and completion), sponsor, testing facility, raw data, quality assurance unit, and study director. Paraphrased versions of these definitions are given in Appendix 9.3, and the reader is advised to review these briefly to best appreciate the paragraphs that follow. Important definitions to keep in mind are those for raw data, where the principle of study reconstruction is introduced, and the role of the study director (the single point of technical control).

This subpart also defines the role of the sponsor, one of the principal players in the GLP orchestra, as the "person who initiates and supports, by provision of financial or other resources, a nonclinical laboratory study." Although not made explicit in the regulations, the sponsor of the study is ultimately responsible for the quality and integrity of that study. This concept is reinforced in Subpart A, where, in Section 58.10, it is stated that "when a sponsor conducting a nonclinical laboratory study intended to be submitted or reviewed by the Food and Drug Administration utilizes the services of a consulting laboratory, contractor or grantee to perform an analysis or other service, it shall notify the consulting laboratory, contractor or grantee that the service is part of a nonclinical laboratory study that must be conducted in compliance with the provisions of this part." Simply put, all contributors to a GLP study have to comply with GLP, and it is the sponsor's responsibility to ensure that all parties are notified to this effect. Sponsor roles in GLP do continue to be the subject of misunderstanding, as the sponsor is not responsible for the study-related scientific decisions unless these are attributed to the sponsor as a contributing scientist in the study protocol. It becomes very easy for a sponsor to undermine the study director's responsibility in a multisite environment, as they may have the advantage of a direct route of communication with the contributing scientists and laboratories. In this situation the sponsor scientists often review study data before they are reviewed by the study director. They can compromise the intent of the GLPs' single point of control by making study-related decisions or by directing the work of the contributing scientists. It is imperative that all parties remember to include the study director when such decisions are being made. Firm understanding as to the communication path desired by the study director may be placed in a contract, in a memo to the file, or in the protocol if appropriate, but should not be left unaddressed.

Inspection Completing Subpart A of the regulations is Part 58.15, "Inspection of a Testing Facility." The first clause in this section states that the FDA can inspect a facility "at reasonable times and in a reasonable manner" to review and copy records and inspect specimens. The subsequent clause warns that if a facility does not permit inspection, the studies conducted in that facility will not be accepted in support of the sponsor's application. Some considerations in planning for a regulatory inspection are given in Appendix 9.4. Importantly, Section 58.15(a) exempts quality assurance records of findings, problems, and recommended actions from the requirement for FDA inspection. This text is a critical part of the GLP structure for quality assurance, allowing QA auditors to write audit reports without any restriction that might be imposed by the thought of an eventual FDA inspection of the report findings. In fact, this clause could be thought of as a "double-edged sword," as without access to QA records, the FDA loses a useful tool for assessing the compliance status of facilities, arguably making their inspection program less effective and impeding their mission to protect public health.

9.3.2 Subpart B: Organization and Personnel

The second subpart of the GLP regulations outlines requirements for organization and personnel and can be visualized as a triangle surrounded by a circle, as illustrated in Figure 9.1. The subpart begins with Section 58.29, general requirements for all personnel involved in the conduct of nonclinical laboratory studies. These requirements can be summarized as follows: "Hire appropriately educated and qualified staff, provide and document all training, and ensure that test articles or test systems are not contaminated through personnel being ill or wearing inadequate protective clothing."

As described earlier, training is a fundamental GLP principle and is a key component of a successful quality system as well as a determining factor in developing a successful business. Resources, time, and planning should therefore be invested in developing a robust training program, made all the more effective when supporting tools are developed to facilitate the scheduling, tracking, and monitoring of training. Designing a system that makes it easy to provide and document training, while making it difficult for personnel to perform operations without having prior training, will return ample dividends on effort invested. It is important to note that training records will need to be accessed and reviewed

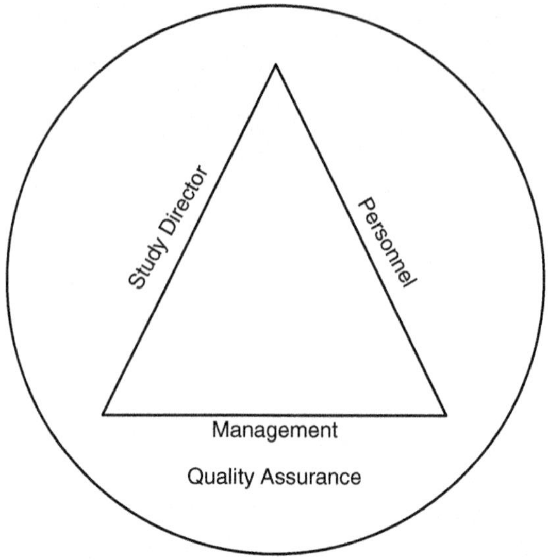

FIGURE 9.1 Personnel triangle.

by several categories of personnel—management and study directors, human resources, quality assurance—so that reduction in the time taken to retrieve and view records will translate into considerable efficiency gains. Apart from their regulatory purpose, training records are also one of the best advertisements for a high-quality company. External auditors and the FDA always review these records, so evidence of comprehensive, thorough training should be evident from even a cursory review.

Management forms the base of the personnel triangle, since this entity controls the corporate resources, and only management can make the decisions affecting staffing, compensation, scheduling, and expectations from each employee that characterize the corporation. Therefore, the GLPs assign functions found in Subpart B, as well as in other subparts, specifically to this corporate foundation. These include the assignment and replacement of study directors, one to each study; the provision for QA functions as well as the communication of problems to the study director; the provision of "appropriately tested" substances and mixtures for use in studies, and the responsibility to assure that all personnel understand and carry out specific job description requirements. The GLPs do not, however, confine expectations of management to subpart B; in addition to procedures affecting personnel, facility operations must be designed and controlled by management. Turning momentarily to Subpart E, "Testing Facilities Operation," Section 58.81(a) requires that SOPs "[set] forth study methods *that management is satisfied are adequate* [emphasis added] to insure the quality and integrity of the data generated in the course of a study." It is important to appreciate that specific points of GLP address single studies, while they direct the operation of the entire facility: hence the need for management to hire, prepare, and constantly evaluate its human resources and to evaluate operations based on their input.

The second panel of the triangle is the *study director*, whose key responsibilities are outlined in Subpart B, Section 58.33. Simply put, this person "represents the single point of study control." GLP definitions declare the starting point of a regulated study to be the date on which the study director signs the protocol (see Subpart G), the *study initiation date*. The study director creates and uses the protocol to guide the operations necessary to conduct the study. It is not possible for the FDA to dictate what an appropriate workload for a given study director should be, but instead, leaves management to apportion its resources accordingly. A facility may conduct studies lasting a few hours, a few days, or several years. The requirements of each may be fairly simple or staggeringly complex, at times needing the services of other scientists or the use of off-site contractors for specific operations. The role of the study director and other principal personnel involved in the multisite study structure is reviewed later in the section.

Although the study director is the single control point, it is rarely possible or desirable for the director to actually carry out the several components of even a single study, so the third panel of the triangle shown in Figure 9.1 is *personnel*. In addition to technical functions, the supporting work of many others is necessary. Subparts C (Facilities) and D (Equipment) both contain several general requirements that must be translated into SOPs or policies appropriate to the corporation's scope. Personnel requirements will relate to persons who are "engaged in the conduct of or responsible for the supervision of a study" but must also consider those engaged in the care of test systems or physical plant or facility operations that could affect one or many studies. SOPs are required for many of these general operations, and all of the associated records must be completed and later archived by yet another specifically trained person, in a manner to satisfy the regulations. Considering these points, it should be seen that all job descriptions have some GLP-related component. Rather than presenting a burden, an opportunity is offered: to achieve that personal investment so crucial to staff morale and commitment to the corporation's overall excellence. In a GLP environment, it must be stressed and repeated that *everybody* is involved in GLP compliance.

Quality Assurance Functions and Responsibilities Encircling the triangle of management, the study director, and "all others" is, of course, the quality assurance unit (QAU). It has been an unfortunate precedent that QA is sometimes classified as the entity responsible for GLP compliance. Instead, QA and management provide the possibility for all other staff and their procedures making up the quality system to be "checked and controlled," not unlike the raw data that are produced in daily operations. Each study must be monitored by the QA unit, which must have its own separate set of written responsibilities and procedures as described in Section 58.35(c). Should a situation arise that could affect study integrity, QA is to report it to the study director and management "immediately." QA staff also view general facility operations, the receipt of test systems, archival procedures, and will serve as valuable aides if any sort of disaster strikes, to ensure that the documentation and approval process is GLP compliant. As explained previously, FDA investigators cannot review "problems and the corrective actions taken" contained in QA audit reports. Rather, the investigators will review a selection of the facility's SOPs, observe procedures during an escorted walking tour of the facility, and conduct interviews with QA and other staff to assure that all is in compliance. Further details on the conduct and management of FDA inspections are given in Appendix 9.4.

Although the regulations refer to a "quality assurance *unit*," their intent is that quality assurance functions must be provided only by personnel who are independent of the activities for a given study. Management staff members have the freedom to decide how this is organized: It may be most appropriate through designation of a separate quality assurance group or be subcontracted at the start. Many competent QA professionals offer services on a contract basis, and when the QA responsibility is thus arranged by management, it is important that qualifications be examined carefully and references checked. Most of the criteria one would normally use for hiring an employee will apply when choosing a contract QA service, but other considerations, such as confidentiality and communication expectations, must also be part of the precontract discussion. As with any other employee, résumés and other records of training and qualifications for the QA professionals should be on file and retained securely. A job description should be prepared despite the contract relationship, to further document expectations. Although it is less desirable to the FDA, separation of QA services can also be achieved by structuring operations such that laboratory personnel provide quality assurance of studies in which they were not personally involved. Regardless of the method adopted, in keeping with the emphasis on education, qualification, and training, management must provide an ongoing program of training for quality assurance. Given regulatory change and new technology, this will ensure that they understand their function and are aware of contemporary concepts of quality assurance.

The responsibilities of quality assurance staff are delineated in the regulations as follows (paraphrased from 21 CFR Part 58):

- *Maintenance of a master schedule sheet.* The master schedule was conceived as a tool to allow assessment of the workload of study directors and other personnel so that management could ensure that adequate staffing is maintained. Further, as studies are indexed by test article, the sheet was envisaged to help management fulfill its responsibility to assure that test and control articles are available and characterized [Section 58.31(d)]. The master schedule is usually maintained using a computerized system, and a variety of personnel may, in practice, have a role in its maintenance. The original intent of the FDA regulations is that the sheet comprises "raw data" that should be archived and available to assist retrospective reconstruction of studies, showing for example when study directors are replaced. Procedures for reviewing, updating, and maintaining the master schedule should be described in an SOP. Given the importance of this schedule (and its visibility to FDA investigators), it is good practice to institute a regular and robust process for review, to ensure that the schedule is up to date and complete. Care should be taken to examine studies that have remained on the master schedule for a prolonged period of time; studies that persist without completion are a "red flag," revealing possible deficiencies in the facility's processes.

- *Maintenance of protocols.* That the QAU should maintain a copy of the protocol (and amendments) emphasizes their responsibility to assure that the protocol is implemented and amended in a compliant fashion as well as their paramount role in assuring management that the protocol is followed during the study. With the use of electronic document management systems, it is no longer necessary, however, for quality assurance personnel to store protocol copies physically within their office areas.
- *Inspection of studies and reporting of these inspections.* Use of the word *inspect* in the regulations underlines the need for QA personnel to actually watch study operations being performed in conjunction with their review of other study, equipment, personnel, and facility records. The intent of the FDA's GLPs is that the QAU will *inspect* every study, even the very shortest, at least once. Inspections should be organized such that the QAU inspects each "critical phase" across a series of studies; further details are given in Appendix 9.5. Whereas the Organization for Economic Cooperation and Development (OECD) GLP regulations permit "process-based inspections" to be performed [13] rather than requiring every study to be inspected, the basis of the FDA's GLP regulations is that nonclinical laboratory studies are "research" studies, which by their nature will have particularities unique to each study, thus requiring QA inspection on a per study basis. The FDA regulations require the QAU to "periodically submit to management and the Study Director written status reports on each study, noting any problems and the corrective actions taken." Of course, if any problems observed during the study are "likely to affect study integrity," the QAU will set aside the reporting schedule and notify the study director "immediately" in accordance with GLPs. An effective system of reporting has to be designed for the QAU to ensure that inspection observations and any corrective actions recommended are communicated and resolved in a timely fashion. Use of an electronic system provides a powerful tool for quality assurance, as in addition to its reporting function, such a system can:

  - Track dates of issue and return of audit reports
  - Track outstanding corrective actions
  - Provide an easy mechanism for writing an accurate QA statement
  - Supply data for metrics on QA performance (e.g., audit reporting turnaround; observation rates)
  - Supply data for metrics on company performance (e.g., problem areas, observation rates per study director)

As discussed earlier, raising the visibility of outstanding items and problem areas through the use of electronic systems reduces the risk of potential hazards lingering without resolution until they become serious concerns for the organization. Further, provision of metrics from QA databases allows targeted process improvement and training to address any adverse trends in compliance.

- *Determining through inspection and audit that all deviations from controlling documents have been properly documented and authorized.* The QAU has the responsibility of ensuring that when noncompliance with controlling documents (e.g., protocol, SOPs, GLP regulations) occurs, the resulting deviation is approved and recorded correctly. The study director should authorize protocol deviations as well as deviations from SOPs that occur during the study. Given management's responsibility to provide SOPs adequate to ensure the quality and integrity of a study, it follows that they should also authorize deviations from these SOPs.
- *Review of the final report and provision of a signed quality assurance statement to be included in the report.* The quality assurance review of study reports should assure that data integrity is maintained: that the report is accurate, complete, and consistent and that it reflects the raw data and controlling documents that were followed in conducting the study. A quality assurance statement should be included in every report, as described later in the chapter.

Multisite Studies The personnel roles described above are easy to envisage when they apply to a single facility where the study director conducts the study and the QAU inspects the study and reviews and reports its findings to management, who provide resources and ensure that corrective actions are taken in response to reported deviations. The research environment has changed, however, since the original FDA GLPs were written, and the majority of nonclinical research is now conducted within a multisite environment, wherein the study director will have to conduct the study by coordinating with a number of different facilities, each charged with performing a specific part of the study. The personnel roles described in the GLP regulations present more challenges in this environment, requiring a larger investment in prestudy planning. For example, we noted earlier that the study director must authorize all deviations from SOPs that occur in the course of the study. In a multisite environment where the study director may be located in a test facility in France, deviations may be occurring in the bioanalytical laboratory in the United States, so a route for communication and authorization of these deviations has to be established. Similarly, quality assurance audit reports of the bioanalytical phase from the American laboratory would have to be sent to France so that the study director and test facility management are aware of any problems found during QA review and subsequent corrective actions.

This multisite structure is addressed in the OECD's revised principles of good laboratory practice, published in 1998 [14]. These more "modern" GLPs were developed by an expert group who revised the original OECD GLP principles from 1981 to take into account changes in the conduct and structure of nonclinical safety studies. *As there can be only one study director*, the OECD principles introduce the concept of a *principal investigator* (PI), appointed when a study is conducted at different test sites or where different geographical locations are involved within the same company. In FDA GLP terminology the principal investigator would be analogous to the "individual scientist" who is responsible for a particular portion of the study. According to the OECD principles, "The principal investigator acts on behalf of the Study Director for the delegated phase and is responsible for ensuring compliance with the Principles of GLP for that phase." This structure is illustrated in Figure 9.2, where the study director resides at one site and relies on other facilities (test sites) to undertake specified study responsibilities (study phases), each test site having a principal investigator as well as management and quality assurance personnel.

The OECD GLP principles are accompanied by a series of consensus and advisory documents, No. 13 of which is entitled "The Application of the OECD Principles of GLP to the Organisation and Management of Multi-site Studies" [15]. This consensus document enlarges on the framework presented in the OECD principles of GLP, and the key success factors for multisite studies are outlined in the introduction: planning, communication, and clear allocation of responsibilities. The guidance recommends the designation of a "lead" QAU which coordinates the overall quality assurance of the study. The lead QAU might be

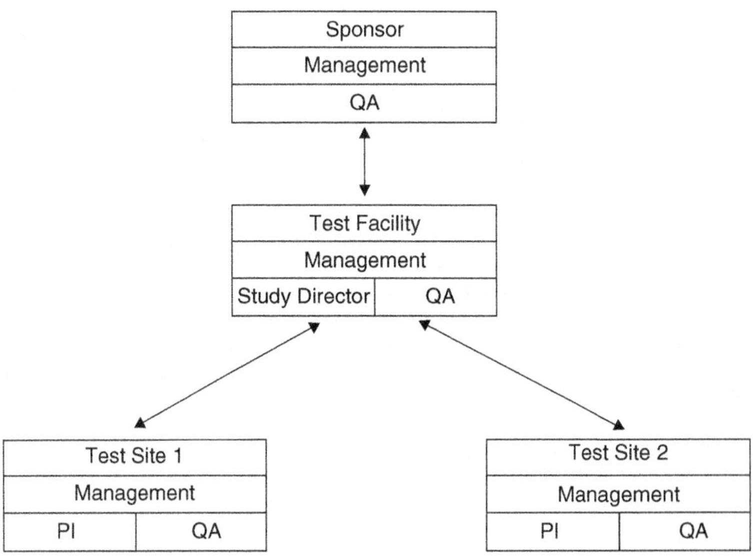

FIGURE 9.2 Multisite studies: Simplified overview of structure.

responsible for receiving all the QA reports of findings issued by the test site QA groups and ensuring that these are addressed properly and routed to the study director and test facility management. The guidance document revisits the various roles within GLP—sponsor, management, study director, principal investigator, quality assurance personnel—from a multisite perspective and provides recommendations for optimizing the conduct of the study. In this environment the protocol (*study plan* in OECD terminology) becomes an even more crucial element in the study: A comprehensive well-written protocol that has been reviewed by all study contributors will be essential to keep all players "playing to the same score." The protocol should specify lead QA, principal investigators, and test site QA personnel, describing their responsibilities and including all contact information necessary to facilitate performance of the study.

9.3.3 Subpart C: Facilities

GLP describes provisions for facilities in general and then gives some instructions specifically for animal care facilities. In general terms, the regulations require that the facilities be of "suitable size and construction" to perform studies and that "separation" is provided where necessary. This requirement for separation is applied to:

- Any function or activity that may have an adverse effect on the study
- Isolation of test and control articles that are biohazardous, volatile, aerosol, radioactive, or infectious
- Separate areas for diseased animals (at the discretion of the study director)
- Areas for feed and bedding separated from housing areas
- Separation of test and control article handling as necessary to prevent contamination
- Separate space for an archive area
- Separate space as needed for the performance of "routine procedures" to minimize the possibility of adverse effects of these procedures on other concurrent studies (For example, the noise and humidity of cage washing should be away from office areas, and buildings housing dogs should be placed out of earshot of rabbit housing areas.)

Note that "separation" in some of the areas above does not apply just to physical separation but also to environmental controls. All heating, ventilating, and air conditioning (HVAC) designs must control airflow and incorporate filtration as necessary to preclude any potential for contamination or hazardous conditions.

9.3.4 Subpart D: Equipment

FDA's GLPs prescribe that equipment be designed appropriately, have adequate capacity, and be suitably located for operation, inspection, cleaning, and maintenance. Further, equipment must:

- Be adequately inspected, maintained, tested, calibrated, and/or standardized, with corresponding records of these operations
- Be described in a written SOP stipulating procedures for routine inspection and maintenance, cleaning, testing, calibration, and remedial action to be taken in the event of failure or malfunction, detailing responsibility for the performance of these functions by naming either a person or an operational unit

In interpreting this part of the FDA GLP regulations, it should be noted that equipment is understood to include computers and computerized systems. Hence, although not stated explicitly, this paragraph requires that computerized systems be validated for their use in nonclinical laboratory studies. The OECD principles of GLP do specifically address the validation of computerized systems, requiring that the study director ensure that any computerized systems used for a study be validated. FDA requirements for computerized systems used in GLP studies are summarized in their compliance program guidance manual [16], wherein Appendix A lists their expectations, section by section of the GLP regulations, in the form of a concise list to guide FDA field investigators.

A comprehensive program of timely and competent equipment maintenance and repair is essential to study data quality and integrity, and records of these events are critical to the reconstruction and evaluation of studies. As such, great care must be taken, especially with nonroutine maintenance records, to document the exact circumstances surrounding the discovery and rectification of any faults. According to the regulations, the "how and when" and a description of the remedial action taken must be recorded to reconstruct the event. Diligent recording allows a retrospective evaluation of the potential impact of any malfunction on the integrity of study data. If a significant problem is uncovered upon subsequent review, such documentation can define its magnitude, allowing the affected data (from a particular instrument/timeframe) to be identified accurately without calling the entire data set into question.

9.3.5 Subpart E: Testing Facilities Operation

The sections in this subpart provide regulations concerning procedures, chemicals under study or used in routine methods, and test system (animal) care. The first section contains the most comprehensive guidance contained in the regulations on FDA expectations for standard operating procedures. As the "score" for harmonizing the facility's operations and study-related activities, special attention is required for the design of an effective SOP system. Some user requirements for an SOP system may include:

- Easy access for all personnel.
- An efficient procedure for writing, reviewing, approving, and revising SOPs. Typically, SOPs are subject to periodic review (commonly on an annual basis) to keep them up to date and pertinent.

- A robust procedure for incorporation of SOPs into training and daily operations that provides documentation of individual dates of SOP reading and/or training. SOP revisions require similar proof of proper circulation and training.
- A common style and format to facilitate comprehension and retention of instructions.
- A system for recording deviations to SOPs that meets requirements for approval and communication.

For more detail on satisfying such requirements, we recommend reviewing Appendix 9.8 and available literature; [17–22] provide guidance on the introduction of a successful GLP SOP system. Clearly, these requirements lend themselves to the adoption of an electronic system in which document control, electronic signatures (for approval, review, and reading), availability, and access control can all be designed and configured to suit business needs.

Labeling and Test Systems The other areas of operation included in Subpart E and mentioned in Subparts C and D are solution labeling and test system (generally, laboratory animal) care. Labels on chemicals, containers of solutions, bench containers, and the like are addressed in Section 58.83. The GLP minimum requirements to be included on the label of all containers are identity, concentration, expiration date, and storage requirements, which can be remembered with the aid of the mnemonic "ICES" (identity, concentration, expiration, storage). In terms of hazard and risk, solution labeling falls into the high hazard category, as errors on a label may affect an entire study or a number of studies. For example, if the incorrect expiration date is shown (where the date exceeds established stability), the reagent may be used for numerous experiments before the error is detected. At this point, additional work will be needed to document the error and support the integrity of data produced using this outdated solution. For this reason it is worth investing time in the labeling process and raising the visibility of labels to allow quality control or other review.

Since the test system may or may not be a laboratory animal, each facility will need to determine appropriate procedures for all required aspects of acquisition, care, and use. Obviously, good science requires test systems that fulfill protocol requirements and are healthy, uniform, and generally available to the scientific community. The use of animals in research and testing is a controversial topic and there are many other regulatory requirements to be met outside the scope of GLP. National organizations such as the American Association for Laboratory Animal Science (AALAS) [23] offer invaluable assistance and support in this area for all levels of staff as well as management.

9.3.6 Subpart F: Test and Control Articles

Subpart F is dedicated to the handling and characterization of test and control articles. This subpart can be condensed to the following simple rules:

- Know the dose!
- Maintain accountability.

Knowing the dose implies that the identity, strength, purity, composition, and stability of the test article have been determined and that the study director has this information in order to manage the study and draw conclusions from the results. If the test article is administered as a mixture with a vehicle, the uniformity of that mixture, the concentration of the test article, and its stability need to be established and communicated to the study director. Further, reserve samples of test and control articles from studies of more than four weeks' duration must be retained for purposes of future evaluation, if necessary. Test facility management is responsible for assuring that all necessary tests have been carried out on these materials.

Stability of test article and resulting mixtures must always be determined (Chapter 5); this can be assessed prior to the study or in an ongoing manner. It is not sufficient to rely on the expiration date of a marketed product (if used as a control article) or to argue that the studies are of such a short duration that stability is irrelevant. On this last point, the OECD principles of GLP recognize in their Consensus Document No. 7 [24] that "if the time interval between the preparation and application of a usually stable substance is only a few minutes, it might not be relevant to determine the stability of the test item." Two key points in this subpart are often misunderstood, concerning the retention of containers and test and reference article characterization:

1. *Storage containers:* Under FDA GLPs, the test and control articles must be maintained in their original containers—they cannot be transferred to other receptacles (e.g., smaller containers that may be warranted as the material is depleted). Although this may seem burdensome in some instances, prohibiting such movement reduces the potential for contamination, deterioration, or mix-up of test and control articles. The intent of this rule is to help avoid accountability problems caused by transfer of materials, several of which had been uncovered during FDA inspections.
2. Characterization has to be GLP compliant, including preparation of a protocol and assignment of a study director, quality assurance oversight, preparation of a report, and archiving of associated raw data. Under FDA GLPs it is not sufficient to characterize the test and control articles under good manufacturing practice (GMP) unless the GMP laboratory also adheres to GLP. If characterization is conducted to GMP standards only, this compliance deficiency should be disclosed in the study report, typically in the compliance statement (as discussed later).

9.3.7 Subpart G: Protocol for and Conduct of a Nonclinical Laboratory Study

Subpart G can be précised as "write and approve a protocol, follow the protocol and collect raw data in a manner that allows reconstruction of the study."

Probably the most important sentence in Subpart G, and possibly in the whole of the GLP regulations, is: "The nonclinical laboratory study shall be conducted in accordance with the protocol." More detailed commentary on the requirements for a study protocol is given in Appendix 9.10. The protocol should be signed and dated by the study director (the study initiation date) and approved by the sponsor, with the date of this approval included in the protocol. All methods to be used in the study—for example, analytical methods or randomization procedures and the records to be maintained for archival at the end of the study—must be specified in the protocol. Subsequent amendments or deviations to the protocol require the signed and dated approval of the study director. Looking briefly at the OECD principles of GLP [14], a *study plan (protocol) amendment* is defined as "an intended change to the study plan after the study initiation date," whereas a *deviation* is defined *as* "an unintended departure from the study plan after the study initiation date." Another way of considering this distinction is to think of deviations as one-time occurrences that are not intended to be repeated, whereas amendments represent changes that will be used in an ongoing fashion, from the date of authorization onward. Similarly, the study director must also prepare a deviation, when appropriate, to a standard operating procedure as a single, corrective measure specific to a study, with raw data documenting the circumstances.

Raw Data Subpart G also contains instructions on how to collect raw data, which are the very crux of a GLP study, as without adequate raw data the study is worthless. Raw data should be captured—on paper or electronically—in a way that ensures data integrity while allowing reconstruction of study activities. Ostensibly, generating high-quality raw data to GLP standards is simple; however, in practice this is one of the biggest challenges faced in conducting GLP studies. This critical success factor for GLP merits careful planning and investment of resource in designing systems and training programs. In considering systems for capturing raw data, it is worthwhile first to review the applicable sections of the FDA GLP regulations:

Subpart A, definitions 58.3(k):

> Raw data means any laboratory worksheets, records, memoranda, notes, or exact copies thereof, that are the result of original observations and activities of a nonclinical laboratory study and are necessary for the reconstruction and evaluation of the report of that study. In the event that exact transcripts of raw data have been prepared (e.g., tapes which have been transcribed verbatim, dated, and verified accurate by signature), the exact copy or exact transcript may be substituted for the original source as raw data. Raw data may include photographs, microfilm or microfiche copies, computer printouts, magnetic media, including dictated observations, and recorded data from automated instruments.

Subpart B, study director responsibilities 58.33(b):

> The Study Director shall assure that. . .all experimental data, including observations of unanticipated responses of the test system are accurately recorded and verified

Subpart G: study conduct 58.130(e):

> All data generated during the conduct of a nonclinical laboratory study, except those that are generated by automated data collection systems, shall be recorded directly, promptly, and legibly in ink. All data entries shall be dated on the date of entry and signed or initialled by the person entering the data. Any change in entries shall be made so as not to obscure the original entry, shall indicate the reason for such change, and shall be dated and signed or identified at the time of the change. In automated data collection systems, the individual responsible for direct data input shall be identified at the time of data input. Any change in automated data entries shall be made so as not to obscure the original entry, shall indicate the reason for the change, shall be dated, and the responsible individual shall be identified.

One critical definition is that of *data integrity*, meaning data that are *accurate, complete*, and *consistent* [6]. Thinking in terms of these three components provides an intuitive way to understand compliance; for example, laboratory reports have to disclose how many assay failures were incurred while producing the final results, as knowledge of all data, not just the desired results, is the only way that rational decisions about public health can be taken. Even if study data can be shown to be very accurate, one does not have data integrity if they are not complete. Similarly, if there are *inconsistencies* between different sections of the raw data, or between the raw data and the controlling documents, data integrity has been compromised. In situations where there is a problem with data integrity, action must be taken (e.g., a deviation, written explanation, or investigation) to address the inconsistency in order to draw meaningful conclusions from the study. Understanding the concept of data integrity provides a basis for individual judgments when particular situations arise during a day's work. Training all staff to "think GLP" results in their asking, "Could this have any effect on study data integrity?" The team of technical staff and study director, at times in consultation with the QAU, can determine which component(s) of data integrity are potentially compromised and provide a guide for subsequent corrective action. Management is then informed if there is a potential shortfall in regulatory compliance so that additional steps can be taken to implement improvements in the quality process.

According to its definition in the regulations, the purpose of recording raw data is to be able to reconstruct and evaluate the study. Raw data, combined with prescriptive documents (SOPs, protocols) and descriptive documents (reports), are central to the ability to assess the study retrospectively to assure its integrity and verify its conclusions. This sounds straightforward, however, the level of reconstruction to be achieved is both a business and a compliance decision; for example, to what level of detail do the study events need to be recorded? Does the technician need to sign for every single action taken in conducting the experiment—the time of putting tubes in the centrifuge, the time of retrieving them, the exact speed of centrifugation—or is it sufficient simply to attest that the procedure was followed? There is no single answer to this question, since each study's design will dictate the amount of detail necessary for reconstruction, however, the following considerations should be kept in mind. Any equipment that needs calibration and maintenance should be referenced specifically to allow reconstruction of the experiment: If the method includes centrifuging samples at a particular temperature, the centrifuge's unique identifier should be included in the raw data. To be able to evaluate the study, it will be necessary to see that the centrifuge was operating correctly and that it was adequately temperature calibrated at the time of the experiment. Conversely, where methods use equipment that does not require special calibration or maintenance (e.g., a vortex mixer or sonicator), it can be argued that knowledge of the exact equipment is not needed to evaluate the study. Recording the identity of the vortex mixer does not enhance the ability to evaluate the data, as there is no further "evaluation trail"; the instrument does not have associated calibration and maintenance records. Another consideration is the criticality of the experimental procedure to the outcome of the experiment. In the centrifuge example above, if the method or SOP being followed requires a specific time and temperature of centrifugation to produce the desired result, this time and temperature should be documented. Clearly, the ability to reconstruct this experimental stage is useful retrospectively to assure the integrity of the experiment. However, if the method or SOP has a nonspecific instruction to "briefly centrifuge" the samples, the level of reconstruction can be scaled down accordingly.

Although a "maximalist" approach, recording every detail, may seem tempting to institute, this can have deleterious effects on the quality of the experiment. A technician who has to stop and record every detail may be interrupted to the point of not being able to maintain good technique. This may even lead to personnel instituting their own, counter-GLP procedures, such as waiting until the entire experiment is complete and then returning to sign all the checkboxes in the comfort of the office.

Consistency in data recording (as a component of data integrity) should be built in to the process through the use of standardized forms or electronic data capture systems. The level of reconstruction can be designed-in, such that forms guide the experimenter to record the exact information deemed necessary for the particular activity being performed. The particular spaces on the form, termed *prompts*, require some sort of entry, either raw data or an assertion of "not necessary." Design of forms and their related procedures can be a valuable tool for staff development and job enhancement. Teamwork in this effort gives all participants in their separate roles a chance to input their thoughts: Can this procedure be done practically by the technical staff? Does the QAU agree that no loss of data integrity will result if some of its stages are not recorded? A form-based raw data capture system will necessarily imply a system of document control, requiring that forms have some link to the controlling procedures, with authorization of changes and withdrawal of previous versions after new versions are implemented. Attention should also be given to the "completeness" component of data integrity by designing forms that allow reviewers to ensure that the data are complete, that no forms are missing, and that there are no blank spaces that are not accounted for in some way.

Data must be legible, clearly recorded, with audit trails (paper and electronic) according to another core principle of GLP, *reconstruction*. Electronically, having a clear audit trail presents technical challenges, but software designers and users are rising to these to provide compliant solutions. For paper-based raw data, *audit trail* means writing clearly and legibly, adding signature and date, and recording reasons for changes without obscuring original entries. To correct an entry error in GLP-regulated data, the entry is struck out with a single line and an explanation provided, then this is initialed and dated prior to entry of the correct data. It takes a lot of practice and coaching to develop this habit. Expect to see QA findings related to this aspect of data reconstruction. Ideally, an end-of-day QC practice of having technicians review each other's work would be instituted to catch these and other lapses, allowing correction on the same calendar date. For explanations of why errors occurred, it is good practice to combine entering a full explanation with codes tied to repeat lapses such as "mislocation (ML)" or "calculation error (CE)" to streamline the process.

Recording raw data sounds easy, but under the stress of performing the study experiments, staff can easily become remiss in their adherence to these instructions. The most common lapses appear to be delay in completing documentation, forgetting initials or date and time, and overuse of certain error codes. In designing a GLP system, techniques to ensure GLP compliance in data collection and documentation should be emphasized heavily in training and oversight. Combined with a rational well-designed system for capturing raw data, this will help guarantee data integrity while increasing productivity by reducing rework.

Training in raw data entry is essential for all personnel to understand why, when, and how to record data. Training must also emphasize the detailed recording of unforeseen events that occur during an experiment. For example, the technician may observe that certain samples do not react in the same way as the others; maybe they form a solid precipitate whereas the others remain liquid. In this instance an entry should be made to this effect so that the study director can assess the effect of the phenomenon on the experiment. If the formation of the precipitate coincides with a trend or discrepancy observed in the data, the study director has a possible assignable cause to explain the observations. Without this level of detail a significant event that could affect study conclusions may be overlooked, yet a reasonable balance has to be found, as overrecording can also detract from clarity of the data. As a general rule, however, it is better to "overdocument" than "underdocument," since data lost by exclusion cannot be retrieved. Taking these points into consideration, the training program should be designed to meet the specific requirements and the challenges faced by the staff.

Quality Control Verification and quality control (QC) activities are also essential to data accuracy. Quality control is not mentioned specifically in the FDA GLP regulations. However, it is explained in the 1987 preamble to the GLP regulations that the GLP requirement for data verification includes *supervisory quality control* as part of the study director's responsibility to ensure accurate recording of data [10]. How this verification is done depends on the nature of the data and

TABLE 9.4 Quality Control Compared with Quality Assurance

Characteristic	QC	QA
Level of involvement with study	Active, direct participation in the study	No direct participation in study
Relationship to study director	Directly involved with study director	Independent of study director
Periodicity of review	Continuous day-to-day involvement	Audit at selected critical phases
Objectives	Verify requirements are met and protocol is executed	Assure that processes are in place, and followed
Level of detail reviewed	Complete detail orientation	Details, but only a subset
Extent of review	100% data check and verification	Sample of data verified
Scientific involvement	Some involvement in day-to-day science with study director	No involvement in day-to-day science
Reporting	Provide assurance to study director and management	Provide assurance to management

the systems in place; if data are collected electronically using a validated system with functionality to reduce possible error to a minimum, further verification may be superfluous. However, where data recording is intensively manual, more scientific review and quality control will be necessary; the human error rate can be notoriously high even under the best circumstances, and this rate can rise dramatically when conducting study procedures, especially when personnel are under stress, fatigued, or distracted. When planning a QC system, the concepts of hazard and risk should be incorporated so that potential high-hazard areas with low visibility and manual processes warrant a more extensive QC process. To define QC clearly, Table 9.4 shows the principal differences between quality assurance and quality control activities. This table shows that quality control is an integral part of study performance, whereas quality assurance constitutes independent study review and audit. QA thereby complements and assesses QC effectiveness but is not engaged in re-reviewing details that have been checked previously.

9.3.8 Subpart J: Reports and Records

There must be a final report for every GLP study, whether completed or not, the concern being that it is not acceptable to "hide" a study that produces unwanted results as a "terminated" study with no further explanation. This subpart contains a list of items required in a study report, including:

- Methods used (a specific reference to a method will suffice).
- Test and control article information, including strength, purity, and composition; the exact dose used in the study has to be disclosed.

- "A description of all circumstances that may have affected the quality or integrity of the data." This statement necessitates a judgment about whether certain circumstances may have affected data integrity. The GLP regulations do not require that every circumstance reflected in a deviation from SOPs, protocol, or regulations be discussed in the study report. However, it pays to have a robust system for recording and tracking deviations, to ensure that they are properly authorized, reviewed, and included in the final report if they constitute situations that may affect the quality or integrity of the study.
- Individual scientist reports signed by the scientists responsible for their portion of the study. These reports have to be included in the final overall study report, typically by inclusion as an appendix. This requirement stems from another completeness concern, the need to disclose all results, not to hide data behind summary statements in a larger report without provision of all information.
- The archive location.
- The dated signature of the study director (the study completion date).

Although the sponsor is not required to approve or sign the study report (the study director is the sole point of technical control), it is good practice for the sponsor to review the report at its draft stage. This review can be documented in the study file: for example, by memo or e-mail correspondence. After the study completion date, changes to the report can only be made by means of a signed and dated (by the study director) amendment to the report. This maintains the ability to reconstruct the progression of the report and minimizes the potential to obscure pertinent information.

One common area of confusion is the GLP compliance statement and its relation to the quality assurance statement. The quality assurance statement is clearly defined in the regulations; Section 58.35(b)(7) states that, quality assurance shall "prepare and sign a statement to be included with the final study report which shall specify the dates inspections were made and findings reported to management and to the Study Director." The OECD principles of GLP include a similar requirement; however, they add that it will also include the phase(s) of the study that were inspected, and that the statement serves to confirm that the report accurately reflects the raw data of the study (a phrase commonly included on quality assurance statements). OECD Advisory Document No. 4 [13] recommends that the QAU sign this statement only if the study director's claim to GLP compliance can be supported, giving quality assurance the power to "veto" a noncompliant study. In contrast, the *compliance statement* has no basis under FDA GLP, although Section 312.23(8)(iii) of the U.S. Food, Drug and Cosmetic Act does require the inclusion of a GLP compliance statement covering all supporting safety studies in an investigational new drug (IND) application. It is standard practice for study reports to include a compliance statement signed by the study director (or principal investigator), listing any instances of noncompliance with GLP regulations. OECD GLP principles state that "the Study Director must sign and date the final report to indicate acceptance of responsibility for the validity of all the data. The extent of compliance with these GLP Principles should be indicated." The OECD Consensus Document No. 13 [15] enlarges on this, recommending that this statement of compliance include "specific reference to the OECD Principles of GLP and Regulations with which compliance is being claimed. This claim of compliance will cover all phases of the study and should be consistent with the information presented in the Principal Investigator claims. Any sites not compliant with the OECD Principles of GLP should be indicated in the final report." Under the multisite model, each principal investigator will indicate the extent to which his or her portion of the study complies with the GLPs; the study director can then review these individual statements and make a final overall statement regarding the compliance of the study, disclosing any compliance deficiencies identified at any of the test sites. Care should be taken with disclosure on the compliance statement; it is very important that all true instances of noncompliance with the regulations be disclosed, and, in case of doubt, all parties involved (including a quality assurance representative) should confer.

Subpart J of the FDA GLP regulations then gives an outline of the requirements for archiving and storage of records and reports. Section 58.190 gives instructions on what should be stored—all raw data, documentation, protocols, final reports, and specimens—and the required characteristics of the archive facility. The archive must be suitably constructed to minimize deterioration of records, it should have access control, and one person (the archivist) must be designated to be responsible for the archives. On the study completion date there is a transfer of responsibility from the study director to the archivist; the study director ensures that the report and all study records are transferred to the archives on this date, after which the archivist is responsible for ensuring the continued security and integrity of the records. In terms of a hazard–risk analysis, the archiving process and the archive facility fall into the "high hazard" (and potentially "high risk") category. The potential hazard is high because if records are lost or damaged, there is no longer a viable study, so all the efforts to date will have been to no avail. There is also a high risk associated with archiving because, by definition, this is a low-visibility process, as it is under the supervision of one person. Those designing GLP-compliant archival systems would do well to recognize this and build a robust archiving process with QC and automated processes to monitor archiving discrepancies and to address emergent problems in a timely manner. Separately, but just as important, are the issues of physical integrity and protection from conditions leading to deterioration. Paper record requirements will therefore differ from those for electronic records, but both share the need for fundamental protection from fire, flood, and other environmental factors. Fireproof file cabinets and nearby fire extinguishers will serve as basic measures. Where rodents or insects are a concern, appropriate measures should be taken. Increasingly, archiving of records means storage of DVDs, CDs, and digital media on hard drives. To serve this electronic component most effectively, systems have to be developed to ensure that all electronic records are securely archived in compliance with GLP principles. Electronic archiving, just as with paper records, is to be performed under the supervision of the archivist, although they may need to delegate some of their responsibility to information technology personnel. Valuable information on this subject can be found in No. 15 of the OECD Series on Principles of Good Laboratory Practice and Compliance [25] and in the guidelines developed by the Working Group on Information Technology [26].

9.3.9 Disqualification of Testing Facilities

The regulations end on a sobering note, with Subpart K addressing disqualification and its consequences. Here the FDA details instances that will lead to disqualification of a test facility: failing to comply with GLP regulations; adverse effects of noncompliance on the validity of study data, and continued lesser regulatory violations. If disqualification is mandated, the FDA will not accept study data from that facility and may choose to reexamine pending or previously approved applications containing data from the party disqualified.

Other scenarios in which a test facility's business is suspended are included in this subpart. When a sponsor suspends or terminates a test facility that is working on an application currently submitted to the FDA, they must notify the FDA of this event within 15 working days of the termination, according to Section 58.217. When a facility conducting nonclinical testing goes out of business, the regulations require that "all raw data, documentation, and other material specified in this section shall be transferred to the archives of the sponsor of the study. The Food and Drug Administration shall be notified in writing of such a transfer." The regulations then conclude with a section on reinstatement of previously disqualified facilities (58.219); such reinstatement is possible at the FDA's discretion after assuring that sufficient corrective action has been taken to address all deficiencies.

9.4 GLPs IN THE BIOANALYTICAL LABORATORY*

The majority of bioanalytical laboratories base their procedures on the requirements of GLPs [9,10,14,28]; however, as GLPs are written primarily to describe the principles that apply to the administration of test drugs to test systems, translating these principles to apply to bioanalysis is not always straightforward. This difficulty in translation is often at the heart of the uncertainties in the profession, as both laboratory and regulatory agency personnel may have different opinions as to how the regulations apply. Nevertheless, the applicable parts of GLP regulations are commonly used as the basis for bioanalytical operations. In setting up a bioanalytical laboratory to perform GLP analyses, consideration needs to be given to other regulations that impinge on bioanalysis, as there are

*Adapted from [27], with permission. Copyright © 2006 John Wiley & Sons, Ltd.

good business reasons to perform work in support of both nonclinical and clinical development studies within the same bioanalytical facility. As discussed in Chapter 4, the cornerstone for bioanalytical laboratories is the FDA's guidance on bioanalytical method validation [29], which was published by the FDA following meetings between the FDA and industry representatives in 1991 and 2000 [30,31]. This guidance contains the FDA's recommendations for method validation, the use of validated methods in bioanalytical studies, and the associated documentation requirements. The guidance states that "the analytical laboratory conducting pharmacology/toxicology and other nonclinical studies for regulatory submissions should adhere to FDA's Good Laboratory Practices" and that "the bioanalytical method for human bioanalytical, bioequivalence, pharmacokinetic and drug interaction studies must meet the criteria in 21 CFR 320.29." The latter reference is to the FDA regulations governing bioavailability and bioequivalence studies [32], where a very general statement is made that an analytical method "shall be demonstrated to be accurate and of sufficient sensitivity to measure, with appropriate precision, the actual concentration of the active drug ingredient or therapeutic moiety, or its active metabolite(s), achieved in the body." This regulation is cited by FDA investigators who review bioavailability and bioequivalence studies at bioanalytical laboratories. Further details of FDA expectations are contained in their "Compliance Program Guidance Manual" for bioequivalence inspections [33].

There are numerous international guidelines and regulations that, to a greater or lesser extent, address bioanalysis; for example, Canada's Health Products and Food Branch has issued comprehensive guidance documents for bioavailability and bioequivalence studies, including guidance on bioanalytical methods [34,35]. The ICH S3A guideline "Toxicokinetics: The Assessment of Systemic Exposure in Toxicity Studies" briefly mentions bioanalysis, stating that analytical methods should be specific and of adequate accuracy and precision, have an appropriate limit of quantification, and be suitably validated [36]. In Europe, the EMEA Committee for Proprietary Medicinal Products (CPMP) adopted a revised "Note for Guidance" on bioavailability and bioequivalence that came into effect in 2002 [37]. This guidance stated that the bioanalytical part of bioequivalence trials should be conducted according to the applicable principles of GLP. Following this, the United Kingdom GLP Monitoring Authority issued a clarifying note to explain that this did not mean that laboratories needed to be included in their country's national GLP program [38]; just that they should adopt "the applicable references from the GLP principles."

The regulations and guidance related to electronic records and electronic signatures [39–41] are very much a part of bioanalysis, as it is a highly automated, data-based environment where electronic records abound.

Next we review briefly the GLP regulations as they apply to bioanalytical laboratories, highlighting areas where interpretation or adaptation of the regulations is necessary.

9.4.1 Organization and Personnel

- The bioanalytical laboratory should have an individual scientist (or principal investigator, using OECD terminology), who acts as the single point of technical control for the bioanalytical portion of the study. As described earlier, mechanisms for communication with the study director will need to be established for the principal investigator and quality assurance unit (QAU).
- The QAU should *inspect* each study at least once in addition to its audit and review activities. The in-process inspection program should be described in an SOP defining the study phases that may be inspected: for example, "sample extraction"; "preparation of quality controls/calibration standards"; "HPLC/MS system setup"; "sample receipt and labeling."

9.4.2 Equipment and Testing Facilities Operation

These sections of the regulations can be related to the bioanalytical laboratory in a straightforward fashion; obviously the clauses related to animal care do not apply; however, other concepts can be applied: for example, the separation of activities (e.g., weighing areas for reference standards should be separate from areas used for analysis of biological specimens).

Test and Control Articles The GLP requirements for test and control articles can be applied to materials used as reference standards for bioanalytical assays; this does, however, present some difficulties, principally the requirement to have characterization performed to GLP standards and the requirements for retention (which is often not possible with the small quantities available). A good starting point is to treat these materials as reference standards as defined by the FDA bioanalytical method validation guidance [29], according to which "the source and lot number, expiration date, certificates of analysis when available and/or internally or externally generated evidence of identity and purity" should be available for each reference standard. The stability of stock solutions of analytes prepared from these reference materials needs to be established, and this is also described in the FDA's guidance [29]. One important concept for a bioanalytical laboratory is *chain of custody* as applied to analytical reference materials or specimens received for analysis. It should be possible to trace materials or specimens from their point of arrival in the laboratory to their eventual disposition, documenting their exact storage conditions, reasons for removal from storage, together with times, dates, locations, and personnel responsible for any handling operations. This can be achieved using paper-based or electronic systems and will serve to demonstrate that the integrity of the materials or specimens was maintained throughout the period of analysis. Information recorded on the chain of custody can be compared to demonstrated stability to prove, for example, that specimens "on the bench" never exceeded their duration of known stability during their analyses.

Protocol for and Conduct of a Nonclinical Laboratory Study According to the GLP regulations, the methods used in a nonclinical study should be described in the study protocol. This means that the protocol should at least contain a specific method reference for the bioanalytical method to be used. As it is not common for the overall study protocol to contain many details of the bioanalytical operations beyond expected sample numbers and matrices to be analyzed, the bioanalytical laboratory will require a more detailed document. This is typically achieved by having a bioanalytical study plan or some form of master document that links the protocol to the laboratory's personnel, SOPs, and methods. The BARQA good clinical laboratory practice document [42] describes use of such a plan, and if used for a GLP study, this can be approved by the study director, not just the sponsor, to comply with GLP principles. The bioanalytical method used must be validated to demonstrate acceptable performance—precision, accuracy, stability, specificity, selectivity—prior to its use in study sample analysis. Details of recommended validation experiments are given in the FDA bioanalytical method validation guidance [29] and the ensuing white papers that have been published following a series of joint meetings between the FDA and pharmaceutical industry scientists, called the Crystal City meetings, named after their Virginia venue [43–48]. A common question is: Does method validation have to be performed under GLP, including quality assurance audit and review? The answer to this question is "no"—validation is clearly not within the scope of the GLP regulations; however, it does present a high hazard activity. Method validation may be the basis for a method that is used in support of multiple studies, and if this is flawed or inaccurate, these studies could all be compromised. There are thus good business reasons to apply GLP principles, including quality assurance, to method validation studies.

Records and Reports Under FDA's GLPs, the bioanalytical individual scientist should prepare and sign a report of the bioanalytical phase of the study. The reporting requirements delineated in the GLP regulations can be used as a guide to the content of the report. More detailed recommendations for reports are contained in the FDA guidance and the 2006 white paper entitled "Quantitative Bioanalytical Methods Validation and Implementation: Best Practices for Chromatographic and Ligand Binding Assays" [43]. This white paper gives very specific advice on best practice for bioanalytical reports, concentrating notably on the "completeness" aspect of data integrity, such that reports contain disclosure of all failed bioanalytical runs and all results from samples that are assayed on more than one occasion.

Archives GLP requirements for archiving are easily applicable to bioanalytical studies; common practice is for the bioanalytical individual scientist (principal investigator) to ensure that data are archived after his or her signature of the final bioanalytical report. The biological samples analyzed are treated as "specimens" in GLP terms and are therefore exempt from the requirement to be archived.

9.4.3 Some Challenges in the Bioanalytical Laboratory

As bioanalysis is an evolving field, new problems, new techniques, and new expectations are continually arising, creating fresh challenges for the bioanalytical laboratory, and despite all the guidelines and regulations, there are still areas in bioanalysis that cause inconsistency, uncertainty, and regulatory citations. These are usually due to technical areas not covered in the guidances or regulations and difficulties in translation and application of the GLP regulations to the bioanalytical environment. Some current challenges for the bioanalytical laboratory are described below.

Carryover and Contamination The FDA's Division of Scientific Investigation's (DSI) scrutiny of bioanalytical analysis in support of bioequivalence studies has generated a number of current issues which apply to bioanalysis at all stages of development, including pre-FIH toxicology. For example, contamination and carryover has gained much attention following FDA untitled letters in 2004 [49,50]. The basis of the problem is the unwanted presence of analyte introduced during the analytical process, either from the extraction procedure or during the chromatographic analyses. The FDA untitled letters demonstrate that this can lead to possible invalidation of studies, widespread investigations of facilities, and reconsideration of a product's therapeutic equivalence rating. Assessment of carryover and contamination are not, however, treated in any detail in regulatory guidelines, leading to a number of different approaches to detecting and addressing this problem.

Site Investigations Many laboratories handle the incidence of contamination or other problems that potentially affect data integrity by performing a formal investigation into the problem. Triggers for investigations include:

- Inconsistent results obtained on reanalysis of samples
- High percentage of run failure
- Chromatographic anomalies not seen during validation, retention time shifts, or atypical chromatography
- Instances of spurious high bias for individual standards or quality controls

This is becoming an expectation in the industry, yet regulations concerning investigation of out-of-specification results reside in the good manufacturing practice arena [51]. Further, it is not clear exactly when such investigations should be conducted.

Reanalysis Situations that require samples to be reassayed have to be treated with care. The larger concern with reanalysis is that it may be indicative of problems with the bioanalytical method, or in the worst case, it is a means by which data can be manipulated—"problem" results can be removed from the data set. Broadly speaking, reanalysis falls into three categories:

1. Reanalysis "for cause," where the first result is clearly not a valid result. Examples include results due to documented laboratory error or failure to meet SOP criteria, and results that are above or below the quantification range of the assay.

2. Reanalysis due to an unexpected result, where the concentration obtained does not fall into the expected pharmacokinetic profile. In these cases it is critical to have a *good* SOP to describe the procedure to be followed. The emphasis is placed on the word *good* to indicate that this SOP should not be "written for convenience," allowing uncertain or inconclusive data to be retained or rejected without sufficient effort invested to understand the cause of the variability. An SOP should describe clearly the circumstances under which a sample can be reanalyzed for pharmacokinetic reasons. The bioanalytical laboratory should have access to this SOP to serve as a justification for repeating a valid measurement. A subsection of this category is where measurable levels of analyte are found in samples from control groups in nonclinical studies, which is the subject of a 2005 guideline published by the European Medicines Evaluation Agency Committee for Medicinal Products for Human Use (CHMP) [52].

3. Reanalysis for incurred sample reproducibility testing. Validation of bioanalytical methods is performed using "spiked"samples, comprising a biological matrix into which a known amount of the intended analyte is introduced. These samples may not necessarily be truly representative of the actual "incurred" samples that the method will be used to assay, notably in the absence of certain drug metabolites or matrix components. When used with incurred samples, the method accuracy and reproducibility are often unknown during validation, and until recently this was not assessed routinely during bioanalytical study analysis. Potential problems that may arise during incurred sample analysis that were not detected during validation are those of analyte stability in the sample or during the analytical process, and effects of metabolites or matrix components on quantification. Following FDA observations of widely differing results occurring upon reanalysis in several studies, this issue has gained a higher profile in the bioanalytical community, being the subject of continuing industry–regulatory agency conferences and discussion. Following the recommendations of the 2007 white paper [43], which states that "a proper evaluation of incurred sample reproducibility and accuracy needs to be performed on each species used for GLP toxicology experiments," a structured approach to systematic reanalysis of a number of samples is now an FDA expectation. This procedure should be defined in an SOP and will apply to both nonclinical and clinical sample analysis.

Despite remaining uncertainty and debate in the bioanalytical community, the FDA bioanalytical guidance, the Crystal City meetings, and related publications and discussion have helped clarify and develop best practices. The process is continuing and there remains healthy debate in the bioanalytical community, a positive indication that this is a profession that intends to continually evolve its understanding and use of scientific and compliance principles.

9.5 MOVING INTO THE FUTURE: A CLOSING OVERVIEW

New York City was graced with a Museum of Holography from 1976 to 1992, and some exhibits produced amusing results, such as a wine glass sitting on a corner shelf, inviting visitors to pick it up. It will never be known how many hands passed right through what was only an image. Not only was the glass with its dregs a hologram, so was the shelf! There are often complaints that the FDA and other regulatory agencies keep "moving the bar" for regulatory compliance, however, like the glass on the shelf, this complaint is little more than illusion. It is *the regulated community* that produces new technology, creates products and devices not dreamed of in past decades, and embraces wholesale advance into electronic collection and storage of data, new hardware designs, and e-signatures. So, more often than not, we are the ones raising the bar, but if you are only just setting up the brackets, where is the starting point? The GLPs are logical and welcome boundaries against intentional fraud as well as innocent mistakes. To begin by instilling motivation for the challenges ahead, management must introduce them not only as a legal obligation, but also as standards that will set an organization apart from those with less integrity and ability. Once this is done, staff on all levels are partners in a communal effort that will raise morale and productivity, not simply profits.

As with any other building project, the GLP foundation must be carefully set, something that can only be achieved by management, the accepted source of corporate direction. In this endeavor it is imperative to get the QAU involved early! The role of QA personnel is to provide management with information, not to conduct "police work." The practical enforcement of SOPs falls under the purveyance of those in the personnel triangle (Figure 9.1)—management, study director, operational personnel (including quality control)—as part of a standardization process. The QAU is to monitor whether or not the processes established initially are sufficient to produce compliance with the regulations at the time of the inspection. In other words, the QAU does not produce quality but, instead, assures its presence or points out its absence, hopefully with some sound solutions. Therefore, involving a QA professional in the earliest stage of any change, be it a first venture into GLP work or the acquisition of new equipment and software, is part of the equation for GLP success.

During the transition into regulated work, it is worth considering use of a non-GLP project or R&D experiment as a training ground to begin the process of getting staff to "live and breathe" the regulatory atmosphere. Remember to begin in a practical, yet thorough way. The definitions given in the regulations are often given scant attention—with predictable results. In particular, that for *raw data* merits much more than a glance since it is this term that underlies documentation and many other quality principles. Raw data are the mortar holding the entire project together and are necessary for reconstruction of what actually happened during the span of time when the study was active. Study activity points are defined by critical dates: the *study initiation date*, when the protocol is signed and thereby effective, and the *experimental completion date* (per OECD GLP), the last day of data collection. The phase of data evaluation and reporting will follow.

The remaining subparts in the GLP table of contents can be viewed as a step-by-step guide for benchmarks in the process. Trained staff is assigned to various roles by competent management; an appropriate facility for the intended scope of operation is set up, the necessary equipment is obtained and prepared, maintained, and calibrated to standards; and a decision is made on how best to operate and set down standard operating procedures. Then, depending on the nature of the business, the organization's proprietary products or those of another facility are delivered to an appropriate test system: animals or other organisms, plants, soils, and the like. "Good" test substances and healthy test systems will be needed for the best results, and all will be done in accordance with protocols. Finally, complete, clear, and concise reports will be prepared for submittal to the regulatory agency.

As this chapter is being written, the FDA is planning a revision to "modernize" its GLP regulations, proving again that compliance is a partnership with industry. Key FDA leaders have been soliciting information from all of their centers and various stakeholders, including professional organizations such as the Pharmaceutical Research and Manufacturers of America (PhRMA) and the Society of Quality Assurance (SQA). Since the original regulations came into effect in 1974, the 35 years since have prepared thousands of professionals to work in tandem with government, to the expected benefit of countless more. Harmonization with the OECD, especially for multisite studies, and a wider evaluation of quality systems' effectiveness outside the QAU, are only two probable areas of focus [53]. Although these efforts are only in the early stages, it is an exciting conclusion to this chapter to think of a new preamble in the *Federal Register* and a possible opportunity to provide input.

To have expected the regulatory agencies to craft regulations to cover every possible contingency for a small company or a multinational firm would have left us all groping in the dark and unable to provide medicine, safe food, and thousands of other products to the world. This is why spokespersons for the regulatory agencies always steer questions back to the regulations, often referring to them as the *predicate rule*. The GLPs will remain the foundation for both the enforcement inspections of raw data, reports, and facilities, and for our corporate practices. They offer sound guidance and a common standard for worldwide corporations and for the smallest of startup companies. The latter stakeholders should study the regulations carefully and show a firm resolve for compliance from the start. They should partner with professional societies and consultants and make regular visits to the FDA Web site to gain advice in structuring their first compliance programs, then allow the mounting experience gained from each study to crystallize their efforts toward excellence. Remember the hologram? Once all staff members begin to "think GLP," the possibility of always being in compliance is a solid objective and not a trick of the light.

Acknowledgments

The authors wish to thank Anastasia Popescu and Kristina Conceicao for their help with the figures used in this chapter.

9.6 APPENDIXES

Appendix 9.1: Preambles—Perspectives on GLP Requirements

One proof of the regulated community's acceptance of GLP is reflected in the two preambles to the FDA's GLP regulations. These preambles were published in the U.S. *Federal Register*, one in 1978 [4] and the second in 1987 [10]. The comments submitted from interested parties on the proposed GLP rule are organized by subpart and responded to comprehensively by the FDA. Anyone involved in instituting, managing, or reviewing GLP systems will need to study them as an invaluable guide to understanding and interpreting GLP. Comparing the arguments against the GLPs as first presented and the depth of consideration given by the FDA in developing each response dispels presumptions that the regulations are either unreasonably inflexible or far too general in their requirements. Given the serious nature of what was found lacking in some laboratories, it was necessary for the FDA to produce regulations—not simply guidelines as some suggested—for *the assurance of the quality and integrity of the safety data submitted to the agency*. Some form of that key phrase appears throughout both preambles. But quality, like freedom, is not free. In fact, some businesses did not survive the post-GLP marketplace, and today's R&D expenses are staggering. Does this support negative perceptions which linger to the present day: for example, that GLP compliance is too costly, overdone, or is a hindrance to research?

Much of the objection to the pending FDA regulation was due to the recognition of the burden already imposed in conducting laboratory animal and other research, evidenced by the high percentage of comments from industry and associations. The GLP requirement for isolation of species, quarantine of ill laboratory animals, or for distinct operation areas translated simply into more cages, bigger facilities, better sanitation equipment, more staff, and increased oversight. Poor choices of ways to meet these costs ranged from attempting fraud to simple corner-cutting, personified by the untrained typist used to transcribe tumor data described in Section 9.1. Today, it is unquestioned that training records be kept and updated periodically, and that employees *expect* regulation, controls, and visits by the QAU. It has just become good business to adhere to GLPs.

Other objections, such as confidentiality issues or constraints on pure research, were assuaged over time. Contracted agreements now spell out confidentiality terms and describe working relationships and expectations that allow global functionality. Internal and external personnel utilize password-protected electronic documents and data just as in the 1980s their peers used locked desk drawers—the same regulations govern the issue of security. R&D scientists learned that the GLPs did not apply until the stage was reached when a promising formula was ready to move into more sophisticated testing to produce a report intended for submittal to the FDA. As experience with the regulations was gained, there was hard proof of benefit to even fundamental research, and more people were won over to GLP.

In the later 1987 preamble, few questions about the need for compliance or suggestions for shortcuts appear. This later public comment reflects a growing body of experience and even creativity emerging in carrying out compliance programs. Compared to "more than 100 comments" in 1978 on the need for quality assurance oversight, by 1987, "eight comments regarding the QA unit" focused on questions about its composition, resource allocation, or job descriptions, not objections to the idea of being audited.

Simply put, good regulatory compliance resulted in better science, and better science led to more diversification, more business. Management must be the driver behind GLP compliance, since it is their commitment—spoken and unspoken—that is first sought by the rest of the staff. Incorporation of parts of the preambles into GLP training content will reinforce the attitude of "thinking GLP," necessary for success in a wide variety of scientific endeavors.

Appendix 9.2: International Regulations

Aside from the FDA's GLPs, two principal international GLP regulations of interest that apply to nonclinical studies of pharmaceutical products are the Organization for Economic Cooperation and Development's (OECD's) "Principles of Good Laboratory Practice" [14] and the Japanese Ministry of Health, Labor, and Welfare's (MHW) "Good Laboratory Practice Standards for Safety Studies on Drugs" [28]. The OECD GLP principles were adopted into law in countries belonging to the European Economic Community (EEC) following a 1986 EEC directive [54]. As of this writing, the 30 member countries of the OECD are Australia, Austria, Belgium, Canada, Czech Republic, Denmark, Finland, France, Germany, Greece, Hungary, Iceland, Ireland, Italy, Japan, Korea, Luxembourg, Mexico, the Netherlands, New Zealand, Norway, Poland, Portugal, the Slovak Republic, Spain, Sweden, Switzerland, Turkey, the United Kingdom, and the United States. The approval in December 2007 of "road maps" marked the start of accession talks with Chile, Estonia, Israel, Russia, and Slovenia. The OECD GLP principles are not legally binding in the United States, despite its membership.

There are differences between these principal GLP regulations and a detailed side-by-side comparison can be found in [55]. The OECD principles omit some of the detail found in the U.S. GLPs, while providing a more "modern" framework for the regulations, encompassing the multisite study structure and addressing validation of computerized systems. The OECD has published a comprehensive set of advisory documents (numbered 1 through 15), which provide very useful sources of information for those wishing to establish, or improve, a GLP program:

No. 1: OECD Series on Principles on Good Laboratory Practice and Compliance Monitoring

No. 2: Revised Guides for Compliance Monitoring Procedures for Good Laboratory Practice
No. 3: Revised Guidance for the Conduct of Laboratory Inspections and Study Audit
No. 4: Quality Assurance and GLP (revised 1999)
No. 5: Compliance of Laboratory Suppliers with GLP Principles (revised 1999)
No. 6: The Application of the GLP Principles to Field Studies (revised 1999)
No. 7: The Application of the GLP Principles to Short Term Studies (revised 1999)
No. 8: The Role and Responsibilities of the Study Director in GLP Studies (revised 1999)
No. 9: Guidance for the Preparation of GLP Inspection Reports
No. 10: The Application of the Principles of GLP to Computerized Systems
No. 11: The Role and Responsibility of the Sponsor in the Application of the Principles of GLP
No. 12: Requesting and Carrying Out Inspections and Study Audits in Another Country
No. 13: The Application of the OECD Principles of GLP to the Organization and Management of Multi-site Studies
No. 14: The Application of the Principles of GLP to in vitro Studies
No. 15: Establishment and Control of Archives that Operate in Compliance with the Principles of GLP

In addition, the OECD has made two position papers available:

- The Use of Laboratory Accreditation with Reference to GLP Compliance Monitoring (1994)
- "Outsourcing" of Inspection Functions by GLP Compliance Monitoring Authorities (2006)

  All these documents are available via the OECD Web site [56].

A GLP program that is compliant with the FDA's GLPs will be, for the most part, compliant with OECD and MHW GLPs. However, compliance with regulations should not be claimed without a detailed review and implementation of all specific requirements. Test sites that are working under a study protocol that claims compliance with multiple regulations must take care to exclude themselves from those that do not apply, either by stating this in the protocol or by a site-specific test plan signed by the study director. Progress has been made on mutual recognition of GLP standards between the United States, other OECD states, and Japan, and memoranda of understanding have been established to document this intent. The "Note Verbal" from 1983 [57] attests to a mutual recognition of nonclinical laboratory data between the United States and Japan.

The document states: "This arrangement is a statement of intent by both parties to implement standards or guidelines of good laboratory practices (GLPs) for laboratories conducting nonclinical safety studies, and to establish national inspection programs to enforce those standards or guidelines in order to promote the mutual acceptance of data between the two countries". Further, "Each party also accepts for regulatory purpose, nonclinical safety studies of pharmaceutical products, which have been carried out in accordance with the GLP standards established by the other party" [57]. A similar document exists between Japan and Europe detailing the acceptance of data generated by confirmed test facilities, including a list of applicable laws in both regions, with their designated competent authorities [58].

Appendix 9.3: Paraphrased FDA GLP Definitions

Test article: any food additive, color additive, drug, biological product, electronic product, medical device for human use, or any other article subject to regulation.

Control article: any food additive, color additive, drug, biological product, electronic product, medical device for human use, or any article other than a test article, feed, or water that is administered to the test system in the course of a nonclinical laboratory study for the purpose of establishing a basis for comparison with the test article.

Nonclinical laboratory study: in vivo or in vitro experiments in which test articles are studied prospectively in test systems under laboratory conditions to determine their safety. The term does not include studies utilizing human subjects or clinical studies or field trials in animals. Basic exploratory studies carried out to determine whether a test article has any potential utility or to determine physical or chemical characteristics of a test article.

Sponsor: A person who initiates and supports, by provision of financial or other resources, a nonclinical laboratory study; a person who submits a nonclinical study to the FDA in support of an application for a research or marketing permit; or a testing facility, if it both initiates and actually conducts the study.

Testing facility: a person who actually conducts a nonclinical laboratory study (i.e., actually uses the test article in a test system).

Person: includes an individual, partnership, corporation, association, scientific or academic establishment, government agency, or organizational unit thereof, and any other legal entity.

Test system: any animal, plant, microorganism, or subparts thereof to which the test or control article is administered or added for study. Test system also includes appropriate groups or components of the system not treated with the test or control articles.

Specimen: any material derived from a test system for examination or analysis.

Raw data: any laboratory worksheets, records, memoranda, notes, or exact copies thereof, which are the result of original observations and activities of a nonclinical laboratory study and are necessary for the reconstruction and evaluation of the report of that study. In the event that exact transcripts of raw data have been prepared (e.g., tapes that have been transcribed verbatim, dated, and verified accurate by signature), the exact copy or exact transcript may be substituted for the original source as raw data. Raw data may include photographs, microfilm or microfiche copies, computer printouts, magnetic media, including dictated observations, and recorded data from automated instruments.

Quality assurance unit: any person or organizational element, except the study director, designated by testing facility management to perform the duties relating to quality assurance of nonclinical laboratory studies.

Study director: the individual responsible for the overall conduct of a nonclinical laboratory study.

Batch: a specific quantity or lot of a test or control article that has been characterized according to Section 58.105(a).

Study initiation date: the date the protocol is signed by the study director.

Study completion date: the date the final report is signed by the study director.

Appendix 9.4: FDA Inspections

A necessary component of any GLP system is the ability to withstand scrutiny by external auditors and regulatory agencies. A facility that has a well-designed GLP system with a high level of compliance, training, and oversight will always be able to satisfy external investigators that they are in compliance with the GLP regulations. However, a high level of inspection readiness should be maintained at all times, such that inspections can be handled effectively, all personnel understand the process, and all records can be produced without delay. Not being prepared for an inspection, even with a first-rate GLP system, can only lead to unnecessary misunderstanding, wasted time, and perhaps even avoidable deficiencies being cited. The FDA has two compliance program guidance manuals, one for good laboratory practice [16] and one for bioequivalence [33]. These manuals, written as a guide for FDA investigators conducting inspections, provide useful insight into the inspectional process and FDA expectations. The GLP manual provides details on the rationale for the FDA's inspection program, the types of inspections conducted, and their possible outcomes.

To be inspection-ready, a facility should consider the following points:

1. Is there a detailed procedure on how to manage an inspection? On the day of inspection there is no time to work out responsibilities and communication routes; these should all be decided in advance, along with assigned deputies for all the key roles. For example, certain features should be defined and agreed to: a single "point person" for the inspection; the person who will communicate inspection

news and requests to staff and sponsors; the responsibilities and procedures for supplying documents.

2. Are all personnel trained in the aims of the inspection, how to act with investigators, and how to respond to questions? It is worth conducting periodic training for all staff members on these points, providing extra training to those categories of staff that will be most responsible for managing an inspection (i.e., study directors, QA personnel).

3. A component of any training should be coaching in interviews with regulatory agency investigators. Although it may seem obvious, explaining the golden rule—"tell the truth"—cannot be overemphasized, as well as providing some basic rules for responding accurately, completely (but not "over-completely"), and clearly to questions. Testing these concepts during training is enlightening; asking selected staff members questions to see how they reply provides an entertaining but useful way of reinforcing the learning objectives.

4. The first three hours count! The outcome of an inspection can be gauged largely by how well the first two to three hours of the inspection are handled. During this time the company should demonstrate its professionalism by presenting an image of calm organization, good communication, and preparedness. To achieve this, details have to be managed: If there is a receptionist (including any temporary replacements) it pays to conduct a separate training and to post clear instructions on what to do when FDA personnel arrive. It creates a very bad first impression if the reception staff appears to lack interest, is slow, or is visibly shocked and worried. A brief, up-to-date summary presentation should be available and easily accessible, remembering that the role of the inspection host is to provide the investigator with all the information needed to assess the facility and the studies performed there. To this end, a clear introduction to the company is invaluable, allowing the investigator to answer some initial questions and providing enough understanding of the company processes to facilitate the inspection. The entire tone of an inspection can be altered if the staff members who greet the investigator do not know what to do or seem disorganized, or if the preliminary meeting is unclear and unstructured.

5. A "mock" inspection can be performed at the company's risk. This tool may serve to test procedures and previous training; however, it should be used carefully, as it can cause misunderstanding and possible loss of trust if the staff is not informed of the mock nature of the inspection within a reasonable time frame.

The FDA's compliance program guidance manual [16] explains the reporting and possible deficiency observations that can be made by the FDA (e.g., FDA Form 483 or Warning Letter) and the post-inspectional process. The FDA is currently using a program called "Turbo EIR" to write their Form 483 observations, a program that requires investigators to preface each observation by a specific citation from the GLP regulations. In this way, this program aims to ensure that an investigator's deficiency observations are specifically linked to the GLP regulations. Further, it provides the FDA with a mechanism for gathering and trending observations, linking them to the associated GLP section. FDA lists of active labs and inspection results (classified as NAI, VAI, or OAI) can be found at the FDA Web site [59].

Appendix 9.5: Critical Phase Inspections—What, Why, How, and When?

What?. *Inspection* implies that a procedure is the subject, whereas an *audit* typically concerns raw data already collected, as well as records and reports. Critical phases in each project are the points reflected in the protocol's experimental design. Depending on the purpose stated in the protocol, a QA target for inspection could be set for one or several phases.

Why?. Study requirements pose hazards and risks in terms of compliance. Critical phase inspections help balance the two by providing "snapshots" of operations for the study director and management's information. They do not comprise the total quality program, but serve as an important tool for assessing the regulatory compliance of systems, personnel, and reports.

How?. A QAU SOP will govern critical phase selection. The method used should combine a documented means of reducing bias (e.g., use of a particular portion of a random number table) with an allowance for discretion based on a known or suspected hazard–risk balance. The QAU must be free to audit and inspect at will. Routine procedures are not exempt from risk, particularly when animals are involved. Consider the risk of rabbits removing wrappings over patches applied to their skin. The dosing period is compromised and there is the possibility of the animals ingesting test substance. To ensure that this risk did not affect a given study, the QAU should include an "end-time" (patch removal) inspection as well as an inspection of the critical phase of dosing (patch application) that is more commonly selected. Since patch removal is timed from application, the QAU gains the chance to carry out an unannounced inspection, always a good test of consistency in operations. The real gain, however, is a more sturdy inspection. By assuring that the full period of exposure to the test material was achieved and that the dose sites were cleaned, any questions concerning the exposure can be answered with surety.

When?. Risk of noncompliance is raised in "new" situations, for example:

- New staff
- A new or infrequently conducted procedure
- New equipment

This risk may also be elevated in circumstances involving:

- Complex procedures, which cause fatigue and loss of concentration.
- Periods when staff is reduced or under stress for other reasons.

- Long procedures, such as the skin-patch example above. There is more risk of patches being disturbed in a 24-hour exposure than in a 4-hour exposure.
- Time lost over the workday due to unforeseen circumstances; the temptation is to hurry or skip documentation until later.

The intention of the GLP inspection requirement in Section 58.35(3) is for the QAU to provide "adequate" oversight in ensuring the integrity of the study. In this endeavor they should assess each study independently and avoid the trap of letting an SOP cause a comfortable routine.

Appendix 9.6: Test System

The protocol is designed to set data-capture points after the test article is administered to the test system. In a primary skin irritation test, for example, a *test article* is applied to the skin of rabbits—the *test system*—and the degree of resulting irritation and its endpoint are assessed. Yet to fully assess unexpected reactions, the animals are also observed as to their daily health and viability.

Since the GLP regulations are broad, it is up to each entity to determine what kinds of conditions must be met for all of the various test systems that are in use at the facility. Beyond GLP, however, are additional regulations and guidelines, such as those from the National Institutes of Health [60] and U.S. Department of Agriculture [61]. Animal welfare represents a significant body of regulatory and physical plant design issues that fall outside the province of GLP. These will require policies and procedures for compliance, as well as specialized training in animal care and use for personnel. Internally, such procedures are governed and assessed periodically by an Institutional Animal Care and Use Committee (IACUC), a group having at least one member *not* associated with the facility. A professional society such as the American Association for Laboratory Animal Science [23] is invaluable to the seeker of guidance in the area of animal welfare, and offers particular guidance regarding the IACUC. For the facility and staff, the Association for Assessment and Accreditation of Laboratory Animal Care International [62] provides guidance on achieving widely recognized certification, especially important for global marketing.

Insofar as the FDA's GLP regulations are concerned, considering the principles for quality and integrity of research, documentation to show satisfaction of the requirements for a test system will be subject to QA and regulatory oversight. Subparts C (Facility), E (Testing Facilities Operation), and G (Protocol, Study Conduct) all contain compliance points for the test system. Whereas the GLP requirements in this area are logical and brief, the measures that will be taken for compliance will usually be extensive, requiring investments in monitoring, control, and refinements over time.

Appendix 9.7: 21 CFR Part 11

21 CFR Part 11, often referred to simply as "Part 11," is the FDA's regulation regarding electronic records and electronic signatures [5] and became effective

in 1997. Part 11 sets forth the circumstances under which the FDA will consider electronic records and electronic signatures equivalent to paper records and handwritten signatures. It applies to records in electronic form under any regulatory records requirements (such as GLPs) or records submitted to the agency. Part 11 does not require that a company use electronic records; rather, it states that electronic records that meet the requirements of the regulation may be used in lieu of paper records. The regulation itself is divided into three subparts: Subpart A, "General Provisions"; Subpart B, "Electronic Records"; and Subpart C, "Electronic Signatures." Subpart A addresses the scope, implementation, and definitions. It is important to note that Part 11 applies to records that the FDA requires to be maintained, not just records submitted to the agency. Subpart B discusses controls for both "open" and "closed" systems, addressing issues such as validation, retention, system requirements, and training.

Subpart C identifies the requirements for electronic signatures and provides details regarding signature components and controls. In this appendix we address key questions and concepts related to these regulations.

What Is an Electronic Record?. The FDA defines an *electronic record* as "any combination of text, graphics, data, audio, pictorial or other information representation in digital form that is created, modified maintained, archived, retrieved, or distributed by a computer system." This definition includes electronic documents. It also includes formats that are not traditionally thought of as records, such as digital images or audio.

Benefits of the Regulation. Part 11 is primarily about building reliable, secure systems. Implementation of these requirements facilitates data security, integrity, and confidentiality. The regulation makes it clear that the agency will accept electronic signatures as being equivalent to handwritten signatures. This eliminates the need to print and sign documents. This assurance that properly executed electronic signatures will be accepted by the agency enables companies to move more easily to a paperless environment and facilitates faster information exchange.

Controls for Closed Systems. The main portion of Part 11 outlines controls required for *closed systems*, which the agency defines as "an environment in which system access is controlled by persons responsible for the content of electronic records that are on the system."

Part 11 requires 11 points of control:

1. Systems must be validated to ensure accuracy, reliability, and consistent intended performance.
2. The system must have the ability to generate accurate and complete copies suitable for inspection by the agency.
3. Records must be maintained in such as way as to be retrievable throughout their full records retention period.

4. System access should be limited to authorized persons.
5. Audit trails must be built into the system to record changes. The audit trails must be maintained for the full records retention period of the subject electronic record.
6. Operational system checks should be built in to enforce sequencing of steps as appropriate.
7. Authority checks should ensure that only authorized persons can use the system.
8. Device checks should determine the validity of the source of data input, as appropriate.
9. Persons who develop, maintain, or use the system are properly trained to perform their assigned tasks.
10. Written policies must be in place to hold people accountable for actions initiated under their electronic signatures.
11. Adequate control over system documentation should be maintained.

These controls can be distilled down to two fundamental types: technical controls, which need to be built into the electronic system, and procedural controls, which must be documented and adhered to. This is important to take into account, particularly when purchasing commercial off-the-shelf systems (COTS). The system developer may have built important technical controls into the system; however, once installed in your organization's environment, it must be validated to ensure its intended performance. Additionally, all of the procedural controls must still be taken into account to ensure that proper policies are in place and that system access is limited to appropriate people who have been properly trained. Fundamentally, these controls are meant to ensure the integrity, reliability, and security of the electronic systems in which we maintain records.

Industry groups have contributed excellent material to assist in implementing and developing good validation and "life-cycle" practices for computerized systems, notably the Drug Information Association and the International Society for Pharmaceutical Engineering/Good Automated Manufacturing Practice. Their respective publications, "Computerized Data Systems for Nonclinical Safety Assessment: Current Concepts and Quality Assurance" [63] and "GAMP 5: A Risk-Based Approach to Compliant GxP Computerized Systems" [64], are recommended for those requiring clear, up-to-date guidance on these topics.

What Is an Open System?. The regulation also addresses controls required for an *open system*, one in which access is not controlled by persons responsible for the content. The best example of an open system is the Internet. Once a record is transmitted via the Internet, the sender no longer controls who has access to the content and can no longer ensure its integrity. Part 11 stipulates that all the requirements for closed systems apply to open systems plus additional controls such as encryption to ensure record authenticity, integrity, and confidentiality. In no instance does Part 11 specify or recommend specific technology.

Electronic Signature Requirements. The agency has outlined some general requirements for electronic signatures and then provides some specific information regarding controls required for implementation. To start the process of using Part 11 compliant electronic signatures, the regulation requires that an organization send a letter to the FDA certifying that electronic signatures in their system are intended to be the "legally binding equivalent of traditional handwritten signatures." Additionally, before allowing the use of electronic signatures, an organization must verify the person's identity. Part 11 requires that each electronic signature be unique to one person. It should not be reused by anyone else at any time. This means that signatures are essentially "attached" to individual employees. If an employee leaves an organization or otherwise should no longer be signing records in a particular system, that electronic signature must be retired permanently. This ensures that from an audit standpoint, there can never be any confusion as to who signed a particular record. For the same reason, electronic signatures should not be shared. The intent of this requirement is to make certain that a signer cannot repudiate a signature executed in his or her name.

Part 11 discusses two types of electronic signatures: biometric and nonbiometric. Because of fundamental differences between the two, they each require different controls. A *biometric signature* is based on a measurement of a person's unique physical feature(s) or repeatable action(s). For example, a fingerprint, a voice print, or a retinal scan could each function as a biometric signature because they are both unique to each person and measurable. Regarding biometric signatures, Part 11 stipulates that they must be "designed to ensure that they cannot be used by anyone other than their genuine owners." Conversely, a *nonbiometric signature* includes no physical characteristic of the user. Its components include something the user knows or has in his or her possession. As you would expect, additional requirements are specified for the use of nonbiometric signatures. The regulation stipulates that nonbiometric signatures use at least two distinct identification components: for example, a user ID and password combination or a user ID and token combination. It is important to note that not every user ID and password combination is considered an electronic signature. Simply logging into a system using a user ID and password is not the execution of an electronic signature. When a signature is required, the user must be aware that he or she is executing a signature on a discrete record.

Systems with electronic signature functionality must be able to produce a human-readable signature manifestation which includes the full name of the signer (not simply a user ID), the date and time when the signature was executed, and the meaning associated with the signature, such as review or approval. Part 11 specifies a number of technical and procedural controls for the use of electronic signatures.

1. No two people should have the same combination of identification code and password.

2. Identification codes and password issuances should be checked, recalled, or revised periodically. This control is most often implemented through the use of password aging, which requires a user to change his or her password after a specified period of time.
3. Loss management procedures must be in place to deactivate lost, stolen, or compromised tokens or passwords.
4. Transaction safeguards must prevent unauthorized use of passwords and detect and report any attempts at unauthorized use. Examples of transaction safeguards include masking the password as it is typed using asterisks, and locking a user out after multiple incorrect password attempts.
5. Devices that generate password information should be tested periodically to ensure that they function correctly.

The rules regarding the use of electronic signatures can be summarized as requirements meant to ensure uniqueness and nonrepudiation.

Does Part 11 Apply Outside the United States?. If the sponsor organization submits records to the FDA or maintains records that are required by the FDA, Part 11 applies.

Applicability of Part 11. Does Part 11 apply to every electronic system used by an organization? Not necessarily. The best way to determine if a system is subject to Part 11 is to ask a few simple questions:

- Does this computerized system create, modify, maintain, archive, retrieve, or transmit any electronic record(s) that are required to demonstrate compliance with FDA regulations or that generate data that are submitted to the FDA? If the answer to this question is "yes," Part 11 applies and your system should be assessed for compliance.
- Does the system require the use of any form of signature that is intended to satisfy any regulatory or company requirement for documenting FDA regulatory compliance (such as a signature, initials, approval, or authorization)? In instances where the regulation does not require a signature but the organization has an SOP in support of regulatory compliance that designates that a signature is required, the signature must be Part 11 compliant. In other words, the SOPs that an organization develops for itself can extend the scope of the regulation.
- Is the computerized system a closed system whereby data and system access are controlled solely by personnel within, or designees of, the organization who are responsible for the content of the electronic records of the system? Answering "no" to this question does not mean that the system is automatically noncompliant. Rather, it means that additional controls are required to maintain the security and integrity of the data.

Records Requirements in GLP Regulations. Written records are specified in several parts of the GLP regulations. Sometimes the reference is subtle, such as in 21 CFR 58.29(b), where the rule says: "Each testing facility shall maintain a current summary of training and experience and job description for each individual engaged in or supervising the conduct of a nonclinical laboratory study." In other cases, it is much more direct, such as in 21 CFR 58.35, where it specifies that "the quality assurance unit shall ... periodically submit to management and the Study Director written status reports. ..."

Even where the GLPs state specifically that a record should be recorded in ink [as it does in 21 CFR 58.130(e)], Part 11 makes it acceptable to use an electronic system if the system is compliant with the stipulations in Part 11. Selected record references in GLP:

- 21 CFR 58.29 Personnel
- 21 CFR 58.35 Quality assurance unit
- 21 CFR 58.51 Specimen and data storage facilities
- 21 CFR 58.63 Maintenance and calibration of equipment
- 21 CFR 58.81 Standard operating procedures
- 21 CFR 58.90 Animal care
- 21 CFR 58.130.e Raw data
- 21 CFR 58.190.e Archived records
- 21 CFR 58.195 Record retention

Regulatory Guidance on Part 11. In September 2003, the FDA released "Guidance for Industry: Part 11, Electronic Records; Electronic Signatures—Scope and Application" [40]. This guidance served to clarify the FDA's current thinking on Part 11. It also stated that the FDA was reexamining Part 11 and that changes to Part 11 are anticipated as a result of this reexamination. [*Author's note:* As of this writing in 2009, changes to the regulation have not been initiated.] It is noteworthy that the regulation remains in place as originally released. However, this guidance has helped to indicate to organizations how best to prioritize resources regarding compliance with the regulation. In the guidance the FDA highlights portions of the regulation for which the agency will exercise enforcement discretion: validation, audit trail, record retention, record copying requirements, and legacy systems.

Critical to an understanding of the implications of this guidance is the awareness that Part 11 remains in effect. The regulation itself has not been eliminated or even changed. The key to maintaining compliance with Part 11 is ensuring that your organization is in compliance with what the FDA refers to as *predicate rules*, in this case, the GLP regulations. In the guidance document, the FDA recommends that organizations document the decision as to which records they consider subject to Part 11 in a specification document or SOP.

Risk-Based Approach. In recognition of the fact that many organizations previously interpreted the scope of the regulation to be unnecessarily broad, and that this broad interpretation led to unreasonably high costs and unnecessary controls, this guidance recommends a risk-based approach to determining the level of compliance necessary for a particular system. Risk assessments should be conducted to determine "the potential of the system to affect product quality and safety and record integrity."

Current Focus. Focus compliance efforts on the highest-risk systems as determined by a documented risk assessment. Ensure that your organization maintains compliance with the underlying predicate rules (GLPs). Systems that most closely affect product quality and safety should be considered to have the highest risk. The overall intention of the regulation remains the same: to maintain the security, integrity, and confidentiality as appropriate for records that support regulatory compliance.

Appendix 9.8: SOP Generation and Review

While the specific operations of a laboratory will depend on the scope and size of the company, any of them can be challenging to set down on paper. However, the task of developing an initial set of SOPs presents a remarkable opportunity for a wise manager. Who knows better what is truly the "standard" procedure for the accomplishment of a given task than the personnel performing the operation? Therefore, as plans proceed to the point of creating initial outlines for common laboratory and facility procedures and equipment maintenance, these staff members should be included in the undertaking.

Where the focus is on review and revision of *existing* procedures, the QAU should be consulted by management for their input on specific procedures. SOP deviations or amendments also indicate a need for change, in order to best produce a "living" set of SOPs that will mirror actual performance of the procedures. In either case, planning and record keeping are keys to success.

To develop the initial SOP set, the list of GLP regulation subparts will serve as a model for the subjects to be addressed. In addition, one or more guidance SOPs (the *SOP on SOPs*) will be the first ones generated and approved, to allow work to proceed. Points for consideration in developing an SOP on SOPs include:

- Development of a numbering system, including indication of the revision (current version) number: for example, SOP 100:01.R00, where 100 is the section number, 01 is the first SOP in the section, and R00 indicates the first edition. If this procedure is subsequently revised, only the final designation changes, from R00 to R01. *Note:* Some facilities conclude this procedure at this stage and begin separate procedures to describe the following several points.

- General format of sections and their headings for uniformity within the SOP set and to provide guidance to authors of new SOPs. Typically used: SOP number, author(s), effective date, title, purpose, scope (who should know the procedure), and procedures (the single steps to be followed). All of these should be explained or defined in this SOP. For example, the effective date may be defined as the date of management's approval signature, or more commonly, a different date upon which each SOP is to be in force (e.g., on the following business day after training).
- Format of the concluding section, which should at least contain the signature and date of management's approval for the single procedure. Some facilities require the primary author to sign as well.
- Preferred font style and size, guidance on margins, and so on.
- Schedule for SOP review: whereas there is no GLP requirement that review be performed annually, this is typically done on a periodicity ranging from one to three years, depending on business practices. Include a provision for review and revision of single procedures should the need arise between formal reviews.

Once SOP formats and authorization details are decided, other general considerations will need to be incorporated into training and document control procedures:

- Person or entity that will arrange for and provide training.
- Appointing a monitor who will be responsible for distribution of new or revised SOPs, to assure that only current versions are available. Where a facility has several identical SOP sets to be placed in distinct areas of the facility, include a numbering system for the set, and designate the location for each. For example, set 1 resides with management, set 2 with Laboratory A, set 3 with the animal care staff, and set 4 with the QAU.
- Procedure for study director notification of SOP amendments or deviations to ensure management's awareness, and communication of the change to appropriate personnel.
- Archiving of the original set of SOPs, as well as revisions, is important for security or reconstruction. Should an FDA investigator wish to inspect raw data from several years past, the SOPs in force at that time will be necessary. SOP sets in the facility are always comprised of copies.

How to Prepare an SOP. Only so much can be done while seated around a conference table gaining input from staff and the QAU. At some point, the actual procedure must be observed, preferably by management and the person who will author the procedure. Each step taken, as well as the materials and equipment required, should be noted and a very detailed outline created as the first draft. This draft should then be circulated for review by those involved in the task as well as the QAU, so that refinements can be made.

The balance between too much and too little detail is tricky at first, but if a careful and inclusive approach is taken from the start, the end result will be a written description of what actually happens in the facility. Management can then peruse the draft with an eye toward necessary additions or improvements.

When created specifically for the SOP, forms provide a way to portray the procedure's requirements and to standardize the collection of data. The left margin should be wide enough to accommodate hole punching if the form will be placed in a notebook, so that information is not lost. In addition:

- Sufficient space should be allowed in columns or cells for a variety of handwriting styles, for the entering of corrections, dates, and explanatory code along with the new data. Testing new forms before actual use is a good practice, allowing refinements that will benefit users and reviewers.
- Consider placing an area for entry of initials and dates for QC, "witnessing," or other documentation.
- On forms for recording daily information, such as temperature records or equipment logs, "force" the placement of at least one entry for the year, along with the calendar date. Where applicable, prompt for units of measure.

Equipment SOP Considerations. Referencing the GLP requirements for equipment is important—a step similar to observation of the actual performance of a procedure. Since each requirement must be addressed, the GLPs serve very well as the format for equipment SOPs. Where any point does not apply, the SOP should state the exception rather than skip the point. For example, it may be more cost-effective to replace less costly equipment annually rather than send it out for service and calibration.

A very important distinction is the concept of *data or duty*, meaning that if the equipment will generate raw data such as a temperature, pH reading, or weight, its SOP will require a higher level of maintenance and calibration than will equipment that does not generate data. Equipment used frequently is typically given *routine* maintenance and calibration as well as *nonroutine* operations such as those occurring after a malfunction. Other equipment, such as that typically found on the laboratory bench or cage-wash area, need only be kept clean and in good repair. However, all operations will require documentation, filing, and eventual archival of records. An annual approach, with information indexed by subject, year, and month, is typically seen in research facilities. It is more useful for equipment logs to be set up for individual pieces rather than "all" balances; if each has its own log, downtime notation and/or retirement of the balance is very simple to accomplish.

An SOP is meant to provide guidance on the proper use of equipment in a GLP-regulated study and to remind users of specific points regarding its operation. The inclusion of equipment manuals is permitted, but as an attachment to the SOP that is referenced in the text as a source of additional information. In other words, an equipment manual is not an SOP.

How to Perform SOP Reviews. When a facility first begins its GLP operation, an SOP set may not be as large as it will become after several years of operation. Management should decide if review of the procedures will best be accomplished in one sitting or if it should be spread out over the year. Whatever means is chosen, it must be documented in the formerly mentioned procedure for SOPs in general.

To create a simple tool for the review, the SOP manual's index can be worked into a checklist. As reviewers read carefully through each procedure, the continued acceptability or potential need for revision is noted on the checklist. Later, the same list can be used to generate the subset of procedures requiring attention so that their revision can be tracked until conclusion. All of these records will be required to document review and management approval of standard operating procedures, so they should eventually be placed in the archives.

Appendix 9.9: Study Director's Responsibilities

FDA's GLP Subpart B, Section 58.33 begins with a general description of acceptable qualifications for a study director: "a scientist or other professional of appropriate education, training and experience, or a combination thereof ...." Note that management has the responsibility to assign the study director, presumably based in part on the qualifications in relation to the type of study. Responsibilities for study oversight remain with the individual study director, regardless of physical location, and include overall responsibility for the technical conduct of the study, including the interpretation, analysis, documentation and reporting of results, and representing the single point of study control. This last responsibility must be constantly reinforced by management and corporate policy. Additionally, although the performance of some of these responsibilities may have to be delegated, such as technical conduct in a multisite situation, some mechanism of providing the study director with a means to examine data and address any questions by staff must be established.

Specifically, the study director must assure that these conditions are met for each study to which they are assigned, as related in this annotated listing of Section 58.33, points (a)–(f):

- The protocol, including any subsequent change (amendment or deviations), is approved as described in Section 58.120, *and is followed*. The emphasis here has been added by the authors, since it is not sufficient that the document simply be approved.
- All experimental data, including observations of unanticipated responses of the test system, are accurately recorded and verified. When the study director is remote, much of the control could be through the use of forms and other means for standardizing data collection.
- Unforeseen circumstances that may affect the quality and integrity of the nonclinical laboratory study are noted when they occur, and corrective action is taken and documented. Obviously, this requires some type of

"presence," with recognition by all participants that there is only one point of control.

- Test systems are as specified in the protocol.
- All applicable GLP regulations are followed. This is important to remember when a protocol lists other regulatory entities, such as the OECD.
- All raw data, documentation, protocols, specimens, and final reports are transferred to the archives during or at the close of the study. Note a distinction in the use of specimens. These typically require types of storage other than paper or electronic records, such as freezer or other secure storage. To assist the study director, appropriate personnel, such as an archivist, and corporate policies for retention duration and control of all data and specimen storage must be in place.

Even under the best of circumstances, unfortunate events occur. Prime examples abound in facility files the world over. The study director should be mindful of the potential for improved study oversight and control that can be gained, and work with management to create better procedures. Here is an interesting case: In a particular raw data package, a protocol deviation form reported a compromise to frozen test sample storage, the result of a power outage. In assessing the impact on the study, the study director noted that since "the samples were described as mushy, they will not be analyzed." This is a serious situation, resulting in rescheduling, economic loss, and overall delay in study completion, but can at least have value in presenting an opportunity for improvement. While the GLPs have been satisfied—the incident was reported and the protocol amended with replacement work under way—there are several important points in this case that should be used to prevent another occurrence.

To analyze the incident with the idea of improving oversight and control, the reason for the outage is first considered. What happened? The deviation states: "A squirrel caused a transformer to blow on the evening of Friday, December 28, 2007. The outage was not discovered until the morning of Monday, December 31, 2007." Clearly, some facility, equipment, and environmental control issues exist. These suggestions should be discussed with management:

- A need for weekend checks of freezer temperatures when samples are present—a reasonable compromise for the extra time compensated.
- If possible, provide protection of the transformer from squirrels and birds (large nests have caused similar problems) using screening mesh.
- An alarm for the freezer, triggered by the internal temperature, could be purchased. Some systems also send a phone or e-mail message to a staff member, possibly a good investment if weekend oversight is not feasible.

The first suggestion could be implemented with little effort, since weekend staff must be present to care for the animals in the vivarium. The last point is typically preferred by FDA investigators, as is freezer security.

Continuing with evaluation of this case, the study director and management can at least be pleased that somebody took the time to provide invaluable information: the condition of the samples when the incident was discovered. This raw data enabled the study director to assess the impact properly and begin remedial action, so recognizing and praising the responsible technician will do much to support future diligence and a focus on improvement. Depending on the proximity of the study director to the testing site, the methods used to accomplish these mandated responsibilities will necessarily vary. But it is clear that the fundamentals include oversight, verification, control, and communication.

In addition to the subsequent preparation of the final report and handling of the raw data and other supporting records, FDA (and OECD) expectations include a clear data trail, timely addressing of situations affecting the protocol, evidence of control over the project, and appropriate response to QA reports. Bearing this in mind, the FDA may be concerned when a person appears to have too many projects listed on the master schedule. During an investigation, one should not be surprised at questions as to the number of studies and the relative complexity of the workload. The investigator may question management about the procedure for study director assignment and replacement, whether or not concerns exist, showing the importance of oversight and control throughout the planning as well as the study process.

Appendix 9.10: Regulatory Requirements for the Study Protocol

The protocol is the controlling document for a study. As such, it serves as a tool for several entities. The setting of schedules, assignment of a study director, and allocation of resources falls to management. The study director will review and finalize the protocol and follow appropriate procedures to maintain control. The QAU will refer to the most current version of the protocol to schedule inspections for studies listed on the master schedule. Later, the protocol will be used during study file review and report preparation, then by the QAU again for the audit of raw data against the report. It is possible that FDA investigators may focus on a study and will begin their review of a particular study file with the protocol. Obviously, the GLPs cannot and should not direct the specifics of a study protocol but must provide its designers with basic requirements. These are listed below, with commentary on each following in a separate section.

Subpart G, Section 58.120

a. Each study shall have an approved written protocol that clearly indicates the objectives and all methods for the conduct of the study. The protocol shall contain, as applicable, the following information:
    1. A descriptive title and statement of the purpose of the study.
    2. Identification of the test and control articles by name, chemical abstract number, or code number.

3. The name of the sponsor and the name and address of the testing facility at which the study is being conducted.
4. The number, body weight range, gender, source of supply, species, strain, substrain, and age of the test system.
5. The procedure for identification of the test system.
6. A description of the experimental design, including the methods for the control of bias.
7. A description and/or identification of the diet used in the study as well as solvents, emulsifiers, and/or other materials used to solubilize or suspend the test or control articles before mixing with the carrier. The description shall include specifications for acceptable levels of contaminants that are reasonably expected to be present in the dietary materials and are known to be capable of interfering with the purpose or conduct of the study if present at levels greater than established by the specifications.
8. Each dosage level, expressed in milligrams per kilogram of body weight or other appropriate units, of the test or control article to be administered and the method and frequency of the administration.
9. The type and frequency of tests, analyses, and measurements to be made.
10. The records to be maintained.
11. The date of approval of the protocol by the sponsor and the dated signature of the study director.
12. A statement of the proposed statistical method to be used.

b. All changes in or revisions of an approved protocol and the reasons therefor shall be documented, signed by the study director, dated, and maintained with the protocol.

Commentary. Point (a) begins with some general requirements. The protocol must be a written document bearing "approval" through the dated signature of the study director. The latter date becomes the study initiation date, bringing all subsequent data, actions, decisions, and outcomes under the control of the regulations specified in the protocol (OECD requirements for the study plan require that a representative of the QAU also sign following protocol review). At a minimum, it is standard practice for the QAU to review periodically all protocols used for regulated research and testing at a given facility, with a report to management of the outcome.

Sections (a) and (b) are appropriate bookends to the requirements, since any change in (1) through (12) necessitate a written, dated record that complements the original written, dated protocol. Approval and control are demonstrated, and the FDA expectation is for this action to be accomplished in a very timely manner. It is no use to complain that the process for drafting and approving protocol changes in one's facility is cumbersome; the response will be a mandate for improvement of the process. As mentioned earlier, handwritten notes or e-mails are often the initial documentation for the preparation of changes to the protocol.

Be sure that the study file contains these raw data, since they (not the formal amendment) demonstrate the degree of control maintained by the study director. Remembering the history of GLPs, this expectation is entirely reasonable.

The published federal guidelines that provide the requirements necessary to design a given study will also generally provide most of the information for the protocol. Using a rabbit skin irritation test as an example, it must be understood that several influential factors come into play, since the use of animals in research and testing is heavily regulated. Federal regulations governing animal husbandry requirements, care and welfare during use, and worker safety are not discussed here but are important, as they influence protocol design.

1. The title would include "Primary Skin Irritation in Rabbits," generally followed by the name of the test material. The purpose would be to assess the potential for human skin irritation using the rabbit as a model.
2. Management will have provided a system for receipt and documentation of all chemicals and materials used. If a compound is experimental, "not applicable" might be recorded for the CAS number.
3. The direction is clear.
4. Testing guidelines will provide the minimum number of animals acceptable for consideration of the results. For our example, all supporting records, such as those from the supplier of the rabbits used in the study (the source), must be maintained in the study file.
5. The most appropriate means for a unique ID of the test system; this is especially important if an animal must be replaced during the study.
6. The direction is fairly clear and will generally be dictated by test guidelines. The "methods for control of bias" in our example could require that skin irritation be evaluated by a technician other than the one applying the test substance. For control of bias, if the word *randomly* is used, there must be a documented method in an SOP, such as the use of lines in a published random numbers table.
7. Long-term rodent studies may deliver the test substance via diet, hence the emphasis on purity of the food source. Where this is not a factor, management may choose to rely on batch evaluations available from the feed manufacturer, conduct an independent laboratory analysis, or a combination of these two methods. Where it is necessary to solubilize a test material, it will be necessary to trace the solvent back to a particular lot, with the expiration date and other details. When considering this GLP point, let the particular situation guide the methods and practices used, always keeping in mind the need for documentation to reconstruct what materials and methods were used.
8. Most of this section will be drawn from the testing guidelines and possibly sponsor requests.
9. The direction is clear.
10. The direction is clear.

11. The direction is clear.
12. The direction is clear; note the use of the word *proposed*, which allows for changes due to actual circumstances.

REFERENCES

1. Jones AB. Principles in quality assurance: Part 2. Don't hide behind the regulations, *Qual Assur J*. 2003;7(1):4–10.
2. Food and Drug Administration. Searle Investigation Task Force. Report of Preclinical (Animal) Studies of G.D. Searle Company, Skokie Illinois, Mar. 1976.
3. 1980 Grand Jury Charges, *United States of America* vs. *J.C. Calandra, M.L. Keplinger, P.L. Wright and J.B. Plank*.
4. Food and Drug Administration, Department of Health, Education and Welfare. *Fed Reg*. 1978;43:59986–60025.
5. U.S. Department of Health and Human Services, Food and Drug Administration. 21 CFR Part 11. Electronic Records; Electronic Signatures; Final Rule Electronic Submissions; Establishment of Public Docket; Notice. *Fed Reg*. 1997;62:13429–13466.
6. Food and Drug Administration, Division of Field Investigations, Office of Regional Operations, Office of Regulatory Affairs. Glossary of Computerized System and Software Development Terminology. Available at: www.fda.gov/ora/Inspect ref/igs/gloss.html.
7. Stoneburner G, Goguen A, Feringa A. *Risk Management Guide for Information Technology Systems*. National Institute of Standards and Technology Special Publication 800–30. Washington, DC: U.S. Government Printing Office; 2001.
8. Guidance for Industry: Quality Systems Approach to Pharmaceutical Current Good Manufacturing Practice Regulations. U.S. Department of Health and Human Services, Food and Drug Administration; 2006.
9. U.S. Department of Health and Human Services, Food and Drug Administration. Title 21, Food and Drugs, Chapter I: Part 58, Good Laboratory Practice for Nonclinical Laboratory Studies. Final Rule. *Fed Reg*. 43:Dec. 22, 1978.
10. U.S. Department of Health and Human Services, Food And Drug Administration. Title 21, Food and Drugs, Chapter I: Part 58, Good Laboratory Practice for Nonclinical Laboratory Studies. Final Rule. *Fed Reg*. 1987;52:33768–33782.
11. World Health Organization, Special Programme for Research and Training in Tropical Diseases. Handbook: Quality Practices in Basic Biomedical Research. Available at: www.who.int/tdr/svc/publications/training-guideline-publications/handbook-quality-practices-biomedical-research.
12. Masson M, Handy L, Volsen SG. *Guidelines for Quality in Non-Regulated Research*. Ipswich, UK: British Association of Research Quality Assurance; 2006.
13. *Quality Assurance and GLP*. OECD Series on Principles of Good Laboratory Practice and Compliance Monitoring, No. 4 (rev.). ENV/JM/MONO(99)20. Paris: Organization for Economic Co-operation and Development; 1999.
14. *OECD Principles of Good Laboratory Practice*. OECD Series on Principles of Good Laboratory Practice and Compliance Monitoring, No. 1. ENV/MC/CHEM(98)17. Paris: Organization for Economic Co-operation and Development; 1998.

15. *The Application of the OECD Principles of GLP to the Organisation and Management of Multi-site Studies*. OECD Series on Principles of Good Laboratory Practice and Compliance Monitoring, No. 13. Consensus Document of the Working Group on Good Laboratory Practice. ENV/JM/MONO(2002)9. Paris: Organisation for Economic Cooperation and Development; 2002.
16. U.S. Food and Drug Administration. *Compliance Program Guidance Manual for FDA Staff*, Chap. 48, Bioresearch Monitoring, Good Laboratory Practice (Nonclinical Laboratories). Compliance Program 7348.808. Implementation Date Feb. 21, 2001.
17. Colligon I, Rosa M. GLP SOPs for equipment calibration and maintenance: Part 1. An overview. *Qual Assur J*., 2006;10(4):107–110.
18. Colligon I, Rosa M. GLP SOPs for equipment calibration and maintenance: Part 2. An organized approach to streamlining procedural documentation. *Qual Assur J*. 2006;10(4):203–207.
19. Colligon I, Rosa M. GLP SOPs for equipment calibration and maintenance: Part 3. Process mapping for SOP development. *Qual Assur J*. 2006;10(4):279–285.
20. Colligon I, Rosa M. GLP SOPs for equipment calibration and maintenance: Part 4. Logistics of SOP writing. *Qual Assur J*., 2007;11(1):60–61.
21. Colligon I, Rosa M. GLP SOPs for equipment calibration and maintenance: Part 5. SOP templates and SOP on SOPs. *Qual Assur J*. 2007;11(3–4):295–301.
22. Colligon I, Rosa M. GLP SOPs for equipment calibration and maintenance: Part 6. Implementation of SOPs. *Qual Assur J*. 2007;11(3–4):302–307.
23. American Association for Laboratory Animal Science. Information available at: www.aalas.org. Accessed Jan. 5, 2009.
24. *Consensus Document: The Application of GLP Principles to Short Term Studies*. OECD Series on Principles of Good Laboratory Practice and Compliance Monitoring, No. 7 (rev.). ENV/JM/MONO(99)23. Paris: Organisation for Economic Co-operation and Development; 1999.
25. *Establishment and Control of Archives that Operate in Compliance with the Principles of GLP*. OECD Series on Principles of Good Laboratory Practice and Compliance Monitoring, No. 15. Advisory Document of the Working Group on Good Laboratory Practice. ENV/JM/MONO(2007)10. Paris: Organisation for Economic Co-operation and Development; 2007.
26. Working Group on Information Technology (AGIT). Good laboratory practice (GLP): guidelines for the archiving of electronic raw data in a GLP environment. *Qual Assur J*. 2003;7(4):262–269.
27. Jones AB. Bioanalytical quality assurance: concepts and concerns. *Qual Assur J*. 2006;10:101–106.
28. Japanese Pharmaceutical Affairs Bureau, Ministry of Health and Welfare. MHW Ordinance 21. Mar. 26, 1997.
29. Guidance for Industry: Bioanalytical Method Validation. U.S. Department of Health and Human Services, Food and Drug Administration; 2001.
30. Shah VP, Midha KK, Dighe S, et al. Analytical methods validation: bioavailability, bioequivalence and pharmacokinetic studies. *J Pharm Sci*. 1992;81(3):309–312.
31. Shah VP, Midha KK, Findlay JWA, et al. Bioanalytical method validation: a revisit with a decade of progress. *Pharm Res*. 2000;17(12):1551–1557.

32. U.S Department of Health and Human Services, Food and Drug Administration. Title 21, Food and Drugs, Chapter I, Subchapter D, Drugs for Human Use. Part 320: Bioavailability and Bioequivalence Requirements.
33. U.S. Food and Drug Administration. *Compliance Program Guidance Manual for FDA Staff*, Chap. 48, Bioresearch Monitoring Human Drugs, In Vivo Bioequivalence. Compliance Program 7348.001.
34. Guidance for Industry: Conduct and Analysis of Bioavailability and Bioequivalence Studies, Part A: Oral Dosage Formulations Used for Systemic Effects. Health Canada, Health Products and Food Branch; 1992.
35. Guidance for Industry: Conduct and Analysis of Bioavailability and Bioequivalence Studies, Part B: Oral Modified Release Formulations. Health Canada, Health Products and Food Branch; 1996.
36. ICH Safety Guideline: Toxicokinetics: A Guidance for Assessing Systemic Exposure in Toxicity Studies. ICH S3A. International Conference on Harmonization; 1995.
37. Guidance on the Investigation of Bioavailability and Bioequivalence. CPMP/EWP/QWP/1401/98. EMEA Committee for Proprietary Medicinal Products. Adopted July 2001.
38. Monk S. Reference to Good Laboratory Practice in EMEA Guidance on the Investigation of Bioavailability and Bioequivalence. United Kingdom Good Laboratory Practice Monitoring Authority; May 2002.
39. U.S. Department of Health and Human Services, Food and Drug Administration. 21 CFR Part 11, Electronic Records; Electronic Signatures; Final Rule Electronic Submissions; Establishment of Public Docket; Notice. *Fed Reg*. 1997;62:13429–13466.
40. Guidance for Industry: Part 11, Electronic Records; Electronic Signatures—Scope and Application. U.S. Department of Health and Human Services, Food and Drug Administration; Aug. 2003.
41. Guidance for Industry: Computerized Systems Used in Clinical Trials. Draft Guidance. U.S. Department of Health and Human Services, Food and Drug Administration; 2004.
42. Stiles T, Grant V, Mawby N. *Good Clinical Laboratory Practice: A Quality System for Laboratories That Undertake the Analyses of Samples from Clinical Trials*. Ipswich, UK: British Association of Research Quality Assurance; 2003.
43. Viswanathan CT, Bansal S, Booth B, et al. Workshop/conference report: Quantitative bioanalytical methods validation and implementation: best practices for chromatographic and ligand binding assays. *AAPS J*. 2007;9(1):E30–E42.
44. Nowatzke W, Woolf E. Best practices during bioanalytical method validation for the characterization of assay reagents and the evaluation of analyte stability in assay standards, quality controls, and study samples. *AAPS J*. 2007;9(2):E117–E122.
45. James CA, Hill HM. Procedural elements involved in maintaining bioanalytical data integrity for good laboratory practices studies and regulated clinical studies. *AAPS J*. 2007;9(2):E123–E127.
46. Kelley M, DeSilva B. Key Elements of bioanalytical method validation for macromolecules. *AAPS J*. 2007;9(2):E156–E163.
47. Rocci ML Jr, Devanarayan V, Haughey DB, Jardieu P. Confirmatory reanalysis of incurred bioanalytical samples. *AAPS J*. 2007;9(3):E336–E343.

48. Hughes NC, Wong EY, Fan J, Bajaj N. Determination of carryover and contamination for mass spectrometry–based chromatographic assays. *AAPS J*. 2007;9(3):E353–E360.
49. U.S. Department of Health and Human Services, Food and Drug Administration. Letter to MDS Pharma Services, Dec. 2004. Available at: www.fda.gov/cder/warn/2004/mdsuntitledltr.pdf. Accessed Jan. 5, 2009.
50. U.S. Department of Health and Human Services Food and Drug Administration. Letter to MDS Pharma Services, Apr. 2004. Available at: www.fda.gov/cder/warn/2004/MDSPharma.pdf. Accessed Jan. 5, 2009.
51. U.S. Department of Health and Human Services, Food and Drug Administration. Title 21, Food and Drugs Chapter I, Subchapter H Medical Devices: Part 820 Quality System Regulation.
52. Guideline on the Evaluation of Control Samples Used in Nonclinical Safety Studies: Checking for Contamination with the Test Substance. CPMP/SWP/1094/04. London: European Medicines Evaluation Agency Committee for Medicinal Products for Human Use (CHMP); Mar. 17, 2005.
53. Gongliewski N. FDA hopes to modernize GLPs. *MARSQA Monitor*. 2008;12(1):3.
54. Directive 87/18/EEC on Harmonization of Laws, Regulations, and Administrative Provisions Relating to the Application of the Principles of Good Laboratory Practice and the Verification of Their Applications for Tests on Chemical Substances. Council of the European Economic Community; Dec. 18, 1986. *Off J Eur Commun. L*. 1987;1S:29–30.
55. Carson PA, Dent NJ. *Good Laboratory and Clinical Practices: Techniques for the Quality Assurance Professional*. Oxford; UK: Heinemann Newnes; 1990.
56. OECD Web site. www.oecd.org/department/0,3355,en 2649 34381 1 1 1 1 1,00.html. Accessed Jan. 6, 2009.
57. Japanese Note Verbal. Subject GLP Mutual Recognition. In: *International Cooperative Agreements Manual*. Washington, DC: U.S. Department of Health and Human Services, Food and Drug Administration; Apr. 15, 1983.
58. Sectoral Annex on Good Laboratory Practice for Chemicals, Part A. Available at: www.mofa.go.jp/region/europe/eu/agreement-glp.pdf. Accessed Jan. 6, 2009.
59. U.S. Department of Health and Human Services Food and Drug Administration. List of active labs. Available at: www.fda.gov/ora/compliance ref/bimo/GLP/wh list intro.htm. Accessed Jan. 6, 2009.
60. Health and Human Services Office of Extramural Research, NIH, Office of Laboratory Animal Welfare (OLAW). Available at: www.hhs.gov. Accessed Jan. 16, 2009.
61. U.S. Department of Agriculture. 9 CFR Part 1, 1989;54:168(Aug 31). See also: www.nal.usda.gov/awic. Accessed Jan. 16, 2009.
62. Association for Assessment and Accreditation of Laboratory Animal Care International. Information available at: www.aaalac.org/. Accessed Jan. 6, 2009.
63. *Computerized Data Systems for Nonclinical Safety Assessment: Current Concepts and Quality Assurance*. Drug Information Association; 2008.
64. *GAMP 5: A Risk-Based Approach to Compliant GxP Computerized Systems*. Tampa, FL: International Society for Pharmaceutical Engineering; 2008.

PART V

PLANNING THE FIRST-IN-HUMAN STUDY AND REGULATORY SUBMISSION

10

ESTIMATION OF HUMAN STARTING DOSE FOR PHASE I CLINICAL PROGRAMS

LORRENE A. BUCKLEY, PARAG GARHYAN, RAFAEL PONCE, AND STANLEY A. ROBERTS

10.1 INTRODUCTION

There is (arguably) no greater leap forward in the development of a novel therapeutic agent than the transition from conducting animal studies to the first phase I trial in humans. Chief among the myriad considerations that must be carefully weighed before this step is taken are the potential risks (e.g., human safety, resource investment) and rewards (e.g., improved patient outcome). In nonclinical development, a variety of investments are made that extend the understanding of the biological properties of the molecule. The decision to administer a first dose to humans is based on the collective experience, scientific knowledge, and judgment from a number of scientific disciplines at the center of this transition, including physicians, toxicologists, and specialists in drug metabolism, pharmacokinetics, and pharmaceutics. The fundamental tenets for establishing a safe starting dose in humans are both simple and rational, and have been applied successfully to the testing of new pharmaceuticals for decades:

- Characterize the exposure–response relationship associated with both the beneficial activity and toxicity of the therapeutic agent in at least two representative animal species, spanning from a no-observed (pharmacologic or

Early Drug Development: Strategies and Routes to First-in-Human Trials, Edited by Mitchell N. Cayen

toxicologic) effect level (NOEL) to a dose associated with some toxicity(ies), and identify potential target organs and safety biomarkers.

- Characterize the absorption, distribution, metabolism, and excretion (ADME) of the molecule and establish the pharmacokinetic profile in representative animal species.
- Identify and consider differences between the toxicology study species and humans that may modify predicted exposure or response in humans.
- Maintain a healthy skepticism regarding the state of knowledge, proceeding with due caution when transitioning from nonclinical to human dosing.

It is not a simple matter to fully integrate all of the information to identify a starting drug dosage and treatment regimen that minimizes risk to the health of the trial participants. The primary complication for this effort is that in many cases there is no prior direct experience with a comparable agent to guide this process. While setting a starting dose too high can present an obvious risk to trial participants, arbitrarily setting a starting dose too low can expend time and resources while administering doses that are far below the therapeutic window, which would slow development of the therapeutic agent and increase costs. This presents a direct risk to the product under development, which could ultimately lead to reduced availability of critical therapies if resources are used inefficiently.

In this chapter we review the various methods and considerations for estimating a safe first-in-human (FIH) dose, including relevant research strategies and regulatory guidance documents that are pertinent to this process. We also discuss how characteristics of the therapeutic agent can influence the projection of safe dosing in phase I clinical trials. Fictionalized versions of actual case histories provide illustrative examples of how nonclinical data are used to support initial dosing in humans and also include the strategies that were implemented to ensure successful transition to phase I human trials. As with most voyages of discovery, safety cannot be guaranteed explicitly, so we also discuss how diligent planning and an unbiased evaluation of the available data can prepare an organization for a successful initiation of the first human trial.

10.2 CHARACTERISTICS OF WELL-BEHAVED THERAPEUTIC CANDIDATES

The biological or chemical platforms used to identify and select promising candidates for clinical development are diverse and involve the infusion of significant financial, scientific, and staff resources early into discovery research, well before the filing of the investigational new drug application (IND; in the United States) or clinical trial application (CTA; in the European Union). Over the last three decades, this investment has resulted in tremendous improvement in physicochemical, pharmacological, drug disposition, and toxicological information to facilitate the identification, optimization, and progression of the best new therapeutic candidates for clinical development and marketing. These efforts have led to the evolution of a tool set of screening assays used during drug discovery to define the potential liabilities for new candidate molecules, culling the least desirable molecules well before the costly FIH-enabling studies are begun.

Current discovery research strategies often focus on defining the rate-limiting characteristics (e.g., target organ toxicity, poor pharmacokinetics) for these new agents, followed by problem solving with experimental methods and assays to select the best compounds. Some of the first successes in utilizing these evolved drug-hunting tool sets were related to improving drug disposition: that is the pharmacokinetics (PK)/ADME attributes of new chemical entities (NCEs; should include small molecules). Development of these tools was facilitated by the increased availability of primary liver, kidney, and gut cells plus cell lines from a variety of animal species (including humans) and increasingly sensitive technologies in analytical chemistry. General criteria desired for optimal PK/ADME properties include a desirable pharmacokinetic and pharmacodynamic (PD) profile, linear and time-invariant pharmacokinetics, low variability of pharmacokinetic characteristics (e.g., no metabolic polymorphisms), good bioavailability, minimal food effects, no postural activities or circadian effect, minimal drug–drug interaction possibilities, low plasma protein binding (e.g., less than 80%), availability of interventions for acute or chronic overdosage, and long-acting pharmacodynamic effect (with reversibility). Using a variety of in silico, in vitro, and in vivo experiments, a number of these characteristics can be determined or predicted to facilitate the selection of a safe dosage in an FIH study. For instance, functionally significant predictions for NCEs can be made for the routes and mechanism(s) of drug absorption, the primary organs of distribution, the routes and mechanism of metabolic clearance and/or renal excretion, the clearance by efflux transporters, and the potential to be either a victim or a perpetrator of drug–drug interactions. New methods have also been, and continue to be, developed to characterize the risk of certain compounds or classes for specific toxicological liabilities. These include a variety of in silico, in vitro, and in vivo assays and application of genomic, proteomic, or metabonomic methods [1–3]. Although not a focus of the current chapter, we recognize the importance of these new, sensitive methods in selecting alternative development candidates and in supplementing more traditional regulatory-based nonclinical toxicology and pathology-based experimentation. This accumulated knowledge typically provides a sound basis for developing a profile of anticipated generalized and target organ toxicity in humans. The relevance of nonclinical models to human safety assessment is evidenced by retrospective analyses of the traditional two-species (rodent and nonrodent) testing paradigm, for which there is over a 70% concordance between animal and human toxicities for compounds that have been clinically tested [4].

10.3 REGULATORY GUIDANCES FOR FIH-ENABLING NONCLINICAL SAFETY ASSESSMENT: GENERAL PRINCIPLES

The International Conference on Harmonization (ICH) M3(R2) and S6 guidance documents provide general expectations for the type and timing of nonclinical data collected to support clinical evaluation of small and large molecules [5,6]. Data from such pivotal nonclinical toxicity studies are used to establish the starting dose for FIH trials. Under current regulatory guidance for the development of novel therapeutic agents, these nonclinical studies are designed to characterize the toxicity of the new drug candidate with respect to target organ, dose-dependency, relationship to exposure and reversibility under conditions that mimic the intended therapeutic application (i.e., dose route, frequency, duration). *Note*: There is an ICH S9 guidance covering the development of certain anticancer drugs in which the use of severely toxic or highest non-severely toxic doses, rather than the NOAEL, is employed to estimate a human starting dose. This special case will not be further discussed in this chapter [80].

The generally accepted paradigm for the nonclinical data required to support FIH trials with small molecules consists of repeated dose toxicity studies in two species (one rodent and one nonrodent) (Chapter 7), safety pharmacology studies (Chapter 6), and an assessment of the potential for genetic toxicity (Chapter 7). As outlined in ICH S6, the design of the nonclinical safety program for biotherapeutics is based on a case-by-case risk-based strategy, due to the specific targeted nature of these molecules; some important differences in the types of studies conducted for small molecules and biotherapeutics have been highlighted separately [7] (Chapter 12). For example, genetic toxicology studies are generally not appropriate for biopharmaceuticals because these large molecular weight molecules generally do not penetrate the cell or interact with the DNA or chromosomal material. In addition, specialized tests such as tissue cross-reactivity studies and immunotoxicology examinations may also be required for biotherapeutics, depending on the nature of the molecule and predicted or observed biological effects.

An important consideration for biotherapeutics, in particular, is the need to conduct nonclinical studies in animal species that exhibit relevant pharmacology [5,8]. This expectation recognizes that animals and humans may differ in the DNA–protein sequence, the availability and distribution of the target, the affinity of the drug for the target, the relative potency for inducing the intended biological response, the modulation capability of the downstream signaling cascades, as well as other potentially unanticipated factors. Thus, there is a need to justify selection of the appropriate animal species used for the nonclinical safety of biotechnology-derived therapeutics by evaluating these parameters using tissues and/or cells from animals and humans. As we demonstrate later, this information also becomes very useful in modeling dose–response effects across species. The expectation that we use relevant species for toxicology testing assumes that data in the test species can be considered meaningful and reduces the potential for a false negative result. In other words, in the absence of biological activity (in an irrelevant species), the toxicity study will probably not be able to detect a truely adverse effect of the molecule and could thus misinform the selection process for the first human dose. Because many biotechnology-derived agents have limited cross-species activity, it is not uncommon for only one species, often the nonhuman primate, to be studied in nonclinical safety assessment studies.

10.4 NONCLINICAL PHARMACOKINETICS AND PHARMACODYNAMICS FOR HUMAN DOSE PROJECTION

Prior to the first human dosing of a new therapeutic candidate, it is important to fully characterize the PK/PD properties of the NCE, which should include the disposition and the relationship between dose (or concentration), efficacy and/or toxicity [9,10]. This characterization is critical in the selection of doses chosen for clinical testing. Various PK/PD modeling and simulation approaches can be undertaken to predict the starting (and efficacious) dose and dosing regimen [11]. These approaches include the establishment of nonclinical pharmacokinetic characteristics, prediction of human pharmacokinetics (e.g., allometric scaling of nonclinical pharmacokinetics, scaling of parameters obtained via in vitro methods or other predictive tools), and empirical scaling of efficacy by using the following:

- Pharmacokinetic data from nonclinical species, including clearance, volume of distribution, elimination half-life, and bioavailability under conditions similar to the intended clinical dosing regimen
- Toxicity studies in nonclinical species to establish dose–response relationships for toxicological/pharmacological activity and tolerable doses
- In vitro data to predict tissue–drug interactions using human and animal cells
- In vivo efficacy models in relevant species to obtain nonclinical pharmacodynamic data
- Pharmacodynamic data from comparator molecules to inform the human efficacy prediction for the therapeutic candidate

In summary, the successful integration and amalgamation of toxicology, pharmacokinetic, and pharmacodynamic data can be used to establish the starting dose for the first human study and to identify dose escalation and study cessation guidelines.

10.5 ESTABLISHING THE FIRST-IN-HUMAN DOSE

At present there exist several different regulatory pathways toward administration of the first human dose [9,12]. The conventional approaches to support phase I dose selection rely on data from studies of nonclinical safety, pharmacokinetics, and pharmacodynamics to define the no observed adverse effects level (NOAEL)

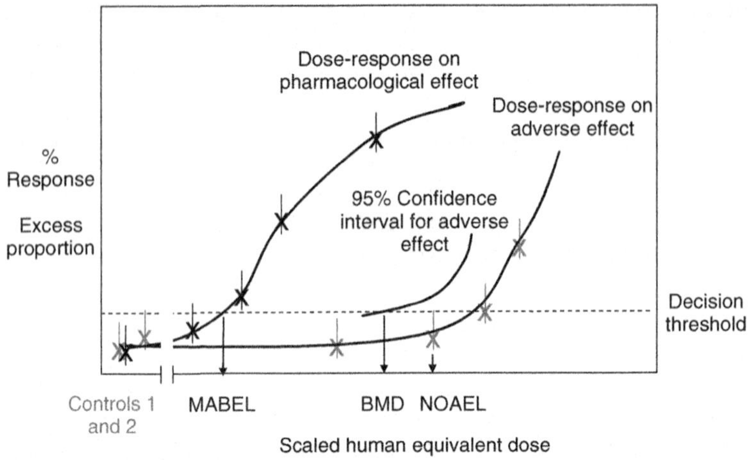

FIGURE 10.1 Derivation of the minimal anticipated biological effect level (MABEL) and the benchmark dose (BMD) in comparison to the no adverse effect level (NOAEL). Dose–response modeling is used to derive the MABEL (based on pharmacology data) and the BMD (based on toxicity data).

or estimates of biological activity, which are termed either the minimal anticipated biological effect level (MABEL) or the pharmacologically active dose (PAD). The first human dose may be estimated to produce a fraction of exposure achieved at either the MABEL or NOAEL. Whereas a conservative approach may derive an initial dose that elicits very low pharmacological activity based on the MABEL, toxicology-driven FIH dose selection relies on the NOAEL established in the most sensitive nonclinical species (see Figure 10.1). Alternatively, under a constrained set of clinical testing conditions, it is also possible to administer a subpharmacological dose (termed a *microdose*) based on a limited set of nonclinical safety and pharmacokinetic data (Chapter 11). We provide an overview for each of these approaches below.

10.5.1 Phase I Clinical Trial Support: Use of the NOAEL-Based Approach

The U.S. Food and Drug Administration (FDA) issued a final guidance to industry in July 2005 that outlined a standardized approach for estimating safe starting doses in FIH clinical trials in normal healthy humans [9]. This approach, as outlined in Figure 10.2, includes identification of a dose associated with the NOAEL in animals; allometric conversion of that dose to a human equivalent dose (HED) and application of a "safety" factor to account for uncertainty in extrapolation of results from nonclinical species to humans. In keeping with the primary emphasis on the safety of clinical trial volunteers, this guidance uses a conservative approach in the definition of a relevant NOAEL, the selection of dose metric, and an appropriate safety factor. Any decisions that represent departures from the guidance require explicit justification.

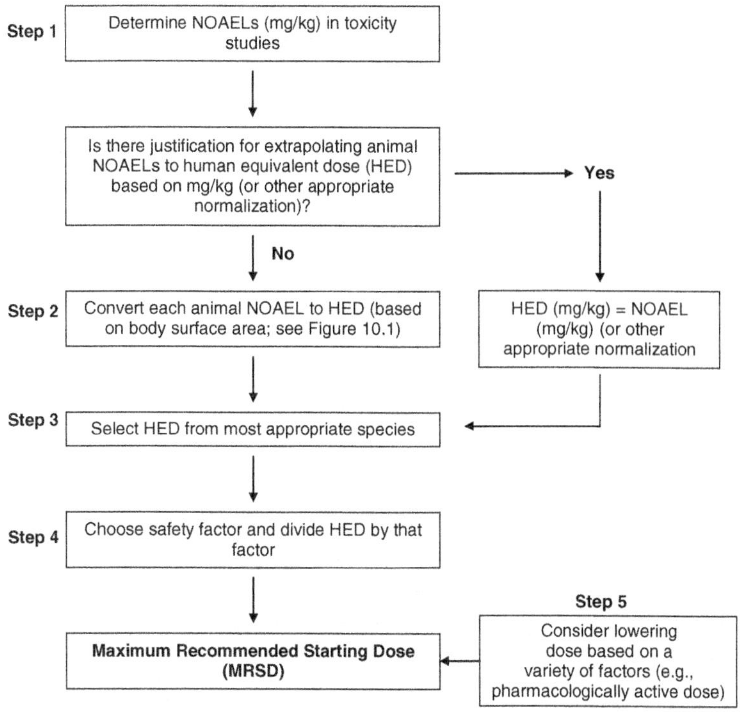

FIGURE 10.2 Selection of the maximum recommended starting dose (MRSD) for drugs administered systemically to normal volunteers. (From [9].)

Characterization of the NOAEL and Toxic Doses As outlined previously, the FIH dose using the current regulatory practice (for novel agents to be tested in healthy human volunteers) is based on animal safety estimates of the NOAEL [9]. By this method, the NOAEL from toxicity studies is used to determine the HED, after which a suitable safety factor is applied. The appropriate application of this general paradigm to specific cases presumes that we will apply our best judgment in designing experiments and then interpreting the data as they become available.

The NOAEL is defined as the highest dose tested in the nonclinical toxicity study that does not produce a biologically relevant increase in adverse effects compared to the control group [9], although other definitions and considerations may apply [13,14]. Adverse effects that are toxicologically relevant, even if they are not statistically significant, should be considered in determining the NOAEL [9]. It is essential that the pivotal animal studies conducted to support an FIH study be designed and conducted to determine doses with and without adverse effects. It is common practice to conduct non-GLP (good laboratory practices) pilot or range-finding studies beforehand, to optimize the design of the pivotal GLP study. When toxicology data are obtained in two or more animal species, the toxicologist will need to identify the species that provides the most relevant basis for FIH dose estimation. Typically, the NOAEL from the most sensitive species is used to establish the starting dose. It should be noted that for biotherapeutics, the most commonly used nonhuman primates are the cynomolgus or rhesus monkeys, which are generally assumed to be the most relevant species (based on target homology or binding/activity similar to humans) for which excellent historical reference data are available. Therefore, these NHP species are typically used unless there are overriding considerations (e.g., the inappropriate expression of the target in normal nonhuman primates, nonrelevant mechanism of toxicity, and/or the presence of antidrug antibodies).

To establish a fully integrated toxicology assessment of a new drug, the toxicologist must carefully consider all the adverse effects produced by the NCE. This process is unique to each therapeutic agent and mechanism of action, although chemical or pharmacological class effects can certainly play a major role in helping to fully understand the potential risk for any specific compound. For biotherapeutics, the toxicity observed often results from exaggerated pharmacology. Such was the case, for example, for mortality and histological evidence of systemic thrombosis and hemorrhage in monkeys associated with the administration of recombinant factor XIII, a thrombin-activated zymogen associated with cross-linking of the fibrin clot [15]. Other examples may include evidence of vascular leak and hepatic injury associated with IL2-mediated immune system activation [16] or lymphocytopenia and reduced serum globulin concentrations following administration of a monoclonal antibody targeting cytokines critical for plasma cell survival [17]. In each of these cases, the toxicologist(s) considered the balance between therapeutic utility and the potential to do harm, sometimes accepting greater risk of adverse events for the opportunity to treat more serious disease conditions for which there are no current treatments. Particularly in cases where the therapeutic window is small, it is critical to evaluate reversibility and to define clear guidelines for patient monitoring and treatment cessation. In such cases the clinical development program may also be limited to studies in patients expressing the disease rather than in healthy volunteers that would probably necessitate the selection of a more "conservative" (i.e., lower) starting dose and dose escalation strategy. Some of the challenges arising from toxicity studies affecting FIH dosing are summarized in Table 10.1.

There are a number of recognized issues with NOAEL-based regulatory strategies [13]. These include the requirement that the NOAEL be one of the doses tested in the nonclinical study, the lack of consideration regarding study power and uncertainty around the NOAEL dose, and the inadequate characterization of the dose–response relationship. For these reasons, interest is growing for use of the benchmark dose (BMD) as an alternative to the NOAEL for establishing regulatory exposure standards, particularly by the U.S. Environment Protection Agency (EPA) [18]. Using the benchmark dose approach, a dose–response model is derived in the range of the data available and a dose estimated for which a low level of adverse response is expected (e.g., 5% response). The uncertainty around this dose is estimated using a confidence limit or Bayesian posterior, and the lower confidence limit of this dose is used as the estimate of the benchmark dose (see Figure 10.1). The EPA currently accepts the benchmark dose for

TABLE 10.1 Toxicity Study Outcomes Affecting the Approach to FIH Dose Estimation

Challenges Arising from Toxicity Studies	Considerations for Proceeding to FIH Study
Identification of a toxicity that is not easily monitored in the clinic	Evaluate whether the toxicity is consistent with the expected pharmacological activity of the molecule Evaluate progression and reversibility of the toxicity in relation to the intended clinical use Perform mechanistic studies (if possible) using in vitro or ex vivo methods to identify possible relevance to treated patients and possible biomarkers suitable for monitoring Evaluate therapeutic window and assess risk to patients Consider clinical studies where risk–benefit is justified and collect human data
An adverse event is identified in each dose group, so it is not possible to define a NOAEL	Evaluate dose–response relationship (incidence and severity) Evaluate frequency of finding in untreated animals Can this be considered a background finding or unrelated to treatment? Consider a MABEL approach to derive a FIH dose with large margin of safety and the inclusion of appropriate monitoring in the clinical protocol
Rodent and nonrodent species reveal different toxicity profiles	Is there a mechanistic basis for difference that would point to which species might be the more relevant species for human risk? Otherwise, select most sensitive species for FIH dose estimation
No toxicity is observed in the nonclinical safety study	Apply MABEL approach to estimate starting dose in the low pharmacologically active dose range

environmental risk assessment, but this approach is not currently used by the FDA in establishing FIH doses, so it is not discussed further in this chapter.

Application of a Safety Factor Under current guidance and by general convention agreement, the default safety factor to be used when establishing the HED is 10. This safety factor is considered a starting point and may be increased or decreased according to the specific circumstances surrounding the therapeutic agent and the patient population. Situations that might lead to a more conservative safety factor (i.e., >10) involve therapeutic agents with novel biology that is poorly understood; data derived from animal models that have limited perceived utility; toxicities that are not easily monitored, irreversible, are judged to be risky (e.g., steep dose–response curve, toxicity without premonitory signs or unexplained mortality), or have perceived unpredictable exposure–response profiles (e.g., large variability of doses or plasma drug levels eliciting toxic effects, nonlinear pharmacokinetics in the therapeutic range, or inadequate dose–response data). Conversely, a decrease in the safety factor (i.e., <10) might be considered for agents in a well-characterized class (and administered by the same route, duration, and treatment schedule), demonstrating similar metabolic and toxicological profiles as preceding agents, or for agents that have limited toxicities that are easily monitored and consistent with the biological properties expected for the molecule.

10.5.2 Estimating a Human Dose

There exist a number of approaches for deriving the first dose and the dosage regimen based on data derived from animal experiments. These include allometric scaling of dose and exposure or modeling to predict human pharmacokinetic parameters. Some of the frequently used methods described in the literature are presented briefly here.

Conversion of Animal Dose to a Human Equivalent Dose Using Allometric Scaling of Dose Several approaches exist for scaling a NOAEL dose in animals to an HED. The most common method relies on allometric scaling using body surface area, although other metrics may be used as appropriate. The basis for this technique is derived from empirical analyses comparing the toxicities of anticancer drugs in animals (based on the LD_{10}, the dose causing lethality in 10% of the animals) to the maximum tolerated dose in humans [19–21]. This research demonstrated a linear correlation across species for relative toxicity when dose was expressed as a function of surface area (or equivalently, as mg/kg$^{0.67}$ per day). Table 10.2 provides the necessary information to convert an animal dose (in mg/kg) to an HED (in mg/kg) using body weight and surface area parameters for common laboratory species, consistent with the FDA guidance [9]. A couple of examples of such conversion follow.

Example 1: Conversion of a 1-mg/kg NOAEL dose in mice to an HED using surface area scaling. Using Table 10.2, a 1-mg/kg dose in mice corresponds to a 2.86-mg/m^2 dose when converted to a surface area–based dose (1 mg/kg $\times$ 0.02 kg $\div$ 0.007 m^2). Under the assumption that doses scale linearly based on surface area, the human equivalent dose would also be equal to 2.86 mg/m^2. Using the conversion factors in Table 10.2, the scaled human equivalent dose in mg/kg would be equal to 0.08 mg/kg for a 60-kg person when converted back to a body weight–based dose (2.86 mg/m^2 $\times$ 1.62 m^2 $\div$ 60 kg). Thus, the HED

TABLE 10.2 Conversion of Dose Based on Body Weight (mg/kg) to a Human Equivalent Dose Using Surface Area Scaling

Species	Weight (kg)	Surface Area (m^2)	Dose Conversion (kg/m^2)	Human Equivalent Dose	
				Multiply[a]	Divide[b]
Mouse	0.02	0.007	2.86	0.08	12.96
Rat	0.15	0.025	6.00	0.16	6.17
Rabbit	1.8	0.15	12.00	0.32	3.09
Monkey	3	0.25	12.00	0.32	3.09
Dog	10	0.5	20.00	0.54	1.85
Human	60	1.62	37.04	1.00	1.00

[a]To derive the human equivalent dose using surface area scaling, multiply the animal dose (mg/kg) by this factor.
[b]To derive the human equivalent dose using surface area scaling, divide the animal dose (mg/kg) by this factor.

TABLE 10.3 Conversion of Dose Based on Body Weight (mg/kg) to a Human Equivalent Dose Using Surface Area Scaling

Species	Weight (kg)	Weight Ratio[a]	Human Equivalent Dose ($b = 0.67$)[b]		Human Equivalent Dose ($b = 0.75$)[b]	
			Multiply[c]	Divide[d]	Multiply[c]	Divide[d]
Mouse	0.02	0.00033	0.07	14.38	0.14	7.40
Rat	0.15	0.0025	0.14	7.35	0.22	4.47
Rabbit	1.8	0.03	0.31	3.21	0.42	2.40
Monkey	3	0.05	0.37	2.71	0.47	2.11
Dog	10	0.167	0.55	1.82	0.64	1.57
Human	60	1	1.00	1.00	1.00	1.00

[a]Animal/human body weight.
[b]b is an exponent of body weight to derive the surface area.
[c]To derive the human equivalent dose using surface area scaling, multiply the animal dose (mg/kg) by this factor.
[d]To derive the human equivalent dose using surface area scaling, divide the animal dose (mg/kg) by this factor.

in human (mg/kg, assuming 60 kg, 1.62 m^2) is approximately equivalent to 0.08 times (or approximately 1/13) the dose in mice (mg/kg, 0.02 kg, 0.007 m^2).

As an alternative approach, Table 10.3 provides the necessary information to convert an animal dose (in mg/kg) for common laboratory species to an HED (in mg/kg) using allometric scaling consistent with FDA guidance [9]. In this approach, the HED is estimated according to

$$\text{HED} = \text{animal dose (mg/kg)} \times \left(\frac{W_{\text{animal}}}{W_{\text{human}}}\right)^{1-b} \tag{10.1}$$

where W represents the weight (in kilograms) and b is the scaling exponent. As discussed below, there exists some debate about the most appropriate scaling exponent, but under current guidelines, the accepted standard exponent is 0.67.

Example 2: Conversion of a 1-mg/kg NOAEL dose in mice to an HED using allometric scaling. Using the parameters listed in Table 10.3, equation (10.1) may be parameterized as

$$\begin{aligned} \text{HED} &= 1 \text{ mg/kg} \times \left(\frac{0.02\text{kg}_{\text{mouse}}}{60\text{kg}_{\text{human}}}\right)^{1-0.67} \\ &= 0.071 \text{ mg/kg} \end{aligned}$$

As shown in Table 10.3 and calculated above, the HED in humans is 0.07 times (or approximately 1/14) the dose in mice (for a 20-g mouse and a 60-kg human, $b = 0.67$). Comparison of the results obtained across species in Tables 10.2 and 10.3 demonstrate a high degree of concordance of results for these two approaches when the allometric scaling factor is equal to 0.67; because surface area varies with body weight $(W)^{0.67}$, these two approaches are considered to be interchangeable [22].

The discussion above demonstrates an empirical approach toward interspecies scaling based on comparative analyses of toxicity data associated with anticancer agents. However, some analyses evaluating alternative scaling metrics support the use of 0.75 rather than 0.67 as the most appropriate value [22]. These include analyses [23–25] that evaluated the allometric relationships governing clearance and dosage at the target tissue for cytotoxic agents, reanalyses of the cancer chemotherapy data sets [26] and analyses supported by the EPA for chemical carcinogens [27]. Analyses comparing the relative effect of using a scaling factor of 0.75 rather than 0.67 are presented in Table 10.3, demonstrating substantial differences in the estimated HED for rodents. Despite the arguments for use of 0.75 as the scaling factor, the FDA maintains use of 0.67 as the default factor based on its inherent conservatism, to maintain consistency with the broader use of surface area scaling by toxicologists and pharmacokineticists, its prevailing experience with this approach, and the absence of definitive data supporting an alternative superior model [9].

FIH Dosing Based on Allometric Scaling of Exposure In contrast to scaling the NOAEL dose as the basis for the FIH dose selection, one may elect to use pharmacokinetic modeling or allometric scaling of exposure as the basis for FIH dose selection. Use of systemic exposure as the basis for interspecies dose extrapolation recognizes the potential differences across species in the pharmacokinetic behavior of a compound, which drives the concentration of the agent at the target tissue. When the toxicity of an agent is related to the target tissue concentration, the use of exposure or pharmacokinetic models can provide a rational basis for dose extrapolation across species. Under such models, drug concentrations at the target tissue have a time-dependent impact across species, so that cross-species comparisons of this effect may be normalized by accounting for species-specific physiologic time [24,28–30].

As described, Travis and co-authors [23,24,30] support the use of allometric scaling using 0.75 as the scaling metric in equation (10.1) by demonstrating that a number of key physiological parameters scale across species in relation to three-fourth power of body weight, including cardiac output, alveolar ventilation, renal clearance, and oxygen consumption (as a measure of metabolic rate). Moreover, use of physiological time (t') as a common metric for scaling physiologic and metabolic rates can be related to chronological time (t) according to the relationship $t' = t/\mathrm{BW}^{0.25}$. Under such a model, the physiologically relevant exposure can be scaled across species using physiologic time ($\mathrm{AUC_{pt}}$) such that $\mathrm{AUC_{pt}} = \mathrm{AUC/BW}^{0.25}$ [24].

Ings [30] conducted separate analyses evaluating the allometric scaling factor (b) for pharmacokinetic parameters relative to body weight (i.e., BW^b). Whereas the scaling metric (b) for volume of distribution was about 1, clearance scaled according to a power of about 0.75, and half-life scaled according to a power of about 0.25 for various drugs [31]. In this analysis, the five small-molecule compounds used for these analyses demonstrated variability around these estimates such that the coefficient of variation ranged from 3% (for volume of distribution) to 18% (for half-life). Because these analyses were limited to a relatively small number of molecules, caution should be used before using general allometric parameters for cross-species predictions of pharmacokinetics for novel compounds.

Hu and Hayton [32] used statistical analysis and Monte Carlo simulation to characterize the uncertainty in the allometric exponent in the estimation of clearance. They used clearance data in nonclinical species and humans for 115 drugs that were reported in the literature. It was concluded that an exponent of 0.75 best described the allometric relation to estimate the clearance, with the exception of drugs that were excreted predominantly through the kidneys having an exponent value of 0.67.

The allometrically scaled exposure and clearance can be used to estimate the FIH dose by regression of clearance in the nonclinical species (preferably using data from three or more species) and using the slope (b) and intercept (a) estimates as follows:

$$\text{dose} = a + b \times \text{predicted clearance in humans} \tag{10.2}$$

Alternatively, one may use the following approaches:

$$\text{dose(mg)} = \text{AUC in animal}(\mu\text{g}\cdot\text{h/mL}) \times \text{clearance predicted in humans(L/h)} \tag{10.3}$$

$$\text{dose(mg)} = \frac{\text{AUC in animal}(\mu\text{g}\cdot\text{h/mL}) \times \text{clearance predicted in humans(L/h)}}{\text{correction factor}} \tag{10.4}$$

TABLE 10.4 Estimated FIH Dosages by Different Calculation Methods for Various Small-Molecule Drugs

Drug	Equation 10.1	Equation 10.2	Equation 10.3	Equation 10.4	Clinical Dose Range (mg total)
Topiramate	175	95	36	44	100–1200
Moxifloxacin	107	86	23	80	84–400
Zonisamide	595	329	265	490	200–800
Troglitazone	90	37	35	85	100–600
Venlafaxine	60	23	22	60	25–150
Morphine	9.3	5.3	2.5	3	7.5–10
Felbamate	145	80	122	183	100–800
Bepridil	400	177	161	176	200–400
Stavudine	243	86	170	134	47–280[a]
Zenarestat	845	460	313	353	150–600

Source: Adapted from [33], with permission.
[a]Given orally based on scaling of i.v. data; the initial i.v. dose was 70 mg.

where the correction factor in equation (10.3) is derived by dividing the clearance in the species closest to the human clearance predicted by the human clearance [33] or bioavailability [34] predicted.

Mahmood et al. [33] compared FIH estimates according to equations (10.1) to (10.4) for 10 small molecules where clearance data were available in at least three species (mouse, rat, rabbit, monkey, or dog) and compared these results against doses administered in clinical trials. Results of these analyses are presented in Table 10.4. These results demonstrate that use of surface area scaling of dose [where $b = 0.67$, equation (10.1)] generally results in a higher FIH dose compared to doses estimated using clearance [equations (10.2) to (10.4)].

The use of allometry of pharmacokinetic parameters presumes conservation of concentration–response relationships across species, which may not always hold, as has been demonstrated for cardiac glycosides [35]. In such cases, the differences in the relative potency may be accounted for by correcting the initial dose by an appropriate potency factor [36].

Several literature methods [37–45] utilize in vitro and/or in vivo nonclinical information to predict human pharmacokinetic parameters, such as volume of distribution, clearance, half-life, and bioavailability for small molecules. As discussed in the preceding paragraph, allometric scaling is used most frequently to scale pharmacokinetic parameters from nonclinical species to humans for biotherapeutics.

Methods for Predicting Human Pharmacokinetic Parameters

Scaling of Intrinsic Clearance Obtained In Vitro Clearance is by far the most important pharmacokinetic parameter that needs to be predicted in humans for reliable estimation of dose selection. Intrinsic clearance values (CL_{int}) are calculated from the in vitro half-life data obtained in an appropriate system (e.g., liver microsomes) and then scaled up to human clearance. The in vitro half-life is used in the following equation (where $f_{u(\mathrm{inc})}$ = fraction unbound in incubation):

$$\mathrm{CL_{int}} = \frac{0.693 \times \text{ liver weight}}{\text{in vitro } t_{1/2} \times \text{liver weight in incubation} \times f_{u(\mathrm{inc})}}$$

The intrinsic clearance above can be converted into plasma clearance (CL_P) using either the well-stirred or parallel tube models of hepatic clearance, respectively [46,47]:

$$\mathrm{CL}_P = \frac{Qf_u \cdot \mathrm{CL_{int}}}{Q + f_u \cdot \mathrm{CL_{int}}} \qquad \text{(well-stirred model)}$$

$$\mathrm{CL}_P = Q(1 - e^{-\mathrm{CL_{int}f_u}/\mathrm{Q}}) \qquad \text{(parallel tube model)}$$

where Q is the hepatic blood flow and f_u is the free fraction in blood.

Allometric Scaling of In Vivo Clearance The following allometric equation can be used with linear regression of nonclinical data to obtain the constants (a and b) in the equation:

$$\log \mathrm{CL} = a \log(\text{body weight}) + b$$

Allometry can be corrected for protein binding where animal clearance values are corrected for plasma protein binding using the following equation to yield the free plasma clearance:

$$\mathrm{CL_{free}} = \frac{\mathrm{CL_{total}}}{f_u}$$

The projected human plasma clearance of the free drug can then be converted into the total plasma clearance by multiplication with $f_{u(\mathrm{human})}$.

Predicting Human Volume of Distribution

Average Fraction Unbound in Tissues Method The volume of distribution (VD) is another key pharmacokinetic parameter that should be estimated in humans with good precision. Using the volume of distribution in conjunction with the estimated clearance value, it is possible to project an estimation of the plasma half-life of the drug in humans.

Experimentally determined values for the volume of distribution at steady state ($\mathrm{VD_{SS}}$ in L/kg) and plasma protein binding for each species are used in the following equation, with standard values for extracellular fluid volumes (V_E), plasma volumes (V_P), "remainder of the fluid" volume (V_R), and the ratio of extracellular to intracellular proteins ($R_{E/I}$), to calculate the average fraction of unbound drug in tissues (f_{ut}) in nonclinical species [48]:

$$f_{ut} = \frac{V_R f_u}{[\mathrm{VD_{SS}} - V_P - (f_u V_E)] - [(1 - f_u) R_{E/I} V_P]}$$

where f_{ut} for each nonclinical species can be calculated and the average f_{ut} for animals may be assumed to be equal to f_{ut} in humans. This, along with the experimentally determined f_u (fraction unbound in plasma/serum), can be used to calculate the human volume of distribution using rearrangement of the equation above as shown in

$$\mathrm{VD}_{\text{human prediction}} = V_P + [f_{u(\text{human})} V_E] + [(1 - f_{u(\text{human})}) R_{E/I} V_P] + V_R \frac{f_{u(\text{human})}}{f_{ut\,(\text{average})}}$$

Proportionality Method Proportionality can be set up between the free fraction of drug in plasma in dog and human and the volume of distribution in these two species. The human volume of distribution can then be calculated using the equation

$$\mathrm{VD}_{(\text{human prediction})} = \frac{f_{u(\text{human})} \mathrm{VD}_{(\text{dog})}}{f_{u(\text{dog})}}$$

Allometry Allometric scaling can also be used to estimate the volume of distribution using total body weight as the physiological parameter for scaling, with linear regression of nonclinical data, to obtain the constants (a and b) in the equation

$$\log \mathrm{VD} = a \log(\text{body weight}) + b$$

The free volume of distribution ($\mathrm{VD}_{\text{free}}$) in animals can be obtained by correcting for protein binding using the equation

$$\mathrm{VD}_{\text{free}} = \frac{\mathrm{VD}_{\text{total}}}{f_u}$$

The projected human free volume of distribution can then be converted into the total volume of distribution by multiplication with $f_{u(\text{human})}$.

Methods for Predicting Human Oral Bioavailability The most common method of predicting human oral bioavailability is to use the average of the oral bioavailability values obtained in nonclinical species. Human oral bioavailabilty (F) can also be predicted by the combined results of the fraction of drug absorbed (F_a), first-pass extraction by the gut wall tissues (F_g), and the hepatic clearance (F_H):

$$F = F_a F_g F_H$$

When F_a and F_g effects are assumed to be negligible, the relationship reduces to

$$F = F_H$$

This can be simplified further to

$$F = 1 - \frac{\mathrm{CL}_P}{Q}$$

CL_P can be estimated by scaling intrinsic clearance as described earlier in the clearance prediction section.

FIH Dosing Based on Physiologically Based Pharmacokinetic Modeling Perhaps the most challenging alternative for cross-species extrapolation of dose is the physiologically based pharmacokinetic model [49,50]. Such models account for species-specific physiology relevant to the pharmacokinetics of a compound by establishing interrelationships between organ systems to characterize the outcome in the whole organism. When such models are available, they allow prediction of target tissue exposure [51,52]. However, such models are parametrically intensive exercises, requiring specification of tissue size, tissue perfusion, permeability of the drug, partitioning of the drug between blood and tissues, metabolism, and excretion [29,30]. As such, physiologically based pharmacokinetic modeling is typically resource demanding and costly and may require access to data that are not available or easily generated. For these reasons, physiologically based models may not be routinely used for drug development [30].

10.6 PHASE I CLINICAL TRIAL SUPPORT: USE OF THE MABEL OR PHARMACOLOGICALLY ACTIVE DOSE

The concept of employing pharmacologic, as opposed to toxicologic, activity to drive safe dose selection for FIH clinical trials is suggested in cases where toxicity may arise from exaggerated pharmacology [9]. This concept is greatly expanded on in the recent European guideline on strategies to identify and mitigate risks for FIH clinical trials [53], which was developed following the devastating toxicity observed in clinical trial subjects exposed to TGN1412 (discussed later in this chapter and in Chapter 12). This guideline emphasizes the need to assess the level of risk associated with testing of any new investigational medicinal product in terms of "knowledge or lack thereof" regarding mode of action, the nature of the target, and the relevance of animal models. Risk factors should be discussed explicitly in applications for FIH trials. Higher risk, defined by a limited extent of knowledge and experience with regard to drug class, pharmacological mechanism of action, dose–response function, and other factors, signals the need for increased caution in clinical trials. Examples characterizing high risk versus more standard therapeutics are provided in Table 10.5.

TABLE 10.5 Characteristics of Standard Versus High-Risk Therapeutics

Property	Standard Therapeutic	High-Risk Therapeutic
Mode of action	Follow-on agent or therapeutic target Well-understood mechanisms Target has limited physiological interactions Target has linear or sublinear dose–response relationship Easily monitored pharmacology/toxicity Toxicity is reversible	Novel Poorly understood mechanism Pleiotropic or systemic activity Bypasses or overwhelms physiological controls Potential for amplification, supralinear, or threshold dose–response Lack of biomarkers of effect/toxicity Irreversible toxicity
Nature of target	Good specificity of therapeutic to target or disease Target is noncritical, has redundancy	Poor specificity of therapeutic to target or disease Inherent risk of targeting specific structures, nonredundant systems Critical biological effect
Relevance of animal models	Good structural homology, target distribution, and signaling pathways Comparable pharmacological effects Animal models established and considered predictive	Poor structural homology, target distribution, signaling pathways, and pharmacological effects Animal models are of limited relevance to study pharmacology and toxicology Disease state alters relevance of studies in normal animals
Basis for first-in-human dose	NOAEL-based approach Healthy volunteers possible Utilize all available in vitro and in vivo data, including receptor binding and occupancy, concentration–response relationships, PK data in relevant species Apply appropriate safety factor	MABEL-based approach Patient population likely Utilize all available in vitro and in vivo data, including receptor binding and occupancy, concentration–response relationships, PK data in relevant species Apply appropriate safety factor

Source: Adapted from [76], with permission.

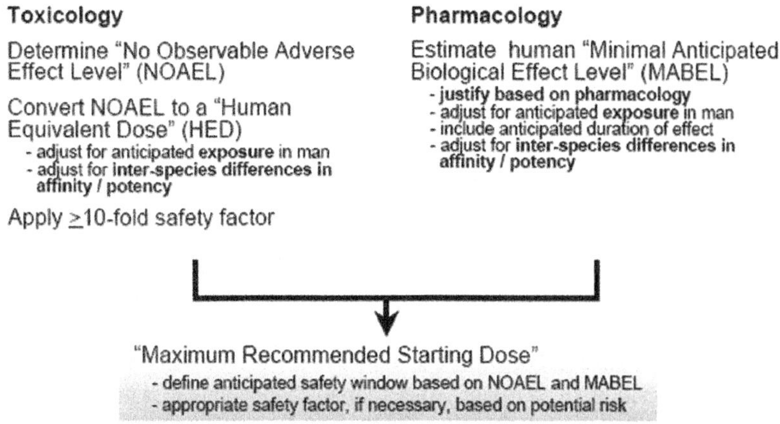

FIGURE 10.3 Toxicology and pharmacology considerations for maximum recommended starting dose for FIH study. (From J. Sims, personal communication.)

With regard to nonclinical aspects in particular, emphasis is placed on the presentation of evidence that demonstrates the relevance of nonclinical models, which may include human and animal comparisons of the following: target expression, distribution, and structure; functional consequences of target activation or deactivation; pharmacokinetics and ADME characteristics; and tissue cross-reactivity (i.e., monoclonal antibodies). Pharmacodynamic studies that characterize the biology of the target, ADME and pharmacokinetic studies, and safety pharmacology data (often obtained from the general toxicology study rather than a separate safety pharmacology study) should be available prior to FIH clinical trials. Additional endpoints may be included in toxicity studies to further define identified risks.

It has been appreciated for many years that exaggerated pharmacological activity can underlie toxicity. This has led the U.S. and EU regulatory agencies to request that initial dosage calculations consider using a minimal anticipated biological effect level (MABEL) or pharmacologically active dose (PAD) since these pharmacodynamic models can be used to predict dosages that would be associated with minimal biological effects in humans. As discussed below, the MABEL integrates in vitro (animal and human) and in vivo (animal) information from PK/PD data, including target binding and receptor occupancy and concentration/dose/exposure–response curves. An illustrative comparison of the concepts of NOAEL and MABEL as they relate to selection of starting doses in clinical trials is provided in Figures 10.1 and 10.3.

10.6.1 Predicting the MABEL and PAD in Humans

Recent experience with a novel biotherapeutic agent has resulted in a much publicized introspection, which has led to a review of current practices surrounding

FIH trials. Specifically, in 2006, a single 0.1-mg/kg dose of TGN1412, a novel superagonist anti-CD28 monoclonal antibody, was administered by intravenous infusion to six healthy volunteers [54]. Within 2 hours after dosing, these patients experienced a cytokine storm involving TNFα, IFNγ, and IL2 that resulted in impairment of the neurological, pulmonary, and renal systems plus a disseminated intravascular coagulation. Immunosuppressive treatment, including use of corticosteroids and/or an IL2R monoclonal antibody therapy, was prescribed to down-regulate the cytokine response.

The nonclinical studies supporting the TGN1412 clinical trial application were conducted in rhesus and cynomolgus monkeys; species selection was based on evidence of CD28 amino acid sequence identity in the critical region associated with TGN1412 contact, and comparison of TGN1412 binding to T-cells from various nonhuman primates and humans; subsequent data evaluating in vitro cytokine induction and T-cell activation and proliferation revealed comparable potency for human and cynomolgus monkey peripheral blood mononuclear cells [55]. Nonclinical safety studies in nonhuman primates did not demonstrate a systemic cytokine release reaction, although there was evidence of cytokine induction in serum, including IL-2, IL-5, and IL-6 [56]. The first human dose had a 500-fold margin of safety against the NOAEL established in cynomolgus monkeys (50 mg/kg) or an approximate 17-fold margin of safety based on a surface area–scaled human equivalent dose.

The basis for the marked difference in response to TGN1412 between monkeys and humans has not been established. Differences in T-cell co-stimulation related to Fc-receptor binding [57–59] or evolutionary differences in T-cell response to stimulation may underlie a relative increased sensitivity among humans compared to nonhuman primates [60]. Alternatively, the first human dose may have been predicated on faulty assumptions during dose extrapolation [61].

The experience with TGN1412 led to intensive review of the nonclinical data, clinical trial design and conduct, and regulatory review, which have been summarized in a number of reviews and editorials [62–69]. In addition, the European Medicines Agency (EMEA) has recently released guidance on requirements for FIH clinical trials [53]. Under this guidance, the potential health risks posed by novel therapeutics may be evaluated according to the proposed mode of action, similarities in the underlying physiology, nature of the dose–response relationship, and relevance of animal models (see Table 10.6). Importantly, this guidance establishes use of the MABEL projected in humans as the basis for FIH dosing for agents considered to pose high potential risk. The concept of a MABEL is captured in the FDA FIH guidance document, wherein a PAD may be considered as an alternative to the NOAEL when it may be a more sensitive indicator of potential toxicity [9].

In principle, the MABEL and PAD rely on experimental pharmacology data to support estimation of the biologically or pharmacologically active dose as the basis for the FIH dose. Conceptually, this should represent a more conservative FIH dose because the starting dose is based on a "low active dose" rather than a "low toxic dose." For novel agents, therefore, the phase I clinician has the

TABLE 10.6 Factors Modifying Cross-Species Predictions of Exposure–Response Profiles in Deriving the MABEL/PAD

Factors Modifying Exposure	Factors Modifying Response
Species differences in drug–target interactions establish exposure distribution at site of action	Species differences in drug–target interactions that drive pharmacodynamic (and toxicologic) response
Binding affinity	Binding affinity
Target density (no./cell)	Target density (no./cell)
Cell abundance	Cell abundance
Species differences in absorption or bioavailability	Species differences in specificity for target
Species differences in specificity for target	Interaction with unintended target elicits unintended pharmacology or toxicity
Off-target or nonspecific binding reduces drug available for target; may act as a depot	Species differences in posttranslational modifications affecting activity
Species differences in rates of metabolism/catabolism or clearance	Species differences in expression/activity of binding partners
Modification/formulation may protect drug, prolong exposure (e.g., PEGylation or sialylation protect protein from catabolism)	Species differences in downstream signaling cascades
Selection/modification of antibody Fc region affects FcRn binding	Species differences in generation of active metabolites

opportunity to follow patient response (and safety) during dose escalation from a low active dose up towards the therapeutic dose rather than risk initiating the trial with a higher active (and potentially toxic) FIH dose based on a relatively arbitrary safety factor to the NOAEL.

Derivation of the MABEL and PAD depends on the unique circumstances surrounding the nature of the intended pharmacological activity, and specific pharmacokinetic and biodistribution data of the molecule. For the simple case of a single target binding a single receptor, an exact solution can be derived, rather than a numerical solution [34]. Derivation of an exact solution in this case is based on the dissociation constant (K_d) for the mAb drug-target complex, total drug (TD), total target (TT), and quadratic solution as follows:

$$K_d = \frac{[\text{mAb}][\text{target}]}{[\text{complex}]} \tag{10.5}$$

$$\text{TD} = \text{mAb} + \text{complex} \qquad \therefore \text{mAb} = \text{TD} - \text{complex} \tag{10.6}$$

$$\text{TT} = \text{target} + \text{complex} \qquad \therefore \text{target} = \text{TT} - \text{complex} \tag{10.7}$$

$$\text{complex} = \frac{(K_d + \text{TD} + \text{TT}) - [(K_d + \text{TD} + \text{TT})^2 - 4 \cdot \text{TT} \cdot \text{TD}]^{0.5}}{2} \quad (10.8)$$

$$\text{receptor occupancy} = \frac{\text{complex}}{\text{TT}} \quad (10.9)$$

Using equations (10.5) to (10.9), an estimated receptor occupancy of 91% for the initial dose of TGN1412 (0.1 mg/kg) was estimated by Lowe et al. [34] using assumptions of T-cell concentration (ca. 1.3×10^9/L blood in an adult human), CD28 receptor abundance (150,000 molecules/cell), number of binding sites for TGN1412 per CD28 (two binding sites/CD28), and knowledge of the equilibrium affinity $K_d(\text{M}) = 1.88 \times 10^{-9}$ and molecular weight (150,000 kDa) as follows:

$$\begin{aligned}[\text{TGN1412}] &= (0.1 \text{ mg/kg dose} \times 70 \text{ kg adult}) \div (150{,}000 \text{ kDa} \times 2.5 \text{ L plasma}) \\ &= 1.867 \times 10^{-8} \text{ M} \\ [\text{CD28}] &= 1.3 \times 10^9 \text{ T-cells/L} \times 150{,}000 \text{ CD28/T-cell} \\ &\quad \times 2 \text{ binding sites/CD28} \div 6.02 \times 10^{23} \text{ molecules/mole} \\ &= 6.48 \times 10^{-10} \text{ M}\end{aligned}$$

This compares well with Mehrishi and coauthors [61], who estimated about 85% receptor occupancy for the initial dose of TGN1412 (0.1 mg/kg) using assumptions of T-cell concentration (ca. 5×10^9/L blood in an adult human), CD28 receptor abundance (30,000 molecules/cell), number of binding sites for TGN1412 per CD28 (two binding sites/CD28), and the same equilibrium affinity and molecular weight. Using similar assumptions, we have estimated a receptor occupancy of about 91%, suggesting that these authors may have used other unspecified assumptions.

Under a strategy based on the MABEL, one might presume that a potent agonist antibody would begin to elicit biological activity at a relatively low percentage receptor occupancy. In such a situation, one could model the receptor occupancy under a range of dosing assumptions using equations (10.5) to (10.9), as shown in Figure 10.4. The pharmaceutical company Novartis has reported an internal policy to limit receptor occupancy to 10% for the first human dose [34]. To this end, animal model or in vitro studies may assist in establishing pharmacological activity as a function of receptor occupancy. Under the conditions evaluated in Figure 10.4, drug/target ratios greater than 0.1 may be associated with 10% receptor occupancy when the affinity is relatively high (0.1 to 1 nM).

In contrast to an agonistic antibody, one might presume that a relatively high percentage receptor occupancy might be required to elicit full antagonistic or "suppressive" therapeutic activity. Such was the case for abciximab (ReoPro) which inhibits platelet aggregation [70]. Review of the U.S. package insert indicates that abciximab inhibits platelet aggregation (as assessed in animal models

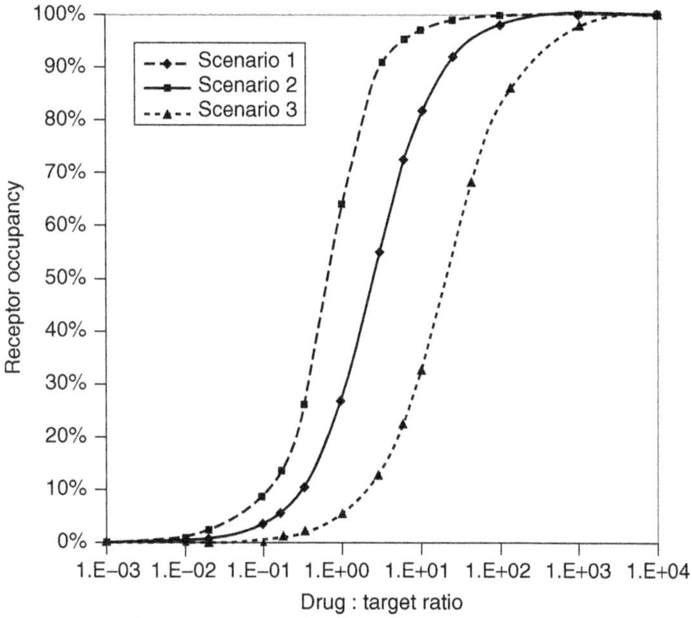

FIGURE 10.4 Sensitivity of receptor occupancy to drug/target ratio and K_d. Receptor occupancy was estimated using equations (10.5) to (10.9) with total target = 5×10^{-10} M and total drug varying from 5×10^{-13} to 5×10^{-6} M. Data are presented for $K_d = 1 \times 10^{-9}$ M (similar to the TGN1412 affinity for CD28, scenario 1), 10-fold stronger (1×10^{-10} M, scenario 2), and 10-fold weaker (1×10^{-8} M, scenario 3).

of thrombosis) with ≥80% saturation of the GPIIb/IIIa receptor (as assessed by a flow cytometric analysis of receptor occupancy); these data allowed correlation of exposure with target tissue concentration and pharmacodynamic activity in the nonclinical safety studies, and provided a basis for estimating the PAD in humans.

As an alternative to these methods, success has been reported in the use of surrogate animal data to support FIH dosing. For example, Mordenti et al. [71] used data derived using a murine monoclonal antibody against vascular endothelial growth factor (VEGF) in a murine tumor model to derive concentration–response data that were used to estimate efficacious doses for the humanized anti-VEGF therapeutic. This approach is a particularly useful strategy for developing an initial dose and dose escalation strategy for antagonistic therapeutic agents that demonstrate no notable biological activity in normal animals.

10.7 SUPPORT OF EXPLORATORY CLINICAL STUDIES

There are various approaches to the design of nonclinical safety programs to support early, "exploratory" clinical studies (e.g., prior to phase I) that are limited in dose and duration [6,53,72,73]. These exploratory IND and CTA studies are described in detail in Chapter 11. The nonclinical package required to support these types of exploratory clinical trials is more limited in scope than that for traditional phase I trials; thus, more conservative assumptions are applied in estimating a maximum safe recommended clinical dose. For example, in a clinical microdose study (i.e., a dose not intended to produce pharmacologic effects) the maximum clinical dose should not exceed 100 μg (or 500 μg total cumulative doses) and is required to be $\leq 1/100$ of the NOAEL and the PAD. For an exploratory trial of up to 14 days into the therapeutic dosage range, predicted exposures for the starting dose should not exceed 1/50 the NOAEL in the more sensitive species on a mg/m^2 basis, and the maximum exposure in humans should not be higher than the AUC (area under the plasma–serum concentration–time curve) at the NOAEL in the nonrodent species or higher than one-half the AUC at the NOAEL in the rodent species, whichever is lower [6].

There is flexibility in the approach prescribed; the rationale for the approach proposed should be fully justified and discussed with the appropriate regulatory authority prior to submission for the FIH study.

10.8 CONSIDERATIONS IN THE DESIGN OF PHASE I TRIALS

10.8.1 Toxicological Considerations

As the concept of *location* is paramount for valuing real estate, the three most important considerations for a phase I trial are: safety, safety, and safety. The phrase *no molecule is without risk* is attributed to the early writings of Paracelsus [74], with the lesson for the practicing toxicologist of today being that risk must be characterized thoroughly so that it can be managed competently in the clinical setting. A toxicology profile should address several basic questions, including the appropriateness of the animal model, the definition of toxic effects and target organs, the dose dependence of the responses, the dose–exposure relationship and other ADME characterization, and the identification of biomarkers [13]. Answers to these questions form the basis for decisions as to whether and how to proceed safely with the first administration of a new drug in humans. The greater the uncertainty and concern around the toxicity profile, the more cautious should be the approach in the design of the clinical trial.

In an ideal world, the following toxicologic characteristics apply for a drug intended for study in humans:

- A scientifically sound expectation that the biology of the nonclinical model is similar to and thus predictive of the human patient
- A well-characterized and preferably shallow dose–response curve with demonstration of a clear and reproducible progression of effect with increasing dose
- Premonitory signs or biomarkers that can be measured in the clinic and serve as “premonitory” signals for potential toxicity

- The reversibility of adverse effect(s)
- A large margin of safety between exposure associated with a serious adverse effect and that expected to result in efficacy

In the real world, deviation from these ideal characteristics occurs frequently and colors the concern for safety and consequent increased caution in approach.

As intimated in the previous discussion, not all toxicity profiles for new candidate drugs are "created equal." Administration of a drug candidate with the potential to elicit a serious adverse or toxic effect that could result in a permanent injury or significant organ dysfunction represents a clear cause for concern that must be manageable within the clinical trial setting. In this situation, there should also be either a very large margin of safety and/or a sufficient warning so as to avoid serious toxicity. Clinical pathology parameters represent classic biomarkers of toxicity: for example, elevations in serum transaminases (e.g., ALT, AST) for hepatic toxicity or peripheral blood cytopenias for hematologic toxicity. Similarly, the appearance of ataxia and tremors may well precede more serious central nervous system (CNS) toxicity. Conversely, lack of premonitory signals prior to actual expression of the injury would generate significant concern for patient safety; for compounds associated with serious, irreversible toxicity, this could result in termination of development. For example, a compound that induced convulsions or other serious CNS toxicities without demonstrating less severe signs at lower doses would be problematic. Damage to an organ with no or limited ability to generate new tissue (e.g., to heart tissue or neurons) must be avoided. Increases in serum troponin may be associated with cardiomyopathy [75,77] and would not necessarily be an acceptable endpoint in the clinical setting. However, if the adverse effect is well understood and the possibility of eliciting a serious toxicity can be managed, then in some cases an effective argument can be built to conduct the FIH trial. For example, if an effective rescue treatment is readily available, such as epinephrine for an anaphylactic response or dilantin for seizures, then it may be possible to establish a plan with the relevant institutional review board (IRB; for a study conducted in the United States) and the clinical investigators to initiate the study. Again, such risk would need to be offset by the potential or real therapeutic benefit, as for example, when the trial is conducted in patients with a life-threatening illness that is currently nontreatable.

10.8.2 Differences Between Animals and Humans That May Modify Exposure or Response

A number of factors may preclude direct comparisons between exposure–response relationships in animals and humans: for example, potential differences affecting systemic drug exposure, potency at the target, and underlying biology of the target therapeutic pathway (see Table 10.6). These and other factors can be accounted for in either the NOAEL- or MABEL-based approach. Specifically, in the NOAEL-based approach, such factors can influence the selection of a larger safety factor when there are noted disparities between PK or PD in the nonclinical animal species and humans. In contrast, the MABEL-based approach can account directly for differences in response between species by comparing the pharmacologic response to a relevant experimental model.

In addition, other considerations, including disease state, individual genetics, or coadministered therapies can influence the design of the FIH study or management of the transition from healthy to diseased patient populations. In vitro–ex vivo evaluations using normal and diseased tissues or cells may provide useful information regarding relative receptor–ligand expression, the presence of splice variants or inactive forms, and other host–environment effects that could influence the dose selection process and/or the potential range of responses in the human subjects.

10.8.3 Healthy Human Subjects or Patients

The decision to conduct human clinical trials with a drug candidate is based on the perceived benefit balanced against the risk of incurring adverse health effects. Most phase I trials are conducted in normal healthy volunteers to facilitate a characterization of the safety and pharmacokinetics of the drug candidate under conditions that are not confounded by variables associated with ill health or disease of the human subject. There is usually little to no benefit to such healthy volunteers; the therapeutic benefit is anticipated in patients, pending later proof-of-concept trials. There are, however, instances when it is preferable or even necessary to conduct phase I trials in patients based on the risk/benefit ratio or other considerations. Among these key decision factors is a risk/benefit assessment relating to the potential risks posed by the novel therapeutic, whether the risk profile is affected by the presence of disease, and the need for adjuvant therapies that may interfere with the main goals of the trial or without which the patient's health may deteriorate. As an example, oncolytic drugs are typically highly toxic in nature, and it is not ethical to expose healthy volunteers who would derive no benefit and who would stand to incur significant toxicity. In the treatment of life-threatening diseases such as some cancers, more risk of adverse events can be tolerated in view of a potentially significant efficacious outcome. Alternatively, in cases involving highly selective targeting (e.g., with a biotherapeutic), enrollment of patients may be considered if the target is not present in healthy human subjects.

10.9 INTERDISCIPLINARY PARTNERSHIPS

10.9.1 Chemistry, Manufacturing, and Control

Early discovery research efforts are directed toward obtaining sufficient systemic exposure in the nonclinical models to allow characterization of toxicity and to provide dose multiples over the intended human exposure. An increasing number of small molecules have characteristics (e.g., limited solubility) that require significant early pharmaceutical development to achieve acceptable bioavailability employing the route of clinical administration. Therefore, the toxicologist must work closely with the formulation chemist to identify a vehicle that is safe (having no toxic liabilities of its own) and which provides adequate systemic exposure. It is important that the absorption characteristics of any formulation should be well described and documented before being used in animal toxicology studies (Chapter 5).

It is also important to note that the quality and characteristics of the test article used in nonclinical studies should be comparable to those used in the clinical trials they support. This may not always be easily achieved, as adjustments to the route of synthesis are not unusual as the development of the new pharmaceutical proceeds. For example, early lots of small molecules may be amorphous or semicrystalline in nature, although the ultimate goal is to have a reproducibly crystalline lot for clinical testing (and for the commercial product). Although use of the clinical lot for nonclinical studies would be optimal, this may result in a delay in conduct of the animal-based toxicology testing. Therefore, to avoid delays in development, it is possible in nonclinical studies to use well-characterized lots of material that are qualitatively and quantitatively similar to those used in the clinic. The situation for biologics can be especially complex. For example, there may be batch-to-batch differences in glycosylation or other differences, due to a change in the cell line used to manufacture the molecule. Any differences in the impurity profiles of the nonclinical and clinical lots of drug may require toxicologic qualification in additional animal studies [78,79]. Again, the opportunity to find successful solutions to these challenges depends on a close collaboration with analytical and pharmaceutical chemistry.

10.9.2 Regulatory Affairs

Approval by a regulatory agency and an IRB is a prerequisite to initiation of clinical trials, and regulatory strategy is an important part of a drug program team's success in initiation of phase I trials (Chapter 14). Despite continuing efforts to harmonize the nonclinical data needed to support clinical trials, significant differences persist between geographies and, in some cases, divisions within a particular regulatory agency. Understanding the expectations and perspectives of regulators improves the chances of a successful submission with minimal approval issues. For example, differences in regulatory opinion regarding acceptable clinical trial designs and dosing paradigms can be anticipated depending on the perceived risk/benefit ratio for various therapeutic areas (e.g., oncology versus obesity) and patient populations (e.g., Japan versus the United States, healthy volunteers versus patients).

10.9.3 Clinical

As discussed previously, the establishment of an FIH dosage regimen depends on a number of nonclinical factors. In addition, selection of the FIH dose is highly dependent on both the specifics and entirety of the clinical program. A close and collaborative working relationship between the toxicologist and the clinical team will ensure development of the appropriate clinical perspective on the pharmacology and toxicology results from the nonclinical animal studies. The investigator's brochure and the clinical protocol should clearly reflect how the nonclinical data support the clinical plan in terms of dose (i.e., margins of safety) and safety monitoring.

10.10 BEYOND THE FIH DOSE

FIH studies provide valuable information regarding the pharmacokinetic behavior, definition of the tolerable dose range, and characterization of the effects and symptoms of the new drug in humans. Nonclinical data are essential for establishing the initial dosing strategy in humans and can even suggest an appropriate approach for dose escalation. Human data from FIH studies can quickly supersede the animal data with regard to progression of dosing in the clinical trial and predictions from pharmacokinetic and pharmacodynamic models derived from animal data. However, when a toxic effect has no readily monitorable biomarker or premonitory sign in humans, the results from the animal data may a priori limit the high dose in clinical trials. For example, dose escalation in humans may be limited to some exposure multiple or margin of safety (based on data derived from animals and humans) until the significance or relevance of the effect in humans is understood more thoroughly. The magnitude of an acceptable margin is also dependent on the degree of the safety concern. Serious, irreversible toxicity that is not predictable, easily monitored, or is associated with significant variability in the exposure response may delay the human phase I program until an appropriate biomarker can be developed or an improved understanding is developed regarding the human relevance of the effect.

10.11 CONCLUDING PERSPECTIVE

The dosage selection process for FIH studies is a complex endeavor that requires the cohesive interaction of a number of professionals in the nonclinical and clinical disciplines. Whether for small-molecule NCEs or large-molecule biotherapeutics, sound scientific principles and an extensive knowledge base are required to develop the FIH dose by holistically integrating all available pharmacodynamic, pharmacokinetic, ADME, and toxicology data. The initial FIH dosage and the escalation strategy can then be determined based on dose–response relationships for pharmacological and toxicological effects (e.g., MABEL, BMD, PAD, or NOAEL) and the use of pharmacokinetic methods (e,g., allometry, exposure). The application of these approaches is generally dependent on the specific characteristics of each new drug candidate, including the nature and type of toxicities seen in nonclinical animal testing, the potential reversibility of these toxicities, the specific pharmacokinetic characteristics, and the nature of the human disease targeted. However, it is not uncommon for a combination of several of these approaches to be used to develop the FIH dosage. Thus, a true interdisciplinary effort is required that includes an extensive discussion of the nonclinical results before a cohesive, integrated, and workable FIH strategy can be built for the clinical plan, which forms the foundation of a successful drug development program.

10.12 FOUR CASE STUDIES

The following case studies represent fictionalized versions of scenarios related to actual nonclinical safety assessment programs in support of FIH clinical trials. Some of the original information and/or data has been altered to emphasize learning points discussed in the chapter.

Case Study 1

Issue: A NOEL for elevation of hepatic enzymes (e.g., ALT) was not identified in the FIH-enabling toxicity studies

Strategy: Advance dosing in the clinic based on ability to monitor toxicity and to predict therapeutic concentrations using scaled PK for FIH dose estimation

Mechanism/target: Hormone receptor modulator

Indication: Endocrine

Toxicology results:

- Repeated dose studies were conducted in rats and cynomolgus monkeys, which were selected based on in vitro metabolic profiles similar to those of humans.
- In both species, administration of the drug was associated with liver toxicity, characterized by elevations in transaminases (ALT, AST) and histopathologic changes (degeneration and necrosis). The monkey was demonstrated to be the most sensitive species for hepatotoxicity. At the lowest dose, 0.5 mg/kg, in a one-month toxicity study, liver effects in the monkey were manifested by an elevation in ALT without associated histopathologic abnormalities. As such, 0.5 mg/kg was considered to be the NOAEL for repeated dose exposure. The lowest observed adverse effect level (LOAEL) in monkeys was 20-fold higher (10 mg/kg per day) and was associated with mild-to-moderate aminotransferase elevation only, without cholestasis or hepatic histopathological abnormalities.
- In pilot single-dose studies in monkeys, aminotransferases were elevated only at higher dose levels of the drug (>300 mg/kg). The single-dose NOAEL was equivalent to 300 mg/kg.

Approach to estimation of a safe starting dose in humans:

- A starting dose for the phase I trial was based on the lowest dose in the monkey (NOAEL of 0.5 mg/kg). This approach was considered appropriate in that the biology of the target was well understood and was conserved across mammalian species so that the nonclinical model was judged appropriate to predict human effects.

- Although the lowest dose was associated with an increase in ALT, the usefulness of this marker for clinical monitoring of potential liver toxicity provided confidence in the ability to detect an effect prior to any serious toxicity.

- According to the algorithm outlined in the FDA guidance (Figure 10.2), the monkey dose of 0.5 mg/kg is expressed in terms of body surface area:

$$(0.5\ \text{mg/kg})(12\ \text{kg/m}^2) = 6\ \text{mg/m}^2$$

- A conventional safety factor of 10 was employed, again based on confidence in the nonclinical model to predict human effects and the monitorability of the effect:

$$\frac{6\ \text{mg/m}^2}{10} = 0.6\ \text{mg/m}^2$$

- The dose is expressed in terms of mg/kg for administration in the clinic:

$$\frac{0.6\ \text{mg/m}^2}{37} = 0.016\ \text{mg/kg}$$

- Finally, the initial FIH dosage is reexpressed in terms of milligrams for a typical female patient weighing 60 kg for administration in the clinic:

$$(0.016\ \text{mg/kg})(60\ \text{kg}) = 1\ \text{mg}$$

  - With regard to the initial human study (single-dose exposure only), an exposure multiple based on a single dose was also derived. In a pilot study in monkeys, elevation of only ALT was observed at single dose of 300 mg/kg which was considered to be the single-dose NOAEL. A single-dose MOS (margin of safety) can be established for the high end of the planned dose range for the FIH single-dose safety study (240 mg) as follows:

$$\text{Monkey}: (300\ \text{mg/kg})(12\ \text{kg/m}^2) = 3600\ \text{mg/m}^2$$

$$\text{Human}: (240\ \text{mg})(1/60\ \text{kg})(37\ \text{kg/m}^2) = 148\ \text{mg/m}^2$$

$$\text{MOS}: \frac{\text{monkey dose}}{\text{human dose}} = \frac{3600}{148} = 24\text{-fold}$$

Clinical trial design:

- With a predefined and carefully administered liver function monitoring plan and with predefined stopping rules for individual subjects and dosing

cohorts, the dose of this drug can be safely escalated in the initial single-dose phase of the study from 1 mg up to 240 mg (i.e., 1/10 of the NOAEL from the one-month monkey toxicity study to 1/24 of the NOAEL from a single-dose monkey toxicity study, respectively).
  - The dose range from 1 to 240 mg was also estimated to encompass the targeted clinical efficacious doses, which were based on animal models of efficacy and PK/PD modeling utilizing predictions of the human pharmacokinetic characteristics and also by comparison to efficacy data from other hormone receptor modulators.
  - Human plasma concentrations following administration of the 1- and 240-mg doses were estimated using allometrically scaled pharmacokinetic parameters based on the dose–exposure relationship in the nonclinical species.
- Once data from a phase Ia dose escalation study are available, a decision can be made concerning the feasibility of proceeding into a multidose study with doses selected based on the data generated in a single-dose escalation study. The decision will be based on liver safety findings and pharmacokinetic monitoring as well as the complete clinical safety package (including all laboratory assessments).

Regulatory outcome:

- Based on the conservative approach described above, initiation of the phase I trial was allowed.
- Dose escalation on the basis of the safety monitoring stopping rules, without planned termination at a dose equivalent to the monkey NOAEL for transaminase elevation, was permitted.
- The multidose phase I clinical trial could be initiated once the single-dose escalation exceeded the multidose study starting dose by at least 10-fold.

Case Study 2

Issue: Serious toxicity (mortality) without premonitory signs was observed in the FIH-enabling toxicology study

Strategy: A conservative phase I study design with an exposure ceiling was proposed

Mechanism/target: Enzyme inhibitor

Indication: Endocrine

Toxicology results:

- Daily oral doses up to 2000 and 1500 mg/kg per day were administered to rats and dogs, respectively, in one-month toxicity studies.
- Whereas no significant adverse effects were observed in rats, doses of 180 and 2000 mg/kg caused extreme morbidity in the dogs on days 18 and 19 such that the animals were euthanized. Thus, the NOAEL dose was identified as the lowest dose (15 mg/mg daily) in dogs.
- The exact cause of death could not be determined, and there were no premonitory signs.

- Morbidity (e.g., decreased body weight and clinical signs of weakness and uncoordination) and mortality in the one-month dog study was not observed until after approximately two weeks of exposure, indicating that severe toxicity is not expected from a single dose.

Approach to estimation of a safe starting dose in humans:

- Due to the severity of the adverse event (death) in dogs and the lack of premonitory signs, a very conservative approach was taken.
  - A starting dose for the phase I trial was based on the NOAEL from the 30-day dog study, which was 15 mg/kg. A proposed starting dose of 1 mg in humans yielded a margin of safety on the order of 500-fold when the body surface area method was utilized.
- According to the algorithm outlined in the FDA guidance (Figure 10.2), the dog dose of 15 mg/kg is expressed in terms of body surface area:

$$(15\ \text{mg/kg})(20\ \text{kg/m}^2) = 300\ \text{mg/m}^2$$

- The human dose of 1 mg (0.014 mg/kg for a 70-kg patient) expressed in terms of mg/m^2 for administration in the clinic:

$$(0.014\ \text{mg/kg})(37\ \text{kg/m}^2) = 0.52\ \text{mg/m}^2$$

- MOS:

$$\frac{\text{AUC dog NOAEL}}{\text{predicted AUC human starting dose}} = \frac{300}{0.52} = 577\text{-fold}$$

  - Using a pharmacokinetic model that assumed linear pharmacokinetics in an allometry model using data from nonclinical species (rat and dog), human exposure was predicted to be 150 ng · h/mL. Based on the exposure of ca. 62,000 ng · h/mL at the NOAEL observed in dogs, the median exposure-based margin of safety was on the order of 400-fold.

Clinical trial design:

- All safety data will be reviewed on an ongoing basis and a washout interval (initially based on extrapolation of pharmacokinetic data in animals) sufficient to eliminate any carryover effects from previous treatments will be employed.
- Pharmacokinetic analysis will be performed after each dosing cohort completion, and exposures at higher dosing levels will be predicted prior to any dose escalation.
  - Reviews of pharmacokinetic data were planned after every dose to estimate the upper 90th percentile of predicted human exposures (and C_{max}) to assist in determining subsequent dosing levels while maintaining a 10-fold margin of safety with respect to the mean exposure and C_{max} at the NOAEL in dogs.

- Dose escalation from dose 1 to dose 2 will be based on the safety and tolerability data (from at least six subjects on at least five days) plus the pharmacokinetic data from dose 1. The trial design will also include a biomarker of efficacy. Predefined stopping rules were put in place to curtail dose escalation in the event of any abnormal pharmacokinetic finding in any subject receiving the experimental drug.

Regulatory outcome:

- Based on the conservative approach described above, initiation and progression of the phase I trial was allowed.

Case Study 3

Issue: A recombinant human cytokine demonstrated cardiac toxicity in mice that was not observed in cynomolgus monkeys

Strategy: Develop a MABEL-based approach using cytokine signaling as a more conservative approach toward FIH dose selection; support the FIH clinical trial with cardiac monitoring

Mechanism/target: Immune system activation

Indication: Infection, cancer

Toxicology results:

- Repeated dose studies were conducted in mice and cynomolgus monkeys, which were selected based on the in vitro and in vivo pharmacological response to the cytokine consistent with that observed with human cells and expected immunological activity.
- Evidence of immune system activation consistent with the expected biological activity of the recombinant human cytokine was observed in cynomolgus monkeys (0.015 to 2.5 mg/kg, twice weekly, s.c.) and mice (0.3 to 30 mg/kg, three times weekly, s.c.). However, a cardiomyopathy was observed histologically in mice but was not observed in monkeys. The histopathology was generally more severe with increasing dose, with a NOAEL dose being seen in mice at the lowest dose tested. The severity and number of animals affected was lower after four drug-free weeks of recovery. Review of the literature on related marketed cytokines of the same class suggested a sensitivity of mice toward this injury that was not observed in monkeys or humans.
- All animals treated demonstrated antidrug antibody responses by the end of four weeks of dosing. In vitro mechanistic toxicology studies using primary cardiomyocytes suggested low potential for direct activity of the cytokine on these cells.

Approach to estimation of a safe starting dose in humans:

- A starting dose for the phase I trial (single escalating dose in healthy subjects) was based on the lowest pharmacologically active dose in the monkey. This approach was considered appropriate since this was a novel cytokine that did not produce consistent toxicities in the two animal species. Further, the mechanism of toxicity could not be established definitively (although there was no apparent functional consequence).

- According to the MABEL/PAD approach, the NOEL in monkeys was based on increased serum concentrations of a biomarker that was thought to be closely linked to the immunological action of the therapeutic:

$$\text{NOEL}_{\text{monkeys}} = 0.015 \text{ mg/kg}$$

- The human equivalent dose (HED) was calculated by allometrically scaling the $\text{NOEL}_{\text{monkeys}}$ using body surface area (Table 10.3):

$$\text{HED} = \frac{\text{NOEL}_{\text{monkeys}}}{3} = 0.005 \text{ mg/kg}$$

- A conventional safety factor of 10 was employed, again based on confidence in the nonclinical model to predict human effects and the monitorability of the effect:

$$\text{FIH dose} = 0.5 \ \mu\text{g/kg}$$

The FIH dose of 0.5 μg/kg estimated using the monkey data is 30,000-fold lower than the mouse NOAEL of 0.3 mg/kg (HED = 0.3 mg/kg/0.02 = 15 mg/kg).

Clinical trial design:

- A single escalating dose range of up to 0.5 to 250 μg/kg was planned in healthy human subjects. In addition to standard evaluations for general health and safety, emphasis was placed on cardiac monitoring.
  - This dose range was defined to encompass the targeted clinical efficacious doses based on using allometry of pharmacokinetic parameters and in vitro pharmacology dose–response modeling.
- Once data from a phase Ia dose escalation study are available, a decision can be made about single- and repeated-dose escalation studies in subjects with disease. The decision will be based on cardiac safety findings, pharmacokinetic monitoring, and the complete clinical safety package (including all laboratory assessments).

Regulatory outcome:

- Based on the conservative approach described above, initiation of the phase I trial was allowed.
- Dose escalation on the basis of the safety monitoring stopping rules was permitted; however, the regulatory agency wanted to review the safety data prior to escalating above the scaled HED associated with cardiac injury in mice.
- The multidose phase I clinical trial could be initiated upon completion of the single-dose escalation study.

Case Study 4

Issue: A NOAEL based on the mortality of a single animal which was conservatively designated as drug related (i.e., it could not be definitively ruled out from being mechanistically related to the consequences of the intended drug action)

Strategy: Establish initial drug dosage and proceed with dose escalation until a maximally tolerated dosage is achieved; in addition to standard assessments, monitor for hematological, clotting, and cardiovascular effects

Mechanism/target: Antiangiogenic

Indication: Oncology

Toxicology results:

- Repeat dose studies were conducted in rats (duration of one month, twice weekly dosing) and cynomolgus monkeys (duration of one and three months, twice weekly dosing). Total weekly dosages were 20, 60, and 200 mg/kg per week for the rats and 4, 20, and 100 mg/kg per week for the monkeys and were designated the low, middle, and high dosages, respectively. Binding of drug to the intended target was observed in both animal species.
- A high-dose (200 mg/kg per week) male rat was euthanized on recovery day 28 as the result of an acute bilateral cerebral hemorrhage (an extremely rare occurrence in normal Sprague–Dawley rats). No other animals at this or any drug dosage exhibited adverse effects for in-life observations, organ weights, clinical pathology (including clotting parameters), and histopathology. Rats were considered to be the most sensitive species, as the single mortality observed could not be precluded from being related to the drug treatment. The 60 mg/kg per week dose was considered to be the NOAEL.

Approach to estimation of a safe starting dose in humans:

- The rationale to establish the initial dosage for the phase I trial was based on the single mortality at the highest dosage in the rat toxicology study. Since this occurred at the end of the recovery period and drug levels were substantially reduced, it was difficult to ascribe this death to the drug. However, this effect was conservatively considered to be drug related because of the severity of this observation and the potential for it to be related mechanistically to the pharmacological action of the drug.
- According to the algorithm outlined in Figure 10.2, the rat NOAEL dosage of 60 mg/kg per week was converted to the HED:

$$(60\ \text{mg/kg/week})(0.16) = 9.6\ \text{mg/kg/week}$$

- A safety factor of 10 was applied based on the low incidence of the finding in rats and the lack of adverse effects in the monkey:

$$\frac{9.6\ \text{mg/kg/week}}{10} = 0.96\ \text{mg/kg/week maximum recommended starting dose}$$

- Due to the serious nature of the finding and the lack of predictive biomarkers, an additional safety factor of three was used resulting in a human starting dose of 0.3 mg/kg/week.

$$\frac{0.96\ \text{mg/kg/week}}{3} = \text{ca. } 0.3\ \text{mg/kg/week}$$

Clinical trial design:

- The study design consisted of standard escalating dose cohorts that incorporated routine clinical examinations and laboratory evaluations with predefined rules for cohort expansion and stopping based on toxicity. Using this design, it was judged that this drug could safely be escalated in the initial phase Ia portion of the study from 0.3 mg/kg up to 12 mg/kg per week (i.e., 1/200 of the NOAEL to 1/5 of the NOAEL from the one-month rat toxicology study).
  - On a body surface area basis, the projected efficacious dosage in humans was projected to be 0.8 mg/kg per week (efficacy in mice seen at 10 mg/kg per week).
  - Safety factor multiples were determined for the toxicity studies in the rat (25, 75, and 250) and monkey (5, 25, and 125) on a mass basis (mg/kg) for the low, middle, and high doses, respectively. Using a body surface dosing (mg/m^2) paradigm, safety multiples were also determined for rats (5, 14, and 46) and monkeys (2, 8, and 40) for the low, middle, and high dosages, respectively.
- Data from each of the phase Ia cohorts will be examined carefully before proceeding to the next-higher dosage cohort.

Regulatory outcome:

- Initiation of the phase I trial was allowed.
- Dose escalation was permitted on the basis of the routine safety monitoring and stopping rules.

Acknowledgments

We thank Judy Henck and Michael Garriott (Eli Lilly) for contributions to the case study examples and Vikram Sinha and David Clarke (Eli Lilly) for their careful review of the manuscript.

REFERENCES

1. Yang Y, Blomme AG, Waring JE. Toxicogenomics in drug discovery: from preclinical studies to clinical trials. *Chem Biol Interact*. 2004;150(1):71–85.
2. Kramer JA, Sagartz JE, Morris DL. The application of discovery toxicology and pathology towards the design of safer pharmaceutical lead candidates. *Nat Rev Drug Discov*. 2007;6(Aug. 1):636–649.
3. Schoonen WGEJ, Kloks CPAM, Ploemen J-PHTM, et al. Sensitivity of ^{1}H NMR analysis of rat urine in relation to toxicometabonomics: Part 1. Dose-dependent toxic effects of bromobenzene and paaracetamol. *Toxicol Sci*. 2007;98(1):271–285.
4. Olson H, Betton G, Robinson D, et al. Concordance of the toxicity of pharmaceuticals in humans and in animals. *Regul Toxicol Pharmacol*. 2000;32:56–67.
5. ICH Safety Guideline: Preclinical Safety Evaluation of Biotechnology-Derived Pharmaceuticals. ICH S6. International Conference on Harmonization; 1998. Available at: www.ich.org.
6. ICH Multidisciplinary Guideline: Nonclinical Safety Studies for the Conduct of Human Clinical Trials and Marketing Authorization for Pharmaceuticals. ICH M3(R2). International Conference on Harmonization; 2008. Available at: www.ich.org.
7. Buckley LA, Benson K, Davis-Bruno K, et al. Nonclinical aspects of biopharmaceutical development: discussion of case studies at a PhRMA-FDA Workshop. *Int J Toxicol*. 2008;27:303–312.
8. Bussiere JL. Species selection considerations for preclinical toxicology studies for biotherapeutics. *Expert Opin Drug Metab Toxicol*. 2008;4(7):871–877.
9. Guidance for Industry: Estimating the Maximum Safe Starting Dose in Initial Clinical Trials for Therapeutics in Adult Healthy Volunteers. U.S. Department of Health and Human Services, Food and Drug Administration, Center for Drug Evaluation; 2005. Available at: www.fda.gov/cder/guidance/5541fnl.pdf.
10. ICH Safety Guideline: Toxicokinetics: A Guidance for Assessing Systemic Exposure in Toxicity Studies. ICH S3A. Center for Drug Evaluation; 1995. Available at: www.ich.org.
11. Chien JY, Friedrich S, Heathman MA, de Alwis DP, Sinha V. Pharmacokinetics/pharmacodynamics and the stages of drug development: role of modeling and simulation. AAPS J. 2005;7(3):E544–E559.
12. Guideline on Strategies to Identify and Mitigate Risks for First-in-Human Clinical Trials with Investigational Medicinal Products. European Medicines Agency, Committee for Medicinal Products for Human Use; 2007. Available at: www.emea.europa.eu/pdfs/human/swp/2836707enfin.pdf.
13. Dorato MA, Engelhart JA. The no-observed-adverse-effect-level in drug safety evaluations: use, issues, and defnition(s). *Regul Toxicol Pharmacol*. 2005;42:265–274.
14. Lewis RW, Billington R, Debryune E, Gamer A, Lang B, Carpanini F. Recognition of adverse and nonadverse effects in toxicity studies. *Toxicol Pathol*. 2002:30(1):66–74.
15. Ponce RA, Visich JE, Heffernan JK, et al. Preclinical safety and pharmacokinetics of recombinant human factor XIII. *Toxicol Pathol*. 2005;33(4):495–506.
16. Harada Y, Yahara I. Pathogenesis of toxicity with human-derived interleukin-2 in experimental animals. *Int Rev Exp Pathol*. 1993;34(Pt A):37–55.

17. Halpern WG, Lappin P, Zanardi T, et al. Chronic administration of belimumab, a BLyS antagonist, decreases tissue and peripheral blood B-lymphocyte populations in cynomolgus monkeys: pharmacokinetic, pharmacodynamic, and toxicologic effects. *Toxicol Sci*. 2006;91(2):586–599.
18. Sand S, Victorin K, Filipsson AF. The current state of knowledge on the use of the benchmark dose concept in risk assessment. *J Appl Toxicol*. 2007;28(4):405–421.
19. Pinkel D. The use of body surface area as a criterion of drug dosage in cancer chemotherapy. *Cancer Res*. 1958;18(7):853–856.
20. Freireich EJ, Gehan EA, Rall DP, Schmidt LH, Skipper HE. Quantitative comparison of toxicity of anticancer agents in mouse, rat, hamster, dog, monkey, and man. *Cancer Chemother Rep*. 1996;50(4):219–244.
21. Schein PS, Davis RD, Carter S, Newman J, Schein DR, Rall DP. The evaluation of anticancer drugs in dogs and monkeys for the prediction of qualitative toxicities in man. *Clin Pharmacol Ther*. 1979;11(1):3–40.
22. Sloan TH. Body surface area misconceptions. *Risk Anal*. 1993;13:375–377.
23. Travis CC, White RK. Interspecific scaling of toxicity data. *Risk Anal*. 1988;8(1):119–125.
24. Travis CC. Interspecies extrapolation in risk assessment. *Ann 1st Super Sanita*. 1991;27(4):581–594.
25. Travis CC, Morris JM. On the use of 0.75 as an interspecies scaling factor. *Risk Anal*. 1992;12(2):311–313.
26. Watanabe K, Bois FY, Zeise L. Interspecies extrapolation: a reexamination of acute toxicity data. *Risk Anal*. 1992;12(2):301–310.
27. Enviromental Protection Agency (EPA). A cross-species scaling factor for carcinogen risk assessment based on equivalence of mg/kg$^{0.75}$/ day. *Fed Reg*. 1992;57:24152–24173.
28. Boxenbaum H. Time concepts in physics, biology, and pharmacokinetics. *J Pharmacol Sci*. 1986;75(11):1053–1062.
29. Mordenti J. Man versus beast: pharmacokinetic scaling in mammals. *J Pharmacol Sci*. 1986;75(11):1028–1040.
30. Ings RMJ. Interspecies scaling and comparisons in drug development and toxicokinetics. *Xenobiotica*. 1990;20(11):1201–1231.
31. Travis CC, White R, Ward RC. Interspecies extrapolation of pharmacokinetics. *J Theor Biol*. 1990;142:285–304.
32. Hu TM, Hayton WL. Allometric scaling of xenobiotic clearance: uncertainty versus universality. *Am Assoc Pharm Sci*. 2001;3(4):art 29.
33. Mahmood I, Green MD, Fisher JE. Selection of the first-time dose in humans: comparison of different approaches based on interspecies scaling of clearance. *J Clin Pharmacol*. 2003;43(7):692–697.
34. Lowe PJ, Hijazi Y, Luttringer O, Yin H, Sarangapani R, Howard D. On the anticipation of the human dose in first-in-man trials from preclinical and prior clinical information in early drug development. *Xenobiotica*. 2007;37(10–11):1331–1354.
35. Smith DA. Integration of animal pharmacokinetic and pharmacodynamic data in drug safety assessment. *Eur J Drug Metab Pharmacokinet*. 1993;18(1):31–39.
36. Reigner BG, Blesch KS. Estimating the starting dose for entry into humans: principles and practice. *Eur J Clin Pharmacol*. 2002;57(12):835–845.

37. Chaturvedi PR, Decker CJ, Odinecs A. Prediction of pharmacokinetic properties using experimental approaches during early drug discovery. *Curr Opin Chem Biol*. 2001;5:452–463.
38. Houston JB, Carlile DJ. Prediction of hepatic clearance from microsomes, hepatocytes, and liver slices. *Drug Metab Rev*. 1997;29(4):891–922.
39. Iwatsubo T, Hirota N, Ooie T, et al. Prediction of in vivo drug metabolism in the human liver from in vitro metabolism data. *Pharmacol Ther*. 1997;73:147–171.
40. Lave T, Coassolo P, Reigner B. Prediction of hepatic metabolic clearance based on interspecies allometric scaling techniques and in vitro–in vivo correlations. *Clin Pharmacokinet*. 1999;36(3):211–231.
41. Lombardo F, Obach RS, Shalaeva MY, Gao F. Prediction of volume of distribution values in humans for neutral and basic drugs using physicochemical measurements and plasma protein binding data. *J Med Chem*. 2002;45(13):2867–2876.
42. Obach RS, Baxter JG, Liston TE, et al. The prediction of human pharmacokinetic parameters from preclinical and in vitro metabolism data. *J Pharmacol Exp Ther*. 1997;283(1):46–58.
43. Obach RS. Prediction of human clearance of twenty-nine drugs from hepatic microsomal intrinsic clearance data: an examination of in vitro half-life approach and nonspecific binding to microsomes. *Drug Metab Dispos*. 1999;27(11):1350–1359.
44. Obach RS. The prediction of human clearance from hepatic microsomal metabolism data. *Curr Opin Drug Discov Dev*. 2001;4(1):36–44.
45. Poulin P, Theil F-P. Prediction of pharmacokinetics prior to in vivo studies: 1. Mechanism based prediction of volume of distribution. *J Pharm Sci*. 2002;91(1):129–156.
46. Pang KS, Rowland M. Hepatic clearance of drugs: 1. Theoretical considerations of a "well-stirred" model and a "parallel tube" model. Influence of hepatic blood flow, plasma and blood cell binding, and the hepatocellular enzymatic activity on hepatic drug clearance. *J Pharmaocokinet Biopharm*. 1977;5:625–653.
47. Wilkinson GR, Shand DG. A physiological approach to hepatic drug clearance. *Clin Pharmacol Ther*. 1975;18:377–390.
48. Oie S, Tozer TN. Effect of altered plasma protein binding on apparent volume of distribution. *J Pharm Sci*. 1979;68(9):1203–1205.
49. Poulin P, Theil F-P. Prediction of pharmacokinetics prior to in vivo studies: II. Generic physiologically based pharmacokinetic models of drug disposition. *J Pharm Sci*. 2003;91(5):1358–1370.
50. Theil FP, Guentert TW, Haddad S, Poulin P. Utility of physiologically based pharmacokinetic models to drug development and rational drug discovery candidate selection. *Toxicol Lett*. 2003;138(1–2):29–49.
51. Kawai R, Lemaire M, Steimer JL, Bruelisauer A, Niederberger W, Rowland M. Physiologically based pharmacokinetic study on a cyclosporine derivative, SDZ IMM 125. *J Pharmacokinet Biopharm*. 1994;22(5):327–365.
52. Charnick SB, Kawai R, Nedelman JR, Lemaire M, Niederberger W, Sato H. Physiologically based pharmacokinetic modeling as a tool for drug development. *J Pharmacokinet Biopharm*. 1995;23(2):217–229.
53. Concept Paper on the Development of a CHMP Guideline on the Nonclinical Requirements to Support Early phase 1 Clinical Trials with Pharmaceutical Compounds. European Medicines Agency; 2006. Available at: www.emea.europa.eu/pdfs/human/swp/9185006en.pdf.

54. Suntharalingam G, Perry MR, Ward S, et al. Cytokine storm in a phase 1 trial of the anti-CD28 monoclonal antibody TGN1412. *N Engl J Med*. 2006;355(10):1018–1028.
55. Duff GC. Expert Scientific Group on Phase 1 Clinical Trials (Interim Report). Available at: www.dh.gov.uk/en/Consultations/Closedconsultations/DH4139038; 2006.
56. Doi F, Kakizaki S, Takagi H, et al. Long-term outcome of interferon-alpha–induced autoimmune thyroid disorders in chronic hepatitis C. *Liver Int*. 2005;25(2):242–246.
57. Colaco CA. T-cell costimulation. *N Engl J Med*. 2006;355(24):2595; author reply 2595.57.
58. Sharpe AH, Abbas AK. T-cell costimulation: biology, therapeutic potential, and challenges. *N Engl J Med*. 2006;355(10):973–975.
59. Wise MP, Gallimore A, Godkin A. T-cell costimulation. *N Engl J Med*. 2006;355(24):2594–2595; author reply 2595.
60. Nguyen DH, Hurtado-Ziola N, Gagneux P, Varki A. Loss of Siglec expression on T lymphocytes during human evolution. *Proc Natl Acad Sci USA*. 2006;103(20):7765–7770.
61. Mehrishi JN, Szabo M, Bakacs T. Some aspects of the recombinantly expressed humanised superagonist anti-CD28 mAb, TGN1412 trial catastrophe lessons to safeguard mAbs and vaccine trials. *Vaccine*. 2007;25(18):3517–3523.
62. Drazen JM. Volunteers at risk. *N Engl J Med*. 2006;355(10):1060–1061.
63. Garcia-Bournissen F, Boragina M, Ito S. Cytokine storm and an anti-CD28 monoclonal antibody. *N Engl J Med*. 2006;355(24):2593; author reply 2593–2594.
64. Goodyear MD. Further lessons from the TGN1412 tragedy. *Br Med J*. 2006;333(7562):270–271.
65. Hanke T. Lessons from TGN1412. *Lancet*. 2006;368(9547):1569–1570; author reply 1570.
66. Hansen S, Leslie RG. TGN1412: Scrutinizing preclinical trials of antibody-based medicines. *Nature*. 2006;441(7091):282.
67. Kenter MJ, Cohen AF. Establishing risk of human experimentation with drugs: lessons from TGN1412. *Lancet*. 2006;368(9544):1387–1391.
68. Schneider CK, Kalinke U, Lower J. TGN1412: a regulator's perspective. *Nat Biotechnol*. 2006;24(5):493–496.
69. Liedert B, Bassus S, Schneider CK, Kalinke U, Lower J. Safety of phase I clinical trials with monoclonal antibodies in Germany: the regulatory requirements viewed in the aftermath of the TGN1412 disaster. *Int J Clin Pharmacol Ther*. 2007;45(1):1–9.
70. ReoPro (abciximab). In PDR Electronic Library. Greenwood Village, CO: Thomson Micromedex. Accessed Aug. 4, 2008.
71. Mordenti J, Thomsen K, Licko V, Chen H, Meng YG, Ferrara N. Efficacy and concentration-response of murine anti-VEGF monoclonal antibody in tumor-bearing mice and extrapolation to humans. *Toxicol Pathol*. 1999;27(1):14–21.
72. Guidance for Industry: Exploratory IND Studies. U.S. Department of Health and Human Services, Food and Drug Administration, Center for Drug Evaluation and Research; 2006.
73. Position Paper on Nonclinical Safety Studies to Support Clinical Trials with a Single Microdose. European Medicines Agency; 2004. Available at: www.emea.europa.eu/pdfs/human/swp/259902en.pdf.

74. Hayes AW. *Principles and Methods of Toxicology*, 5th ed. Boca Raton, FL: CRC Press; 2008:18–20.

75. O'Brien PJ, Smith DEC, Knechtel TJ, et al. Cardiac troponin I is a sensitive, specific biomarker of cardiac injury in laboratory animals. *Lab Anim*. 2005;40:153–171.

76. Visich J, Ponce R. Science and judgment in establishing a safe starting dose for first-in-human trials of biopharmaceuticals. In: Cavagnaro JA, ed. *Preclinical Safety Evaluation of Biopharmaceuticals*. Hoboken, NJ: Wiley; 2008:971–984.

77. Berridge BR, Pettit S, Walker DB, et al. A translational approach to detecting drug-induced cardiac injury with cardiac troponins: Consensus and recommendations from the Cardiac Troponins Biomarker Working Group of the Health and Environmental Sciences Institute. *Am Heart J*. 2009;158:21–29.

78. ICH Quality Guideline: Impurities in New Drug Substances. ICH Q3A(R2). International Conference on Harmonization; 2006. Available at: www.ich.org.

79. ICH Quality Guideline: Impurities in New Drug Products. ICH Q3B(R2). International Conference on Harmonization; 2006. Available at: www.ich.org.

80. ICH Safety Guideline: Nonclinical Evaluation for Anticancer Pharmaceuticals. ICH S9. International Conference on Harmonization; 2009. Available at ich.org.

11

EXPLORATORY INDs/CTAs

MITCHELL N. CAYEN

11.1 INTRODUCTION

Some contemporary challenges in drug discovery and development are outlined in Chapter 1. For example, the resource commitment for a new chemical entity (NCE) to reach the market—approximately 15 years and about $1 billion in research and development [1]—is well appreciated by those involved directly or indirectly in various aspects of drug discovery and development. Much of this expense is lost on drugs that fail at various stages of development, with only about one in 10 drugs that enter phase I clinical testing attaining regulatory approval [2]. Even more disturbing is the approximately 50% attrition rate of drugs that fail in phase III after demonstrating sufficient efficacy and safety in phase II clinical trials [3].

Pharmaceutical companies of all sizes are looking for ways to reduce the attrition of compounds that seem promising initially. Numerous efforts are under way to shift this high failure rate from late stages to earlier stages of drug development. A major initiative was the report issued in 2004 by the U.S. Food and Drug Administration (FDA) entitled "Innovation or Stagnation: Challenge and Opportunity on the Critical Path to New Medical Products" [4]. One of the main conclusions from this report, called the *critical path initiative*, was that a major cause of inefficiency in the development of successful drugs was the absence of innovative new approaches to the nonclinical and clinical testing of new drug candidates. Such an innovation was the 2006 FDA guidance entitled "Exploratory IND Studies" [5], wherein approaches are described that provide opportunities for streamlining nonclinical testing in support of a small-scale first-in-human (FIH) study with specifically defined goals.

Early Drug Development: Strategies and Routes to First-in-Human Trials, Edited by Mitchell N. Cayen

In contrast to traditional investigational new drug applications (INDs), whereby one NCE can be investigated, an exploratory IND or exploratory clinical trial application (*expIND* or *expCTA*) provides the sponsor with an opportunity to perform a clinical study with an NCE or a series of chemically related drug candidates under the same IND. Some potential advantages of this nontraditional approach are as follows:

- Enables sponsors to select the most promising molecule for further development.
- Creates a potential for an earlier go/no go decision, resulting in earlier termination in the development of an unsuccessful entity. With the identification of compounds likely to fail earlier, wasted resource (time, cost, and staff) investment can be reduced.
- The requirements for toxicity studies are less than those for a traditional IND, due to limits set for human exposure to the NCE.
- As a result, smaller amounts of drug substance are required.
- There is minimal risk to human subjects, as the dose regimens selected are designed to target pharmacokinetics and/or pharmacodynamics, and are not as high as those in a traditional phase I study, in which clinical safety is also a primary endpoint.
- The initial evaluation of the NCE in humans is more rapid.

It is important to note that regulatory initiatives and experiences to date have been principally with small-molecule NCEs. As biotherapeutics have their unique challenges, the perspectives discussed below may not apply to these drugs.

Primarily two categories of studies are contained within the eIND framework, based on dose level: microdose and pharmacological dose. A *microdose study* involves the administration of a single subpharmacological dose of an NCE or several NCEs, and is designed to obtain an early assessment of the pharmacokinetics and/or distribution (based on an appropriate imaging technique) in human subjects. A *pharmacological dose study* within an expIND involves "doses expected to produce a pharmacological, but not a toxic, effect; the potential risk to human subjects is less than for a traditional phase I study that, for example, seeks to establish a maximally tolerated dose" [5].

In this chapter we describe the regulatory background that supports expIND (and/or expCTA for European submissions) submissions, the nonclinical studies necessary to conduct an FIH study under the expIND or expCTA, the advantages and disadvantages of the different types of studies that can comprise an expIND, and the current perspectives of the initiative based on meeting presentations by various industry and regulatory specialists as well as two industry surveys conducted by the author. Aside from *expIND* or *expCTA*, the terminology sometimes employed for these early stage clinical studies has included *eIND/eCTA*, *phase 0*, *prephase I*, and *exploratory phase I studies*.

11.2 REGULATORY BACKGROUND

Regulatory agencies in Europe and the United States have been encouraging the use of an abbreviated nonclinical program to enable rapid initiation of a short-term human trial with an NCE. The purpose is rapid determination of whether a targeted property of an NCE obtains in human subjects, thereby enabling an early decision as to whether a compound has the potential of being developed further via a traditional clinical program.

11.2.1 FDA Single-Dose Toxicity Guidance

The first regulatory guidance which theoretically offered a nontraditional approach to early clinical testing was the 1996 FDA guidance on single-dose toxicity testing [6]. This approach, sometimes called a *screening IND*, allows for single-dose studies in humans up to a maximum tolerated dose to be supported by appropriate single-dose acute toxicity studies in a rodent and a nonrodent species. However, this strategy has not been utilized sufficiently in the 14+ years since the guidance was released.

11.2.2 European Position Paper on Microdose Clinical Trials

In 2004 the European Medicines Agency (EMEA) published a position paper that described nonclinical GLP safety studies that can support a single microdose trial in human subjects [7]. A microdose was defined as "less than 1/100th of the dose calculated to yield a pharmacological effect of the test substance based on primary pharmacodynamic data obtained in vitro and in vivo—and at a maximum dose of $\leq$100 μg." The position paper further stated that "an example of such a clinical trial is the early characterisation of a substance's pharmacokinetic-/distribution properties or receptor selectivity profile using positron-emission tomography (PET) imaging, accelerator mass spectrometry (AMS) or other very sensitive analytical techniques."

The EMEA toxicity studies required to support such a clinical microdose trial are as follows:

1. *Extended single-dose toxicity studies* (the term *extended* means that separate groups of animals are divided into different groups with different sacrifice times: for this guidance, on days 2 and 14)
   - *Number of species:* one, choice based on comparative in vitro metabolism and/or in vitro pharmacodynamics/biological activity as compared to humans.
   - *Number of dose levels:* sufficient to assess minimal toxic effect; include placebo.
   - *Highest dose:* based on allometric scaling from animal species to humans using a safety factor of 1000; if a toxic effect is observed at this dose, the nontoxic dose level should be established.

- *Dose route:* therapeutic route + (possibly) intravenous ("allow assessment of local tolerance").
- *Observation period:* 14 days, to include an interim sacrifice on day 2.
- *Hematology and clinical chemistry:* at a minimum of two time points (at least on days 2 and 14).

2. *Genotoxicity studies:* in vitro studies, as recommended in the relevant International Conference on Harmonization (ICH) guidances
   - Bacterial mutations (Ames test)
   - Chromosomal aberration
   - Mouse lymphoma or in vitro micronucleus

The genotoxicity studies may be shortened should the NCE be shown to belong to a chemical class for which genotoxicity data are available for other relevant NCEs in the class. Should the microdose study be planned to compare specific properties of several NCEs, the safety studies described above, as well as relevant pharmacodynamics, are required for each test substance. The position paper points out that the approach describes expectations for small molecules and may not apply for biopharmaceutics; the latter should be considered on a case-by-case basis. The position paper also emphasizes that the abbreviated nonclinical requirements apply only to microdose studies, not to higher doses (as described in the 2006 FDA guidance) or for dose escalation studies.

11.2.3 FDA Critical Path Initiative

In 2004 the FDA raised an alarm on the state of drug development when they launched their *critical path initiative* [4], designed to stimulate and facilitate a national effort to better modernize the use of emerging techniques to streamline the development of successful drugs. The report diagnosed the scientific reasons for the decrease in the approval of successful medicinal products, which had become and still remains a disappointing trend given the increased sophistication in recent technological and biomedical advances. A surprising statistic was the 50% decline in new product submissions to the FDA compared to the preceding decade, this despite a 250% increase in research and development expenditures. The report also emphasized the increasing failure rate of drugs entering the various phases of clinical drug development. The principal conclusion from this FDA wake-up call was that the inefficiency in drug development was due to the insufficient use of innovative approaches in the nonclinical and clinical testing of new drug candidates: "Often, developers are forced to use the tools of the last century to evaluate this century's advances." The report called for enhanced creativity in the utilization of available and emerging tools, such as in vitro tests, computer models, qualified biomarkers, and innovative study designs, in order to better predict safety and efficacy.

This was followed in 2006 by the critical path opportunities list [8], developed with extensive public input, describing areas of opportunity for improved product development. The list comprised some 76 examples of how new discoveries (e.g., in fields such as genomics and proteomics, imaging, bioinformatics) could be applied to enhance the rate of successful prediction of clinical safety and efficacy of investigational medical products, and fell into the following six topic areas:

1. Biomarker development
2. *Streamlining clinical trials*
3. Bioinformatics
4. Manufacturing
5. Antibiotics and countermeasures to combat infection and bioterrorism
6. Therapies for children and adolescents

It has been pointed out that to take advantage of this initiative, collaboration is needed between scientists from the FDA, industry, and academia in order to develop improved testing methods for candidate drugs [9]. Thus, another topic cited in the opportunities list document was the need for improved nonclinical testing of drugs. This topic, coupled with the critical path challenges for innovative study designs [4] and streamlining clinical trials [8], was followed by publication of the FDA exploratory IND guidance discussed below.

11.2.4 FDA Guidance on Exploratory IND Studies

In 2006 the FDA released a guidance entitled "Exploratory IND Studies" [5]. Unlike the EMEA position paper of 2004, which focused solely on microdose studies, the FDA guidance provided three examples (including microdosing) on how the IND process could be used with greater flexibility to advance several compounds into humans in parallel (or rapidly evaluate a single NCE) by testing specific pharmacologic and/or pharmacokinetic hypotheses, with the goal of potentially generating critical information that would enable the selection of a single candidate with properties that would optimize its chance of becoming a successful drug. An interesting comment in the guidance was the FDA's assertion that most traditional IND submissions contain too much information for the scope of the clinical plan proposed. The guidance provides the following three examples of the types of studies that can be conducted under an expIND, along with a description of the recommended supporting nonclinical studies:

1. Microdose studies
2. Clinical trials to study pharmacological effects
3. Clinical trials to evaluate the mechanism of action (MOA)

Microdose Studies A *microdose* is defined as "less than 1/100th of the dose calculated to yield a pharmacological effect of a test substance and a maximum dose of <100 micrograms" and is designed to evaluate the pharmacokinetics of the drug and/or its distribution in imaging studies. The maximum dose limit for biopharmaceutics is 30 nm [5]. The microdose approach in the FDA guidance evolved basically from the EMEA guidance issued two years earlier. Because of the small dose levels (which are not intended to induce a pharmacological effect), the nonclinical supporting data required are relatively limited (Table 11.1).

Similar to the FDA 1996 guidance on support for single-dose clinical studies, a single-dose microdose study in humans can be supported by an extended single-dose GLP (good laboratory practice) toxicity study in laboratory animals; however, only a single mammalian species (both genders) is required, the choice of which is "justified by in vitro metabolism data and by comparative data on in vitro pharmacodynamic effects." The study should be designed such that a minimum toxic dose is determined. Also, "the sponsor should demonstrate that a large multiple (e.g., 100×) of the proposed human does not induce adverse effects in the experimental animals" (based on scaling mg/m^2). The route of administration should be the same as that intended for the clinical trial. Because of the very low planned clinical exposure to the drug for microdose studies, the standard battery of genotoxicity and safety pharmacology studies are not required.

Clinical Trials to Study Pharmacological Effects The second approach permitted under an expIND is a clinical trial using higher doses that enable evaluation of a pharmacological endpoint or biomarker as long as the study goal does not encompass definition of a maximum tolerated dose (MTD). Herein, because of the higher doses, more extensive nonclinical safety data are required than for microdose studies (Table 11.1). The studies required are, however, still substantially fewer than required for a traditional IND, thus resulting in significant resource savings, depending on the study goal(s).

The guidance states that "Repeat dose clinical trials lasting up to 7 days can be supported by a 2 week repeat dose toxicology study in a sensitive species accompanied by toxicokinetic evaluations. The goal of such a study would be to select safe starting and maximum doses for the clinical trial. The rat is the usual species chosen for this purpose, but other species might be selected" if sufficient justification is provided. If the rodent is the species selected, a confirmatory study should be conducted in a nonrodent (typically, a dog or a nonhuman primate) with a limited number of animals [fewer than in a standard pre-FIH (first-in-human) study, but sufficient to identify a toxic response] at one dose level [i.e., the rodent NOAEL (no observed adverse effect level) calculated on the basis of body surface area]. This confirmatory study may be conducted in a single gender (presumably males) if there were no gender differences in the rodent study, and only a single gender is planned for the expIND clinical trial. "If the data from the confirmatory study suggest that the rodent is not the more sensitive species, then a 2 week *repeat* dose toxicity study should be performed in the second species to select doses for human trials." Genotoxicity and safety pharmacology studies are also required. For the latter, the central nervous system (CNS) and respiratory effects can be evaluated as part of the two-week rodent study, while the effect of

TABLE 11.1 Characteristics of and Requirements for Exploratory IND Studies with Common Classes of NCEs

Characteristic or Nonclinical Requirement	Microdose Study	Pharmacological Effect Study	Mechanism of Action Study
Description	Single administration of subpharmacologic or pharmacologic dose to a limited number of subjects	Single or repeat dose administration for a maximum of 7 days; can be escalating dose study	Single or repeat dose administration for a maximum of 7 days
Study goal(s)	Collecting PK data and/or performing imaging (e.g., PET) studies	PK and/or pharmacological or PD endpoints	Mechanism of action of NCE(s)
Clinical dose	Less than 1/100 of dose calculated to yield a pharmacological effect to a maximum of 100 μg	Starting dose is no more than 1/50 of NOAEL in sensitive species (mg/m^2 basis); maximum (stopping) dose is lowest of four doses (Section 11.2.4)	Case by case, based on target PD endpoint
In vivo toxicity[a]	Extended single dose in single species (both genders), selected based on in vitro metabolism + in vitro PD; similar to EMEA, observations on days 2 and 14	Two-week repeat dose in a single sensitive species (both genders) (+ TK), usually rat; also confirmatory study in a nonrodent species (may be one gender)	One or two species, based on dosing strategy to achieve a clinical PD endpoint; discuss with FDA
Toxicity doses[a]	Selected to establish minimal toxic effect or a margin of safety (latter at least 100× of expIND human dose, based on scaling)	Selected to establish safe starting and maximum doses for the clinical trial; second species can be single-dose level at the rat NOAEL	Based on PD in sensitive species, and not necessarily designed to produce frank toxicity; however, need hematology and histopathology
Safety pharmacology	Not required	Required; can be included in toxicity studies except for CV safety, which should be tested separately	Required; can be included in toxicity studies except for CV safety, which should be tested separately
Genotoxicity	Not required (unlike EMEA)	Required (except for biopharmaceutics or NCEs targeted for terminal patients)	Presumed to be required, although not stated in guidance
Bioanalytical technology for PK	Probably AMS for low LLOQ	LC-MS/MS or similar technique	LC-MS/MS or similar technique

[a] Actual program should be designed based on an appropriate case-by-case basis, pending consultation with regulatory authorities.

the NCE on the cardiovascular system can be assessed in the confirmatory study, generally using a dog.

The guidance addresses calculations of the human lowest (starting) and highest (stop) doses as follows:

- *Starting dose:* no greater than 1/50 the NOAEL from the two-week toxicity study in the more sensitive species, based on mg/m^2.
- *Stop dose:* the lowest of one of the following:
  1. One-fourth of the two-week NOAEL.
  2. One-half of the plasma AUC (area under the concentration–time curve) at the NOAEL in the two-week rodent study, or the AUC in the nonrodent at the rodent NOAEL, whichever is lower.
  3. The dose that produces a pharmacological response or at which target modulation is observed in the clinical trial.
  4. The dose at which an adverse clinical response is observed.

Clinical Trials to Evaluate the Mechanism of Action The third approach under the FDA's expIND umbrella is the determination of whether a MOA defined in vitro or in vivo in animals can be observed in humans (e.g., based on a receptor binding property, inhibition of target enzyme, relevant biomarker). The nonclinical requirements for an expIND designed to evaluate the MOA of an NCE is less clearly defined in the guidance. The guidance appropriately allows the sponsor to propose a scientifically rational nonclinical safety program that would support the clinical expIND goal. "The FDA will accept alternative, or modified, pharmacological and toxicological studies to select clinical starting doses and dose escalation schemes." Safety studies in two animal species (one species may be acceptable if scientific evidence supports this to be the more relevant species) can be designed to attain endpoints that may be considered indicative of the clinical efficacy of the NCE. "The dose and dosing regimen determined in the animal study would be extrapolated for use in the clinical investigation." Although not stated in the guidance, the planned clinical dose and dosing regimen would be expected to be determinants as to whether genetic toxicity and safety pharmacology studies would be desirable as part of the nonclinical package.

11.2.5 Belgium National Guidance on Exploratory Trials

In 2007 a working paper was issued by the Federal Agency for Medicines and Health Products in Belgium which described the conduct of what were termed *exploratory trials* in Belgium, "while awaiting the development of guidelines at the European level" [10,11]. Among the exploratory trials described, the document incorporated many of the principles of the first two examples in the FDA guidance (microdosing and pharmacological dose), with some exceptions. Also, unlike previous such documents, this paper addressed the specific challenges with biopharmaceutics and pointed out that "repeated daily administration to animals and humans may not be acceptable and a dosing schedule adapted to the product may be required." The paper outlines the toxicological and CPD [chemical and pharmaceutical data; the European counterpart to CMC (chemistry, manufacturing, and controls) in the United States] information recommended to support such studies. Probably as a result of the TeGenero incident with the monoclonal antibody TGN1412 in Europe (see Chapter 12), the Belgium paper uses the minimum anticipated biological effect level (MABEL) as the maximum starting dose for both small molecules and biopharmaceutics, or 1/50 of the NOAEL in the most sensitive species. Another difference from the FDA guidance is that human dosing up to two weeks is permitted. The paper also described additional approaches that enabled flexibility in the human clinical trial. For example, the document permits microdoses of 100 μg to be administered not once but up to five times, with appropriate washout between doses, an approach that would, however, require a seven-day multiple-dose rodent toxicity study. This new microdosing alternative is considered an important step forward for conducting imaging studies [12].

11.2.6 The ExpIND (or ExpCTA) Submission

The content of an expIND is similar in principle to that of traditional IND, but with the major exception that the supporting toxicology data are less extensive and more flexible. This also applies to CMC information. The extent of information provided by the sponsor will depend on the clinical study proposed and the extent of exposure of human subjects to the NCE(s). As with a traditional IND, the expIND submission must include (1) a clinical development plan, (2) CMC information, and (3) pharmacology and toxicology data. In contrast to a traditional IND, an expIND application must articulate the rationale for the compound(s) selected and the reason for the clinical study proposed. It should also be clear in the application that the expIND will be withdrawn after completion of the study.

Sufficient CMC information should be provided in a summary report "to enable the agency to make the necessary safety assessment." For example, "the sponsor must state in the beginning of the exploratory IND application whether it believes the chemistry of the candidate product presents any signals of potential risk (e.g., specific findings in nonclinical studies associated with known risks of related compounds)." Should the chemistry or manufacturing of the product create a potential for human risk, the sponsor should propose how such risk will be monitored in the clinical trial.

Much of the CMC section within an expIND is similar to that of a traditional IND, but with several exceptions described in the guidance [5]. The CMC information should include sufficient data on the stability of the test substance during the duration of the toxicity studies and a description as to how stability will be monitored during the clinical trial.

Regarding analytical characterization, if the same batch of NCE is used in both the toxicology and clinical trial, the material will be qualified for human use based on other CMC information, and thus not all impurities may need to be characterized at the expIND stage; this would be recommended as the most resource-sparing approach. However, if the clinical batch will not be same as the toxicology batch, "the sponsor should demonstrate by analytical testing that the batch to be used is *representative* of batches used in the nonclinical toxicology studies." Thus, the following analytical quality tests would be required:

- Identity
- Structure
- Assay for purity
- Impurity profile
- Assay for potency (biologic)
- Physical characteristics, as appropriate

It should be emphasized that once the clinical portion has been completed, the expIND is withdrawn, and any further study that would involve the NCE that has been selected would require submission of a traditional IND, wherein the applicant would cite the expIND in the investigational plan section of the new IND.

Some specific characteristics and nonclinical requirements for the three types of expIND studies are listed in Table 11.1. This guidance allows significant flexibility in the amount of nonclinical data to be included in the expIND submission. The amount of supporting data depends on the design of the clinical study proposed. In general, the expIND sets limits on dose level, duration of treatment, and number of subjects exposed to the test drug. The microdose approach is limited to evaluating relevant pharmacokinetic or imaging parameters and is not designed to induce pharmacological effects. The pharmacological effect and MOA studies involve the use of higher doses and possibly longer treatment times than do microdose studies, but they are not designed to establish an MTD.

11.3 EXPERIENCE AND VARIOUS PERSPECTIVES ON ExpINDs OR ExpCTAs

Based on the theoretical approaches and limited experience to date by drug sponsors on the various types of expINDs (or expCTAs), information is emerging on the pros and cons of the various accelerated IND/CTA paradigms. The real utility is based on the whether the effort in this approach is useful in the selection of a drug candidate for further development and whether the data generated within an expIND is predicable regarding a specific safety and/or efficacy and/or pharmacokinetic endpoint under conditions of the therapeutic use of the NCE in patients.

11.3.1 Microdose Studies

Technical and Bioanalytical Challenges As a result of the 100-μg maximum dose allowable in microdose studies, ultrahigh-sensitivity analytical methodology is required to enable sufficient characterization of the targeted pharmacokinetic (PK) parameter. Initially, an ultrasensitive liquid chromatography-mass spectrometry (LC-MS/MS) method should be attempted to attain the anticipated lower limit of quantification (LLOQ) (anticipated in the low-pg/mL range), since it is a relatively standard technique that does not require the availability of radiolabeled drug. PET is capable of measuring distribution as long as the results are interpreted appropriately.

For compounds with limited oral bioavailability, high apparent volume of distribution, and/or rapid clearance, it might be impossible to quantify some key PK parameters, such as elimination half-life, with widely available bioanalytical techniques, and thus the bioanalytical methodology to assess plasma exposure after such a low dose may be feasible only with AMS methodology after administration of a radioactive dose [13]. It is noted that the microdose definition is based on a maximum of 1/100 the anticipated pharmacological effect rather than of the expected *therapeutic dose* as derived from animal and in vitro models. It is unfortunate that the FDA guidance did not select the fraction of the therapeutic dose instead of the pharmacological dose since, for example, drugs that act by enzyme inhibition work at IC_{90}, and thus 1/100 of this value may be at the lower plateau of pharmacological activity. With a wide safety margin in a sensitive toxicology species coupled with an acceptable gradient slope of the dose–response curve of pharmacological activity, the fraction based on the anticipated therapeutic dose should still be safe, and thus more conducive to detection of plasma drug concentrations.

As discussed above, AMS is currently the bioanalytical tool of choice for measurement of the low concentrations [down to zeptogram/mL (10^{-21} g/mL)] of drug-derived material in plasma which are inherent in microdose studies. AMS is not a new technology, and the low radioactive dose inherent in a microdose study does not necessitate the laboratory to have a radioactivity license. In a microdose study with AMS measurement, a single dose of trace-enriched ^{14}C-labeled drug is administered to a small number ($n = 3$ to 6) of human volunteers at a dose of 0.5 to 100 μg. As with a typical human radiolabeled metabolic disposition study, blood (and possibly urine) samples are collected at prescribed intervals for a sufficient length of time after dosing, based on the goals described in the protocol, and radioactivity concentrations are measured in the targeted matrices. Although this involves the synthesis of radiolabeled drug, the low amounts of radioactivity required for AMS permits the clinical microdose study to be conducted without dosimetry assessments in support of the typical regulatory approvals for radiation required for typical radiolabeled human mass balance studies. Because the technique is specific for atoms but not for molecules (thus, radioactivity), it does not distinguish between parent drug and its putative metabolites without accompanying chromatography. However, the approach can be utilized in an early traditional phase I ADME (absorption, distribution, metabolism, and excretion) study by coadministration of a microdose of the ^{14}C-labeled drug with an unlabeled pharmacological dose, resulting in reduced radiation exposure and, in most instances, the need to precede such a study with animal mass balance studies for dosimetry calculations.

Experience to Date A critical determinant of the utility of the microdose approach is whether it indeed can predict pharmacokinetics at therapeutic dose regimens. An important contribution to this question was the CREAM (Consortium for Resourcing and Evaluating AMS Microdosing) trial conducted by a group of European and U.S. industrial institutions, for which the results with five drugs were reported by Lappin et al. [14]. In a three-way crossover design, each with warfarin, diazepam, midazolam, erythromycin, or the experimental drug ZK253 (Schering AG), healthy subjects were administered a microdose (100 μg) of the ^{14}C-labeled drug, a therapeutic dose of the ^{14}C-labeled drug, or a simultaneous intravenous microdose of the ^{14}C-labeled drug + an oral therapeutic dose of the same drug. A combination of LC-MS/MS and AMS was used to evaluate the pharmacokinetics and the absolute bioavailability of each compound. There was a good concordance between the microdose and therapeutic dose pharmacokinetics for diazepam, midazolam, and ZK253, but not for warfarin or erythromycin. Based on the known properties of the respective drugs, the discrepancy in warfarin volume of distribution was attributed to the high-affinity, low-capacity tissue binding, while the negligible bioavailability of the erythromycin (even with the ultrasensitive AMS analytical methodology) was concluded to be due to its possible acid liability in the stomach. Although the authors concluded that "when used appropriately, microdosing offers the potential to aid in early drug candidate selection," the results still showed that predictability was observed with only 60% of the drugs tested (albeit with only five drugs), and thus the prospective use of microdosing for new drug candidates for which its PK properties have not yet been established remains debatable.

In a companion report [15], microdosing was used to evaluate the distribution and pharmacokinetics of an investigational carbon-11 antiamyloid drug 1,1′-methylenedi(2-naphthol) (ST1859), using PET imaging and plasma radioactivity/HPLC analyses in healthy volunteers and patients with Alzheimer's disease. Following intravenous administration of 3.4 μg of a mixture of ^{11}C-labeled and unlabeled ST1859, peripheral metabolism was rapid in both groups of subjects, with only 20% of the plasma radioactivity due to unchanged drug at 10 minutes. Based on PET imaging up to 90 minutes after dosing, there was a relatively uniform distribution of radioactivity in the brain, including both amyloid-beta-rich and amyloid-beta-poor regions, in both healthy volunteers and patients. The authors concluded that "these data provide important information on the blood–brain barrier penetration and metabolism of an investigational antiamyloid drug and suggest that the PET microdosing approach is a useful method to describe the target-organ pharmacokinetics of radiolabeled drugs in humans." However, with the demonstration of such rapid biotransformation, the question can be raised as to how much of the radioactivity penetrating the blood–brain barrier was parent drug versus metabolite(s). Also, it would have been predicted that there should have been a significantly higher association of radioactivity in the amyloid-beta-rich area of the brain, particularly in the Alzheimer's patients. Accordingly, although an interesting study, the utility of microdosing for this type of drug for this purpose remains an open question.

Although many drug sponsors appear to be studying the utility of microdosing, relatively few reports have appeared in peer-reviewed journals [16, and personal communications], probably because studies conducted at such early stages of clinical developed are often not submitted for publication, and sponsors may prefer to retain the results only in corporate archives. In 2007 the American College of Clinical Pharmacology (ACCP) issued a position paper on microdosing in the drug development process and concluded that "from the paucity of reported data describing the strengths, but more important, the limitations of this evolving paradigm, it would appear that more validation of the technique, along with the specific focus on its limitations, needs to be addressed," but that, after appropriate refinement and validation, it "may have an impact on the new drug development process" [16]. This was followed by further commentary [17]. A Japanese initiative entitled "Establishment of Evolutional Drug Development with the Use of Microdosing Clinical Trial, Based on the Quantitative Prediction Technology of ADME" organized by the New Energy and Industry Technology Development Organization is currently ongoing, with one of its goals to determine the conditions whereby microdosing can accurately predict human therapeutic dose and respons [18].

Pros and Cons of Microdose Studies Based on reports and initiatives to date, the following appear to be some potential advantages of a microdose study:

1. Such a study can be used to evaluate the pharmacokinetics of one or more backup compounds to an original NCE with a well-established pharmacokinetic profile, but may have an undesirable property related to its pharmacokinetics (e.g., high variability). For backups with similar potencies (thus similar anticipated therapeutic doses), a microdose study wherein both backup(s) and original NCE are compared may be useful.
2. As mentioned above, the concept can be employed, though not within an expIND paradigm, but as part of an early traditional phase I clinical AME (absorption, metabolism, and excretion) study wherein a microdose of the ^{14}C-labeled drug is coadministered with a pharmacological dose of the drug. As AMS itself measures only radioactivity, the metabolite profile portion of such a study can be determined by splitting high-performance liquid chromatographic (HPLC) fractions between classical MS and AMS. Since an unlabeled amount of a pharmacological dose would be coadministered with the microdose of the radiolabeled drug, sufficient "bulk" is present to enable HPLC analyses for putative metabolites. In this manner, information can be obtained on both metabolite structure and concentration.

Because of the very low amount of radioactivity required, this would not create a need to determine radiation exposure based on animal mass balance data.

3. Certain PET studies can be amenable to an appropriately designed and interpreted microdose protocol.

Several years have passed since issuance of the EMEA and FDA documents describing microdosing, and it is understandable why the initiative has not had a significant impact on drug development strategies [11,19]. The key to success is for drug sponsors to feel confident that a carefully designed microdose study will indeed be predictive of the target human endpoint (i.e., that the method is prospectively predictive). Some of the reasons why, both in theory and in practice, microdose studies have not yet had, and arguably may not have, a significant impact on overall drug development strategies are as follows:

1. *Problematic extrapolation of PK from microdose to therapeutic dose.* Many xenobiotics do not obey linear kinetics, for various reasons (Chapter 2): saturation of absorption and/or clearance, enzyme inhibition, enzyme induction, and so on. As a first cut, a microdose study should not even be considered if there is already information available that (1) dissolution rate limitation is suspected at oral therapeutic doses, (2) saturable first-pass metabolism is anticipated at therapeutic doses, (3) the extent of plasma protein binding is concentration dependent, or (4) if dose-dependent kinetics is anticipated within the normal therapeutic range. Since, by definition, an expIND study is the first exposure of the NCE in human subjects, there is usually insufficient information available to anticipate prospectively whether the PK at the microdose can be extrapolated to the ultimate therapeutic dose. This would also apply to the evaluation of several compounds within the same expIND, insofar that a rank order of a targeted PK endpoint at the microdose may not be the same rank order at higher doses if there are between-compound differences in the dose-related PK among human subjects. This is probably the major critique of microdosing, and was borne out with the five compounds tested in the CREAM study reported by Lappin et al. [14].

2. *Reduction in clinical failures due to PK.* Due to improved technology (such as LC-MS/MS as a routine bioanalytical tool) as well as in vitro and in vivo testing methods utilized pre-FIH (Chapters 2 and 4), attrition due to clinical bioavailability and pharmacokinetics has been declining steadily. For example, the attrition due to these variables was about 40% of the drugs entering the clinic in 1991 compared to less than 10% in 2000 [2], and this decline appears to be continuing, whereas attrition due to toxicology, clinical safety, and commercialization of new drugs is on the rise.

3. *Highly sensitive bioanalytical assay.* Due to the low dose, another limitation of the microdosing approach is the requirement for a bioanalytical assay which is much more sensitive than techniques considered standard and is available in most bioanalytical laboratories. LC-MS/MS may be insufficient to characterize the PK of a drug administered at 1/100 the anticipated therapeutic dose. If AMS is

planned, there is a relatively large resource commitment involved in the synthesis of radiolabeled compound and use of this highly sensitive instrumentation. Several vendors have made AMS instrumentation available to drug sponsors, but this technology has yet to reach the stage where it can be considered to be routine. Should the highest dose allowed for a microdose study (100 μg, unless agreement with a regulatory agency would permit a dose up to 1 mg) be employed, and based on accumulated bioanalytical and pharmacokinetic data in laboratory animals, it is advisable to attempt to develop an LC-MS/MS assay for human plasma with an LLOQ in the low-pg/mL range, with the hope that this would be sufficiently sensitive to enable PK assessment in a clinical microdose study. Such a feasibility approach was used for fluconazole and tolbutamide, each of which has a similar pharmacokinetic profile in rats and humans, where sensitive LC-MS/MS assays (LLOQ = 0.1 nM) were shown to be sufficient to evaluate the pharmacokinetics of the drugs after an oral microdose (1 μg/kg) administration to rats [20]. Although this strategy was used for established drugs with known rat and human pharmacokinetics, it demonstrates that, on a prospective basis, if an NCE shows similarity, for example, in its profile of hepatic in vitro metabolism both in a laboratory species and human, a feasibility study in the animal species administered a microdose may help determine the potential success of a sufficiently sensitive LC-MS/MS assay for evaluation of the human pharmacokinetics in a microdose study.

11.3.2 Pharmacological Dose and MOA Studies

Experience to Date Exploratory IND or CTA studies at pharmacological doses and for MOA studies offer the sponsor more advantages than microdose studies and can probably better help reduce attrition rates in clinical drug development. Although more nonclinical testing is required for these studies under the expIND umbrella than for microdose studies, the extent is still less than that for a traditional IND. The Drug Information Association (DIA) recently held a workshop in Lisbon on expCTAs, and it appears that the initiative may become more popular in Europe as well as in the United States [21].

Pros and Cons of Pharmacological Dose and MOA Studies Some of the potential advantages of pharmacological dose and MOA studies are as follows:

1. Given the higher dose for such studies than for microdose studies, and with a properly focused protocol design, the sponsor can monitor pharmacokinetics using standard bioanalytical technologies such as LC-MS/MS, without the need to synthesize radiolabeled compound and the utilization of more sophisticated instrumentation, such as AMS. Since the dose level would be within the pharmacological range, the resulting pharmacokinetic variables are likely to be predictive of those under therapeutic conditions. Similarly, with the possibility of daily dosing up to seven days and the use of different dose levels, the resulting pharmacokinetic data can provide significant early information on the relationship of dose level and dose

duration on plasma exposure to the drug [and/or if appropriate, relevant metabolite(s)].

2. In addition to pharmacokinetics likely to be representative of the therapeutic dose regimen, the dose levels used in these studies also enable the sponsor to target a specific pharmacodynamic (PD) endpoint using a relevant biomarker or pharmacological target. With a daily dose regimen of up to seven days, a pharmacological response that develops over time can be evaluated.
3. Based on the totality of pharmacokinetic and pharmacodynamic endpoints potentially available with a pharmacological dose or MOA study, the sponsor can determine whether the NCE is worth pursuing via a traditional IND. If several compounds are included in such an expIND/expCTA, such PK and PD data can help select the best NCE for further development.
4. Some situations in which an expIND at pharmacological doses has been used by pharma companies to date and which may be considered are as follows:
   a. For compounds that show poor solubility or high clearance but may still be considered based on in vitro activity/potency or animal in vivo biological data.
   b. In evaluation of the absolute bioavailability of an oral pharmacological dose of a compound compared with concomitant intravenous administration of a microdose of the ^{13}C-labeled compound.
   c. In evaluation of the pharmacokinetics and/or pharmacodynamics of a pharmacological dose of backup NCEs compared to a compound undergoing clinical testing.
   d. In evaluation of the relative bioavailability of a compound administered with different drug formulations or as different salt forms.
   e. In initial evaluation of plasma metabolites, due to the higher analyte concentrations at pharmacological doses than with microdosing, thereby enabling an earlier comparison with metabolites observed in animal species in vivo and/or to compare with data obtained after in vitro metabolism with human liver preparations.

11.4 SOME REACTIONS AND PERSPECTIVES ON THE ExpIND/ExpCTA INITIATIVE

Regulatory authorities in the United States and Europe have provided drug sponsors with admirable flexibility in planning a rapid nontraditional approach for NCEs to be tested in human subjects more rapidly. However, the use of this initiative has not been as extensive as anticipated. This enthusiasm has been concentrated mainly within a few (but not all) big pharma companies, whereas the reaction from smaller companies has initially been hesitant and guarded.

However, smaller drug sponsor companies in Europe currently appear to be more enthusiastic about the initiative than are those in North America. Currently, the expIND/expCTA paradigms have been brought to the attention of the ICH for a possible rewrite of the ICH M3 guideline. There is no doubt that the expIND/expCTA approach can offer substantial resource savings in time, animal use, and other associated costs. The extent of such savings has been calculated by various major pharma sponsors and, as expected, varies between institutions and bases for calculations. Feedback to the author from various sponsors representing big pharma, small pharma, biotech companies, virtual companies, industry consultants, and regulatory colleagues has painted a picture of guarded optimism for expIND/expCTA studies, and drug sponsors should be aware of a number of considerations, discussed below.

11.4.1 What an ExpIND/ExpCTA Can Do

1. An expIND/CTA can help select the most promising new drug candidate among several NCE molecules (same pharmacological target but different scaffold). In a similar manner, it can help select the most appropriate salt form of the same molecule, or different formulations of the test substance.
2. A more rapid go/no go decision can be made on a single molecule, thereby preventing failure at a later stage in clinical drug development. A target decision can be based on pharmacokinetics (e.g., to determine feasibility of once-daily dosing) and/or pharmacodynamics with a relevant biomarker.
3. The approach will save time, cost, animal use, and bulk material by taking advantage of the abbreviated toxicology requirements and flexibility in the CMC requirements for clinical supplies. The savings regarding drug substance may be substantial, as the bulk drug requirements for an expIND program may still be amenable to a small-scale synthesis process and may not involve significant scale-up issues.
4. Although the time to FIH is shortened, there is no sacrifice regarding the safety of human subjects, given the strict limits of dose level and dose duration.
5. The expIND can enable the selection of a potential backup compound to a lead candidate which has shown some liability during a later stage of clinical development, or which has no apparent liability, but a backup is strategically desirable for "insurance" as a possible lead replacement. In this manner, the identification of a putative backup is accelerated.
6. The approach can help to rapidly identify a potential biomarker.

11.4.2 What an ExpIND/ExpCTA Cannot Do

1. An expIND/expCTA can be the first entry of a drug candidate into humans, but it cannot represent the beginning of a typical phase I clinical program.

This is not a replacement of a phase I study. At the end of an expIND/CTA clinical study, the IND is withdrawn, and a traditional IND for the targeted NCE needs to be prepared, and thus the normal process of product development needs to take place. Accordingly, this will delay submission of the traditional IND. The expIND cannot be considered to be a shortcut to drug development.

2. Regarding clinical efficacy, an expIND is not amenable to a therapeutic or diagnostic goal, as the dose limitations do not enable a therapeutic regimen to be evaluated. The purpose of the study is limited to a PK and/or PD endpoint, and there are no benefits of the study to patients.
3. Regarding clinical safety, the limited dose regimen is not intended to establish an MTD.

11.4.3 Some Potential Drawbacks or Challenges in the Conduct of an ExpIND/ExpCTA Program

The following are some potential issues in the conduct of an expIND/expCTA program, in addition to those cited specifically for microdose studies:

1. If the rodent is not a sensitive species, FDA/regulatory concurrence is advisable as to the maximum feasible dose and/or NOAEL margin for the clinical study.
2. Following a "go" decision in the expIND/expCTA study, the delay in initiating bulk drug synthesis for the traditional IND may be substantial. Similarly, the standard time allowance for the traditional nonclinical program (toxicology and CMC) needs to be factored into the time lines. Thus, the overall time line for development of the lead candidate is longer.
3. Some big pharma sponsors have noted that the various FDA divisions may treat an expIND submission differently: for example, requests to submit data typically within a traditional IND submission (in vitro metabolism across species, plans for clinical AME study, different interpretations of animal NOAEL in support of the highest clinical dose). Also, the sponsor is advised to clearly indicate that the submission is indeed an expIND, as these have not consistently been identified as such at the FDA.
4. ExpIND/expCTA experience to date with biopharmaceutics is very limited compared to that with small-molecule NCEs. The time gain for biologics with long half-lives may not be substantial, since delayed toxic effects may first need to be investigated nonclinically. The specific issues for expIND/CTA studies with biopharmaceutics need to be evolved and may require more of a case-by-case consideration than do small molecules.
5. Although the FDA and EMEA guidelines describe specific requirements for expIND/expCTA studies, sponsors have found that some (although not all) regulatory agencies or divisions have been flexible regarding the design

of animal and human studies. As with any development study, the protocol proposed should be based on sufficient background data and a sound scientific rationale.

6. The maximum clinical dose may be too restrictive for many drugs. However, regulatory agencies appear amenable for discussion on this restriction, also on a case-by-case basis.

Some additional feedback to the author from drug sponsors is as follows:

- Some companies, in particular smaller pharma and biotech in North America, much prefer the traditional route, as they are uncomfortable with the delay in submitting a standard IND after data have been generated in an expIND. Smaller companies generally have fewer compounds under consideration and may be looking to more rapid successful clinical outcomes for potential out-licensing as early as possible. Two INDs are needed to initiate phase I, thus representing a longer path to the NDA.
- Smaller companies may find the approach useful as a licensing strategy (i.e., to attain a targeted PK and/or PD result with minimal resources as the only clinical study).
- There is generally much more enthusiasm about the pharmacological approach than for microdosing, due to the inherent limitations of the latter in projecting to therapeutic dose regimens.
- The approach works for small molecules but not for biopharmaceutics.
- One company used the approach to determine absolute bioavailability based on simultaneous administration of an intravenous ^{14}C microdose and an oral pharmacodynamic dose. However, the caveat is that the oral and intravenons milligram doses were different; thus, absolute bioavailability calculation was based on the unproven assumption of linear kinetics.
- There is uncertainty that a failed microdosing result necessarily means a "no go" decision, so why do it?
- PK is best done at a PD dose, not at a microdose.
- It is best to consult the regulatory agency regarding the expIND/expCTA plan, but this in itself causes delays in the time necessary to schedule and implement the study.
- The lower bulk drug requirement (ca. 300 to 400 g instead of 1 to 2 kg) is a major advantage, as are other resource savings in toxicology and CMC, although some companies believe that the major resource savings is with API and is minimal with toxicology and CMC.
- Pharmacodynamic effects in the expIND/expCTA program are rarely explored in the manner desired.
- The approach can generate a faster answer to a specific question.
- Since, upon completion of the expIND, there is the need to move to a traditional IND, the following needs to be repeated: toxicology (expIND

toxicity study was too short), safety pharmacology (in separate studies), bulk synthesis (probably new route), and CMC (more extensive testing of a new API batch).

- ExpIND/expCTA is "a good path for unsuccessful candidates."
- "The total amount of resource savings is not enough to justify routine use of the expIND strategy when weighed against the risks and opportunity costs for most drug programs."
- For biologics, "the pharmacodynamic approach has been done for years." However, microdosing is not realistic, as a small unnoticeable difference in the pharmacokinetics of a biopharmaceutic can result in a completely different biological response.

It is thus apparent from the commentary above that the current impression and utility of expIND/expCTA varies widely and that there remains some misinterpretation about the initiative.

11.5 WHAT IS AN IDEAL CANDIDATE FOR AN ExpIND/ExpCTA?

When considering the option of an expIND/expCTA for a single NCE or a series of closely related compounds, the properties listed in Table 11.2 will enable a decision as to the likelihood of success for this approach. Input from all relevant disciplines (chemistry, CMC, biology/pharmacology, toxicology, drug metabolism, bioanalytical, clinical, management) is required in order to develop a team decision as to whether this approach is advantageous for the specific project and therapeutic goal.

11.6 CONCLUSIONS

Several nontraditional approaches are now available for sponsors to attain an early assessment of relevant pharmacokinetic and/or pharmacodynamic properties of an NCE in an FIH study. However, to attain optimal return (i.e., a targeted early development decision) from the effort involved in conducting an expIND/expCTA study, the sponsor must assure that such a study will be considered and conducted under the right circumstances. Study designs must be such that the results will enable a go/no go decision regarding whether an NCE should proceed through a traditional IND/CTA path. If the various possible anticipated results are equivocal, the effort will be wasted.

One such nontraditional approach is microdosing, which in theory has the potential of attaining early pharmacokinetic and/or imaging data, with the hope of determining whether a single candidate, or one of several NCEs, has the appropriate property to enable a go/no go decision regarding further development. The most unavoidable caveat is the prospective ability to project in a microdose the pharmacokinetics that would be attained under therapeutic conditions. Herein

TABLE 11.2 Ideal NCE Candidate for an expIND or expCTA Study

Drug Property or Study Goal	Advantages/Considerations
High-potency drug	Efficacy at low-mg/kg doses limits bulk drug requirement
Good oral bioavailability in laboratory animals	Better likelihood that there will also be good bioavailability in human subjects
Large-scale synthesis is difficult and/or resource intensive	Can prevent time and cost of large-scale synthesis for NCEs ultimately eliminated by results of expIND/expCTA study
Single-targeted PK and/or PD goal	Better enables a go/no go decision
Detectable clinical efficacy marker or biomarker attainable within expIND/expCTA	PK can be the only goal, but PD is the major driver for success; reduced time to initial clinical evaluation
Resource and project considerations are amenable to an expIND/expCTA	Too much or too little can kill an expIND Cost to next decision point Cost to full development Potential outsourcing or licensing plans
Management understanding of issues, limitations, and predictability	Potential cost savings should not be overly optimistic; needs an internal champion
Overall portfolio strategy	Candidate(s) for expIND/expCTA should be considered based on the pharmaceutical company's portfolio management strategy regarding risk for delays to phase I and other resource commitments

lies a "catch-22." For microdosing to be successful regarding such predictability, fairly extensive pharmacokinetic information (e.g., animal data that show linear kinetics and similar in vitro metabolism as in humans) should be available to assess if the NCEs are good candidates for such a study, but the timing of an expIND/expCTA is such that these data are usually generated at a later stage of development. The study by Lappin and Garner [13] showed only a 60% success rate with known drugs. With the possible exception of imaging biomarker targets, it would appear that microdosing for pharmacokinetics assessment has very limited capacity to have an impact on the decision-making process of candidate selection, and it is therefore recommended that this technique be considered only in those rare instances where it is known in advance that such subpharmacological doses would generate reliable data that would enable a go/no go decision.

It would appear that the use of a pharmacological dose level as an expIND/expCTA study has significantly more advantages than does microdosing. A single compound or a series of compounds can be evaluated in parallel in order to test specific pharmacokinetic or pharmacodynamic hypotheses, and potentially to generate critical information that would enable selection of the best compound having the highest likelihood of therapeutic and commercial success.

This option has already been proven to be a valuable option for several pharmaceutical companies. It is important to consider advantages and disadvantages of this option. The primary advantage is that a properly designed pharmacological dose study is amenable to both pharmacodynamics and predictable pharmacokinetics (at least much more predictable than microdosing) of one or more NCEs. Should a readily detectable pharmacodynamic endpoint or biomarker be identifiable upon the short-term administration inherent in an expIND/expCTA, the approach can be most valuable. If the goal is pharmacokinetic assessment alone (without a pharmacodynamic component), such as in comparing several compounds, several salts, or formulations of a single NCE, or determination of the half-life with a goal of evaluating whether the NCE is a candidate for once daily administration, it is recommended that the expIND/expCTA comprise administration of a pharmacological dose rather than a microdose.

There is no doubt that appropriate use of an expIND/expCTA study involves the use of significantly fewer resources (e.g., bulk drug, animals, time) than traditional INDs or CTAs and can be a valuable tool in the early clinical assessment of some NCEs. Its primary goal is to allow early attrition of poor candidate drugs or drug (drug substance or drug product) forms. Such a study should not be conducted unless the results permit a clear go/no go decision to be made. The initiative is still undergoing growing pains and remains a work in progress. Time will tell whether the approach becomes a major part of the early drug development armamentarium.

Acknowledgments

The author is grateful to William T. Robinson (consultant, Novartis Pharmaceutical Corporation) for helpful discussion, commentary, and critiques during the preparation of this chapter. The author also wishes to thank Frank Bullock (drug development consultant), Joy Cavagnaro (AccessBio), James Green (BiogenIdec), Howard Hill (Covance, UK), Lew Klunk (BiogenIdec), James Keirns (Astellas Pharma, U.S.), James MacDonald (Chrysalis Pharma), Check Quon (iNDa Consulting), and Alfred Tonelli (Johnson & Johnson) for their perspectives on the expIND/expCTA initiative.

REFERENCES

1. DiMasi JA, Hansen RW, Grabowski HG. The price of innovation: new estimates of drug development costs. *J Health Econ*. 2003;22:151–185.
2. Kola I, Landis J. Can the pharmaceutical industry reduce attrition rates? *Nat Rev Drug Discov*. 2004;3:711–715.
3. Melvis J. Productivity counts—but the definition is key. *Science*. 2005;309:26.
4. Innovation or Stagnation: Challenges and Opportunities on the Critical Path to New Medical Products. U.S. Food and Drug Administration; 2004. Available at: www.fda.gov/oc/initiatives/criticalpath/whitepaper.html.

5. Guidance for Industry: Exploratory IND Studies. U.S. Department of Health and Human Services, Food and Drug Administration, Center for Drug Evaluation and Research; 2006.
6. Guidance for Industry: Single Dose Acute Toxicity Testing of Pharmaceuticals. U.S. Department of Health and Human Services, Food and Drug Administration; 1996.
7. Position Paper on Nonclinical Safety Studies to Support Clinical Trials with a Single Microdose. CPMP/SWP/2599/02/Rev 1. European Medicines Agency; 2004. Available at: www.emea.eu.int/pdfs/human/swp/259902en.pdf.
8. Critical Path Opportunity Report. U.S. Department of Health and Human Services, Food and Drug Administration; 2006. Available at: www.fda.gov/oc/initiatives/criticalpath/reports/opp list.pdf
9. Woosley RL, Cossman J. Drug development and the FDA's critical path initiative. *Clin Pharmacol Ther*. 2007;81:129–133.
10. Guidance to the Conduct of Exploratory Trials in Belgium. Federal Agency for Medicines and Health Products in Belgium; June 2007.
11. Attarchi F. Exploratory IND studies: A review of the Food and Drug Administration guidance and similar provision in Europe. *Drug Inf J*. 2007;41:309–314.
12. Robinson WT. Innovative early development regulatory approaches: expIND, expCTA, microdosing. *Clin Pharmacol Ther*. 2008;83:358–360.
13. Lappin G, Garner RC. Big physics, small doses: the use of AMS and PET in human microdosing of development drugs. *Nat Rev Drug Discov*. 2003;2:233–240.
14. Lappin G, Kuhnz W, Jochemsen R, et al. Use of microdosing to predict pharmacokinetics at the therapeutic dose: experience with 5 drugs. *Clin Pharmacol Ther*. 2006;80:203–215.
15. Bauer M, Langer O, Dal-Bianco P, et al. A positron emission tomography microdosing study with a potential antiamyloid drug in healthy volunteers and patients with Alzheimer's disease. *Clin Pharmacol Ther*. 2006;80:216–227.
16. Bertino JS Jr, Greenberg HE, Reed MD. American College of Clinical Pharmacology position statement on the use of microdosing in the drug development process. *J Clin Pharmacol*. 2007;47:418–422.
17. Bertino JS Jr, Greenberg HE, Reed MD. Response to comments on ACCP position statement on microdosing. *J Clin Pharmacol*. 2007;47:1597–1598.
18. Sugiyama Y. Effective use of microdosing and positron emission tomography (PET) studies on new drug discovery and development. *Drug Metab Pharmacokinet*. 2009;24:127–129.
19. Boyd RA, Lalonde RL. Nontraditional approaches to first-in-human studies to increase efficiency of drug development: Will microdose studies make a significant impact? *Clin Pharmacol Ther*. 2007;81:24–26.
20. Balani SK, Nagaraja NV, Qian MG, et al. Evaluation of microdosing to assess pharmacokinetic linearity in rats using liquid chromatography–tandem mass spectrometry. *Drug Metab Dispos*. 2006;34:384–388.
21. Silva-Lima B, Laurie D, Robinson WT. The European and American use of exploratory approaches for first-in-human studies. *Clin Translational Sci* (in press).

12

UNIQUE CONSIDERATIONS FOR BIOPHARMACEUTICS

LAURA P. ANDREWS AND JAMES D. GREEN

12.1 INTRODUCTION AND BACKGROUND

Drug development scientists have generated an extensive experience base with a wide range of product classes of biopharmaceutics over the last two decades. These product classes have included molecules that are diverse in origin and biological activity and have been produced by a variety of production methods. For example, host cells [e.g., *Escherichia coli*, yeast, Chinese hamster ovary (CHO) cells] are used in the production of antibodies and proteins; solid- and liquid-state chemical syntheses have been used for the production of oligonucleotides, and a variety of vectors (e.g., retrovirus, AAV) have been used to produce gene therapy products. It is impossible to remain contemporary in a nonclinical approach with new products and new indications being developed and addressed every day. However, in this chapter we review the historical information that has established the groundwork for current practices, identify crucial global regulatory documents that should be considered collectively, and highlight unique considerations for the variety of product classes during pre-FIH (first-in-human) development. These considerations and the challenges behind the diversity of products and approaches should be addressed in the design of nonclinical safety evaluation and pharmacokinetics programs to support FIH studies.

Early Drug Development: Strategies and Routes to First-in-Human Trials, Edited by Mitchell N. Cayen

12.2 SELECTION OF THE MOLECULE: CONTRASTS TO SMALL-MOLECULE CONSIDERATIONS

The compound selection paradigm for a protein or monoclonal antibody, for example, is very different from that utilized for a small-molecule drug. For a typical small-molecule program [1], nonclinical development comprises a complex triage whereby literally thousands of new chemical entities' (NCEs) are considered. On the basis of a combination of potency, selectivity to a target receptor, drug metabolism and pharmacokinetic properties, and biological characteristics, a small-molecule candidate drug is selected for comprehensive nonclinical safety assessments that are most often conducted in two species (one rodent and one nonrodent). For most biopharmaceutics that are considered for development, the drug candidate (e.g., protein, antibody, fusion construct) is selected on the basis of potency, specificity, molecular characteristics, formulation stability, and isotype (for antibodies). In some instances, specific target identification (i.e., for vaccines) will drive the product selection decision.

For programs that involve proteins or monoclonal antibodies, two other very important decisions that are required during the early nonclinical phase of a biopharmaceutic are: (1) the type of host cell that is selected to be transfected with the gene construct, and (2) the degree of characterization required of what are typically referred to as *key product attributes* for the biopharmaceutic. By definition, these are important molecular features of the biopharmaceutic that determine potency and activity under conditions of intended use. For example, if glycosylation is an important product attribute and necessary for the compound to be active or to have desired pharmacokinetic properties, CHO cells are often used in lieu of *E. coli* [2–5]. One very common issue that is often encountered by development scientists is the fact that much of the early data generated by scientists working in discovery and research groups utilize test material or a form of the molecule (sometimes called prototype material) that is not the intended clinical candidate. If this is the case, it is important that key discovery potency and receptor occupancy experiments be repeated with the clinical candidate to confirm the observations made with the early prototype materials. If biologically significant discrepancies are observed between different sources or forms of the biopharmaceutic, it is important to understand the reason for the presumed differences. One of the key learning lessons from the TeGenero incident (discussed later in the chapter), which involved the development of a humanized agonist antibody that caused severe adverse drug reactions in the first clinical trial, involved exactly this point [6]. That is, at the pre-FIH stage of development, safety data or signals generated with all forms of the biopharmaceutic need to be considered in determining initial human doses and conditions. It is very important that the cell line and production process used to produce the test material that is utilized for the pivotal nonclinical toxicology and pharmacokinetic studies be the same as that utilized to generate the clinical material. If for some reason this is not possible, appropriate comparative laboratory and bridging nonclinical safety studies should be performed.

12.2.1 Utility of Animal Efficacy Models

Nonclinical data generated in animal models of disease coupled with data that demonstrate specificity to the target receptor are relevant for understanding the pharmacology and perhaps dose response as they relate to exaggerated pharmacology. Most animal models of disease are imperfect replicas of the human disease conditions [7,8]; however, in some cases they may help determine whether or not a selected form of the molecule retains suitable activity. For example, in consideration of the development of a monoclonal antibody candidate, an animal model may show whether or not the presence or absence of an Fc effector function is necessary for in vivo activity. These data may sometimes be important in determining the choice of the production cell line. In addition, the demonstration of pharmacological activity in animal models may provide the development scientist with insight into which species to consider for use in subsequent safety assessment studies.

12.2.2 In Vitro Activity Profiling, Sequence Homology, and the Use of Homologous Molecules for nonclinical Efficacy and Safety Assessments

During the discovery phase, data that demonstrate in vitro binding to the target receptor and an ability of this binding to either antagonize or turn on the targeted molecular pathway are typically available. If there is more than one molecular construct or form of the biopharmaceutic available, comparative data should be generated if there are theoretical advantages of one form over another. Potency, usually expressed as IC_{50}/EC_{50} (inhibitory or effective concentration giving a 50% response) or binding affinity can be used as a basis for selecting one form of the molecule over another. In addition to in vitro activity, conservation of sequence homology to the human form of the biopharmaceutic is important and should be known during the pre-FIH phase. The latter information can sometimes help to inform discussions related to the likely conservation of biology and target responsiveness across species, which is extremely valuable when trying to extrapolate to the clinic observations made in the animal setting.

Sometimes one may encounter a situation where the human form of the biopharmaceutic is not biologically active in typical animal species that are used for nonclinical safety assessment (mouse, rat, dog, or commonly used primates). In this case, the biopharmaceutic is referred to as *human specific*. This designation must be used with caution, as it has been shown that many biopharmaceutics considered to be human specific early in discovery or research were, when more thoroughly tested, demonstrated to be biologically active in rodents and nonrodents. However, when working with a molecule that is thought to be truly human specific, it is sometimes reasonable to perform nonclinical work with a homologous form of the molecule, the homologous form being defined as the species-specific form of the molecule being tested in that host species (e.g., a murine monoclonal antibody tested in various mouse strains). This is not an unusual situation to encounter in a discovery or research setting. Initial observations of interesting biological activity are often made with a murine form of a protein or antibody in murine models of disease. In a situation where the human form of the biopharmaceutic is not active in the rodent or nonrodent species that are typically used for nonclinical safety assessment, it may be necessary and valuable to perform IND-enabling safety studies with the homologous form of the biopharmaceutic to identify the range of potential human toxicities related to exaggerated pharmacology. In reality, for the development scientist this is a difficult situation pre-IND (investigational new drug application), because in this case only very limited data would be generated with the clinical form of the molecule. The latter studies may be limited to pharmacokinetic estimates. This is not an optimal situation and renders more difficult the prediction of expected human toxicities and human dosimetry calculations with the human form of the molecule.

12.2.3 In Vivo Profiling of Biopharmaceutical Activity

Once the candidate biopharmaceutic is selected, data should be generated in a suitable animal model of disease that might represent key features of the targeted clinical indication. In this animal model a dose–response curve should be generated over a range of doses that would be expected to demonstrate a range of biological activities encompassing minimal, moderate, and full pharmacological activity. The key data that need to be gleaned from any animal model are those that delineate the dose–response activity range. The expression of the active dose range on a mg/kg basis is suitable for most biopharmaceutics that distribute primarily to the plasma compartment; however, it is important to recognize that many regulators and physicians working in the oncology area are accustomed to seeing dose units also expressed on a mg/m^2 basis. Whichever dose unit form is viewed as most appropriate should be scientifically justified by the development scientist in the expression of therapeutic ratios used to support the initial clinical trial application. In cases where possible, activity over this dose range should be correlated with receptor occupancy. In addition, these animal model dose–response data should be correlated with plasma or serum exposure data over the range of doses studied.

After a working dose range is established in one or two animal models, this range should be studied in the animal species that are selected for use in the nonclinical safety evaluation program. This will allow initial comparisons to be made between doses and exposures expected to be active in the disease setting to be compared with ranges of activity that are shown to be active in a nondiseased setting. This may provide some initial insights into any differential sensitivity that might exist between the diseased and normal animal models. Once the presumed active dose range can be bracketed, this information can be considered in discussions involving suitable toxicology doses and the projected range of clinical doses likely to be studied in early clinical trials. Interspecies pharmacokinetic scaling techniques have been shown to be useful in certain situations for projecting clinical pharmacokinetic parameters [9,10].

12.3 PRODUCTION AND PROCESS CONSIDERATIONS IN PRE-FIH DEVELOPMENT

The process by which a biopharmaceutic is made can undergo many changes during the pre-FIH and phase I, II, and III clinical phases. In some instances, these process changes can extend well into the postmarketing setting. The major driving force behind the need to change a specific process fermentation or purification scheme is often related to the desire to improve product quality characteristics and to improve the cost-of-goods structure. A typical process evolution is depicted in Figure 12.1. As shown in the figure, a process can change in size and scope between the various stages of drug development. During the course of these stages, it is not unusual for changes to occur to the cell line, formulation, and various components of the production of purification scheme. Typical changes that often occur are shown in Table 12.1.

How a biopharmaceutic is made affects the key product attributes of the biopharmaceutic. Examples of these attributes which are sometimes encountered for proteins and antibodies include the necessity for amino acid sequence(s) required for binding or folding, the importance of specific glycosylation patterns of forms for biological activity, the relative importance of truncated or clipped forms of the biopharmaceutic, the importance of incorrectly folded disulfide linkages, and changes in the nature of aggregates. These will differ for each product and each product class. This is an important concept for the development scientist to be familiar with because key product attributes govern potency, safety, efficacy, therapeutic ratio, and risk estimates made for the biopharmaceutic. Furthermore, important host- and process-related impurities are related to the production process used to make the drug product, and these need to be studied adequately in the nonclinical phase. The relationship between how a biopharmaceutic is made and its key product attributes is sometimes referred to by process scientists as "product = process" [11].

TABLE 12.1 Example of Changes that Occur to a Manufacturing Process of a Biopharmaceutic During Development and After Approval

Process or Stage of Development	Types of Changes
Formulation and filling	Excipient, equipment, change in manufacturing protocol, scale, site change, shipping
Drug product	Batch definition, shelf life, container/closure, shipping, storage
Expression system	Master cell blank; working cell blank
Fermentation/culture process	Raw materials, cell culture conditions, scale, equipment, site change
Purification process	Column/resin, reagents, scale, site, equipment

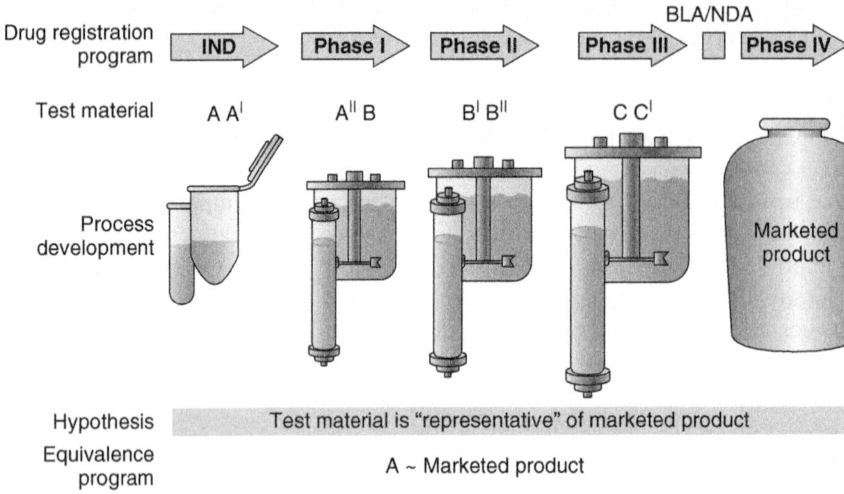

FIGURE 12.1 Typical life cycle of a biologic production process.

During the pre-FIH phase, the development scientist should be as diligent as possible to assure that the test material used in the pivotal IND-enabling studies is derived from a production process that is very similar to or, ideally, identical to that intended to produce the initial clinical batches. In this case, the pivotal studies are those that are relied upon to establish the initial therapeutic ratio and safety margin used to determine safe use conditions. In some cases this requirement may reasonably be extended to include pivotal pharmacology studies that defined in vivo pharmacologically active doses. If changes are made to the process between the pre-FIH period and Phase I, it is imperative that the development scientist see data from a well-designed product comparability program of study in which the test material that was used in the pivotal pharmacologic, pharmacokinetic, and toxicity studies is demonstrated to be highly similar (comparable) to that intended to be used in the phase I clinical program. Product comparability studies typically include a tiered approach, but can include biochemical, bioactivity, and pharmacokinetic studies. If major differences in the comparability profile are discovered between the pre-FIH and clinical material, it may be necessary to repeat the pivotal IND-enabling safety studies to assure that safe use conditions are supported [12,13].

When significant portions of the nonclinical data are generated with a homologous form of the clinical product, the challenge of establishing product comparability to the clinical material is much greater. Sometimes, unexpected safety findings are observed which were not predicted from studies completed with the homologous form of the biopharmaceutic. For this reason, many companies will try to avoid development and selection of biopharmaceutics that are characterized as human specific because they cannot be studied adequately in nonclinical safety assessment studies for which a large history of experience exists.

12.4 BIOANALYTICAL ASSAY CONSIDERATIONS

As discussed for small-molecule drug candidates (Chapters 7 and 8), toxicological assessments with biopharmaceutics must be accompanied by assessments of exposure, and accordingly, an appropriate bioanalytical assay needs to be developed for the measurement of concentrations of the biopharmaceutic in serum or plasma. The technical approaches to such development and validation of these assays are discussed in Chapter 4.

Several considerations surround the development and qualification of such assays for biopharmaceutics to support the nonclinical program. Certainly, early in development the assays may not be sufficiently developed to address limits of quantification, sensitivity, and challenges of different matrices. It is recognized that early in the development program, during proof-of-concept studies and early safety assessment, the assays may only be useful for product quantification in the dosage form or formulation. However, as the development program moves toward IND-enabling studies, it is necessary to address issues of sensitivity, species and matrix variability, and general robustness of the assays being developed. The assays to be designed should be developed to identify a specific component in the matrix. Components to be identified include the active drug product, antibodies against the drug product, and if required, any impurities that may affect the safety and efficacy of the product. Typically, the bioanalytical assays should be developed to address as many validation criteria as possible, but certainly should be designed to demonstrate accuracy, precision, specificity, detection limit, quantification limit, linearity, and range. Furthermore, reevaluation of these characteristics will need to be considered if there are changes in the manufacturing processes, changes in the composition of the final product, and/or changes in the analytical procedures themselves. It is important to understand that assays also need to be developed and qualified for any homologous proteins that are being used for safety evaluation. The need to requalify an assay will depend on the magnitude of the change and where in the process of the development of the product the change is occurring.

The biggest challenge faced in qualifying assays for both in vivo evaluations and bioanalytical validation is establishing assays with sufficient sensitivity and precision to detect small differences following manufacturing or scale-up changes and to distinguish the impact of such factors as antibody titers on exposure assessment. With increased product complexity (heterogeneity and higher structures) than is the case for small molecules, it is important that the analytical techniques be sufficient to distinguish relevant differences within the product development cycle. The possible presence of endogenous proteins or clipped forms of the protein that may be detected in the assay format utilized must also be considered.

With respect to development of antibodies, it is recognized in International Conference on Harmonization (ICH) S6 [15] that "most biotechnology-derived pharmaceuticals intended for humans are immunogenic in animals." It is important, therefore, that these antibodies be measured and characterized as to their effect on the pharmacodynamics and pharmacokinetics in the animal models that are utilized to support safety predictions. It may be important to characterize the antibodies as to their clinical relevance and to determine if the antibodies are clearing antibodies, sustaining antibodies, neutralizing antibodies, or antibodies that cross-react with an endogenous protein. Any of these antibodies could have an effect on the safety profile of the product in development.

Many platforms are currently available to detect the presence of antibodies, and the choice may be user and product specific. However, as with all assays, the bioanalytical assay must be sensitive, specific, and able to detect low-affinity antibodies. It is important to fully characterize the immune response. It may be necessary to develop and implement immunoassays to detect antibodies that bind to the drug, biopharmaceutical assays to identify neutralizing antibodies, and the utilization of FACS (flow-automated cell sorting) analyses to evaluate or quantify populations of circulating immune effector cell types. These assays may need to be developed early in the nonclinical process to provide important endpoint analysis to support FIH dose consideration.

During the development program of a therapeutic protein for use in humans, an antibody-monitoring strategy for nonclinical studies is highly recommended. This strategy should include development and thorough validation of a reliable antibody screening assay capable of detecting high- and low-affinity antibodies. It is recommended that a sensitivity of 1 μg/mL in neat serum or better be considered a sensitive endpoint analysis. In addition, it may be necessary to develop and validate a neutralizing antibody assay, preferably cell based, and to employ this assay to analyze samples positive in a screening assay.

During the conduct of nonclinical studies in which both rodents and nonhuman primates are used, it is suggested that a neutralizing antibody assay should be applied at least in nonhuman primate studies. It is critical to understand and evaluate drug interference in the assays as well as establishing the antibody incidence and level at various time points after drug administration. If applicable, cross-reactivity with the endogenous counterpart molecule should be explored.

The choice and characterization of assays for nonclinical development will differ for each product class. Specific guidance documents addressing the quality and robustness of the assay criteria are available for consideration, and contemporary reviews can enhance the analytical process [14].

12.5 OBJECTIVES AND IMPLEMENTATION OF PRE-FIH SAFETY ASSESSMENT PROGRAMS

12.5.1 ICH S6 Guideline

Over the last two decades, development scientists have built an extensive experience base with a wide range of product classes of biopharmaceutics. Prior to the release of the ICH S6 guideline document in 1997 [15], there was no international consensus on what would be key considerations for the design of nonclinical safety evaluation programs of biopharmaceutics. Today it is well recognized that each class of biopharmaceutic represents unique product-specific features, and as a result, one nonclinical program for a biopharmaceutic (as opposed to more standardized programs for small-molecule drugs) may not appear identical to another nonclinical program design for a similar biopharmaceutic of the same product class. For this reason, the term *case-by-case program design* has been adopted.

The main objective for nonclinical safety evaluation programs in the pre-FIH phase is to define safe use conditions and to predict potential untoward effects in humans (hazard identification and hazard characterization). To accomplish this, general product testing paradigms for nonclinical pharmacology, toxicology, and pharmacokinetic studies have been established for biopharmaceutics. These testing paradigms have some similarities to those typically employed for small-molecule drug development; however, for program designs to be successful, many important differences must be recognized.

12.5.2 Considerations and Typical Program Designs for Nonclinical Safety Assessment of Biopharmaceutics

The nonclinical safety evaluation program for a given biopharmaceutic is specifically designed based on the properties of the product and the intended clinical use. However, based on collective experience, there are many common components that cut across a wide variety of product classes. The nonclinical development program needs to be developed in consideration of ICH S6, with justifications relevant to the individual product as needed. In comments below, key considerations for each product class are addressed.

Monoclonal Antibody and Related (FAb′, FAb′2, Fusion Constructs) Strategies The most important nonclinical criteria for the design of safety evaluation programs for a monoclonal antibody are receptor distribution in the animal model of disease, animal models chosen for the establishment of the therapeutic ratio and starting dose, and the relationship of these data to the human condition. This is true regardless of whether a humanized antibody, a fusion construct, or a FAb′ or FAb′2 is being developed. It is imperative that a good understanding of the intended target tissue or site of action is determined.

Receptor distribution is evaluated by conducting a tissue cross-reactivity study. In this study, the clinical antibody or another form known to target the receptor is incubated with a comprehensive list of animal and human tissues affixed to slides. The tissues are then evaluated for binding the antibody to membrane and cytosol. The intent of this study is to determine what tissues from typical animal models that are used in safety assessment bind or do not bind to the test antibody, and to estimate the degree of binding. This binding profile can then be compared to the binding profile of human tissues that are prepared in a similar way. Based on what is understood regarding the presumed target of the antibody, if the study is conducted properly and reagents are appropriate, the antibody should be demonstrated to target those tissues in which binding is expected and not to bind to those tissues in which the receptor is believed not be present. In addition, it is possible to identify heretofore new binding sites in other tissues due to unexpected cross-reactivity of the antibody. The totality of the binding profile between the animal models can be compared to that observed with human tissue and correlations can be made. Binding sites identified should be evaluated carefully for potential functional or toxicological significance in subsequent in vivo safety studies that employ functional and histopathological endpoints and in subsequent clinical phase I studies.

Discovery research and nonclinical development studies conducted to establish a pharmacologically relevant species are extremely important. Based on the identification of receptor distribution and a pharmacologically responsive animal model, an initial impression of potential toxicological effects can be predicted. If, for example, the profile would show a potential for the molecule to induce a direct or indirect biological response on a given organ system, specific safety pharmacology studies (e.g., cardiovascular) may be designed to evaluate the dose and exposure conditions under which this organ system might be adversely affected. Complete pharmacokinetic profiles should be determined over the dose range that is intended to be used in the pivotal toxicology studies. These studies should employ the formulation and route of administration used in the toxicology studies. One or two repeat dose toxicology studies in pharmacologically responsive species of up to four weeks' duration may be conducted to support the initial IND; however, alternative program designs are acceptable to regulatory agencies. For example, comprehensive single-dose toxicology studies may support a single-dose patient study. In these studies the intended clinical route and frequency of administration should be used. These studies should include adequate clinical, gross, and histopathological evaluations to afford a comprehensive assessment. Furthermore, these studies should be conducted in a manner to be compliant with good laboratory practices (GLPs) (Chapter 9) and designed to be consistent with prevailing global ICH regulatory requirements. For the IND application, mutagenicity studies are not relevant unless the antibody construct contains an organic linker or conjugate or if there is an organic impurity of concern identified as part of the production process.

Protein Therapeutics Several recombinant human proteins have been approved over the past decade for use as long-term therapy in patients [16]. The successful development of a protein therapeutic is often predicated on the choice of relevant animal species, dose selection, and length of administration. The dosing of recombinant human proteins is often difficult, due to the paucity of pharmacologically relevant species and the likelihood of antibody development to a human protein with long-term administration. The nonclinical development program needs to be conducted in consideration of the most pharmacologically relevant species, if one is available, and the species most likely to be predictive for human safety assessments. As with development programs for monoclonal antibodies, studies for recombinant human proteins are designed to establish a safety margin above the clinical dosing regimen and to identify any possible adverse effects of the protein administered. Since these products are naturally occurring human proteins, the likelihood of severe, adverse side effects are low for many (e.g., growth hormone, enzyme replacement therapies); however, proteins with pleotrophic biological effects can induce severe toxicities in animals and humans (e.g., interferons, interleukins). Understanding the pharmacokinetics, tissue distribution, and exposure are key to establishing the safety profile of the product.

With acceptance and implementation of the ICH S6 guidance document, more consistent development of recombinant human proteins is possible. Similar studies are performed to assess the short- and long-term safety of proteins administered. Challenges induced by immunogenicity can limit the duration of toxicology studies, due to the development of a neutralizing antibody response to the administered protein. A classic example of this is the protein interferon β-1a. This molecule is biologically active only in nonhuman primates, and treatment for durations beyond three or four weeks does not produce any useful toxicological information, because all animals have developed an antibody response that completely blocks the pharmacological activity of the protein administered. In this case, the utility of long-term dosing in animals is questionable, due to the generation of antibodies to the recombinant human protein. All drug sponsors of biopharmaceutics should be aware of the lessons presented by the interferon examples.

As noted above, a major consideration is the relevance of the animal model and which study would enable prediction of safety outcomes in patients. As more and more recombinant proteins reach the development phase, the best studies and relevant endpoints are increasingly challenged. It is necessary to conduct studies for appropriate lengths of time, but also to deliver the protein in a manner similar to that used in the clinical program. For many recombinant proteins this means hour-long infusions in an animal considered likely to display the appropriate safety signals without exhibiting the hypersensitivity response sometimes associated with administration of a human protein.

Due to the specificity of the individual proteins for particular cellular targets, demonstration of a clear pharmacodynamic effect may only be performed in genetically modified animal models lacking the endogenous protein (or, in rare naturally occurring disease models). Many genetically induced animal models are embryonically lethal or have alternative compensatory mechanisms such that the pathology of the disease is not consistent with the human disorder. In addition, as a result of significant antibody responses in some knockout mouse models, administration of recombinant human proteins may preclude meaningful interpretation. Long-term studies of the human protein are often not achievable in these animal models. Unfortunately, toxicology studies in normal animals are limited by the presence of native protein and the absence of relevant pathologic features: both attributes that we now recognize can significantly affect the safety of the product. Although development programs for some of the protein therapies were conducted prior to the ICH S6 document, many were nonetheless consistent with the guideline.

Myozyme as an Example of a Protein Development Program In 2006, recombinant alglucosidase α (Myozyme) received approval in the United States and Europe for the treatment of Pompe disease. Although the development program of alglucosidase α was in consideration of the ICH S6 document, and with further consideration to conduct studies in the most relevant species with the greatest predictability, additional pressure was placed on this program for the establishment of safety in animal studies.

The GAA knockout mice used for the nonclinical program were generated by Raben et al. [17,18]. The model was produced by inserting a neomycin-resistance (neo) gene into exon 6 of the murine GAA gene, resulting in disruption of the coding region. Mice homozygous for this disruption ($6^{neo}/6^{neo}$) lack enzyme activity and accumulate lysosomal glycogen. By three weeks of age, homozygous $6^{neo}/6^{neo}$ mice begin to accumulate glycogen in cardiac and skeletal muscle lysosomes, due to the lack of GAA enzyme activity. However, they grow normally, reach adulthood, and remain fertile. By eight to nine months of age, obvious muscle wasting and a weak and waddling gait develop, and by 18 to 19 months of age they have severe progressive muscle wasting, resembling advanced late-onset Pompe disease. At this age they have pronounced glycogen accumulation in multiple organs (including skeletal muscle, diaphragm, heart, and brain), as well as cardiomyopathy, hypotonia, severe motor disability, and profound muscle weakness and wasting [17].

Glycogen accumulation and the extent of muscle pathology in GAA knockout mice is not as striking as that noted in infantile-onset Pompe patients. Based on life span, $6^{neo}/6^{neo}$ GAA mice more closely resemble late-onset Pompe disease in humans. Despite these differences, GAA knockout mice provided a valuable tool for nonclinical studies. Since they lack GAA enzyme activity, they can be used to evaluate the pharmacokinetics and biodistribution of GAA activity following the administration of clinically relevant doses of rhGAA. Moreover, since the heart and skeletal muscle of GAA knockout mice contain accumulated glycogen, they can also be used to evaluate the pharmacodynamic effects of rhGAA dose and dosing regimens on glycogen depletion. Since most pharmacodynamic studies were conducted on asymptomatic mice less than six months of age, we were unable to determine if rhGAA could reverse or stabilize the clinical phenotype.

Although useful for evaluating substrate reduction and tissue distribution, the knockout mouse also presented specific challenges to the nonclinical development program. After repeated administration of rhGAA, a predictable hypersensitivity response to the recombinant human protein was observed. Frequently, this reaction resulted in morbidity and mortality associated with test article administration. This hypersensitivity reaction responded to diphenhydramine prior to and, as necessary, during dosing, however, such intervention complicated interpretation of the toxicity studies.

In Vivo, single- and repeat-dose pharmacodynamic studies were conducted in GAA knockout mice to evaluate the efficacy of rhGAA. Most of these studies were designed to assess depletion of glycogen from target tissues, while others assessed the time course of glycogen depletion and reaccumulation following administration of rhGAA. Tissue glycogen content was measured by biochemical assay and histomorphometric analysis. In addition, a safety pharmacology study was also performed in beagle dogs. A series of pharmacokinetic studies were performed to assess absorption of rhGAA across single- and repeat-dose administration, species (mouse, rat, dog, and monkey), dose, formulation, and process scale. Process scale-up to larger reactors to accommodate the high dose and rapid expansion of patient numbers has placed an especially demanding pharmacokinetic burden on this program, even postapproval. Tissue distribution studies were performed in GAA knockout mice to assess the uptake and tissue residence time of rhGAA in target organs.

In addition, more traditional toxicity studies were designed to establish a maximum tolerated dose and safety profile in mice, rats, dogs, and cynomolgus monkeys. Two single-dose acute toxicity studies in rats and dogs, two repeat-dose subchronic toxicity studies in rats, one repeat-dose subchronic toxicity study in mice, and two repeat-dose chronic toxicity studies in cynomolgus monkeys were performed to evaluate the safety of rhGAA administered intravenously. Furthermore, three reproductive toxicity studies were conducted in mice to assess the effect of rhGAA on fertility, early embryonic development, and embryo–fetal development. The Myozyme example highlights the importance of using all appropriate animal data, including an animal model of disease (i.e., the GAA knockout) to produce clinically relevant nonclinical safety data.

Gene Therapy Gene therapy as a platform for a therapeutic product has been considered for decades with little success as it relates to an approved product. Despite the promise of the potential for a vast impact of gene therapy on diseases, slow progress has been made, due to long-term intractable effects associated in part with the administration of therapy [19,20]. As much of the progress has been hindered due to specific safety signals, a more extensive and long-term safety evaluation is often needed due to the extended nature of the therapy. A single administration study might require a year of follow-up in an animal model, as persistence of the viral vector and/or long-term expression of the transgene need to be considered and evaluated.

The gene therapy environment has been challenged by successes and setbacks as well as the emergence of many viral and nonviral gene transfer vectors [19,20]. These vectors include liposomes, plasmids, retroviruses, adenoviruses, and adeno-associated viruses. The development of safer and more efficient vectors had led to a renaissance of the potential for successful gene therapy. The newer and safer vectors, a more rigorous review process, and a more thorough and scientifically relevant nonclinical program give hope to the promise that gene therapy may become an effective treatment for specific diseases.

In 2002 a gene therapy trial was initiated for the correction of X-linked SCID in humans. This is the most common genetic type of SCID (ca. 40%). It is the result of a defective common cytokine receptor gamma chain (gC) (component of receptors for IL2, IL4, IL7, IL9, IL15, and IL21) with the result of absent T and NK cells and defective B cells. In this disease, opportunistic infections often lead to early death. The trial involved retroviral-mediated transfer of normal human gC cDNA into bone marrow cells of 10 infants with X-SCID. Following administration of the gene therapy there was rapid development of T-cells with normal or nearly normal counts, phenotype, subset distribution, and function. Also notable was the development of T-dependent B-cell immune response. However, serious adverse events in two X-SCID were reported at 30 and 34 months' posttreatment. The adverse events consisted of splenomegaly and a 300,000 white blood cell count/mm^3 with >80% blasts.

It was determined that there was an integration of recombinant provirus into and near the LM02 proto-oncogene, resulting in a severe B-cell lymphoma. These patients were required to undergo chemotherapy and an allogeneic bone marrow transplant. The late onset of the adverse event, and the likelihood that nonclinical programs did not evaluate long-term administration of a gene therapy, point to the potential challenges of identifying long-term sequelae in a gene therapy trial [21].

An additional clinical trial of gene therapy clearly points to the importance of understanding the relevance of safety findings in relevant animal models and the relationship of underlying disease (or lack thereof) to safety signals. This event was a fatal systemic inflammatory response syndrome in an ornithine transcarbamylase–deficient patient following adenoviral gene transfer. The gene therapy treatment was to address an X-linked inborn error of urea synthesis in the liver, resulting in hyperammonemia. In September 1999, an 18-year-old patient received 6×10^{11} particles/kg of a recombinant adenoviral vector encoding human ornithine transcarbamylase. Eighteen hours later, the patient presented with jaundice, systemic inflammatory response syndrome, disseminated intravascular coagulation, and multiple organ failure, resulting in his death 98 hours following treatment. The outcome in this clinical trial resulted in significant changes to the safety evaluation programs to support gene therapy programs [19].

Despite the challenges in the clinical setting with gene therapies, there are still significant benefits to developing a safe gene therapy product. Notably, there is a good safety profile of AAV vectors nonclinically in numerous animal models, including dogs and monkeys. The longevity of therapeutic gene expression is measured in years. There is clinical experience by several routes of administration, and there is proven and long-lasting expression from a single administration. The benefits of these factors alone make gene therapy an attractive product for many biotechnology companies.

Research has been ongoing into the generation and characterization of more specific vectors and serotypes, and there is a significant potential to exploit the serological differences between the various serotypes for more specific targeting and systemic exposure. As an example, AAV1 and AAV6 have greater muscle gene transfer, AAV2 has greater human experience and neuronal specificity, AAV4 has selective gene transfer of ependymal cell layer in the central nervous system, and AAV8 may generate a higher level of gene expression via the intrahepatic route.

In developing a nonclinical program for gene therapies, there are a few unique considerations to acknowledge. It is important to recognize that the product is a combination of the protein (transgene) and the vector. It is also important to consider that specific toxicities and safety concerns may apply to the vector, the therapeutic protein, or both, and that nonclinical studies need to be designed to address the components individually and collectively. As mentioned previously, the development of robust and reliable assays applies to gene therapy products as well. Development of appropriate assays in multiple matrices for the detection of vector, product, and antibodies to both is essential early in development. This can be an extensive exercise and should be initiated early in the nonclinical program in order to have appropriate assays in place during the totality of the nonclinical program.

A significant issue in the conduct of nonclinical studies in nonhuman primates is the presence of preexisting cross-reactive antibodies to the vector and/or the development of specific anti-AAV antibodies during conduct of the study. These antibodies may inhibit gene transfer and the assessment of efficacy and safety and may limit the opportunity for re-dosing and therefore limit chronic safety assessments. Potential resolution to the effect of these antibodies on the efficacy of the product might include passive transfer of anti-AAV antibodies in rodents followed by vector administration. This may help address the impact of antibodies on the efficacy. In choosing animals for toxicity studies, it is prudent to prescreen animals for cross-reactivity antibodies to AAV to eliminate animals that might add significant variability to the interpretation of the study.

It is possible that there may be the presence of AAV capsid-specific memory cytotoxic T cells, and these T lymphocytes directed against AAV capsid proteins may eliminate infected cells, decreasing the efficacy. It may be essential to evaluate this by conducting nonclinical rodent studies where a robust anti-AAV capsid cytotoxic T-lymphocyte response in rodents is generated, and then challenged with therapeutic vector. Efficacy under these conditions is then assessed.

As with all therapeutic products, it is certainly appropriate to understand and evaluate the kinetics of the therapeutic gene expression. This can be complicated by the fact that maximum expression of the therapeutic protein may not be achieved for several days or weeks, expression may last for an extended period of time, and later time points may be required to properly determine the kinetic profile of the transgene. It is therefore essential to design nonclinical studies to measure kinetics of expression at appropriate time points and for appropriate duration to assess safety accurately.

It is also important to assess the biodistribution and persistence of the vector in the body by a formal evaluation of tissue distribution. This evaluation should be evaluated by polymerase chain reaction (PCR), and to rule out inappropriate administration to control animals, it could be valuable to assess by PCR the vector presence in a small number of control tissues. These studies may not be necessary if not justified scientifically. It is, however, important to assess the potential for the vector to infect cells of nontargeted tissues (especially gonads), and biodistribution studies can adequately address this question.

Despite many of the challenges outlined in the development of gene therapies and many considerations that must be given to the design of nonclinical studies, there remains a great deal of optimism in this field. There have been some impressive achievements despite some setbacks. These setbacks have resulted in the development of safer vectors, greater regulatory oversight, and better nonclinical safety assessment. The unique challenges that exist in developing a gene therapy product may be overcome by appropriately designed nonclinical safety studies and successful clinical applications of a long anticipated safe and effective therapy.

Vaccines Despite the fact that vaccines are one of the oldest regulated pharmaceutical classes, there are new and emerging technologies that require a more specific approach to the nonclinical development program. With new vaccine technologies and new adjuvant technologies, it is important to consider the appropriate safety program to assure patient safety. Many of the toxicities associated with vaccine therapy are related to an indirect immune response not associated with the action of the vaccine, including vaccine-specific antibodies and/or T cells that are responding inappropriately. Recent advances in vaccine technology that may have novel pharmacological properties or in the case of live viruses, are attenuated by novel genetic mechanisms require nonclinical studies aimed at identifying possible causes of toxicity prior to FIH dosing.

The nonclinical safety evaluation program should consider both the vaccine and the adjuvant under development, as they can have individual effects as well as combined effects. The programs will certainly need to be developed with respect to the product and the particular clinical application. As with other biopharmaceutic products, the manufacture, characterization of the product, specificity, and purity need to be well understood prior to initiating the nonclinical program. A number of guidance documents exist to guide in the design and implementation of a nonclinical program for a vaccine and should be reviewed for the individual needs of the product [22]. In general, the same considerations hold true as have previously been discussed to identifying a relevant species and administration consistent with the clinical dose and dosing regimen. In the case of the vaccines, however, the goal is to elicit an immune response that is measurable and is predictive to humans.

Some of the unique considerations for vaccine development include using only one species for safety assessment, or when there is not a relevant species (e.g., a vaccine against a pathogen nonexistent in a particular animal model) using a homologous protein, as has been noted for other biopharmaceutic therapeutics. As has been mentioned, the use of homologous proteins requires extensive consideration to the characterization and comparison to the human reagent and could add significant time and cost to the development program. Following the establishment of a relevant species and the choice of an appropriate reagent, the nonclinical development plan should largely address the clinical regimen and be consistent with the guidance documents. Studies should include acute and chronic studies as well as pharmacokinetic and pharmacodynamic assessments. Tissue distribution studies are useful to help predict target organ toxicity and residence time and to support long-term chronic studies. Studies of immunotoxicity and immunopharmacology are useful in defining the potential for the development of vaccine-specific immune responses. Additional safety studies need to be considered and conducted when relevant to the clinical population and the clinical regimen. These studies will be designed on a product-specific case-by-case approach.

Other Nonprotein Biopharmaceutics: Oligos, siRNA, Aptamers, and Cell Therapies Development programs for oligonucleotide therapeutics, which include aptamers, antisense, siRNA products, and cell therapies, are often specific as to disease indication and product. With relatively few approved products in this area, the development programs are specific and targeted to the therapy. Certain guidance documents help to guide the development programs [23], but in this area more than any others, the approach is on a case-by-case basis. Each particular therapy warrants its own consideration with respect to a safety assessment; however, as with all other biopharmaceutics the goal is to establish a relevant safety profile for administration to humans.

One of the unique attributes of the oligonucleotides is the ability to prepare a homologous product for use in rodents and nonhuman primates for the safety evaluation program. Although each of this class of therapeutics has a slightly different mechanism of action, the overall nonclinical strategy can be similar. Because of the similarities among the classes of oligonucleotide drugs, it is possible to leverage the knowledge from previous nonclinical and clinical development approaches [24,25].

The antisense and siRNA therapeutics are hybridization dependent. Their activities will be proportional to the concentration in the tissue or target cell type with a gradual onset of effect, but the duration of effect should be proportional to the elimination half-life from tissues or target cells. For the nonclinical development program, specific active analogs can be synthesized that may have differences in mRNA target sequences due to the differences in the specificity across species. However, there is utility in this approach for nonclinical safety evaluation. In considering aptamers, the onset of effects is much more rapid, and the circulating concentrations are often important for the effect of the aptamers. The species specificity is, however, less well understood for the class of therapeutics.

In the assessment of safety, much of the process is consistent with small-molecule evaluation in the understanding of the disposition, pharmacokinetics, and metabolite profile of the oligonucleotide products. The metabolism and pharmacokinetic program is often driven by the chemical characteristics and is often similar between sequences of a given chemistry. For all but the aptamers, the tissues are the active sites and activity is related to the tissue concentration. In the nonclinical assessment it should be noted that for this class of product, the doses scale better with body weight than with surface area. Plasma protein binding is essential for transport and uptake, and oligonucleotide binding to plasma proteins does not compete with smaller molecular weight drugs. The liver and the kidneys are often the sites of the most accumulation. The tissues are cleared of the product slowly by nuclease-dependent mechanisms and not by cytochrome P450s. In addition, the metabolite patterns among species are similar, and urinary excretion of shortened oligonucleotides is the route of drug elimination.

In general, activity of the oligonucleotide therapies is sequence dependent and related to concentrations in target tissues, except siRNA, which may have prolonged effects. The pharmacokinetics is described as first order and, except for mice, is predictable from animals to humans on the basis of body weight. Additionally, the pharmacokinetics is often predictable from sequence to sequence. In considering the safety profile, often many toxicities have been described, but these are usually related to the chemical class and are generally predictable from sequence to sequence. It is notable, though, that sequence-dependent toxicities do occur and it is only through cumulative understanding of species differences in toxicity that a strong basis for predicting clinical relevance of findings can be achieved. Finally, understanding the clinical relevance of animal data is promoted by the cumulative body of information available as to class effects.

Cell Therapies There are unique considerations for a nonclinical program for a cell therapy. The nonclinical program will depend not only on the source of the cell therapy, whether autologous or donor cells, but also on the route and location of administration. Direct administration of a cell therapy into a specific organ site or in conjunction with a matrix or scaffold makes the nonclinical safety program a bit more targeted versus a cell therapy that may be administered systemically, and thus multiple considerations need to be taken into account with respect to safety. Certainly, the more localized that a cell therapy can be administered, the more traceable and evaluable the product is with respect to safety. Cell therapies that are administered systemically have an opportunity to track and migrate to multiple locations, where in some instances differentiation factors may influence the cells' ultimate outcome. One of the most critical evaluations is understanding total cell retention in the tissue of interest as well as the percentage of viable, differentiated cells that are relevant to the organ and therapy. Many of these cell therapies require very specialized species evaluation, as the outcome of route and safety depends on the specifics of the therapy. In addition, multiple-species evaluation is usually not useful for establishing safety margins, as one species is usually the most relevant. In many cases the cells that are used are generated in an autologous manner and therefore may not be consistent with the clinical candidate. True nonclinical safety assessment of the human product is often not achievable. As relevant to the clinical indication, additional nonclinical safety pharmacology studies may or may not be warranted. These studies may be unnecessary if it can be assured that cells remain at the site of administration and do not suggest a risk to other organ systems. Much work is continuing to evolve on the specifics, strategies, and specifications for the development of a cell therapy product [26].

12.6 POST-IND CONSIDERATIONS: SUPPORT OF PHASES II AND III AND REGISTRATION

As clinical indications for biopharmaceutics have moved to patient populations that are intended to be treated chronically, often involve the treatment of women of childbearing age, or are intended for patients who are treated with multiple biopharmaceutics, the complexity of nonclinical development safety programs has increased. The most significant nonclinical issue that can affect the design of post-IND studies is the availability of a pharmacologically responsive toxicology species that can be treated by the clinical route of administration for a period equivalent to the planned duration of phase II clinical studies. This study should be able to be conducted in the absence of confounding antibody response in that it would render the species to be not pharmacologically responsive. The classic example of this is the case with interferons described earlier. For most biopharmaceutics developed for chronic use, this would involve some form of repeat-dose treatment for periods of up to six months duration [16]; however, in certain instances, regulatory agencies still require chronic toxicity studies between nine and 12 months' duration, as stated in the ICH M3 guidance [27].

For chronic-use biopharmaceutics, the sponsor may be asked to consider a plan to assess carcinogenic potential and the potential for deleterious developmental and reproductive toxicity in the intended patient population. The toxicologic assessment of both of these endpoints is the subject of much debate, and there is no clear scientific or regulatory consensus as to the most appropriate approach to take in every case. At present, the recommendation is to develop a scientifically defensible plan which may involve a combination of laboratory and animal toxicology assessments to define risk. This plan should be proposed in regulatory submissions at the earliest possible point, certainly before or at end of phase II discussions with regulatory authorities. At this point, an agreement on the assessment strategy should be obtained so that the approach taken will be deemed acceptable at the time of registration. ICH S6 provides some general guidance on these topics that is still very relevant and useful today. The S6 guidance document has just been approved to undergo "maintenance" within the ICH process. It is anticipated that addendums will be added to the original document to provide additional guidance in the areas of species relevance, carcinogenicity, and reproductive/developmental assessments based on additional experience that has been accumulated in these areas.

12.6.1 Changes in Production and Process, and Impact on Completed Studies

In Section 12.3 we described the reason for carefully evaluating the manufacturing process, whereby the biopharmaceutic is made to produce test material for use in what are referred to as definitive nonclinical safety studies that define initial safe use conditions. As programs progress into phases I, II, and II of clinical development, the ongoing toxicity studies that are conducted to support chronic drug administration should utilize test material identical to that used for the clinic; this will assure the highest degree of relevancy of these ongoing studies to support clinical safety. Most sponsors will try to avoid making any significant changes in the production process, purification process, or formulation after completion of pivotal proof-of-concept phase I/II studies. These components of the process will, in fact, be locked down and not changed until phase III is completed and registration is achieved. Even at that point, changes made to licensed production processes postregistration are made only for well-justified reasons (e.g., to move to a completely serum-free process devoid of animal components, which significantly reduces viral contamination risks). If significant process changes are made postregistration, it may be necessary to support these changes with a significant comparability program. Product comparability studies at this stage of development typically include biochemical, bioactivity, and nonclinical and clinical pharmacokinetic studies. If major differences in the comparability profile are discovered between the phase III and IV test materials, it may be necessary to repeat the pivotal IND-enabling safety and clinical studies to assure that the efficacy and safety profile of the biopharmaceutic has not changed. For these reasons, these process changes should only made after careful consideration of all possible ramifications, including the need to repeat a substantial portion of the clinical program.

12.7 THE TEGENERO INCIDENT AND IMPLICATIONS FOR BIOPHARMACEUTIC NONCLINICAL SAFETY EVALUATION PROGRAMS

Nonclinical testing paradigms for all types of biopharmaceutics, including humanized antibodies, have proven to be adequate to support the determination of safe use conditions for the overwhelming majority of clinical trials. Additional scrutiny, however, on ICH S6 and related guidance documents has come recently on the heels of the TeGenero incident, in which a cohort of phase I normal volunteers treated with a single dose of TGN1412 (an anti-CD28 humanized antibody) developed severe adverse drug reactions [6,28]. Some critics have considered this outcome to reflect a failure of the adequacy of current nonclinical program designs. This is an unfortunate conclusion because the adverse events observed were predictable and consistent with some of the nonclinical data that were available for consideration. A review of published data with surrogate antibody and redacted data, which was released by the UK regulatory authorities for public review shortly after the incident, supported the following conclusions: (1) administration of a surrogate agonist anti-CD28 to rodents led to a quick, dramatic polyclonal stimulation and lymphocytosis—this is activation-induced cell death in vivo and is an observation that is consistent with that observed with other agonist antibodies (anti-CD3 and anti-CD2); (2) cynomolgus monkeys' PBMCs (peripheral blood mononuclear cells) were relatively nonresponsive to

TGN1412-evoked activation and stimulation compared to human PBMCs; and (3) the sponsor (TeGenero) in fact reported that the kinetics of the T-cell expansion were delayed in vivo in the nonhuman primate compared to the mouse. In this case, the cynomolgus monkey was chosen by the sponsor as a pharmacologically relevant animal model upon which to base predictions for human safety. To experienced development scientists, this species discrepancy is a major pharmacodynamic difference and is a notable red flag. In many settings, this would prompt additional work and/or caution. At a minimum, basic safety implications of large pharmacodynamic species discrepancies emphasize that the biology of the primate and that of the rodent differ, or there is something technical that needs to be better understood in order to explain the pharmacodynamic difference. Both of these points should have raised major safety flags that would have warranted a high degree of caution in defining the development path forward. Unfortunately, the human starting dose was based on doses used in the primate model, which in this case was not pharmacologically sensitive to the clinical antibody. The lesson from this experience is that all the data need to be considered at this early stage of development to set FIH dosing conditions. A critical review of the TeGenero incident and its impact on pharmaceutical development has recently been published [29–31].

As noted earlier, nonclinical testing paradigms for all types of biopharmaceutics, including humanized antibodies, have proven to be adequate to support the determination of safe use conditions for clinical trials. The TGN1412 event is an unfortunate outlier from this experience and should not, in itself, warrant a complete redesign of nonclinical development program requirements for biopharmaceutics. From public documents alone, a conclusion of increased caution with this antibody construct should have been evident. If nonclinical programs are well designed and all data are considered carefully by experienced nonclinical scientists, the vast history of experience to date supports the conclusions that laboratory and robust toxicology assessments can provide sufficiently predictive information regarding human toxicities. The TeGenero incident prompted the expeditious development and release of a new guidance document in the European Union that specifically addresses in a comprehensive manner nonclinical program design considerations for FIH trials for new chemical and biopharmaceutic products [32]. This guidance is discussed in Chapter 3. We believe this recent guidance document to be extremely well written and it should also be consulted by sponsors developing biopharmaceutics.

12.8 CONCLUSIONS

Nonclinical testing paradigms based on ICH S6 guidance for all types of biopharmaceutics have proven to be adequate to support the determination of safe use conditions for clinical trials. We have reviewed what are considered to be the most important unique considerations that drug sponsors must be aware of as they design pre-FIH safety assessment programs that are specific to the properties and indication of their product. Program designs that consider these aspects and in which data are evaluated by experienced drug development scientists will be successful in supporting the safe conduct of first-in-human studies and subsequent clinical development.

REFERENCES

1. Kramer JA, Sagartz JE, Morris DL. The application of discovery toxicology and pathology towards the design of safer pharmaceutical lead candidates. *Nat Rev Drug Discov*. 2007;6:636–649.
2. Goochee CF, Gramer MJ, Andersen DC, Bahr JB, Rasmussen JR, The oligosaccharides of glycoproteins: bioprocess factors affecting oligosaccharide structure and their effect on glycoprotein properties. *Biotechnology*. 1991;9:1347–1355.
3. Jefferis R. Glycosylation of recombinant antibody therapeutics. *Biotechnol Prog*. 2005;21:11–16.
4. Jefferis R. Criteria for selection of IgG isotype and glycoform of antibody therapeutics. *BioProcess Int*. 2006;Oct., pp. 40–43.
5. Roque ACA, Lowe CR, Taipa MA. Antibodies and genetically engineered related molecules: production and purification. *Biotechnol Prog*. 2004;20:639–654.
6. Expert Scientific Group on Phase One Clinical Trials. Final Report. Nov. 30, 2006. Available at: http://www.tsoshop.co.uk.
7. Kips JC, Anderson JJ, Fredberg JJ, et al. Murine models of asthma. *Eur Respir J* 2003;22:374–383.
8. Perel, P, Roberts, I, Sena, E, et al. Comparison of treatment effects between animal experiments and clinical trials: systematic review. *BMJ*. Dec. 15, 2006.
9. Mordenti J, Chen SA, Moore JA, Ferraiolo BL, Green JD. Interspecies scaling of clearance and volume of distribution data for five therapeutic proteins. *Pharm Res*. 1991;8(11):1351–1359.
10. Mahmood I. *Interspecies Pharmacokinetic Scaling: Principles and Application of Allometric Scaling*. Rockville, MD: Pine House Publishers; 2005.
11. Copmann T, Davis G, Garnick R, et al. One product, one process, one set of specifications: a proven quality paradigm for the safety and efficacy of biopharmaceutic drugs. *Biopharm Int*. 2001;14(3):14–24.
12. Guidance for Industry: Note for Guidance on Comparability of Medicinal Products Containing Biotechnology-Derived Proteins as Drug Substance. CPMP/BWP/3207/00. European Medicines Agency; effective Mar. 2002.
13. Note for Guidance of Biotechnological/Biopharmaceutical Products Subject to Changes in Their Manufacturing Process. CHMP/ICH/5721/03. International Conference on Harmonization; effective June 2005.
14. Gupta S, Indelicato SR, Jethwa V, et al. Recommendations for the design, optimization, and qualification of cell-based assays used for the detection of neutralizing antibody responses elicited to biopharmaceutical therapeutics. J Immunol Methods. 2007;321(1–2):1–18.
15. Guidance for Industry: ICH S6 Preclinical Safety Evaluation of Biotechnology-Derived Products. CPMP/ICH/302/95. International Conference on Harmonization.

16. Clarke J, Hurst C, Martin P, et al. Duration of chronic toxicity studies for biotechnology-derived pharmaceuticals: Is 6 months still appropriate? *Regul Toxicol Pharmacol*. 2007;50(1):2–22.
17. Raben N, Nagaraju K, Lee E, et al. Targeted disruption of the acid alpha-glucosidase gene in mice causes an illness with critical features of both infantile and adult human glycogen storage disease type II. *J Biol Chem*. 1998;273(30):19086–19092.
18. Raben N, Nagaraju K, Lee E, Plotz P. Modulation of disease severity in mice with targeted disruption of the acid alpha-glucosidase gene. *Neuromuscul Disord*. 2000;10(4–5):283–291.
19. Raper SE, Chirmule N, Lee FS, et al. Fatal systemic inflammatory response syndrome in a ornithine transcarbamylase deficient patient following adenoviral gene transfer. *Mol Genet Metab*. 2003;80(1–2):148–158.
20. Cavazzana-Calvo M, Hacein-Bey S, de Saint Basile G, et al. Gene therapy of human severe combined immunodeficiency (SCID)-X1 disease. Science. 2000;288(5466):669–672.
21. Hacein-Bey-Abina S, Le Deist F, Carlier F, et al. Sustained correction of X-linked severe combined immunodeficiency by ex vivo gene therapy. *N Engl J Med*. 2002;346(16):1185–1193.
22. Brennan F, Dugan G. 2005. Non-clinical safety evaluation of novel vaccines and adjuvants: new products, new strategies. *Vaccine*. 2005;23:3210–3222.
23. Black LE, Farrelly JG, Cavagnaro JA, et al. Regulatory considerations for oligonucleotide drugs: updated recommendations for pharmacology and toxicology studies. *Antisense Res Dev*. 1994;4(4):299–301.
24. Henry SP, Kim T-W, Kramer-Stickland K, Zanardi TA, Fey RA, Levin A. Toxicologic properties of 2α-*O*-methoxyethyl chimeric antisense inhibitors in animals and man. In: *Antisense Drug Technology*, 2nd ed. Boca Raton, FL: CRC Press; 2007:327–357.
25. Levin A, Yu RZ, Geary RS. Basic principles of the pharmacokinetics of antisense oligonucleotide drugs. In: *Antisense Drug Technology*, 2nd ed. Boca Raton, FL: CRC Press; 2007:184–211.
26. Guidance for Industry: Guideline for Human Cell-Based Medicinal Products. EMEA/CHMP/410869/2006. European Medicines Agency; 2006.
27. ICH Multidisciplinary Guideline: Nonclinical Safety Studies for the Conduct of Human Clinical Trials and Marketing Authorization for Pharmaceuticals. ICH M3 (R2). International Conference on Harmonization; 2008.
28. Suntharalingam G, Perry MR, Ward S, et al. Cytokine storm in a phase 1 trial of the anti-CD28 monoclonal antibody TGN1412. *N Engl J Med*. 2006;355:1018–1028.
29. Green JD. Regulatory affairs introduction. *Toxicol Pathol*. 2009;37:361–362.
30. Horvath CJ, Milton MN. The TeGenero incident and the Duff report conclusions: a series of unfortunate events or an avoidable event? *Toxicol Pathol*. 2009;37:372–383.
31. Milton MN, Horvath CJ. The EMEA guideline on first in human trials and Its impact on pharmaceutical development. *Toxicol Pathol*. 2009;37:363–361.
32. Guidance for Industry: Guideline on Strategies to Identify and Mitigate Risks for First-in-Human Clinical Trials with Investigational Medicinal Products. EMEA/CHMP/SWP/28367/07. European Medicines Agency; effective Sept. 1, 2007.

13

PROJECT MANAGEMENT AND INTERNATIONAL REGULATORY REQUIREMENTS AND STRATEGIES FOR FIRST-IN-HUMAN TRIALS

Carolyn D. Finkle and Judith Atkins

13.1 INTRODUCTION: INITIATE PRODUCT DEVELOPMENT WITH THE END IN MIND

Product development requires careful planning and strategizing, without which, untimely and poorly designed studies may result. A document that can be termed a *strategic product development plan* (or similar designation) serves as a blueprint for the development of the product, analogous to a blueprint for the construction of a house. The best product development planning from the beginning involves designing the path with the end in mind. Indeed, a useful exercise is to design the product label first and then embark on a development plan that will meet the key goals contained in the label. A product development plan incorporates all aspects of the development, including the clinical plan, the nonclinical program to support the clinical plan, and the manufacturing plans to support the nonclinical and clinical plans. These plans ultimately support the market application and commercial distribution of the approved product. Often, in our effort to design a scientifically robust clinical development plan, we fail to consider carefully our ultimate targeted label claim. Are we designing the product to be used as a first- or second-line treatment? Are we intending to demonstrate superiority (safety and/or efficacy) over a competitor product, or are we developing a first-in-class product? Are we designing the development for a new molecular entity leading to

Early Drug Development: Strategies and Routes to First-in-Human Trials, Edited by Mitchell N. Cayen

a 505(b)1 new drug application (NDA), an application that contains full reports of investigations of safety and effectiveness, or a follow-on product leading to a 505(b)2 NDA, an application that contains full reports of investigations of safety and effectiveness but where some of the information comes from studies not conducted by the sponsor? Is it a single drug or a combination product (e.g., drug–drug or drug–device)? Targeted product planning may be valuable when used to clarify the desired label statements resulting from the proposed development program and can be modified in light of evolving scientific and regulatory issues. Elements of the target product plan may also be useful when meeting with the U.S. Food and Drug Administration (FDA) (or other regulatory agency) to discuss the label concepts and whether the currently designed clinical development plan supports the label claim desired. The purpose is to enhance clinical development planning to lower the risk of a failure in late-stage development or a nonapprovable NDA.

When drafting the product development plan, the sponsor should consider the therapeutic indication, target patient population, disease prevalence, standard of care, and size of market. The plan should include a description of the mechanism of action of the product, any pharmacology studies conducted to date, and the possible clinical indications. If there are a number of possible indications, the sponsor should look at the prevalence of the disease or affliction and determine the competitive landscape and the problems associated with the current standard of care. For example, Company X is developing a therapeutic product for the treatment of cancer. If the mechanism of action suggests that the product may be effective in breast cancer, the product plan should include the following:

- In vitro and in vivo pharmacology evaluations such as IC_{50} determination in a variety of cancer cell lines
- Xenograft studies (e.g., human breast cancer tumor implanted in nude mice)
- Appropriate pharmacokinetic studies (mouse, rat, and nonrodent species used in the toxicity studies)
- Toxicity studies [dose ranging, single- and multiple-dose (14 to 28 days) studies in rodent and nonrodent]
- Safety pharmacology
- Chemistry, manufacturing, and controls (CMC)
- Drug substance and drug product manufacturing (master operating instructions, establishment of test attributes and specifications, stability protocols)
- Regulatory strategy (plans for a pre-IND meeting to obtain FDA feedback on a development plan and reduce the risk of an IND hold, IND/regulatory filing strategy)
- Clinical phase I study in cancer patients who have failed conventional therapy (protocol outline, including estimated number of patients, safety exclusions, dosing plan, sampling and monitoring plan, and stopping rules)
- Outline of plans for phase II studies in breast cancer patients

Many of these disciplines and activities have been described in detail in earlier chapters. The plan should include the number and type of nonclinical studies required to support the clinical development, based on two major considerations: (1) FDA [and International Conference on Harmonization (ICH)] requirements for rodent and nonrodent toxicity studies, and (2) a study design that best models the clinical trial design.

The product development plan should be comprehensive and include all aspects of development, the nonclinical plan, the clinical plan, and CMC activities. Outlined below is a sample table of contents of a product development plan:

1.0 Introduction and Product Background
  Product Description
  Indication for Use and Therapeutic Potential
2.0 Scope of Work
2.1 Nonclinical Studies
2.2 Manufacturing Development
  2.2.1 Drug Substance Manufacture
  2.2.2 Drug Product Manufacture
  2.2.3 GMP Compliance
2.3 IND-Related Regulatory Support
  2.3.1 Pre-IND Activities
  2.3.2 IND Preparation, Submission, and Maintenance
  2.3.3 General Clinical Regulatory Support
2.4 Clinical Development
  2.4.1 Overview
  2.4.2 Phase I Clinical Trial Synopses
  2.4.3 Rationale for Selection of Clinical Target for Phase II Trials
  2.4.4 Phase II Clinical Trial Synopses
  2.4.5 Clinical Scope of Work
  2.4.6 Phase III Clinical Trial Synopses
2.5 Program Management
3.0 Proposed Time Line
4.0 Budget
5.0 Appendixes
6.0 References

The product development plan is a comprehensive document outlining the CMC, nonclinical, and clinical steps involved in the investigation of the product. However, the plan is also a living document, requiring revisions based on new information as it becomes available during development.

13.2 IMPORTANCE OF PROJECT MANAGEMENT

To be assured that product development milestones will be met, the project should be well managed. Project management is utilized as a means of achieving the goals of the strategic product development plan and requires integration of numerous disciplines, resources, skills, and development activity tools to meet ultimate therapeutic goals. Managing a development project involves establishing a clear and achievable goal (target product label), identifying tasks (CMC, nonclinical, clinical), balancing the competing demands for quality [good manufacturing, laboratory, and clinical practices (GMP, GLP, GCP)], scope, time [pre-IND, INDs/CTAs (clinical trial applications) end of phase II, pre-NDA, NDA/MAA], staff (operations, regulatory, management) and cost (up to $1 billion for product development), adapting the plan and approach to the different concerns and expectations of the various stakeholders. Managing the triple constraint—project scope, time, and cost—is a challenge for all project managers.

The framework of project development management involves the following structure: project life cycle and organization, project management processes, integration management, scope management, time management, cost management, quality management, human resources management, communication management, risk management, and procurement management [1]. A possible paradigm for project management can consist of the following steps. It is noted that the terminology used and specifics of project management functions vary among drug sponsors, and the terminology used herein is based on the experience of the authors and various collaborators:

1. Developing the project charter
2. Defining the project scope
3. Outlining the project management plan
4. Executing the project
5. Monitoring and controlling the project work
6. Integrating change control
7. Closing the project and undergoing a "lessons learned" exercise

Project scope management is the process involved in determining that a project includes any and all of the work required to complete the project successfully. It consists of (1) scope planning, (2) scope definition, (3) creating a work breakdown structure, (4) scope verification, and (5) scope control.

Project time management is the process concerning the timely completion of the project, consisting of (1) defining the tasks, (2) sequence of tasks, (3) task resource estimation, (4) task duration, and (5) schedule control. To control costs during the project, the following financial planning is involved: (1) planning, (2) estimating, (3) budgeting, and (4) controlling costs. By understanding and monitoring these attributes, the project can be completed within the budget approved.

Project management is the process concerning the assurance that the project will satisfy the objectives for which it was undertaken. Decision-making points are incorporated in the project plan (e.g., at the end of phase IIA or proof-of-concept study, a go/no go point). As information is gathered at these defined steps in the drug development process, the sponsor can make determinations of risk and benefit of the product and whether additional resources should be invested to continue development. The project can be halted for a variety of reasons: lack of clinical efficacy, poor safety profile, undesirable pharmacokinetics or metabolism, unfavorable pharmacoeconomics, emerging favorable competitor profile, emergence of a more promising backup investigational drug, lack of resources, and so on.

Project quality management consists of the following: (1) quality planning, (2) quality assurance, and (3) quality control project management.

Project human resource management is the process involved in organizing and managing the project team. It consists of (1) human resource planning, (2) acquiring the project team, (3) development of the project team, and (4) management of the project team. The team composition changes with the emerging needs of the development program. For example, in the early development stage or pre-IND [prior to first-in-human (FIH) studies], the team will consist of discovery scientists, pharmacologists, chemists/biochemists, toxicologists, drug metabolism specialists, and regulatory personnel, although it is often advisable to include clinical staff even at the early development stages. As the development program progresses, the team composition will adapt to include medical and clinical development specialists, clinical pharmacologists, biostatisticians and data management specialists, manufacturing operations (drug substance and drug products), and a regulatory specialist. In the case of small pharma or biotechnology companies without resources within all relevant disciplines, external consultants should be included as team members. These consultants may act as the development team, consisting of nonclinical specialists [pharmacology/toxicology/pharmacokinetics/ADME (absorption, distribution, metabolism, excretion)], CMC (GMP experts, chemists, and formulation scientists), clinical/medical, and regulatory experts. Also, smaller companies may not have in-house manufacturing capabilities and will need to use contract manufacturing organizations (CMOs) to produce the active pharmaceutical ingredient (API) and dosage form (drug products). Contract research organizations (CROs) with the full clinical operational staff, including medical monitors, clinical project managers, clinical research associates, data managers, and clinical supplies coordinators, may be used to conduct the clinical trials (phases I to III) on behalf of smaller sponsor organizations. GLP toxicology studies may be contracted to a CRO which has internal toxicology experts and controlled animal facilities. In such cases, these external institutions become an extension of the sponsor's development program and must be managed appropriately.

As a case study, let us consider the example of planning the development of a chemotherapeutic agent to treat breast cancer. To reiterate, it is wise to start with the end in mind, as outlined in Section 13.1. The example involves a small biotechnology company with plans to develop their breast cancer drug to a proof-of-concept phase II stage (i.e., demonstration of human efficacy). The sponsor plans to license the product to a major pharmaceutical company, which would then develop the product through to market entry. The first step is to start with the end in mind—the completion of phase II. The major milestones would be to outline the development plans to the FDA at a pre-IND meeting, followed by filing the IND, then completing the phase I safety and pharmacokinetic study followed by the phase II safety and efficacy study. The milestone dates may be estimated or may have been determined previously, and the plan would be fleshed out with the nonclinical, clinical, and manufacturing tasks required. The project plan would outline all the required tasks, the resource requirements, and the costs. Once the tasks, durations, and linked dependencies were determined, the critical path would emerge. Such dependencies include drug product manufacturing, which is linked to the date on which the API preparation is completed, or the initiation date of the FIH study, which is linked to the completion of the pre-FIH toxicity studies and IND filing. The critical path is the sequence of linked tasks that lead to the overall milestone. Any tasks that are delayed along the critical path will delay the project in reaching the milestone. For example, if the drug substance batch fails specifications, the drug product production will be delayed awaiting the production of the new drug substance batch, and this will delay the IND filing and the start of phase I.

13.3 FDA INPUT EARLY AND OFTEN

Obtaining FDA input on the strategic product development plan is an important first step in development. The FDA sincerely wishes to be a partner with the sponsor, and the sponsor has the right to obtain FDA's input on their development plans. By doing so, the company can reduce the risk of a clinical hold if the FDA has concerns. The company can also initiate the relationship with the FDA by virtue of the pre-IND meeting authorized by the Prescription Drug User Fee Act (PDUFA) of 1992 and reauthorization in 1997 (PDUFA II), in 2002 (PDUFA III), and in 2007 (PDUFA IV).

The steps to a successful pre-IND meeting and outcome are as follows:

Step 1: Establishing *objectives*. Establish objectives for the meeting and outline the key questions for the FDA regarding product development.

Step 2: *Drafting the letter of request*. After the sponsor has identified the key questions, they should submit a letter to request a pre-IND meeting with the FDA. The agency will review the request and key questions to determine if a meeting is required. Within two weeks, the FDA will acknowledge receipt of the letter and suggest a date for a meeting, which could be as soon as six weeks or as late as four to five months.

Step 3: *Crafting the briefing document*. The sponsor should draft a briefing document, which will include the necessary background information on the manufacturing plans (drug substance and drug product), pharmacology, toxicology, and ADME/pharmacokinetic data to date, clinical plans, and clinical trial outlines.

Step 4: *Identifying the key meeting participants*. The list of anticipated meeting participants should be included in the letter of request and the briefing document.

Step 5: *Preparing pre-meeting*. It is imperative that the company prepare and rehearse for the meeting with the FDA. The questions and the FDA responses (which should be received by the sponsor at least one day before the meeting) should be planned carefully.

Step 6: *Holding a mock meeting*. The company should identify a person who will coordinate the responses from the company meeting participants and capture the meeting minutes. Practicing the desired meeting behavior is key; this will include emphasis on listening skills, planning clear and concise responses to FDA questions, and anticipation of other questions or comments that may be raised by the agency during the meeting.

Step 7: *Drafting meeting minutes*. The company representative should draft the meeting minutes and send them to the FDA regulatory project manager.

PDUFA meetings are also allowed at the end of phase I, phase II, and before filing the NDA (pre-NDA) or BLA (pre-BLA). In addition to formal meetings with the FDA, depending on the types of questions and the division within the Center for Drug Evaluation and Research (CDER), it may also be possible to contact the reviewers by way of the sponsor's regulatory project manager.

13.4 IND SUBMISSION IN THE UNITED STATES

The IND consists of information on the chemistry, manufacturing, and controls, pharmacology and toxicology studies, investigational plan, investigator's brochure, clinical protocol, and previous human experience. The content and format of the IND are described in detail in the *Code of Federal Regulations* (21 CFR 312.23) ["Content and Format of Investigational New Drug Applications (INDs) for Phase 1 Studies of Drugs, Including Well-Characterized Therapeutic, Biotechnology-Derived Products"] and in an FDA guidance [2], as outlined below.

U.S. IND Content and Format

1. Cover letter and FDA forms 1571 and 3674
2. Table of contents
3. Introductory statement
4. General investigational plan

5. Investigator's brochure
6. Protocol(s)
7. Chemistry, manufacturing, and controls information
8. Pharmacology and toxicology information
9. Previous human experience
10. Other information

The FDA requires a 30-day review period before initiation of the FIH trial. Questions may be asked any time during this period and most often will be forwarded within the last week of review. Amendments may be filed with chemistry, pharmacology and/or toxicology data, new protocols, new investigators, and/or safety reports.

The IND can be submitted in the common technical document (CTD) format for the registration of pharmaceuticals for human use. This common format will reduce the time and resources used to compile applications for the registration of pharmaceuticals. The CTD can be added to as development progresses, leading to the final NDA submission in CTD format. The CTD format [3] is outlined below.

Module 1: Administrative Information and Prescribing Information This module contains documents specific to each region: for example, application forms or the label proposed for use in the region.

Module 2: Common Technical Document Summaries Module 2 begins with a general introduction to the drug candidate, including its pharmacological class, mode of action, and clinical use proposed. In general, the introduction should not exceed one page.

Module 2 contains the following seven sections:

- CTD Table of Contents
- CTD Introduction
- Quality Overall Summary
- Nonclinical Overview
- Clinical Overview
- Nonclinical Written and Tabulated Summaries
- Clinical Summary

Because Module 2 contains information from the quality, efficacy, and safety sections of the CTD, the individual summaries are discussed in three separate ICH guideline documents:

- M4Q: The CTD—Quality
- M4S: The CTD—Safety
- M4E: The CTD—Efficacy

Module 3: Quality Information on quality is presented in the structured format described in ICH guidance M4Q.

Module 4: Nonclinical Study Reports The nonclinical study reports are presented in the order described in ICH guidance M4S.

Module 5: Clinical Study Reports The human study reports and related information are presented in the order described in the ICH guidance M4E.

13.5 GLOBAL CLINICAL TRIALS

Numerous pharmaceutical companies are increasingly conducting their FDA-regulated clinical trials outside the United States and Western Europe. The primary reasons are less expensive labor and the availability of treatment-naive subject populations. In addition, such subjects tend to be more trusting of researchers and in many cases more willing to participate in trials. In fact, some drug companies project that as much as 65% of their trials will be based abroad by 2010, according to research from the Tufts Center for the Study of Drug Development [4].

As global competition grows for clinical trial business, some developing countries are also offering tax breaks. India, for example, announced a 12.24% tax exemption in early 2007 on all services carried out by its contract research and clinical trials industry. The current consensus is that conducting trials outside North America and Western Europe is less expensive and that well-trained physicians are available to serve as investigators. Drug shipment issues have largely been overcome, and the adoption of electronic clinical trial technology solutions has helped alleviate operating support issues.

The percentage of FDA form 1572s, which is essentially the contract between the investigator and the FDA stipulating the GCP responsibilities of the investigator, filed by investigators abroad nearly doubled between 2001 and 2006, indicating a dramatic increase in global clinical trial participation by non-U.S. investigators. Asia, Latin America, Eastern Europe, and South Africa have now either adopted ICH-GCP as a guideline or formally made ICH-GCP law, paving the way for international research and drug development even for small and midsized sponsor companies. The FDA requires no minimum number of U.S. patients for an NDA. Sponsors may design and conduct studies in any manner provided that they demonstrate that subjects are similar to U.S. patients both in terms of pretreatment disease characteristics and treatment outcomes.

Some clinical trials for certain disease types may remain solely within the United States within the foreseeable future, given the wide variations in diet, lifestyle, and health care consumption. Diseases most sensitive to these variations include age-related illnesses such as Alzheimer's disease, Parkinson's disease, and ALS and gastrointestinal, central nervous system, and endocrine disorders.

Despite these promising signs, some risk still accompanies clinical trials conducted outside North America and Western Europe. Kearney [5] notes that decisions to locate clinical trials are often based on the location of key partners, internal facilities, and future product launches. It estimates that cost savings can range from 30 to 65% compared with sites in the United States or Western Europe. In low-cost countries, pharmaceutical companies can often complete phase III clinical trials up to six to seven months sooner than in domestic markets. In 2006, a Kearney study ranked China, India, Russia, and Brazil as the most attractive of the low-cost countries, based on the five factors of its country attractiveness index: patient pool, cost efficiency, regulatory conditions, relevant expertise, and infrastructure and environment [5].

China provides both a vast patient pool and a large infrastructure of hospitals. The relatively low salaries of medical professionals translate into clinical trials that cost about half that of a comparable U.S. trial. Principal investigators from the Chinese State Food and Drug Administration often have extensive experience with Western companies. However, bureaucracy and government regulations pose risks. Getting the necessary approval to conduct a trial in China can take nine to 12 months, according to Kearney [5], and companies must acquire a drug import license for every shipment that enters the country rather than one for each type of drug. Cultural and language differences can also slow the process.

Like China, India offers a large population with a growing market. Expertise of scientists is on a par with the highest international standards. Clinical trial data from India are accepted at major conferences, English is the primary language for education and research, and strong economic growth is driving improvements in the health care infrastructure. On the downside, intellectual property protection has been weak in India and the country has not permitted foreign companies to conduct phase I trials. There are some bureaucratic headaches as well. It is mandatory for pharmaceutical companies to coordinate their efforts with local physicians and hospitals and to perform toxicology tests between phases II and III, leading to delays.

Russia also provides lower costs and an appealing patient pool. Patient recruitment is facilitated by the country's centralized medical system, in which patients with similar symptoms receive treatment in the same ward. Many patients are also treatment naive. Kearney reports that patient recruitment can be 10 times faster than in the United States [5]. Problems in Russia are similar to those in China and India: weak intellectual property protection and government intervention. Ethics in patient recruitment is also a concern. Doctors can make 10 times their salary by performing clinical trials, so some sponsors fear that doctors may neglect to inform patients of potential study risks [6].

Brazil, Argentina, Mexico, and Colombia are the most popular clinical trial locations in Latin America, and Colombia is expected to undergo a period of rapid growth over the next few years, along with Peru and Chile. Many of these countries have now put internationally acceptable legislation and regulations in place in regard to clinical research and have acceptable facilities, infrastructure, and access to large patient populations. On the other hand, Latin America is said to be reaching a saturation point in its number of experienced investigators. Brazil is the dominant Latin American country for clinical trials, with a population of 180 million who display both Western and developing world diseases. The Brazilian regulatory authority, ANVISA, logged 923 CTAs and 56 NDA trial approvals in 2006. The clinical trial industry in Brazil began to evolve in 1996, when it established regulations that adhered more closely to ICH guidelines, along with the establishment of a national bioethical committee that investigates institutional review boards (IRBs). Argentina, with a population of 38 million, boasts a more developed regulatory system, yet approved only 223 clinical trial protocols in 2006. Although Argentina is the most advanced Latin American country in terms of regulatory processes, trial approval times are still slow, officially taking around 90 days but realistically requiring 120 days.

Knowledge of regional regulatory requirements is fundamental in any clinical trial. Drug approval processes vary between countries, and in many cases guidelines are not clear. The FDA relies largely on sponsors to conduct clinical trials that adhere to their own high standards and periodically inspects offshore sites. In 2004, the FDA found that researchers did not follow the protocol sufficiently in 30% of the sites inspected. However, an increasing number of countries are improving their standards for clinical trials. In addition to national regulatory guidelines, international GCP guidelines provide a common platform that all drug sponsors, local professionals, and CROs should follow.

13.6 CLINICAL TRIAL APPLICATIONS

13.6.1 Europe

General Organization of the Regulatory Authority The European Union (EU) currently comprises 27 member states: Austria, Belgium, Bulgaria, Cyprus, the Czech Republic, Denmark, Estonia, Finland, France, Germany, Greece, Hungary, Ireland, Italy, Latvia, Lithuania, Luxembourg, Malta, the Netherlands, Poland, Portugal, Romania, Slovakia, Slovenia, Spain, Sweden, and the United Kingdom. The European Medicines Agency (EMEA) is a decentralized body responsible for protecting and promoting the health of EU citizens through the evaluation and supervision of medicines. A centralized procedure allows companies to submit one marketing application to the EMEA for eventual marketing throughout the member states.

Unfortunately, clinical trial applications (CTAs) do not enjoy the same mechanism of review as marketing applications. CTAs must be submitted to each national authority responsible for the conduct of clinical trials in that country. However, the European parliament issued a directive in 2001 on "the approximation of the laws, regulations and administrative provisions of the member states relating to the implementation of good clinical practice in the conduct of clinical trials on medicinal products for human use." Under the rules of membership of the EU, each state is obliged to pass a version of this directive into the laws of the state. The directive enshrines patient rights and protection and provides a framework for the content of a CTA. Moreover, it states that valid CTAs should be authorized within 60 days by the respective competent authority. A shorter review period may be used by member states if this is in compliance with current practice. Information on the pharmaceutical data required in a CTA is available in EMEA document CHMP/QWP/185401/2004 [7]. Additional information can be found in Attachment 1 of ENTR/F2/BL D (2003), revision 2, published by the EC [8].

Prior to submitting a CTA, sponsors are required to register the trial in the European clinical trials database (Eudract), which assigns a unique number for each trial. European regulatory authorities use this database to provide themselves with an overview of clinical trials being conducted in the EU. The database facilitates communication among the various regulatory authorities.

Two examples of requirements for CTAs are given below for a Western European (UK) and an Eastern European (Czech Republic) country. These country-specific regulatory requirements apply not only to FIH but also to later-stage clinical trials.

Western European Example: United Kingdom The main governmental body that regulates small-molecule pharmaceuticals, biopharmaceutics, and medical devices in the UK is the Licensing Division of the Medicines and Healthcare Products Regulatory Agency (MHRA). In general, the MHRA is responsible for assessing and approving applications for marketing authorizations and clinical trials for pharmaceuticals, biologicals, generic drugs, homeopathics, and herbals. The activities include both national licensing (mutual recognition system) and European licensing (centralized system). The division is also responsible for answering inquiries made by the pharmaceutical industry, the EMEA, and external regulatory agencies.

One copy of the request for a clinical trial authorization, consisting of the following, should be submitted in English to the MHRA:

- Covering letter
- The completed clinical trial application form (including the signature page, which, for electronic submissions, has been signed and scanned onto the submission disk)
- Protocol
- Investigational medicinal product dossier (IMPD) or summary of product characteristics, where relevant
- Supporting data documents
- The Extensible Markup Language (XML) file of the application form (complete data set)
- Applicable fee

All files should be provided in electronic format with one portable document format (PDF) file for each document. If the sponsor is not established in the European Community, it must have a local legal representative. Either the sponsor or the representative may submit the clinical trial application. The application form should be completed using the EudraCT database, EudraCT: European Clinical Trials Database [external link], and saved as an XML file. Information on the pharmaceutical data required in a CTA is available in the EMEA documents listed above. The contents of a CTA for a generic product differs from that of an NCE in that the applicant can refer to the reference product, thereby diminishing (or eliminating) the need for nonclinical and previous clinical information (the sponsor may submit a simplified IMPD). Requirements for a generic biologic are currently the same as for a new biologic.

In addition to approval by the MHRA, all clinical trials must also be approved by an ethics committee. Ethics committee approval generally takes 60 days and can occur in parallel with MHRA approval. The main human ethics committee will send its decision to the MHRA. The Gene Therapy Advisory Committee is the ethics committee for gene therapy in the UK. Depending on the type of product [such as trials with genetically modified organism(s), radioactive substances or involving medical devices], an application may be required to be reviewed by other bodies.

Once received by the MHRA, all CTAs, including those for FIH clinical studies, will be validated, an acknowledgment letter will be sent, and an assessment period of 30 days will begin. If the application is not valid, a deficiencies notice will be sent to the applicant. An assessment of the application will not occur until the missing components are provided. If the MHRA finds grounds to reject the application, the applicant has 15 days to respond to the deficiencies and submit an amended application. The MHRA then has an additional 60 days to review and approve the application.

Eastern European Example: Czech Republic The Czech Republic is presented as an example of clinical trial requirements in Eastern Europe. The main governmental body that regulates pharmaceuticals, biologicals, and medical devices in the Czech Republic is the State Institute for Drug Control (Státní ústav pro kontrolu léčiv; SÚKL). In general, this agency is responsible for assessing and approving applications for marketing authorizations and clinical trials for all small molecule pharmaceuticals, biopharmaceutics, and devices [9].

Clinical trials in the Czech Republic are regulated under the Medical Products and Good Clinical Praxis and Clinical Trials legislation. This regulation describes the contents of a CTA and specifies that a CTA form must be included, signed and dated by the sponsor's representative established in the Czech Republic [10]. The CTA, consisting of the following, should be submitted in Czech or English to the SÚKL. (*Note:* Some sections of the application may be submitted only in Czech.)

- Covering letter
- The completed CTA form (including the signature page, which for electronic submissions has been signed and scanned onto the submission disk)
- Completed form "Confirmation of the Approval/Notification of a Clinical Trial for the Customs Clearance"

- A letter of authorization enabling a representative to act on behalf of the sponsor (if necessary, i.e., someone who is residing or established within the territory of the Czech Republic or an EU member state)
- Protocol
- Investigator's brochure
- Investigational medicinal product dossier or summary of product characteristics where relevant
- List of competent authorities within the community to which the application has been submitted, and details of decisions
- A copy of the ethics committee opinion, if available
- Outline of all active clinical trials with the same medicinal product
- The XML file of application form (complete data set)
- Applicable fee

The number of copies of each section varies, based on whether the applicant is applying for a phase I (including FIH) to phase IV clinical trial versus a bioequivalence study, and the Czech Republic Web site should be consulted prior to submission. All files should be provided in printed form as well as electronically in XML format on a disk. Information on the pharmaceutical data required in a CTA is available in the EMEA documents listed above. A simplified IMPD can be submitted for products already known to the SÚKL.

In addition to approval by the SÚKL, clinical trials must also be approved by an ethics committee. Review by the ethics committee generally takes 60 days and may occur in parallel with the SÚKL review. There is a fee for ethics committee reviews. Following their review of the CTA, the SÚKL will issue an opinion. For gene therapy products or products obtained by biotechnological processing, the review time can be 90 days, and in some cases the assessment period may be extended by an additional 90 days. There is no time limit for the SÚKL to assess a CTA for xenogenic cell therapy. If the SÚKL requires clarifications or has questions during their review, further information or revised documents will be requested. The applicant has one chance to correct or submit the requested information within a specified time frame, usually within several days of the request [11–15].

13.6.2 Canada

The section of the Canadian government that is responsible for health care is called Health Canada. Its Health Products and Food Branch is responsible for managing the health-related risks and benefits of health products and food. It is organized into directorates. The main directorates that deal with clinical trials for human medicines are the therapeutic products directorate (for pharmaceuticals and devices) and biologics and genetic therapies directorate (for biologics, biotechnology, and radiopharmaceuticals).

Clinical trials in Canada are regulated under the Food and Drugs Act, specifically Part C, Division 5, Section C.05.005 [16]. This section describes the contents of a clinical trial application and specifies that a CTA must be included, signed and dated by the sponsor's senior medical or scientific officer established in Canada.

Health Canada has also issued guidance documents that clarify the regulations and provide more detailed instructions on the format and content of the CTA [17,18]. A CTA is not required to conduct trials with marketed products within the approved parameters of the notice of compliance (NOC) or drug identification number (DIN) application. However, the CTA is required for clinical trials involving products that have received a notice of compliance with conditions (NOC/c). One advantage of filing a CTA in Canada versus filing an IND in the United States is that the content of the Canadian CTA is abbreviated compared to the IND.

The Canadian CTA loosely follows the format of the common technical document (CTD) as outlined by ICH and may be submitted in either French or English. Module 1 contains country-specific information and such key clinical documents as the investigator's brochure, protocol, and informed consent form. In Module 2, only the quality overall summary (QOS) is required. The U.S. IND requires that all sections be submitted. The quality overall summary is not required if the drug product to be used in the clinical trial has received a notice of compliance or a DIN from Health Canada. Module 3 is required in an IND; however, it is optional in a CTA and needs to be submitted only if there is a large amount of detailed information that does not fit within the QOS. For biopharmaceutics and radiopharmaceuticals, only the following additional information should be provided in both the QOS and Module 3:

- Production documentation
- Executed batch records
- Literature references related to quality

Modules 4 (nonclinical information) and 5 (clinical information) are not required in a Canadian CTA, unlike in a U.S. IND. The CTA requirements are similar for pharmaceutical and biological products, but there are some specific differences. Appropriate Canadian guidance documents, found on the Health Canada Web site, should be consulted.

The following electronic review documents must be submitted in the CTA in hard copy and in electronic editable format accepted by Health Canada (e.g., Microsoft Word or editable PDF files on a CD-ROM):

- Investigator's brochure
- Protocol synopsis (pharmaceuticals only)
- Study protocol(s)
- Quality overall summary

Clinical trial regulations and guidelines for generic pharmaceuticals are the same as those for NCEs. However, the applicant can refer to a reference product, thereby diminishing (or eliminating) the need for nonclinical and previous clinical information. Currently, Canada has no separate regulations or guidelines for clinical trials investigating follow-on biologics (or generic biologic products). There are no fees for clinical trial applications.

In addition to approval by Health Canada, clinical trials must also be approved by an ethics committee. There are no legislated time lines for ethics reviews. Each ethics committee sets its own. Therefore, each site should consult with its ethics committee to determine review time lines. Ethics review may occur in parallel to the review by Health Canada, However, most ethics committees will not give final approval until the CTA is approved by Health Canada. Fees vary for ethics committee reviews.

Sponsors are requested to send CTAs to the appropriate regulatory body: the Office of Clinical Trials for pharmaceutical products or the Office of Regulatory Affairs, Submission Management Division, for biopharmaceutics and radiopharmaceuticals. Health Canada must review the application within seven to 30 days and notify the sponsor if the application is found to be deficient. Sponsors generally have two calendar days to provide clarifications. Health Canada targets to review the CTA for comparative bioavailability trials and phase I trials in healthy adult volunteers (with the exceptions noted below) within seven days. All other CTAs have a 30-day default review, including phase I clinical trials with somatic cell therapies, xenografts, gene therapies, prophylactic vaccines, or reproductive and genetic technologies (even if healthy volunteers are used). The clinical trial proposed can proceed only when a no objection letter is received from Health Canada prior to the 30-day default period, or if within 30 days of official receipt of the application by authorities the sponsor has received no notice indicating that it may not proceed (i.e., the CTA has not been declined or rejected). Prior to receiving its stamp of the official date of receipt, the CTA is screened to ensure that all appropriate documents are included. The screening time is included in the review time lines unless screening deficiencies are found. Health Canada will usually send the sponsors an acknowledgment letter indicating the official date of receipt [17–26].

13.6.3 Australia

The regulatory authority in Australia responsible for overseeing drugs and clinical trials is the Therapeutic Goods Administration (TGA). It is composed of a number of branches, offices, and units. The Drug Safety and Evaluation Branch evaluates clinical trials for small-molecule NCEs and biopharmaceuticals that are not covered by the Office of Devices, Blood and Tissues.

The format and administration of clinical trials in Australia is now unique among Western nations. Australia has two formats under which clinical trials can be conducted: the clinical trial exemption (CTX) scheme and the clinical trial notification (CTN) scheme. However, the types of products requiring clinical trial approval are similar to those of other Western nations, specifically:

- A product not already approved or listed by the TGA
- An approved or listed product being used outside the conditions of its marketing approval

Clinical trial medicines or medical devices that are used within the conditions of their Australian marketing approval require no approval under a CTN or CTX scheme but still require approval by a human research ethics committee (HREC). All CTN and CTX trials must have an Australian sponsor (or a local representative when the sponsor is from outside Australia). In addition, the sponsor's medical or scientific advisor must attest to the veracity of the information submitted.

The sponsor can propose which scheme (CTN or CTX) governs the conduct of a clinical trial, but the ethics committee makes the final decision, based on whether it has the scientific and technical expertise to assess the safety of the proposed trial. An ethics committee may refuse to approve a trial under a CTN. Under the CTX scheme, the TGA reviews all data submitted (Part 1 of the CTX application) to support a clinical trial and must approve the proposed usage guidelines for the drug or device. Once the guidelines are approved, the sponsor can conduct multiple trials without prior approval under the same CTX as long as the parameters fit the guidelines; however, a notification for each trial must be submitted to the TGA. In addition to TGA approval, sponsors must obtain approval from the Human Research Ethics Committee and the approving authority of the clinical trial site. The last step before initiating the trial involves paying the fees.

Part 2 of a CTX application is used to notify the TGA of each new trial conducted under the CTX and addition of new sites in ongoing trials. The Part 2 form must be submitted within 28 days of initiation of the trial or site. There are no fees when submitting Part 2 of the CTX application.

Under the CTN umbrella, the TGA reviews no data, even for FIH clinical trials. The Human Resources Ethics Committee receives all information about the proposed trial, including the protocol, directly from the sponsor. It is the responsibility of the HREC to evaluate the safety of the investigational drug or device, proposed trial design, and the ethical acceptability of the trial process. The HREC also approves the trial protocol. The approving authority of the clinical trial site gives the final approval, taking into consideration advice from the HREC. The last steps before initiating the trial include submitting a notification to the TGA and paying the appropriate fees.

As one can see, applying for clinical trial approval via the CTN route may save a large amount of time, for FIH and other phase clinical trials, as a review by the TGA is not required. This may provide an advantage to conducting clinical trials in Australia versus other Western countries where review and approval are required by both the regulatory authority and ethics committee(s) [27].

The formats of the Australian CTN and CTX do not follow the CTD format and do not resemble the CTA submissions of Western nations. However, the CTD format may be followed within each of the summaries (Parts 2, 3, and 4) of the CTX scheme. The CTX comprises six parts:

1. Administrative and additional information, such as the protocol proposed
2. Summary of quality information
3. Summary of nonclinical information
4. Summary of clinical information
5. Summary of adverse events
6. Information for human research ethics committees, which includes the investigator's brochure and usage guidelines

Unlike the CTX, the format and content of a CTN are dictated by the HREC and usually contains the CTN application form, the protocol(s), the investigator's brochure, and supporting information.

The TGA will send an acknowledgment of receipt of the CTX. A CTX is reviewed within 30 working days if it contains only chemical, pharmaceutical, and biological information. It is reviewed within 50 working days if it also contains nonclinical and clinical information. If a notice is issued that the file is found deficient, or a clarification is requested by the reviewer, the review clock stops and the sponsor has 30 working days to provide a complete response. The TGA will review the response within 20 working days, assuming a minimal amount of new data. Greater quantities of new data may require longer reviews. Clinical trials cannot start without written approval from the TGA and an HREC.

A CTN is submitted directly to the HREC. Each HREC sets its own time line. A CTN must be approved by both the HREC and the approving authority. Both must sign the CTN form. The principal investigator must also sign the CTN form, which is then submitted to the TGA with the appropriate fee. Unlike the case with the CTX scheme, sponsors do not need to wait for an acknowledgment letter from the TGA before initiating the clinical trial [28,29].

13.6.4 Latin America

No central authority governs clinical trials across Latin America, so each country has its own procedures. However, some countries—Chile, for example—have received support from such organizations as the Pan-American Health Organization (PAHO) and the World Health Organization (WHO). Most of the countries in the Latin American region have some type of legislation or Ministry of Health regulations covering the conduct of clinical trials. With the proper level of preparation and knowledge of each country's requirements, it is possible to undertake successful studies in nontraditional locations. Three examples of Latin American country requirements for clinical trial applications (from Argentina, Colombia, and Chile) follow.

Argentina The Health Authority of the National Administration of Drugs, Food and Medical Technology (Administración Nacional de Medicamentos, Alimentos y Tecnología Medica: ANMAT) oversees clinical studies in Argentina, ensuring that they are conducted according to standards for good clinical practices [30]. To carry out clinical investigations in phases I (including FIH), II, and III, sponsors should submit a clinical trial application to ANMAT that meets the requirements detailed below. The following clinical investigations will require ANMAT approval:

- Studies for a new indication
- Studies for a new dosage
- Studies of bioavailability, bioequivalence, and other pharmacokinetics studies
- Studies of specific incidence of adverse effects
- Studies using a placebo group as a control
- Studies in special populations, such as neonates, infants, adolescents, and the elderly.

Documents required in all clinical trial applications, including FIH, to ANMAT are as follows:

- Protocol
- Investigator brochure containing relevant nonclinical and clinical information
- Informed consent form
- Monitoring plan
- Power of attorney
- Case report form

In addition, approvals from the appropriate ethics committees must be included in the application. Documents should be provided in Spanish.

There are no specific regulations or guidelines for submission of a clinical trial application for biopharmaceuticals. However, every biological product should have a clear methodology of investigation and assessment that assures the uniformity of the preparation to be studied.

The first site approved by IRB/IEC is submitted to ANMAT. Once approved, the approval of the remainder of the sites takes 15 working days after each submission (more than one site can be submitted at the same time). If ANMAT questions the protocol, there is a delay. The time line for the first site is as follows:

- *IEC:* two weeks
- *MoJ:* one week
- *IRB:* six weeks

- *Ministry of Health:* 12 weeks
- *Import license:* one week

Colombia In Colombia, the Instituto Nacional de Vigilancia de Medicamentos y Alimentos (INVIMA) is responsible for the review and approval of clinical trial applications. Within the national health system, this Ministry of Health (MOH) sets policies and establishes scientific and administrative standards for clinical trials [31].

Similar to the procedure in Argentina, clinical trial applications in Colombia should be submitted in Spanish and usually contain:

- Cover letter
- Protocol
- Investigator's brochure, containing relevant nonclinical and clinical information
- Information on the investigators
- Patient information and informed consent form
- Local IRB approvals and institutional director's authorization
- Study design and monitoring plan

There are no official application forms. If the investigator's brochure is not available, documents containing nonclinical information and any information on previous human experience should be submitted.

Institutions that carry out research with pathogenic microorganisms or biological materials that may contain pathogenic microorganisms are required to have facilities, equipment, and safe handling procedures in accordance with MOH technical standards. They are required to prepare a procedure manual for microbiology labs and make it available for professional, technical, service, and maintenance personnel, and to train personnel in the handling, transportation, use, decontamination, and disposal of waste. Such institutions are also required to determine the need for medical monitoring of the personnel who participate in the research.

The regulatory process in Colombia is sequential: IRB approval is required prior to MOH approval. After that, the import license process takes about three weeks. IRB approval requires an average of five weeks and depends on the IRB internal time lines. The MOH sets monthly deadlines for submissions to evaluate the protocol the following month. The results of the evaluation are published on the Internet (www.invima.gov.co/). Additional sites do not require MOH approval; once study approval is granted for at least the first site, remaining sites can be initiated after their IRB approval. MOH notification may then follow.

Chile Chilean authorities include the Health Ministry's Public Health Institute (ISP), which approves protocols and drug importation. The MOH has separated the country into regions; more than 10 MOH ethics committees or regional ethics committees (RECs) operate within the country.

Recent process improvements include development of a checklist for inspection of sponsors, investigation sites, and the management and distribution of products in the investigation sites. In addition, OPS/OMS coordination helps harmonize regional regulations, and an effort has been made to coordinate the MOH Bioethical Unit activities with those of the Public Health Institute. Supreme Decree No. 494 of the Ministry of Health, 1999, created the Ethical and Scientific Evaluation Committee (Comité de Evaluación Ético-Científico), which reviews clinical research protocols. This committee is separate from the existing hospital ethics committees. The decree also established a procedure for the receipt, study, and conclusions on clinical research projects submitted, as well as for considering appeals based on unfavorable judgments.

The Clinical Trials Unit is part of the Department of Drug Regulation. The unit reviews and authorizes clinical trials conducted in order to allow entry into the country of nonregistered products. The MOH ethics committee reviews and authorizes clinical trials, or vaccination trials, in which three or more health services participate. The scientific ethics committee of the health service reviews and authorizes trials that are made in its geographical area.

Documents to be submitted to health authorities include the following:

- Protocol and amendments (English and Spanish versions)
- Investigator's brochure (English and Spanish versions)
- EC approval letter
- Informed consent form, patient diary, etc.
- Hospital director authorization letter
- Insurance certificate
- Letter of delegation of responsibilities/power of attorney
- Principal investigator's résumé
- Protocol signature page signed by the principal investigator

Sponsors are expected to propose the trial and the responsible investigator, and must support and supervise the entire trial (insurance, information, approval proceedings, and permanent monitoring).

For phase III and IV trials, data analysis is expanded in the protocol to include a statistical evaluation of the minimal sample size for the results to be conclusive. Pharmacological and economic analysis and/or quality of life analysis, if relevant, is also required.

Sponsors are required to obtain the protocol approval from each regional ethics committee and to apply to obtain drug importation approval from the ISP. Approvals from the LEC are not mandatory according to current legislation; nevertheless, the institution's directors do not give the approval to carry out the study in their sites when the LEC was omitted. LEC and REC submissions can be done in parallel.

According to the terms established by the regulation, the process should last no more than 120 calendar days from the moment the project is formally received by the chairman of the corresponding committee until it is finally accepted or rejected by the director of the Institute of Public Health.

13.6.5 China

The State Food and Drug Authority (SFDA) of China includes the Department of Drug Registration (which in turn includes the Division of Pharmaceuticals and the Division of Biological Products) and the Department of Drug Safety and Inspection (including the Division of Drug Reevaluation and the Division of Research Supervision). The Division of Pharmaceuticals and the Division of Biological Products are each responsible for evaluating, approving, and registering drugs and clinical trials in their respective domains, with the latter also responsible for biological diagnostic reagents and in vitro and biologic clinical trials. Both divisions also draft and revise national standards and research guidelines for drugs [32].

The Department of Drug Safety and Inspection oversees the adverse drug reaction monitoring system, setting GLP and GCP, and reviewing clinical study institutions. Its Division of Drug Reevaluation creates and reviews national formularies, verifies drug reevaluation, and regulates adverse drug monitoring. The Division of Research Supervision, by contrast, assesses the qualifications of institutions conducting clinical trials, drafts and revises GCP and GLP; supervises implementation of regulations, and investigates and punishes GCP and GLP violations.

In 2007, the State Food and Drug Authority revised Order No. 28, directing regulators to be strict with drug safety requirements and marketing permission and to "upgrade the review and approval standards, encourage innovation, and restrict low-level repetition." The State Food and Drug Authority also solicited opinions on guidelines for ethics committees to intensify the supervision of drug clinical trials and ensure the rights and benefits of trial subjects. Regulators now have draft fast-track and approved non-fast-track procedures.

The draft fast-track procedures cover the registration of drugs in four key categories:

1. Those involving active plant, animal, or mineral-based ingredients new to Chinese markets
2. Modern drugs, active pharmaceutical ingredients, or biological products that have not been approved previously in China or a foreign country
3. New treatments for AIDS, cancer, or other serious illnesses
4. New drugs targeting diseases without effective cures

Eligible drug sponsors may apply to the State Food and Drug Authority for special approval procedures and the agency's Center for Drug Evaluation (CDE) would have five days to decide whether to accept applications based on new ingredients. For drugs that target AIDS, cancer, and diseases without effective treatments, a Center for Drug Evaluation expert panel would have 20 days to make a decision.

In addition, the time frame for the CDE technical evaluation would be shortened, and the new draft rules allow sponsors to request meetings, including pre-IND and pre-NDA meetings, with SDFA and CDE experts. In addition, SFDA could approve fast-track drugs based on surrogate markers; approved drugs would be required to have postmarket risk control plans in place. The new special approval procedure replaces the rapid approval procedure and will involve a different procedure with regard to new drug registration, which will provide for the innovation of new drugs and improve efficiency in the approval system. For non-fast-track drug development, the CDE remains responsible for reviewing technical documents. The National Institute for the Control of Pharmaceutical and Biological Product is responsible for sample testing, and SFDA makes final decisions.

Documentation required for CTAs in China includes the following:

- *Part I:* Administrative information, including:
  - Certificate of pharmaceutical product (import)
  - Patent certificate (import)
  - Applicant authorization letter (import)
  - Summary of the research, study, and product characteristics
  - Package and label design
  - Insert sheet design
  - Introduction of the R&D
- *Part II:* Quality information
- *Part III:* Nonclinical information
- *Part IV:* Clinical information, including the protocol

The general review process and time line for non-fast-track drugs is as follows:

- *Technical documents review:* five to six months
- *Sample testing:* four to five months, in parallel with technical documents review
- *SFDA approval:* one to two months
- *IRB approval:* one to two months

13.6.6 India

In India, the Central Drugs Standard Control Organization (CDSCO) sets product standards, regulatory measures, and amendments. It also regulates clinical research and work relating to the Drugs Technical Advisory Board and Drugs Consultative Committee. Drug control functions are divided between the central government and state governments. The central government is responsible for setting standards for drugs, cosmetics, diagnostics, and devices; establishing regulatory measures; regulating market authorization of new drugs and clinical research; approving licenses to manufacture certain categories of drugs; and regulating the standards of imported drugs [33]. The state, by contrast, handles the licensing of drug manufacturing and sales establishments, licensing of drug testing laboratories, approval of drug formulations for manufacture, and monitoring of quality for drugs and cosmetics.

CDSCO Schedule Y, Good Clinical Practices for Clinical Research in India, amended in 2005, governs clinical studies, whether prior or subsequent to product registration in India. The guidelines were developed with consideration of the World Health Organization, ICH, U.S. FDA, and European GCP guidelines as well as the Ethical Guidelines for Biomedical Research on Human Subjects issued by the Indian Council of Medical Research.

Applications for clinical trials require the following information, as well as required fees:

- Regulatory status of the drug and ongoing studies in other countries
- Objective of the study
- Regulatory/IRB approvals from participating countries
- Suspected unexpected serious adverse reaction data from other participating countries

Data to be submitted include the following:

- Chemical and pharmaceutical data (generic name and chemical name, dosage form, composition)
- Animal pharmacology and toxicology data
- Clinical data
- Rationale for selecting the proposed dose(s) and indication(s)

Documents to be submitted include the following:

- Form 44, Application for Grant of Permission to Import or Manufacture a New Drug or to Undertake Clinical Trial, and Treasury chalan
- Form 12, Application for License for Examination, Test or Analysis, and Treasury chalan
- Details of biological specimens to be exported
- Protocol
- Informed consent documents
- Case report form
- Investigator's brochure and affidavit

- Undertakings by the investigators
- Ethics committee approvals

Clinical trials are classified into two categories. Category A includes those trials whose protocols are approved by developed countries: the United States, the UK, Switzerland, Australia, Canada, Germany, South Africa, Japan, and EMEA countries. Permission is granted for such trials based on approval of protocols by these countries. The time frame for such clearances, based on the current load of 20 applications per month, is two to four weeks. Category B comprises all other clinical trials. They require more time for approval because the adequacy of the protocol must be verified to protect the subjects. The approximate time for such approval is eight to 12 weeks. Once an application is considered under category B it will not be shifted to category A, even if the applicant produces an approval from a developed country.

13.6.7 Japan

The Pharmaceutical and Food Safety Bureau (PFSB) is one of 11 bureaus within Japan's Ministry of Health, Labor, and Welfare (MHLW). In addition to policies to assure the efficacy and safety of drugs, quasidrugs, cosmetics, and medical devices, and policies for safety in medical institutions, the PFSB tackles problems related to the lives and health of the general public, including policies related to blood supplies and blood products, and narcotics and stimulant drugs. This bureau consists of a secretary-general, a councilor in charge of drugs, five divisions, and one office.

The Pharmaceutical and Medical Devices Agency (PDMA), an independent administrative organization established in 2004, handles all consultation and review work from the nonclinical stage to approvals and postmarketing surveillance [34]. The PDMA Office of New Drugs confirms clinical trial notifications and adverse drug reactions and conducts reviews required for approval, reexamination, and reevaluation of drugs, as follows:

- *The Office of New Drugs I:* gastrointestinal, dermatologic, new antimalignant neoplasm, antibacterial, and anti-HIV or AIDS agents.
- *The Office of New Drugs II:* new cardiovascular drugs, urological and anal drugs, reproductive system drugs, metabolism-improvement drugs, in vivo diagnostics, and radiopharmaceuticals.
- *The Office of New Drugs III:* new gastrointestinal drugs, metabolic disease drugs (other than combination drugs), hormone products, dermatologic agents, central nervous system drugs, sensory organ drugs, respiratory tract drugs, antiallergy drugs, and narcotics.

The Office of Biologics confirms clinical trial notifications and adverse drug reactions of biological products and cell- and tissue-derived drugs and medical devices and performs the reviews required for approval, reexamination, and reevaluation. It also conducts reviews required for the approval of generic biological products. Reviews on the properties of biological products are also conducted for drugs and medical devices handled by the office of New Drugs III and the Office of Medical Devices.

The MHLW Ordinance on Standards for Implementation of Clinical Studies on Drugs specifies requirements for the planning, conduct, and reporting of clinical studies performed to collect data to be submitted with applications for approval to manufacture and distribute drugs. The Evaluation and Licensing Division issued a notification in 2000 on the topic of monitoring and audits to promote and establish GCP. The document emphasizes two points: (1) time points of monitoring and auditing should be agreed on between the two parties, and (2) a designated area for monitoring and auditing activities (e.g., comparing information contained in the patient records with data entered on case report forms) must be provided to the sponsor by the medical institution. Electronic retention of some documents is approved. Guidelines on the methodology for clinical studies and the evaluation criteria have been published as guidelines for clinical evaluation. The results from ICH are also introduced into Japanese regulation as ICH guidelines. Some 28 guidelines for clinical evaluations have been published based on therapeutic category. Regarding the conduct of clinical trials, the MHLW must be notified of the study protocol beforehand. The scope of the GCP has been extended to cover postmarketing clinical trials, and the role and responsibility of the sponsor has been clarified and strengthened.

Documentation required for a clinical trial notification includes the following:

- Notification form with SGML format
- Reason that the clinical trial is judged to be scientifically appropriate
- Draft protocol and ICF
- The most recent investigator's brochure
- A sample of the case report form

Pharmaceutical manufacturers outside Japan can apply for marketing approval directly under their own name if they perform studies regarding quality, efficacy, and safety required for the drugs they intend to export to Japan. In such cases, the overseas manufacturer appoints a marketer in Japan from among those licensed. In general, the process and timelines for consultation and approval of clinical trial notification are as follows:

- *Consultation application to consultation meeting:* four months
- *Meeting to clinical trial notification* (CTN): one to two months
- *CTN to approval:* one month
- *IRB approval:* one to two months

13.7 CONCLUSIONS

Product development requires a focused strategy and careful planning to ensure that appropriate studies are designed to support the desired target product profile. The strategic product development plan involves designing the path from the beginning with the end in mind and serves as a blueprint for the development of the product. It incorporates all aspects of the development, including the clinical plan, the pharmacology/toxicology program to support the clinical plan, and the manufacturing (CMC) plans to support the nonclinical and clinical studies. These plans ultimately support the market application and commercial distribution of the approved product.

To be assured that product development milestones are met, a project needs to be well managed. Project management involves the application of knowledge, skills, and tools to project activities to meet therapeutic goals. Managing a project involves establishing a clear and achievable goal, identifying tasks, balancing the competing demands for quality, scope, time, and cost, and adapting the plan and approach to the different concerns and expectations of the various stakeholders.

Obtaining regulatory input on the specific development plan is an important first step in development. In the United States the FDA sincerely wishes to be a partner in the sponsor's development, and the sponsor has the right to obtain the agency's input on their development plans. Early FDA input on the IND plans will help the sponsor reduce the risk of a clinical hold.

Many pharmaceutical companies are increasingly conducting their FDA-regulated clinical trials outside the United States and Western Europe. In fact, some drug companies indicate that as many as 65% of their trials will be based abroad by 2010. Less expensive labor and the availability of treatment-naive subject populations are the chief reasons for conducting trials outside the United States.

Clinical trial applications are required outside the United States for the investigation of new drugs. The successful investigation of new drugs requires strategic planning, clear communication with health authorities, solid project management, and the submission of INDs/CTAs prior to initiating clinical trials. Strategic development and compelling data supporting the drug's benefits with acceptable risks will allow sponsors to file market applications to gain access to global markets.

REFERENCES

1. Project Management Institute. *A Guide to the Project Management Body of Knowledge: PMBOK Guide*, 3rd ed.: PMI; 2004.
2. Guidance for Industry: Content and Format of Investigational New Drug Applications (INDs) for Phase 1 Studies of Drugs, Including Well-Characterized Therapeutic, Biotechnology-Derived Products. U.S. Department of Health and Human Services, Food and Drug Administration; 1995.

3. Guidance for Industry: Submitting Marketing Applications According to the ICH/CTD Format: General Considerations. U.S. Department of Health and Human Services, Food and Drug Administration; 2001.
4. Getz KA. A swift predominance of ex-U.S. sites. *Appl Clin Trials*. 2005. Available at: www.actmagazine.com/appliedclinicaltrials/article/articleDetail.jsp?id = 261633.
5. Kearney AT. Make your move: taking clinical trials to the best location, *Executive Agenda*, 2006.
6. Tassignon J. Setting the Russian record straight. *GCP J*. 2006;13(1):21–23.
7. CHMP Quality Working Party Guideline: Requirements to the Chemical and Pharmaceutical Quality Documentation Concerning Investigational Medicinal Products in Clinical Trials. QWP 18540. European Commission; 2006.
8. Detailed Guidance for the Request for Authorization of a Clinical Trial Product for Human Use to the Competent Authorities; Notification of Substantial Amendments and Declaration of the End of the Trial. European Commission, Enterprise Directorate-General, Pharmaceuticals Unit; 2004.
9. Wichary JM. A magnet for trials? *GCP J*. 2007;14(3):17–18.
10. Law 79/1997 on Medical Products and Its Amendments, Regulation 228/2008 on Good Clinical Praxis and Clinical Trials, SUKL regulations KLH 19 (documentation required for an approval of a clinical trial on a human pharmaceutical) and KLH 20 (application for approval or notification of a clinical trial).
11. CHMP Guideline: Requirements to the Chemical and Pharmaceutical Quality Documentation Concerning Investigational Medicinal Products in Clinical Trials, Attachment 1. QWP 185401/2004. European Commission; 2006.
12. Clinical Trial Authorisations: Applying for Authorisation to Conduct a Clinical Trial—Initial Application. Medicines and Healthcare Products Regulatory Agency. Available at: www.mhra.gov.uk/home/idcplg?IdcService=SS GET PAGE& nodeId=723
13. CHMP Guideline: European clinical trials database (EUDRACT database). ENTR/CT 5. European Commission; 2003.
14. European Parliament Directive: European Parliament and of the Council on "the approximation of the laws, regulations and administrative provisions of the Member States relating to the implementation of good clinical practice in the conduct of clinical trials on medicinal products for human use." Directive 2001/20/EC. European Commission; 2001.
15. State Institute for Drug Control [Státní ústav pro kontrolu léčiv, Skul] Web sites: www.sukl.cz/en03/en03.htm; www.sukl.cz/ download/en08/klh/klh20a.rtf.
16. Food and Drugs Act, *Code of Federal Regulations*, Title 21, Part C (Drugs, Division 1 to Division 10): Administrative Practices and Procedures.
17. Ministry of Health Canada Guidance: Management of Drug Submissions. 2005.
18. Ministry of Health Canada Guidance: Clinical Trial Sponsors; Clinical Trial Applications. 2003.
19. Ministry of Health Canada Guidance: Sponsors of Clinical Trial Applications: Quality (Chemistry and Manufacturing). 2003.
20. Ministry of Health Canada Guidance: Quality (Chemistry and Manufacturing), Draft. 2001.

21. Ministry of Health Canada Guidance: Quality Overall Summary—Chemical Entities (Clinical Trial Applications—Phase I). 2004.
22. Ministry of Health Canada Guidance: Quality overall summary—Chemical Entities (Clinical Trial Applications—Phase II/III). 2004.
23. Ministry of Health Canada Guidance: Preparation of the Quality Information for Drug Submissions in the CTD Format: Biotechnological/Biological (Biotech) Products. 2004.
24. Ministry of Health Canada Guidance: Preparation of the Quality Information for Drug Submissions in the CTD Format: Vaccines. 2004.
25. Ministry of Health Canada Guidance: Preparation of the Quality Information for Drug Submissions in the CTD Format: Blood Products. 2004.
26. Ministry of Health Canada Guidance: Industry: Preparation of the Quality Information for Drug Submissions in the CTD Format: Conventional Biotherapeutic Products. 2004.
27. Mansell P. Australia courts clinical investment. *PharmaTimes*. Apr. 2007.
28. National Statement on Ethical Conduct in Human Research. National Health and Medical Research Council, Government of Australia; 2007. Available at: www.tga.gov.au/unapp/ctglance.htm.
29. Access to Unapproved Goods. Department of Health and Ageing, Government of Australia. Available at: www.tga.gov.au/docs/pdf/unapproved/clintrials.pdf.
30. Barnes K. PAREXEL Talks Clinical Research in Latin America. 2007. Available at: www.outsourcing-pharma.com/news/ng.asp?n=78007-parexel-latin-america-clinical-research.
31. Hurley D. Leveraging Latin assets in clinical trials. *GCP J*. 2006;13(3):16–19.
32. McVean S, Zborovski S. China remains untapped market for conducting trials. In: *Clinical Trials Advisor*. Washington, DC: Washington Business Information Inc.; Dec. 15, 2005.
33. Anon. A new era begins for India's clinical research market. *CenterWatch Mon*. 2006;13(7).
34. Sugii H. Japan rides a wave of globalization. *GCP J* 2006;10:18–21.

14

FIRST-IN-HUMAN REGULATORY SUBMISSIONS

MARY M. SOMMER, MARK AMMANN, ULF B. HILLGREN, KATHLEEN J. KOVACS, AND KEITH WILNER

14.1 INTRODUCTION

The purpose of this chapter is to enable the reader to successfully position, prepare, and submit a high-quality dossier to regulatory authorities to support a first-in-human (FIH) clinical trial. In the preceding chapters, the course of investigational drug discovery and selection, drug metabolism, formulation, nonclinical safety and toxicity testing, and regional requirements and expectations for initial clinical trials have been described. The culmination of these early development efforts is application and authorization for the first use of the investigational drug in humans. Authorization is based on the review of the written dossier by regulatory and medical authorities. In this final chapter on FIH submissions we address the preparation and submission of dossiers, including the general context and strategic considerations, relevant regulatory guidances, and organization, content, and written presentation.

In the first sections of the chapter we describe the regulatory and clinical considerations for the location of the FIH clinical trial, the dossier preparation, and the submission process in the three major regulator regions: the United States, the European Union (EU), and Japan. The situation in the United States is described in detail first, including the relevant regulatory guidance and general process and teamwork considerations. Submissions for the EU and Japan are then discussed, mainly from the perspective of how they differ from the U.S. submission preparation and process, including differences in regulatory guidance and expectation. A

Early Drug Development: Strategies and Routes to First-in-Human Trials, Edited by Mitchell N. Cayen

separate section follows on the unique aspects for biotechnology-derived products. In the final sections we address emerging regions and final submission considerations.

For a successful submission, the design of the investigational drug development program and the data generated should be presented effectively in the dossier and consistent with the intended use in the initial clinical trials. In general terms, the basic constituents of FIH submissions are the same for most pharmaceuticals. However, the regulatory authorities' expectations for the specific types of pharmacology and toxicity studies, types of toxicities, and doses and systemic drug exposures relative to those projected for humans will depend on the type of pharmaceutical, therapeutic indication, human subjects (patient or volunteer), and phase I trial design. Most phase I programs are conducted in healthy human volunteers, with the goal of safely determining the maximum tolerated dose (MTD) and characterizing the adverse effects (see Section 14.2.2).

To support testing in humans, evaluation of the safety data in the dossier should assess the risks and their relevance for the first subjects and determine appropriately that the potential adverse effects of the investigational drug are manageable. Sufficient information in in vitro and in vivo biologic test systems must be presented to support robustly the safety of use in humans, as described in the clinical protocols proposed. The toxicity profile in animals should be characterized as to the types of toxicities, associated doses, and systemic drug concentrations [including the no-observed-adverse-effect levels (NOAELs)], biomarkers and monitoring mechanisms for toxicities, and reversibility. These data are critical to justify the initial starting dose and escalation plan for the FIH trial. The appropriate assessments of human risk and risk management must be communicated in the dossier clearly and thoroughly.

In addition, the organization of the dossier and process for submission must meet the expectations of the regulatory authorities, as published in regulations and regulatory guidance documents and as expressed less formally in actual day-to-day practices. Expectations can vary significantly from region to region and country to country. Knowledge of the relevant guidance for the specific type of investigational new drug and the recent trends in regulatory expectations across regions greatly facilitates a successful and uneventful review by the regulatory authority. For efficient continuation of development in subsequent trials leading to market authorization, the initial activities should be the strategic start of an overall clinical and regulatory plan for development of the investigational drug. The patients and conditions studied and the designs of the supporting nonclinical studies ultimately will determine the indications and label that a regulatory authority will approve.

14.2 SUBMISSION STRATEGIES

The factors guiding the choice of geographic location for the FIH trial and submission of the dossier are primarily regulatory and clinical. The decision regarding the location for an investigational drug FIH clinical trial should be made after considering the regional regulatory environment, review time lines, dossier requirements, available clinical trial sites, subjects, and investigators, and medical review board processes and time lines. Because most FIH trials involve healthy volunteers in fairly standard trial designs, many sponsors consistently use only a few specific sites with which they have established relationships and working practices.

14.2.1 Regulatory Environment

The regulatory process and documentation required by the local regulatory authorities across different regions can influence the region chosen for the initial trial. The key variables to consider include regulatory authority review time lines, extent and type of dossier components and time lines for creating those components, requirements for shipping drug product from manufacturing sites to clinical sites, and regional regulatory authority concerns and unique restrictions.

Review time lines for an initial clinical trial application can vary significantly across regions (Table 14.1). Usually, the approval of both a government regulatory agency and a medical review board is required prior to initiation of a clinical trial. In some countries, for example the United States, there are explicit time lines associated with review of the application. Regulations stipulate that review of an application to initiate trials in humans must be completed within 30 calendar days. Similar time lines exist in many developed countries and regions, but it should be noted that some countries do not have specific review time lines for clinical trial applications, and durations of three to six months are not uncommon.

The documentation needed to support an initial clinical trial also varies from providing a copy of the investigator's brochure (IB) and the proposed clinical protocol to producing a complex dossier containing these documents plus

TABLE 14.1 Approval Time Lines for Selected Countries

Country	Regulatory Authority Time Line	IRB/IEC[a] Review Relative to Regulatory Authority
Australia	Notification after IEC approval	IEC approval first
Canada	30 days	In parallel
China	270 days	30–60 days; regulatory authority approval first
India	90 days	28 days, in parallel
Japan	30 days	Regulatory authority approval first
South Korea	30–60 days	40 days, in parallel
United States	30 days	IND number required prior to IRB approval, in parallel
European Union	60 days[b]	Varies by country

[a]IRB, institutional review board; IEC, independent ethics committee.
[b]Maximum is 60 days; for some countries the review time may be shorter.

toxicology, pharmacology and pharmacokinetic summaries and reports, an integrated nonclinical summary, a detailed description of the manufacturing process and analytical testing, and explanation of the overall clinical development plan.

The site for manufacturing of clinical trial supplies can influence the selection of the location for initial human testing. The requirements for both import and export of the investigational product should be evaluated. In some cases, import authorizations are integrated with clinical trial authorizations; in other cases, the authorizations are managed separately. Although it is fairly clear why regulatory authorities would control the import of investigational products into their country, some countries, notably the United States, also carefully control export. As an example, a sponsor manufacturing supplies in the United States for a clinical trial in Europe needs to satisfy both the import requirements in the clinical trial country as well as the U.S. requirements for export. In most cases, the latter is now a relatively simple notification, but neglecting this step can lead to lengthy delays in U.S. customs. Such delays can be especially problematic for investigational drugs with special handling requirements (e.g., temperature control).

The review of the dossier submitted is facilitated if the regulatory authority has prior experience with similar investigational drugs (i.e., comparable chemistry and/or mechanism of action) and indications (e.g., HIV, oncology). In some cases, prior experience is a significant consideration in the choice of the region for submission. For example, emerging safety concerns may significantly affect the review of subsequent submissions, as occurred in March 2006, when six patients developed multiorgan failure in a phase I clinical trial conducted in the UK (Chapter 12). As a result, significant additional scrutiny has been given to clinical trials with (1) biological molecules with novel mechanisms of action, (2) new agents with a highly species-specific action, and (3) new drugs directed toward immune system targets. As this situation unfolded, clinical trial applications were delayed for a wide range of biologic agents in Europe. Although the greatest impact was in Europe, where this trial occurred, similar effects were observed in other regions. As such, safety issues for related products need to be considered carefully when selecting the location for clinical trials. Investigation of these factors, and those described below for selection of the clinical site, well ahead of the submission permits anticipation and accommodation of the effects on the process, timing, and deliverables.

14.2.2 Clinical Considerations

Clinical Trial Facilities The selection of the appropriate clinical site is critical to successful execution of the FIH study. The following are considered critical factors in determining the appropriate clinical trial facility for the FIH study:

- Competent clinical, scientific, management, and support staff
- Management and storage of biological samples
- Motivated and experienced investigators

- Prior phase I experience
- Record of high subject recruitment rate
- High data quality and low error rate
- Electronic data management capability
- Timely medical board review
- Efficient contract and budget process
- Reasonable costs per subject
- Other capabilities specific to the particular trial design or subject population (e.g., imaging capability)

The clinical site must have competent staff, including experienced research nurses and study coordinators. It is particularly important that the study coordinator be knowledgeable and experienced in clinical trial research, as this person is the primary contact between the clinical site and the sponsor. The sponsor relies on the study coordinator to oversee all aspects of the clinical study. It is also important that the investigator and staff have prior phase I experience and a good understanding of the nuances of phase I clinical trials. Because one of the major objectives of the FIH study is to evaluate the pharmacokinetics of the investigational drug, the clinical site must be capable of collecting, handling, and storing plasma and/or serum and other required specimens. Since the FIH study is on the critical path to drug registration, subject recruitment rate is important to the time lines and the overall cost of the program. As part of a pretrial assessment, it should be determined that the investigator has access to the protocol-defined subject population and a record of efficient subject recruitment. The sponsor can best follow the progress of the trial if the subject data are available in real time. This is best accomplished by some type of electronic data-entry system, where the data are entered directly into the clinical database rather than being transcribed from paper case report forms, and can be accessed remotely. Direct electronic data entry avoids the additional resources and time required for transcription of the hard-copy case reports and review for and correction of transcription errors and associated delays in data review. High-quality safety data are important, since these data support the decisions to go forward with development of the investigational drug. Selected clinical sites should have a reputation for quality and timeliness of data entry. Reliable data that are delivered when expected enable rapid assessment of the investigational drug program.

Oversight of clinical trial design is the responsibility of a medical review board, such as the institutional review boards (IRBs) in the United States and independent ethics committees (IECs) in the EU. The approval of such a medical review board is required to start a clinical trial. Some sites use a central board, that is, one that reviews clinical trial proposals for several clinical sites, as opposed to a local body that is responsible for only a single site. Due to the relatively large volume of proposals, central boards usually meet more frequently (perhaps once a week) than local ones (perhaps once a month). The general process for review and approval is very similar across countries. Most review boards require that the sponsor submit the protocol and consent form two weeks prior to the meeting date. As part of the pretrial assessment, the sponsor should be aware of the exact dates of board meetings and protocol and consent form submission deadlines. The law in some countries may require regulatory authority approval prior to submission to the medical review board (see Table 14.1). Other factors being equal, selection of a clinical site might be based on the frequency at which the review board meets and whether the regulatory authority review and medical review board review can be done in parallel.

Finally, in this time of cost containment, subject costs are important. The subject costs are related to the number and type of parameters evaluated and the time lines set to start and complete the study. Additional subject costs can be a reasonable trade-off for faster delivery of a higher-quality clinical trial.

In addition to evaluating the safety and pharmacokinetics in the FIH study, the pharmacologic properties can also be evaluated, often by the use of biomarkers or imaging techniques. If this is a primary objective of the FIH study, the investigator's knowledge and capabilities in this area are important factors in selection of the clinical site.

Clinical Site Relationships If the clinical site is to be used repeatedly, the sponsor should consider the advantages of a master research agreement with the site. A master research agreement specifies contract language between the sponsor and site for all new studies with the clinical site and often reduces the time it takes to negotiate contract language. In addition to a master research agreement, the sponsor can establish an accepted budget template with set costs for various potential protocol-required procedures, which saves time on budget negotiations. If the sponsor plans to use the site extensively, it can be helpful to set up a preferred provider contract. This type of contract gives preference to the sponsor's studies. Although the preferred provider status is usually more costly, the sponsor's studies are given a high priority by the clinical site and can be better conducted according to the sponsor's needs. Such an agreement enhances smooth communication lines between the sponsor and clinical site and facilitates study scheduling and startup.

Healthy Volunteers or Patients In most instances, healthy volunteers are selected for FIH studies. Healthy volunteers are usually recruited very rapidly and their evaluation is not complicated by concomitant medication or concurrent diseases. They are a more homogeneous population than patients and generally, fewer need to be enrolled in the FIH study to evaluate safety and pharmacokinetics effectively. For example, the pharmacokinetic data from a healthy volunteer study are often less variable than data from patients, due to exclusion of disease factors or interactions with other medications. Healthy volunteers are also considered less vulnerable to potential ill effects of investigational drugs. However, since healthy volunteers derive no medical benefit from receiving the investigational drug, there should be every expectation that the drug can be given safely with little risk of serious adverse effects. In some therapeutic areas, such as oncology and ophthalmology, patients rather than healthy volunteers are often the first clinical trial subjects, because the relatively high risk of adverse effects can be balanced by potential benefit to the patients. Patients are also the population targeted when the critical endpoints to be evaluated can only be measured in the disease state. Starting a first-in-patient (FIP) study is often much more complicated than starting an FIH study in healthy volunteers. To recruit sufficient patients, the studies tend to involve multiple clinical trial centers and generally require multiple committee approvals at each clinical site: for instance, scientific committee review in addition to IRB review. Where a healthy volunteer study is possible and will meet some of the objectives of a patient study, the sponsor should balance the advantages of the relative ease of healthy volunteer studies versus those of generating potentially more relevant safety and efficacy data in the patient population.

14.3 FIRST-IN-HUMAN DOSSIERS

14.3.1 Introduction

The dossier prepared must meet the requirements of that regional regulatory authority where the submission is planned. The FIH dossiers of the major global regions—the United States, the EU, and Japan—are described in this section. The FIH dossiers for other countries are very similar to those required in the major global regions. Depending on the country, English may not be an acceptable submission language. If the requirements are not clear from published guidance, the regulatory authority should be contacted to determine in advance whether the documents submitted need to be translated to the local language, as this may have a significant impact on the submission time lines and therefore the country selection.

14.3.2 General Considerations for Dossier Preparations

The International Conference on Harmonisation of Technical Requirements for Registration of Pharmaceuticals for Human Use guidelines have been developed by regulatory authorities and industry trade groups from the United States, the EU, and Japan. ICH was formed in 1990 specifically to provide uniform guidelines across these three major markets for pharmaceuticals. Prior to this effort, guidelines varied greatly across the globe and, as a result, drug sponsors were often required to conduct different, often redundant or scientifically unjustified, studies for a given program. This situation was inefficient for the sponsors and for the regulatory authorities reviewing and approving new medicines for their patient populations. The ICH guidelines are the best source of general expectations for development program content and dossier format and organization. These guidelines are categorized into four groups, consistent with the

TABLE 14.2 ICH Guidelines Relevant for FIH Submissions

Guideline Designation	Title
ICH M4	Organization of the Common Technical Document for the Registration of Pharmaceuticals for Human Use
ICH M4Q	The Common Technical Document for the Registration of Pharmaceuticals for Human Use: Quality
ICH M4S	The Common Technical Document for the Registration of Pharmaceuticals for Human Use: Safety
ICH M4E	The Common Technical Document for the Registration of Pharmaceuticals for Human Use: Efficacy
ICH M2	The Electronic Common Technical Document Specification
ICH M3	Nonclinical Safety Studies for the Conduct of Human Clinical Trials for Pharmaceuticals
ICH E6	Good Clinical Practice: Consolidated Guideline
ICH S6	Nonclinical Safety Evaluation of the Biotechnology-Derived Pharmaceuticals

three areas of relevant scientific expertise: (1) quality (chemistry), (2) safety (pharmacology/toxicology), (3) efficacy (clinical), and (4) multidisciplinary (for those guidelines affecting a combination of disciplines). The guidance designations are ICH Q, S, E, and M. The relevant ICH guidelines are listed in Table 14.2.

Historically, each country/region has had its own unique content and format for marketing applications and clinical trial applications. The ICH M4 guideline, "Organization of the Common Technical Document," presents an accepted organization and format for registration dossiers and is the required standard for marketing applications in the major regions. Although this guideline was developed for marketing applications, the format and organization of the common technical document (CTD) provide the regulators with a familiar and broadly accepted dossier organization that can be applied to clinical trial applications (e.g., FIH) earlier in the drug development process. The key benefit of the CTD is the constant structure for multiple regions that minimizes duplication when submitting clinical trial applications in more than one region, although regionally specific formats may still be acceptable to those regions. Since the data generated by the time that clinical development is completed are much greater than for an initial FIH submission, several of the CTD template sections will have limited or no data in an FIH dossier. Therefore, when applying the CTD guidance to an FIH submission, the dossier should be modeled according to the general order and content as is reasonable for the information that is available and as is suitable for the specific region's expectations for FIH submissions. The table of contents for the CTD is presented in Table 14.3.

ICH M4 provides for a structure of five basic modules (see Figure 14.1). Module 1 (administrative and prescribing information) contains the regionally

TABLE 14.3 Common Technical Document Contents

Organization of the Common Technical Document for the Registration of Pharmaceuticals for Human Use

Module 1: Administrative Information and Prescribing Information[a]
- 1.1 Table of Contents of the Submission including Module 1
- 1.2 Documents Specific to Each Region (e.g., application forms, prescribing information)

Module 2: Common Technical Document Summaries
- 2.1 Common Technical Document Table of Contents[a] (Modules 2 to 5)
- 2.2 CTC Introduction[a]
- 2.3 Quality Overall Summary[a]
- 2.4 Nonclinical Overview[a]
- 2.5 Clinical Overview
- 2.6 Nonclinical Written and Tabulated Summaries[a]
  - Pharmacology
  - Pharmacokinetics
  - Toxicology
- 2.7 Clinical Summary
  - Biopharmaceutic Studies and Associated Analytical Methods
  - Clinical Pharmacology Studies
  - Clinical Efficacy
  - Clinical Safety
  - Literature References
  - Synopses of Individual Studies

Module 3: Quality[a]
- 3.1 Table of Contents of Module 3
- 3.2 Body of Data
- 3.3 Literature References

Module 4: Nonclinical Study Reports[a]
- 4.1 Table of Contents of Module 4
- 4.2 Study Reports
- 4.3 Literature References

Module 5: Clinical Study Reports[b]
- 5.1 Table of Contents of Module 5
- 5.2 Tabular Listing of All Clinical Studies
- 5.3 Clinical Study Reports
- 5.4 Literature References

[a] For FIH submissions.
[b] The only documents included for FIH are the initial clinical protocol and investigator information.

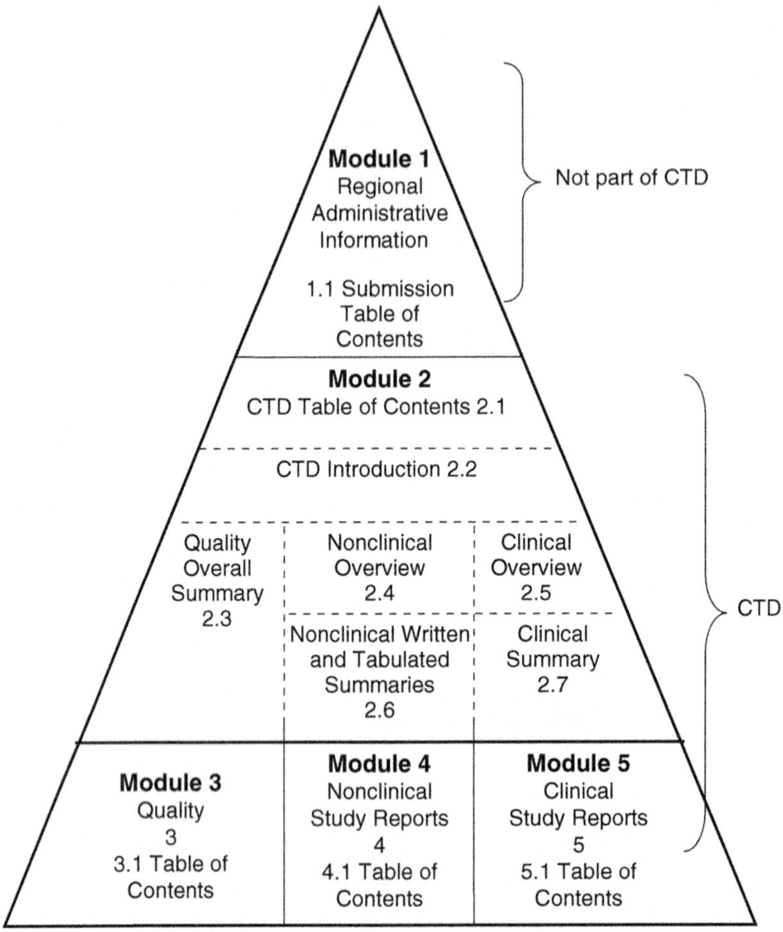

FIGURE 14.1 Common technical document modules.

specific application documentation (i.e., application forms, cover letter, investigator's brochure); Module 2 (common technical document summaries) includes overviews and summaries for quality, nonclinical (nonclinical) and clinical information; Module 3 (quality) provides more details on description of the drug substance, drug product, and analytical testing; and Modules 4 (nonclinical study reports) and 5 (clinical study reports) contain the study reports indicated. Additional guidance for the content and organization in modules 2 through 5 is provided in ICH M4Q, M4S, and M4E.

At the time of FIH submission, no clinical data are available. The clinical components will be limited to the proposed clinical protocol and associated investigator documentation. Human dose, target therapeutic systemic drug concentrations, clearance, and metabolism are projected from in vivo animal data and in vitro metabolism data with human liver microsomes or hepatocytes. Relative to a drug registration dossier, the dossier for an FIH submission will contain only the relatively limited data that have been generated to support the first trials, and as a result, some sections contain no data or text because the supporting studies are not conducted until later in clinical development. Other sections contain only a fraction of the information that is generated by the time a drug candidate dossier is submitted for registration.

Building a CTD document from the start of development has the advantages of being acceptable to many regions and serving as the first version of what can be a living document that grows with the progress of the investigational drug, accommodating subsequently acquired data and eventually supporting the marketing application. In addition to the various ICH guidelines, each region or country has regulations and guidances that are relevant to the conduct of clinical trials for pharmaceuticals. Regulations, guidances, and regulatory Web sites relevant to preparation and submission of an FIH dossier for the United States and the EU are outlined in Table 14.4.

14.3.3 Coordination of the Disciplines

Expertise in several disciplines is required to design the investigational drug development program, interpret the data, and write the submission documents. Successful submission of an FIH dossier requires that experts in the various subjects work together to coordinate production of the dossier components. Although much of the content of the quality (in the United States termed chemistry, manufacturing, and controls [CMC]), nonclinical, and clinical components is independent, related areas should be appropriately cross-referenced and the perspectives of the different sections should present unified support for the use intended. To draft and assemble an FIH submission, the following must occur:

1. An appropriate FIH-supporting development program is designed and executed.
2. Expert data summaries and scientific assessments are written for the quality and nonclinical sections of the dossier.
3. Clinical protocols are written to define the FIH trial(s) and an IB (see Section 14.4.6) is written to provide the investigator and regulator with background information for the clinical trial.
4. Components are unified into a single dossier compatible with regulatory expectations.

The project manager for the dossier preparation process establishes the project plan and time lines and identifies the interdependencies and hand-offs among the discipline experts. The contributing experts must understand their contribution and the relationships among the contributions. The important elements to capture in the project plan include the following:

TABLE 14.4 Legislation and Guidance Documents for FIH Submissions in the United States and the European Union

Title	Topic
FDA Requirements and Guidance (www.fda.gov)	
Title 21 CFR Part 50	Protection of Human Subjects
Title 21 CFR Part 56	Institutional Review Boards
Title 21 CFR Part 58	Good Laboratory Practice for Nonclinical Laboratory Studies
Title 21 CFR Part 312	Investigational New Drug Application
Guidance for Industry, November 1995	Content and Format for Investigational New Drug Applications for Phase 1 Studies of Drugs
Guidance for Industry, February 2000	Formal Meetings with Sponsors and Applicants for PDUFA Products
Guidance for Industry, May 2001	IND Meetings for Human Drugs and Biologics, Chemistry, Manufacturing, and Controls Information
Guidance for Industry, November 1995	Submission of Environmental Assessments for Human Drug Applications and Supplements
EU Requirements and Guidance: The Rules Governing Medicinal Products in the European Union ec.europa.eu/enterprise/sectors/pharmaceuticals/documents/eudralex/index_en.htm	
Directive 2001/20/EC	Good Clinical Practice
Directive 2005/28/EC	Good Clinical Practice
Directive 2003/94/EC	Good Manufacturing Practice
Eudralex, Vol. 10, Chapter 1	Application and Application Form
ENTR/F2/BL D (2003) CT1, Revision 2, Oct. 2005	Request for Authorization of a Clinical Trial
Eudralex, Vol. 10, Chapter 1 ENTR/CT2, Feb. 2006	Application for Ethic Committee Opinion
Eudralex, Vol. 4, Annex 13	Manufacture of Investigational Medicinal Products
ENTR/F/2/AM/on D(2010) 3374	
EMEA Guidance for Human Medicines www.emea.europa.eu/index/indexh1.htm	
EMEA/267187/2005	New Framework for Scientific Advice and Protocol Assistance
EMEA-H-4260-01-Rev. 5	EMEA Guidance for Companies Requesting Scientific Advice or Protocol Assistance
CHMP/QWP/185401/2004	Chemical and Pharmaceutical Quality Documentation
CHMP/SWP/28367/07	Strategies to Identify and Mitigate Risk in FIH Clinical Trials
EU Clinical Trial System	eudract.emea.europa.eu/

- A list of the necessary deliverables and the content, style, and format expectations
- The duration required to complete each deliverable
- The interdependencies of the activities
- A project plan with the calendar dates that each activity can actually be scheduled and completed
- The person accountable to complete each activity or ensure that it is completed
- A process to compile, review, and approve the dossier

The plan should have at least two levels of granularity: a high level that links the main deliverables from each discipline, and a detailed level for the activities and interdependencies for each deliverable for each discipline. The team managing the high-level plan should be kept small, limited to a size just large enough to accommodate those accountable for the overall progress of the major deliverables for a discipline. Within each discipline there should also be a team to monitor the details of each activity and the specific materials they need from other lines to complete their tasks. The teams should meet regularly, monitor progress, and troubleshoot issues that arise. The earlier an unexpected issue is identified, the earlier the impact can be assessed and the greater the likelihood that it can be resolved without affecting project time lines. Outsourcing of work to another company or to a contract research organization (CRO) transfers the management of those specific deliverables. This makes the CRO part of the team working to deliver the dossier. In these cases, extending the partnership to the CRO and establishing clear expectations and good communication will better ensure timely deliverables of the quality expected.

In each case, the team of expert contributors should clarify the process for completing the submission, such as expectations for time lines, document completion dates, document quality and characteristics, responsibilities for deliverables, and mechanisms for issue resolution. Lack of clarity can lead to misunderstandings. Misunderstandings can lead to delays, repeat work, poor dossier quality, and erosion of the sponsor's relationship with the regulatory agency.

Careful forward planning of the deliverables and time lines required for the various components and the clinical trial start date offers the best opportunity for a well-written and complete dossier. A contrasting, but common approach consists of setting the clinical trial start date and then attempting to complete all the needed activities in the time available. In the latter approach, the time allotted is often inadequate, resulting in a poorly written, unintegrated dossier. General considerations for the most common rate-limiting FIH-supporting activities are presented in Table 14.5. The duration required to complete the activities will depend on the number and complexity of the studies and the results of the studies. Exploratory FIH programs (Chapter 11) that are supported with fewer, shorter studies than those supporting a traditional FIH will, in general, take less time to write and compile. The best-laid time lines can be disrupted if unanticipated findings cannot

TABLE 14.5 Example of Approximate Relationships and Durations for Common Rate-Limiting FIH-Supporting Activities

Activity	Duration
Start to end of in-life of rate-limiting pharmacology or toxicity studies[a]	>5–8 weeks
Data analysis and interpretation of rate-limiting studies, including histopathology	
Compilation and drafting of remaining pharmacology, ADME, and toxicology study reports	∼2–12 weeks
Writing of CTD written and tabular summaries of individual reports	
Scientific and managerial review of reports	
QA/QC audit of study reports and data files	
Writing of CTD summary sections, such as nonclinical and quality overviews	∼1–4 weeks
Writing of clinical protocol	
Writing of regional administrative dossier components	
Compilation of IB	
Reconciliation of QA audits and study reports	
Review and QC of CTD summary sections	
Compilation of CTD Modules 1, 2, 3, and 4	1–6 weeks
Review of complete FIH dossier	
Incorporating edits subsequent to dossier review	
Formatting for submission-ready electronic dossier preparation	
Submit dossier to regulatory authority	
Approximate total duration range	∼9–30 weeks

[a] One-month studies are an example of the rate-limiting study duration for this table, and the time frame includes predosing study preparation time and in-life dosing. Studies may be of shorter or longer durations.

be explained adequately and additional studies need to be conducted for the data package and risk assessment to support human safety. The rate-limiting activities are usually the safety pharmacology or toxicity studies. Activities such as dose-range-finding toxicity studies and pharmacology efficacy studies, protein-binding assays, and in vitro metabolism assays that are conducted earlier than the final toxicity studies are best documented in study reports as they are completed. In that way the data from those early studies are appropriately evaluated and available for robust data-based internal development decisions along the course of development, and final comprehensive data evaluation is less likely to identify gaps in the assessments and result in dossier submission delays. Activities conducted in parallel with toxicity studies include preparation of the clinical trial protocol, investigator's brochure, and quality sections. Particular attention should be paid to these activities to ensure that they can be completed in the same time frame. If not, they should be tracked as rate-limiting activities that will determine the earliest submission date. Unexpected delays should be identified and rectified as early as possible to prevent delay of the submission and clinical trial.

Completed reports are not necessary for inclusion in the submission except for the toxicity studies, and even then only for the United States. Those pharmacology and toxicity studies providing the key data for projecting human safety, called the pivotal or definitive studies, should be conducted according to good laboratory practices (GLPs). GLP compliance includes quality assurance (QA) inspections during the study data collection and audits of the reports and data files. GLPs are described in the documentation cited in Table 14.4. Draft reports for which the QA audit has not been completed are acceptable for submission in the United States but are subject to additional reporting, as described in Section 14.4.1.

14.3.4 Document Preparation

There are several aspects of document preparation that should be considered when planning a regulatory submission for an FIH study. These considerations should include the following:

- Who is to write each section of the dossier?
- Is the submission to be electronic or paper? If electronic, who is to create the bookmarks, cross-references, and hyperlinks and ensure compliance to electronic guidance standards?
- Is a template to be used?
- Does the template comply with regulatory guidelines?
- Is a style guide available for the authors (i.e., standard headers, document formatting, section numbering, standard font)?
- Who is to review and/or approve each section of the dossier?
- Have the primary source documents, meaning the reports of those studies that generated the data characterizing the safety profile of the candidate drug, such as GLP toxicology reports, received the QA inspections and audits required?
- Is each section to undergo quality control (QC) review to ensure correctness of each submission document? If so, who will perform the QC evaluation?
- Who is responsible for ensuring that the documents for the dossier are "submission ready"?
- Who is to submit the dossier to the regulatory authority and the appropriate components to the medical review boards?
- Who is responsible for dealing with the communication or issues related to the submission review by the regulatory authority?

All sections should follow regulatory guidelines for style, format, and quality, and therefore be ready to incorporate into a single dossier. The expression *submission-ready* refers to the ultimate state of all submission components, such that the documents are fit for purpose and error-free. Formatting standards are defined in ICH and U.S. Food and Drug Administration (FDA) guidelines for the United States and in ICH and European Medicines Agency (EMEA) guidelines for the EU and must be met for a document to be acceptable to these regulatory authorities. Failure to adhere to these specifications could result in a "clinical hold" based solely on format (e.g., incorrectly located information or inadequate navigational tools such as table of contents, table headers, and bookmarks). Although Health Canada accepts the formatting standards set out for the quality section by ICH, they prefer that the quality data be summarized using a specific quality overall summary tabular format, available from the Health Canada Web site. For Health Canada, use of their specific form promotes review efficiencies by serving as the basis for the quality assessment report and provides additional guidance with respect to technical content requirements. Any sponsor style guide and dossier templates should incorporate submission-ready standards. See Table 14.4 for the relevant Web sites.

An important step in preparing the dossier is ensuring that the components are accurate and complete. Each component should be evaluated carefully against the expectations for format, style, accuracy, and completeness. This process is called quality control (QC). Established consistent standards and process for QC should be specified and applied. Interpretive and summary sections should be checked for accuracy against the original data sources. Each section should have all the necessary parts and should be labeled appropriately. Literature and report references for the summary sections should be correct, and copies should be available within the dossier. References cited in study reports must be available upon request. Internal dossier components such as the table of contents and cross-references should be checked. If the dossier is an electronic submission, bookmarks and hyperlinks should be correct. In general, QC is conducted most effectively by someone other than the author, as the author is too familiar with the contents and will often "read over" errors or omissions.

A submission-ready dossier provides several benefits to the sponsor company:

- All documents are structured in accordance with the current FDA and ICH CTD and electronic common technical document (eCTD) guidance to reduce the risk of a "clinical hold."
- Reopening of approved components or documents for administrative corrections is reduced and rework is eliminated.
- The final stages of document preparation, process, and submission time lines are predictable and streamlined.

If the dossier submission is to be electronic, there are special considerations for the preparation. Electronic submissions can expedite submission of data and documentation (i.e., through electronic gateways managed by regulatory authorities) and facilitate the review of complex interdependent data through bookmarks, hyperlinks, and so on. The electronic format laid out in ICH M2 specifies file structure and relationships based on the CTD structure. Bookmarks allow navigation through the tables of contents and hyperlinks facilitate transitions to reports, tables, and appendixes within the dossier. If a dossier is submitted in the United States in eCTD format, all subsequent submissions for that drug program must also be in electronic format. As electronic submissions are accepted more broadly by other regions, similar requirements are likely to apply. ICH M2 specifications were designed with the complexity of life-cycle management in mind, that is, the continued integration of subsequent material to that application over the course of development of the investigational drug.

14.4 UNITED STATES: INVESTIGATIONAL NEW DRUG APPLICATION

14.4.1 Regulatory Perspective

The regulatory authority in the United States is the Food and Drug Administration (FDA). The document submitted to the FDA for the initial clinical studies of a new candidate drug is called an investigational new drug application (IND). The submission of an IND to the FDA is required to support human testing of any drug product not previously authorized for marketing in the United States. Once an IND is opened, subsequent study reports, safety reports, manufacturing changes, and clinical protocols are submitted as "amendments" to that IND. The exception is the exploratory IND (eIND) (Chapter 11), which is closed after completion of the clinical study described therein. The relevant legal requirements for pharmaceutical development are captured in Title 21 of the *Code of Federal Regulations* (CFR), and those specific to INDs are in Title 21 CFR Part 312 (Table 14.4). In addition, the FDA issues guidance documents that provide interpretation of the regulations and the FDA perspective on various aspects of pharmaceutical development and registration. The guidances are theoretically not binding, but do represent the FDA's current thinking and expectations. The regulations and guidances can be accessed at the FDA Web site (Table 14.4). The approval of a medical review board, called an institution review board (IRB), is required prior to initiation of a clinical trial. IRB review and approval are mandated for all biomedical research by Title 45 CFR Part 46. The charge of the IRBs is to safeguard the rights, safety, and well-being of all trial subjects.

A good place to start in understanding the requirements for the FIH dossier is with the FDA guidances titled "Guidance for Industry: Content and Format of Investigational New Drug Applications for Phase 1 Studies of Drugs" (November 1995) and "Guidance for Industry Q & A Content and Format of INDs for Phase 1 Studies of Drugs" (October 2000). These guidances were written as clarification to the Title 21 CFR Parts 312.22 and 312.23. Currently, the FDA accepts INDs in either the structure stipulated in Title 21 CFR Part 312.23 or the CTD format.

The dossier components are FDA form 1571; table of contents; description of the general investigative plan; IB; planned clinical study protocols; name, CV, and address of the investigator and IRB; chemistry, manufacturing, and controls (CMC) information; and pharmacology and toxicology information, including an integrated summary of the findings with full tabulation of data suitable for detailed

TABLE 14.6 Investigational New Drug Application Contents

Cover letter from sponsor contact to relevant division head at the FDA
FDA form 1571
Table of contents
Introduction
General investigational plan
Investigator's brochure
Protocol and related information
Protocol
Informed consent document
Investigator CV
Chemistry, manufacturing, and controls
Pharmacology and toxicology data
Previous human experience (no data for FIH)
Additional information
Appendixes
Literature references
Pharmacology study reports
Pharmacokinetic and toxicokinetic study reports (latter may be part of toxicology study reports)
Toxicology study reports

review (Table 14.6). The purpose of the information presented within the initial IND is to inform the FDA so they can determine whether or not the proposed FIH study can proceed safely. The general investigative plan is included so that the FDA can provide guidance and facilitate the intended course of development. As such, the document should be a general overview of the company's plans for the next year or so. Guidance for the CMC section (called "quality" in the ICH guidance) is also included in the FDA IND guidance.

The main requirement for the CMC section is to present information that demonstrates convincingly that the clinical test material is safe to use. Any signal of potential human risk is stated in the introduction to this section and discussed in detail in the relevant subsections. The data generated from testing the drug substance in the nonclinical studies are key to demonstrating safety. Any differences among batches are discussed, particularly those between the batches used in the toxicity studies and the batch to be used in the clinical trials. Of particular concern are impurities present in the clinical batch that are at higher levels than those in the batches testing in the toxicity studies. In general, there is an expectation that the impurity profile of material used in human testing is the same or better than material used in the animal studies. The safety of the drug substance and impurities are presented as evaluated in the safety pharmacology and toxicity studies. Excipients in the drug substance and drug product should also be shown to be safe at the levels given used either by animal testing, by precedented use in similarly administered products, or by listing the accepted pharmacopeia (Table 14.7).

TABLE 14.7 Major Pharmacopeia and Web Sites

Pharmacopoeia	Web Site
USP-NF (*United States Pharmacopeia-National Formulary*)	www.usp.org/USPNF; www.uspnf.com/uspnf/login
European Pharmacopeia	online.pheur.org/entry.htm
Japanese Pharmacopeia	jpdb.nihs.go.jp/jp14e/

The nonclinical contributions to the IND include abstracts or summaries of the pharmacology and ADME data, an integrated summary of the toxicology data, and complete data listings for all of the toxicity studies. The integrated toxicology summary is composed of a brief description of the design and results of the toxicity studies supporting the proposed clinical trial, an integration of the findings, and a critical assessment of the findings and relevance for human risk. The GLP status of the studies, the location of study conduct and data archive, and nonclinical expert(s) are also specified. Generally, final study reports should be included in the original IND. However, the guidance makes the provision that "unaudited draft" reports can be submitted if final reports are not available. If the IND is submitted with draft reports, the final reports are to be available and a summary provided to describe any changes from the initially submitted information within 120 days of receipt of the IND. Although the original guidance states that "120 days from the start of the human study for which the animal study formed part of the safety conclusion basis," the subsequent Q and A clarification specifies that "the Agency measures the 120-day period based on the Agency's receipt (date of receipt stamped on the IND submission) of the *integrated summary report* including the toxicology information." The guidance also seems to indicate that instead of a draft or final study report, individual data points and the study protocols and amendments can be submitted, but this interpretation makes assessment of the toxicology section of the dossier studies more difficult for the pharmacology/toxicology regulatory reviewer and in practice can result in difficulties for the submission.

In the United States, the format and organization of the IND submission can either follow the structure outlined in Title 21 CFR, Part 312.23 or ICH M4. The sections of the CTD that appropriately support an IND submission are discussed later in the chapter (Figure 14.2). The FDA guidance "Formal Meetings with Sponsor and Applicants for PDUFA Products" (February 2000) details the types of meetings that the FDA grants to sponsors, the procedures for requesting meetings, and the recommended contents of the information package that is prepared for such meetings. Meetings with the FDA are classified into one of three categories (type A, B, or C) (Table 14.8) based on the issues to be discussed and the status of the drug development program. An important difference among these categories is the time line for FDA to grant a meeting, following receipt of a request. The primary meeting related to FIH studies is the pre-IND meeting, a type B meetings that is generally granted within 60 days of request. Pre-IND

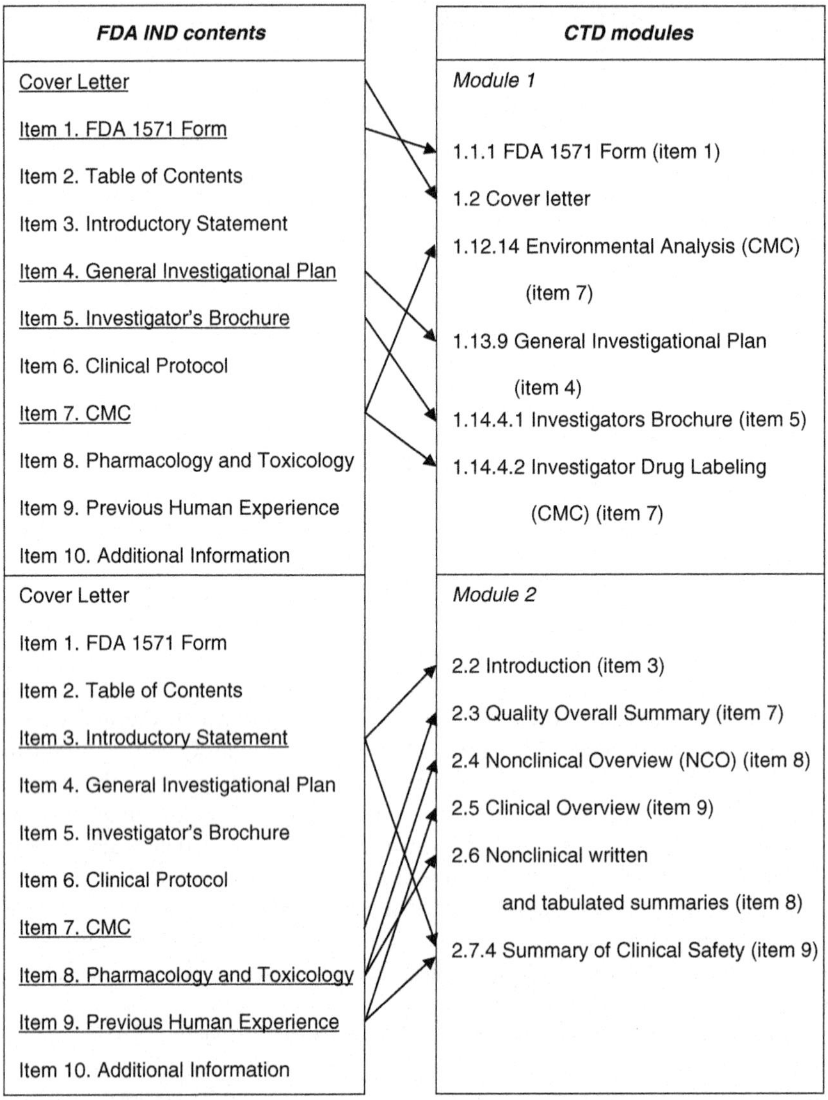

FIGURE 14.2 FDA IND content mapped to ICH CTD modules.

meetings are not required, but can be requested by the sponsor to obtain guidance from the FDA on an investigational drug development program prior to submitting an IND. For example, a sponsor might request FDA input on a nonclinical testing strategy for a novel mechanism or chemical construct or input into the sponsor's plans to monitor for specific safety concerns in the clinical trial. The particular issue of concern drives the targeted timing of the discussion with the FDA. For input on the design of an untraditional nonclinical package such as

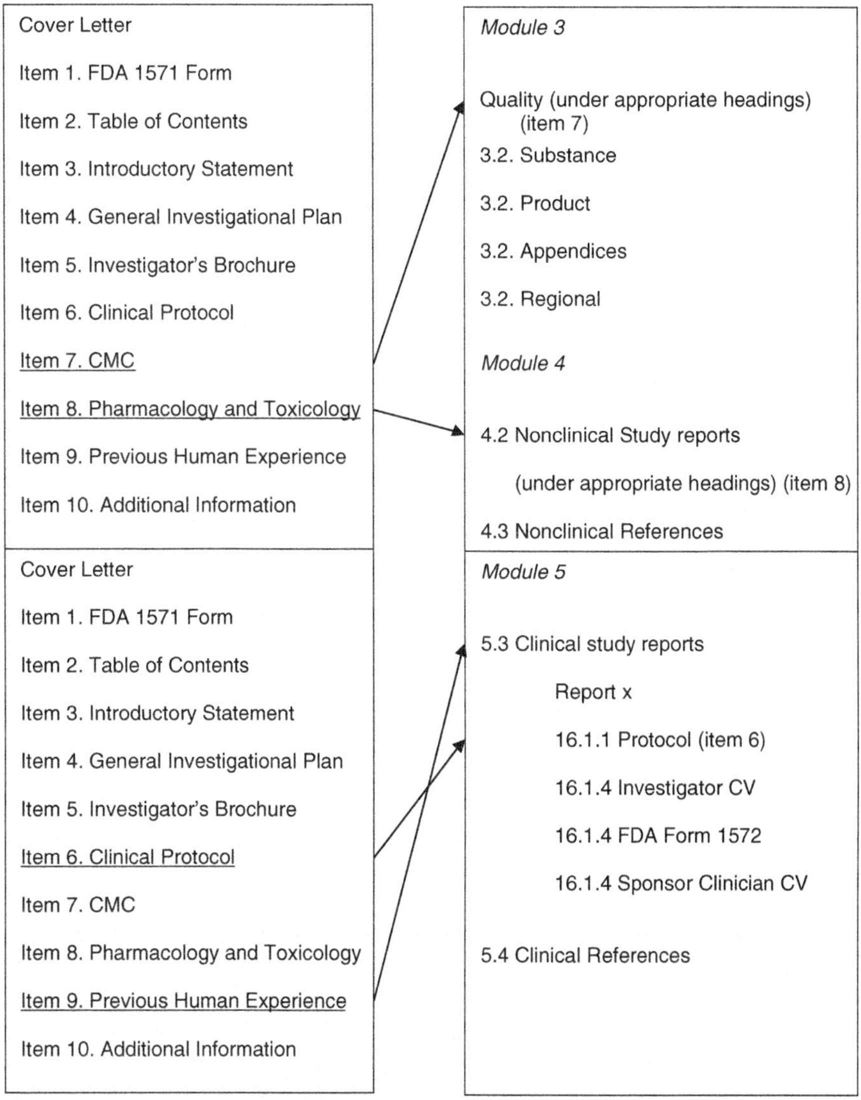

FIGURE 14.2 (*Continued*)

exploratory INDs (Chapter 11), the pre-IND meeting with the FDA should be scheduled prior to execution of the toxicity studies. Alternatively, to obtain input on clinical trial dosing or safety monitoring, it is appropriate for toxicity studies to be complete and for the data to be available. To request a pre-IND meeting, the sponsor submits a meeting request to the reviewing division to which the IND is to be submitted. Upon receiving the request, the reviewing division has 14 days to respond. The reviewing division is not under any obligation to grant a

TABLE 14.8 Types of FDA Meetings with Sponsors

Meeting Designation	Meeting Purpose	Time Lines
Type A: "Stalled" development program	Dispute resolution Resolve FDA-imposed "clinical hold" Address questions on special protocol assessment	Responds to meeting request within 14 days Schedules meeting within 30 days Briefing book due 2 weeks in advance
Type B: "Milestone" meetings	Pre-IND (21 CFR 312.82) Certain end of phase I (21 CFR 312.82) End of phase II/pre-phase III meetings (21 CFR 312.47) Pre-NDA/BLA meetings (21 CFR 312.47)	Responds to meeting request within 21 days Schedules meeting within 60 days Briefing book due 4 weeks in advance
Type C: All other meetings during development	General guidance	Responds to meeting request within 21 days Schedules meeting within 75 days Briefing book 2 to 4 weeks due in advance

meeting. If a meeting is granted, the reviewing division responds to the sponsor with a proposed meeting date. The FDA can propose a teleconference instead of a face-to-face meeting.

Upon receipt of an IND, the reviewing division assigned designates an internal review team. This team consists of clinical, pharmacology/toxicology, and chemistry reviewers and a project manager. By regulation, the FDA must complete their review of an original IND within 30 calendar days of receipt of the application. In the United States, as a default, an IND goes into effect and clinical trials can begin when the 30-day review period elapses, if no objections have been cited by the reviewing division. In practice, it is rare that a 30-day review period concludes without communication from the FDA to the sponsor. In most cases, reviewing divisions assign an internal meeting date during the last week of the review to discuss their conclusions with the full FDA team. Shortly following this meeting (and before the end of day 30) the FDA usually contacts the sponsor either (1) to notify them that it is acceptable to proceed with the trial, (2) to request modifications to the trial or to request additional data, or (3) to place the study on *clinical hold* (either partial or full). A clinical hold delays or suspends part or all of a proposed study, and/or future clinical studies, until the issues cited are resolved. Even if the FDA allows the FIH trial to begin, they can impose a clinical hold at any time during development.

14.4.2 Chemistry, Manufacturing, and Controls

The CMC section of the IND describes the chemical properties, manufacturing materials and process, and characteristics of the drug substance and drug product. The term CMC is the U.S. terminology for this section and is synonymous with the term *quality* in international use. Guidance for the CMC section content and organization is provided in ICH M4Q, which includes a brief overview and more detailed content in Modules 2 and 3, respectively (Table 14.3). The two major subjects of the CMC section are drug substance and drug product. *Drug substance* is the investigational drug, that is, the active pharmaceutical ingredient (API). *Drug product* is the formulation of the drug substance in the form that it is to be dosed to human subjects. Since many of the subsection headers are the same for both drug substance and drug product, the CTD avoids the potential for confusion between the sections with numerical headings that contain the letter S or P according to whether the section pertains to drug substance or drug product (Table 14.9).

For an FIH dossier, because of the relatively limited data available at this early stage of development, many sections contain appropriately little or no data. Sections with no data can be included with a note of explanation.

The data presented in the various sections are related, in that different aspects of the same constituents are evaluated. The presentation and order of the data need to be consistent across the sections. The sponsor should be familiar with the industry's use of CMC terms and apply them consistently throughout the dossier.

Reference to sources may help simplify the presentation of some sections. Each of the three regions—the United States, the EU, and Japan—has published a pharmacopeia (Table 14.7). Pharmacopeias are compendia of accepted standards for drug substance, dosage forms, excipients, reagents, packaging, and medical devices. The monographs in a pharmacopeia summarize the information on each product, including the identity of the material, labeling and storage, and specifications. The specifications, consisting of a series of tests, test methods, and acceptance criteria and descriptions of general methodology for chemical and physical tests, are provided. Critical characteristics define the reference standard for a particular substance.

When these materials or tests are used, the appropriate monograph or compendial standard can be referenced. These references support the appropriateness of the analytical tests and materials, such as process materials, excipients, and packaging. Citing the pharmacopeia simplifies the presentation and the review by the regulators, because the standards are familiar and accepted and the reference replaces otherwise long descriptions of testing methods.

Specific guidance from the FDA, "Guidance for Industry: IND Meetings for Human Drugs and Biologics Chemistry, Manufacturing, and Controls Information" (May 2001), provides a perspective on the preparations for IND meetings specific to the CMC. If the sponsor requests a pre-IND meeting, the questions, if any, regarding the CMC section should be clearly articulated and should pertain to the planned clinical trials. The narrative sections below and in Table 14.10 provide

TABLE 14.9 Headers for Content of CMC Section in CTD Format

Heading	Subheadings
Introduction	
S. Drug Substance	
S.1 General Information[a]	S.1.1 Nomenclature S.1.2 Structure S.1.3 General Properties
S.2 Manufacture[a]	S.2.1 Manufacturer(s) S.2.2 Description of Manufacturing Process and Process Controls S.2.3 Control of Materials S.2.4 Control of Critical Steps and Intermediates S.2.5 Process Validation and/or Evaluation S.2.6 Manufacturing Process Development
S.3 Characterization[a]	S.3.1 Elucidation of Structure and Other Characteristics S.3.2 Impurities
S.4 Control of the Drug Substance[a]	S.4.1 Specification(s) S.4.2 Analytical Procedures S.4.3 Validation of Analytical Procedures S.4.4 Batch Analyses S.4.5 Justification of Specification(s)
S.5 Reference Standards or Materials[a]	
S.6 Container Closure System[a]	
S.7 Stability[a]	
P. Drug Product	
P.1 Description and Composition[a]	
P.2 Pharmaceutical Development[a]	P.2.3 Manufacturing Process Development
P.3 Manufacture	P.3.1 Manufacturer(s)[a] P.3.2 Batch Formula[a] P.3.3 Description of Manufacturing Process and Process Controls[a] P.3.4 Controls of Critical Steps and Intermediates P.3.5 Process Validation and/or Evaluation
P.4 Control of Excipients	P.4.1 Specifications[a] P.4.2 Analytical Procedures[a] P.4.3 Validation of Analytical Procedures P.4.4 Justification of Specifications P.4.5 Excipients of Animal or Human Origin[a] P.4.6 Novel Excipients[a]
P.5 Control of the Drug Product or Investigational Medinicinal Product[a]	P.5.1 Specifications P.5.2 Analytical Procedures P.5.3 Validation of Analytical Procedures

TABLE 14.9 ***(Continued)***

Heading	Subheadings
	P.5.4 Batch Analyses P.5.5 Characterization of Impurities P.5.6 Justification of Specification(s)
P.6 Reference Standards or Materials[a]	
P.7 Container Closure System[a]	
P.8 Stability[a]	

[a]Applies to FIH submissions.

guidance on how to write the CMC section. Although the CMC section is not presented in the tabular format in the submission dossier, Table 14.10 is arranged in tabular format to highlight the relationships of the drug substance and drug product sections.

Introduction to the CMC Section The introduction to the CMC section provides an overview and context for the CMC information. The drug substance and formulation are presented briefly, and major conclusions about the suitability of the investigational drug product for use in humans are given. The introduction may be located in the CMC section of the IND format (Table 14.6) or in Section 2.3, Quality Overall Summary, as indicated for the CTD organization (Table 14.3). Table 14.9 contains the order of the CMC section contents.

Drug Substance and Drug Product The drug substance section presents the structure and characteristics, manufacturing process and process controls, the analytical and validation tests and results, stability, and drug process development. These sections are completed in the order and with the content indicated in Table 14.10. The manufacturing materials and drug substance and drug product constituents are identified, characterized, quantified, and assigned specifications. To facilitate regulatory review, the materials should be listed in a consistent order across all sections. Appropriate cross-references to related data in other sections should be included. The focus should be on those aspects important to the safety of the investigational drug (i.e., structure, quality, stability, and performance of the drug substance and product). The data are limited at this early stage of development, so many sections are quite short.

Other CMC Documentation In addition to the drug substance and drug product sections as outlined in Table 14.10, the FDA requires a request for categorical exclusion from environmental assessment and information on the label that is going to be used on the immediate package of the clinical trial drug supplies. These components can be included as appendixes at the end of the CMC section or in the administrative part of the submission.

TABLE 14.10 Comparison of Listings and Content of Drug Substance and Drug Product in the CMC Sections

Drug Substance	Drug Product
S.1 General Information	*P.1 Description and Composition*
S.1.2 Nomenclature Drug substance generic, chemical, and laboratory names *S.1.2 Structure* Structural formula with designations of stereochemistry, molecular formula, molecular mass by IUPAC convention for atomic weight; refer to S.3.1 as appropriate Chemical structure diagram with stereochemistry, chiral centers, hydrates *S.1.3 General Properties* Description of physicochemical characteristics relevant to activity, solubility, such as pK_a, polymorphism, isomerism, log P, permeability, crystallinity, moisture sorption	Composition of drug product dosage forms List of all components used in the manufacture, whether or not they appear in the final drug product (e.g., water, nitrogen), with component name, function, unit formula, and compendial standard,[a] if applicable List of acronyms and definitions
	P.2 Pharmaceutical Development Description of the methods preformed to develop the formulation of the drug product Description of the appropriate and compatible solvents, diluents, and admixtures
S.2 Manufacture	*P.3 Manufacture*
S.2.1 Manufacturer(s) List of manufacturer(s) of drug substance with addresses For EU, indicate function performed by each site	*P.3.1 Manufacturer(s)* List of manufacturers of drug product (manufacture, testing, release, and labeling) and addresses For EU, indicate function performed by each site and include the site of the QP release
S.2.2. Description of Manufacturing Process and Process Controls Brief narrative description and flow diagram of manufacturing process and process controls for clinical batch, with starting materials, intermediates, solvents, reagents (see also S.2.3)	*P.3.2. Batch Formula* Formula for the batch to be used in the clinical trial List of all components of the dosage form, amounts per batch, and quality standard

TABLE 14.10 (*Continued*)

Drug Substance	Drug Product
Reference to S.2.6 for alternative description of nonclinical batches, if different Details on critical steps,[b] if known For EU, specify production scale or range of batch size	Reference to the quality standard, if possible a major pharmacopeia, for the United States, EU, or Japan[a] Batch size range, if appropriate
S.2.3 Control of Materials List of all materials, including raw materials, reagents, solvents, catalysts Description of analytical procedures for control of starting raw and process materials; details of tests are not expected at this stage of development Emphasis on key raw materials and intermediates contributing to structure of the drug substance Chromatographic procedures accepted at FIH For EU, list of items of human or animal origin and reference and provide more information in Appendix 1	*P.3.3 Description of Manufacturing Process and Process Controls* Process flow diagram with an explanatory narrative, to include materials, equipment, important process aspects, and process controls
S.2.4 Control of Critical Steps and Intermediates Description of critical synthetic steps and intermediates, if known For EU, tests and acceptance criteria also	*P.3.4 Controls of Critical Steps and Intermediates* No information for FIH, except for process for sterile drug product and nonstandard manufacturing processes[c] for the EU
S.2.5 Process Validation and/or Evaluation Statement that drug substance is not intended to be sterile or description of process to ensure sterility For EU, process validation and/or evaluation to be conducted at a later stage	*P.3.5 Process Validation and Evaluation* No information for FIH
S.2.6 Manufacturing Process Development Brief description of synthetic route of nonclinical batches, if different from clinical batch described in S.2.2	

(*Continued overleaf*)

TABLE 14.10 (*Continued*)

Drug Substance	Drug Product
S.3 Characterization	
S.3.1 Elucidation of Structure and Other Characteristics Spectroscopic or other study data that established the structure and physicochemical characteristics Discussion of proof of structure, configuration, and conformation of molecule Spectra and associated interpretations, polymorphisms, and stereoisomerism	
S.3.2 Impurities List of all known impurities, including organic and inorganic process impurities, residual solvents, intermediates, by-products, ligands, catalysts, inactive enantiomers, and degradation products Structures of impurities, if known Evaluation of impurities relative to the impurity levels in batches qualified by use in nonclinical toxicology studies Recognition of structural alerts for toxicity, especially genotoxicity	
	P.4 Control of Excipients
	P.4.1 Specifications List of specifications for excipients with tests and limits Compendial and/or DMF[d] references, as available
	P.4.2 Analytical Procedures Statement of tests that are compendial Name and brief description of noncompendial tests
	P.4.3 Validation of the Analytical Procedures No information for FIH
	P.4.4 Justification of Specifications No information for FIH
	P.4.5 Excipients of Animal or Human Origin

TABLE 14.10 (*Continued*)

Drug Substance	Drug Product
	Reference of DMFs For EU, reference Appendix 2 and certificates of suitability
	P.4.6 Novel Excipients Manufacturing process, characterization, stability, and control information for novel excipients Evaluation of safety, based on literature or studies done to evaluate the excipient Appendix for detailed information For EU, detail in Appendix A.3
S.4 Control of Drug Substance	*P.5 Control of the Drug Product*
S.4.1 Specifications Description of acceptable limits for appearance, identity, strength, purity, quality, chiral identity, counter ion identity, and impurities Analytical test methods regarding identity, strength, quality, and purity Analytical test limit of quantitation List of upper limits of impurities considering the impurity levels present in the toxicology studies Discussion of special considerations for the levels of impurities with structural alerts relative to recommended limits	*P.5.1 Specifications* Specifications, including test methods and acceptance criteria covering both release and shelf life of the drug product Upper limits for individual and total degradation products Limits for each impurity in the batches of drug substance and/or drug product used in the nonclinical studies For EU, specifications for both release and shelf life; specified accordingly
S.4.2 Analytical Procedures Description in general terms of the analytical methods for all tests to determine the specifications List of methods in the same order as the specifications listed in preceding section Reference to compendial tests, if used	*P.5.2 Analytical Procedures* Description in general terms of the analytical methods for all tests to determine the specifications Reference to compendia
S.4.3 Validation of Analytical Procedures Validation procedures for the analytical methods and description of the suitability of the analytical methods for the various endpoints For EU, parameters for performing validation of the analytical procedures and the acceptance limits in a tabulated form	*P.5.3 Validation of Analytical Procedures* Validation procedures for the analytical methods and description of the suitability of the analytical methods for the endpoints. For EU, parameters for performing validation of the analytical procedures and the acceptance limits in a tabulated form

(*Continued overleaf*)

TABLE 14.10 ***(Continued)***

Drug Substance	Drug Product
S.4.4 Batch Analysis Analysis data of the batches used in both the nonclinical and clinical studies, unless the batches are the same Analysis of representative batches, if the clinical batch analysis is not available Data organized in the same order as in other sections: S.4.1, S.4.2, S.4.3, and comparable section for drug product List of batch number, batch size, batch usage, manufacturing site, manufacturing date, control methods, acceptance criteria, and test results	*P.5.4 Batch Analysis* Results or certificates of analysis for the clinical batch of drug product or representative batches, if clinical batch analysis is not available List of batch number, batch size, batch usage, manufacturing site, manufacturing date, control methods, acceptance criteria, and test results
	P.5.5 Characterization of Impurities Cross-referenced to S.3.2, if drug product impurities are the same as drug substance impurities Brief text summary of the critical impurities specific to the formulation, if any
S.4.5 Justification of Specification(s) Brief justification of the specifications and acceptance criteria of impurities and other aspects of the drug substance considering the nonclinical data and analytical methods Cross-referenced to S.3.2, if appropriate	*P.5.6 Justification of Specification(s)* Brief justification of the specifications and acceptance criteria for degradation products and aspects relevant to the performance of the drug product
S.5 Reference Standards or Materials Key characteristics that establish the reference standard of the drug substance Description of additional processes, if used, for the preparation of the reference or current working standard Cross-referenced to S.3.1 for additional information	*P.6 Reference Standards or Materials* Cross-referenced to S.5, where appropriate Clarification of the reference standard, if the drug product standards differ from the drug substance Description of additional processes, if used, for the working reference and materials used for testing drug product
S.6 Container Closure System Description of all container closure systems for packaging for drug substance	*P.7 Container Closure System* Description of all container closure systems of packaging for drug product Identification of the materials of each primary packaging component

TABLE 14.10 ***(Continued)***

Drug Substance	Drug Product
Identification of materials of each primary packaging component Identification of secondary or outer packaging included, if relevant to drug substance quality	Identification of secondary or outer packaging, if relevant to drug product safety Reference to compendia, as appropriate Descriptions and specifications for nonstandard administration devices or noncompendial materials used Additional details for situations with interaction potential between the drug product and container closure system (e.g., parenterals, ophthalmics, oral solutions) Description of packaging for "blinding," if appropriate
S.7 Stability Brief description of the stability studies and test methods used to evaluate the stability of the drug substance Data summarized in tables Representative batch analysis, if the data for the clinical batch not available Aspects critical to stability, such as chemical and physical sensitivity (e.g., light or moisture)	*P.8 Stability* Description of stability studies and test methods used to evaluate the stability of the drug product Data on the clinical batch, if available, or representative batches If the latter, data on stability under conditions of accelerated and long-term storage and proposal that stability studies for the clinical batch be conducted in parallel with the clinical trials and tested at regular intervals For those drug products intended for multiple uses after reconstitution, data for stability under these conditions and proposed conclusion for appropriate handling and storage conditions For EU, proposed shelf life of the drug product; data from development studies supporting stability presented in tabular format
	Appendixes Detailed information on the specific topics if applicable
	A.1 Not Applicable
	A.2 Adventitious Agents Safety Evaluation

(*Continued overleaf*)

TABLE 14.10 ***(Continued)***

Drug Substance	Drug Product
	A.3 Novel Excipients *A.4 Solvents for Reconstitution and Diluents* For United States (regional) R.1 Labeling R.2 Environmental assessment, claim for a categorical exclusion R.3 DMF letter of authorization (if relevant)

[a]Compendial substance and methods: compendial status refers to inclusion in major pharmacopeia, reference databases of constituents, and procedures that support similar or related purposes (see Table 14.7).
[b]Critical step: ICH Q7A definition as "process step, condition, test requirement or other relevant parameter or item that must be controlled within predetermined criteria to ensure that the API meets its specification."
[c]Nonstandard manufacturing processes: for definition of these processes, see note for "Guidance on Process Validation, Non Standard Processes," CPMP/QWP/2054/03.
[d]DMF: drug master file, a dossier containing chemistry and safety information on a chemical entity appropriate for U.S. submissions; see www.fda.gov/cder/dmf.

Clinical Supply Label A preliminary representation of the proposed package label for an investigational drug for the planned clinical trial is submitted. This is not to be confused with the package insert or other labeling for approved or marketed drugs. In the United States investigational labels must carry a precautionary statement: "Caution: New Drug—Limited by Federal (or United States) Law to Investigational Use (Title 21 CFR Part 312.06)".

Environmental Assessment Certification By law, the FDA is also required to assess the impact of drugs on the quality of the human environment. Therefore, all INDs include an environmental assessment or a claim for categorical exclusion from an environmental assessment. Investigational drugs at IND usually qualify for a categorical exclusion. A request for categorical exclusion from environmental assessment must state that the IND submission meets the exclusion requirements and that to the applicant's knowledge, no extraordinary circumstances exist (Title 21 CFR Part 25). For more information on environmental assessments, see "Guidance for Industry for the Submission of Environmental Assessments for Human Drug Applications and Supplements" (November 1995).

14.4.3 Nonclinical Sections

The FDA's guidance on IND nonclinical content specifies an integrated summary, written summaries of the pharmacology, pharmacokinetics and ADME

TABLE 14.11 Headings for Nonclinical Overview

1. Overview of nonclinical testing strategy
2. Pharmacology
3. Pharmacokinetics
4. Toxicology
5. Integrated overview and conclusions
6. List of literature references

data, and complete data listings for all of the toxicity studies. These expectations are satisfied by following the specific FDA guidance "Content and Format of Investigational New Drug Applications for Phase I Studies of Drugs Including Well-Characterized, Therapeutic, Biotechnology-Derived Products" (November 1995) or by including the corresponding sections of the CTD. The FDA-specified integrated summary is analogous to the Nonclinical Overview, Section 2.4 of the CTD (Table 14.11), in that it specifies brief descriptions of the studies, a systematic review of the findings, and an evaluation of the relevance of the findings for humans. The summaries of the pharmacology and ADME data can be satisfied by the written and tabular summaries described in Module 2.6.2/3 and 2.6.4/5 of the CTD. The draft or final toxicity study reports meet the requirements for complete data listings and can be organized according to the order for reports in Module 4 of the CTD.

The data and assessments in these sections provide the basis of safety and efficacy for human clinical trials. The FDA evaluates the information relative to the proposed indications and population in the initial clinical trials. FIH trials are usually designed to evaluate the safety, tolerability, and pharmacokinetics at single, and/or multiple, escalating doses. Therefore, the nonclinical package submitted needs to provide data that are sufficiently compelling to support the risk of exposing humans to the doses of the drug proposed.

Nonclinical data appear in other clinical and administrative documents of the submission, including the IB, the clinical protocol, and the general investigational plan. In general, the information for these documents can be excerpted from the nonclinical overview. Using the nonclinical overview as the source document for the other dossier components saves time and effort and avoids the possibility of conflicting presentations or interpretations of nonclinical information across the FIH dossier that can occur if the sections are written independently.

To ensure that the appropriate studies have been conducted, a careful review of ICH M3, "Nonclinical Safety Studies for the Conduct of Human Clinical Trials for Pharmaceuticals," is recommended (Table 14.2). This guideline outlines in general terms those nonclinical studies needed to support clinical trials, including FIH trials. A revised version was issued in 2009. The combined purpose of these studies remains the same: to characterize the toxicity and target organs, to provide the foundation for safe initial dose selection in humans, and to identify relevant safety endpoints to monitor for the detection of adverse effects in humans. For

TABLE 14.12 Order of Nonclinical Studies for CTD Module 4

- 4.1 Table of contents
- 4.2 Study reports
  - 4.2.1 Pharmacology
    - 4.2.1.1 Primary pharmacodynamics
    - 4.2.1.2 Secondary pharmacodynamics
    - 4.2.1.3 Safety pharmacology
    - 4.2.1.4 Pharmacodynamic drug interactions
  - 4.2.2 Pharmacokinetics
    - 4.2.2.1 Analytical methods and validation reports
    - 4.2.2.2 Absorption
    - 4.2.2.3 Distribution
    - 4.2.2.4 Metabolism
    - 4.2.2.5 Excretion
    - 4.2.2.6 Pharmacodynamic drug interactions (nonclinical)
  - 4.2.3 Toxicology (in order of route, species, and duration according to ICH M4S)
    - 4.2.3.1 Single dose toxicity
    - 4.2.3.2 Repeat dose toxicity
    - 4.2.3.3 Genotoxicity
      - 4.2.3.3.1 In vitro
      - 4.2.3.3.2 In vivo
    - 4.2.3.4 Carcinogenicity
    - 4.2.3.5 Reproductive
    - 4.2.3.6 Local tolerance
    - 4.2.3.7 Other toxicity studies
- 4.3 Literature references

an FIH, the guideline recommends the conduct of safety pharmacology, general toxicity studies in two species (one rodent and one nonrodent), and evaluation of in vitro bacterial reverse mutation and chromosomal injury. For a traditional IND, the duration of the repeat-dose studies is to be at least 14 days of dosing or the length of dosing proposed for the clinical phase 1 studies, whichever is longer. Exploratory INDs, as explained in Chapter 11, are also detailed. Drug exposure data in the nonclinical animal studies and basic information on ADME data should be included. The usual expectation is that these studies evaluate doses and systemic or local drug concentrations that produce toxicity, demonstrate a dose response, and identify a low dose or exposure at which no adverse effects were observed. These data contribute to the basis of the starting dose and the range to be explored in the initial clinical trials.

Nonclinical Overview In general, the guidance supplied for the CTD nonclinical overview is appropriate to meet the expectations of the FIH for the integrated summary of the nonclinical safety described in the FDA IND guidance. The relevant contents of this document are described below.

Overview of the Nonclinical Testing Strategy In the introduction section of the nonclinical overview, a short rationale of the pharmacology, ADME (absorption, distribution, metabolism, and excretion), and toxicology program is described, including the basis for the selected design and duration of studies, species selected, and route and frequency of dosing relative to the initial trials and use in humans. Providing a list of the studies conducted and indicating the relationship among studies is helpful to orient the regulators. For example, it is useful to clarify which studies were conducted as standard studies as expected for the program based on regulatory guidances and which studies were conducted to further characterize or investigate findings in prior studies. The order of the topics should be organized as prescribed in the ICH M4S guidance (Tables 14.2 and 14.11).

Pharmacology The pharmacology section contains a brief summary of the in vitro and in vivo studies that demonstrate selectivity, specificity, and efficacy of the investigational drug for the intended target. The models and methods used will vary depending on the therapeutic indication and type of molecule. Data should be included on the specific interactions of the target molecule and affected physiology, such as measures of affinity, residence time, type of pathway affected and functional cascade, and evidence of the absence of activity in other off-target biological systems. These studies provide information on the primary pharmacology. Secondary (unintended) and safety pharmacology evaluations (Chapter 6) are also usually required. Secondary pharmacologic effects occur due to activity at an unintended molecular target or due to intended molecular action on an off-target organ or pathway. Safety pharmacology studies are conducted as standard studies that evaluate aspects of primary and secondary pharmacologic properties. The studies generally required are neurobehavioral studies and pulmonary function in rodents, cardiovascular evaluations in nonrodents, and in vitro studies to evaluate ion channel effects, such as hERG.

Pharmacokinetics and Metabolism The pharmacokinetics and metabolism section summarizes the ADME data accumulated. At this early stage of development, most of the definitive work to determine ADME endpoints has not been conducted. For the FIH submission, the data expected consist of the systemic exposure data of the pharmacology and general toxicity studies and in vitro metabolism data from microsome and/or hepatocytes from animal and human liver (Chapter 2). The pharmacokinetic and toxicokinetic data, such as C_{max}, t_{max}, AUC (the area under the plasma–serum concentration–time curve), and possibly $t_{1/2}$, are best summarized in tables. Graphs can be used to present dose–exposure relationships or relationships of exposures over time. The data available on routes of metabolism, metabolites, and activity of metabolites should be presented in diagrams or tables. Usually, no data have been generated on elimination.

In addition, regulators may expect to see protein-binding data across species and calculations of the unbound fraction in the systemic circulation if the efficacy or toxicity is thought to be driven by unbound drug levels. If indicated by the data, sponsors can also include information on hepatic enzyme induction as a result of repeated exposure to the investigational drug and an assessment of the potential for drug–drug interactions.

In summary, the pharmacokinetic, toxicokinetic, and metabolic profile of the investigational drug should be described, noting key features, such as pharmacokinetic characteristics across species and between genders, potential for interactions with other drugs, and relationship of the characteristics to the targeted characteristics for humans. Aspects such as species differences in potency, protein binding, half-life, and dosing regimen, which are considerations for the relevance of the effects and the safety margins for human pharmacokinetics and dynamics should be included if available.

Toxicology Information In this section of the nonclinical overview, the toxicity studies are summarized briefly. The studies are discussed according to study type and species in the order specified in the CTD M4S guidance (Table 14.2). Information is provided on species, strain, doses, route, duration, and major endpoints. The findings of significance should be highlighted and sufficient detail provided for the regulatory reviewer to get a clear picture of the toxicity profile and understand the relationships of the findings. The toxicology program for an FIH submission will usually include GLP multiple-dose studies in two species and genetic toxicology studies (Chapter 7). Single-dose or non-GLP dose-range-finding studies are usually conducted to provide dose-setting information for the GLP multiple-dose studies. Because higher doses are often used in the range-finding studies than in the definitive GLP studies, the information from these studies is often included to support the dose selection of the GLP studies and to provide additional perspective on the safety of the new drug candidate.

Integrated Summary and Conclusions The integrated summary of the nonclinical overview incorporates the nonclinical findings across all of the studies and species, identifies and addresses apparent conflicts in data points, provides an assessment of relevance and potential risk of the nonclinical findings for humans, and finally, affords a conclusion as to the suitability of the investigational drug for the clinical trial. The presentation should be clear, concise, and based on the data. The presentation should not be promotional; regulators expect an open and objective assessment of the data.

Related findings across systems and species should be identified and a comprehensive system-by-system evaluation provided. For example, findings in the cardiovascular system can be seen in the safety pharmacology or general toxicology cardiovascular evaluations, clinical signs, and gross and histopathological evaluations. The findings should be integrated across the studies and the relationships among them described, including their relationship to the dose and the pharmacokinetic or toxicokinetic measures. The dose–response curve, that is, the progression of the effects as related to dose, should be presented and comparisons made among the species studied. Tables or graphs comparing the systemic drug exposures of key pharmacologic and toxicologic findings with the projected exposure for humans at the efficacious dose expected or at the maximum dose to be studied is useful to regulators in assessing projected safety margins.

Observations should be made as to initial effects, progression of effects with continued dosing, and regression of effects when dosing is discontinued or lowered, if that information is available. An evaluation should be provided of the relevance of the findings and risks posed for humans based on anatomic and physiologic comparisons and expected differences and similarities in doses and exposure. The impurity profile of nonclinical drug batches should be compared to the batch intended for clinical use and the safety of the clinical batch justified. This justification is more straightforward when the nonclinical batch is the same as that intended for use in the clinic.

Finally, based on the analysis of the integrated summary, a conclusion is drawn as to the suitability of the investigational drug for the use intended in the FIH trial.

Pharmacology and ADME Summary As stated in the FDA guidance "Content and Format of Investigational New Drug Applications for Phase 1 Studies of Drugs" (November 1995), summaries of the pharmacology and ADME studies are required. The requirement can be met by following the specifics of this guidance or those of ICH M4S. The FDA guidance says that the section should include "(1) the description of the pharmacologic effects and mechanism(s) of actions of the drug in animals, and (2) information on the absorption, distribution, metabolism, and excretion of the drug. . . . A summary report, without individual animal records or individual study results, usually suffices. In most circumstances, five pages or less should suffice for this summary." ICH M4S detailed written and tabular summaries are both accepted by the FDA. Study results are often represented more succinctly in tabular format, and as mentioned in Section 14.5.3, tabular format is preferred by EU regulators, so particularly if submissions are contemplated for the EU, the CTD written and tabular formats are recommended (Table 14.2). The order of the topics in the summaries should be consistent with the order in which the studies are discussed in the NCO or integrated summary.

Toxicology Full Data Tabulation Complete data listings for toxicology studies are expected in an IND dossier and are best included in the form of complete draft or final study reports. Separate summaries for the toxicity studies, as for the pharmacology and ADME program, are not required, as the NCO or integrated summary and study reports provide all the information needed. Although the reviewers will examine the data themselves and draw their own conclusions, the study report narrative aids the reviewer in understanding the sponsor's view of how the study supports the clinical trial. The reports also supply details of the methods, which provide insight into the standards and rigor of the study conduct. The reports are best organized in the order in which they are discussed and presented elsewhere in the dossier, such as indicated in ICH M4S (Table 14.12).

14.4.4 Clinical Components

Clinical Protocol The contents of the clinical trial protocol are described in 21 CFR Part 312.23(a)(6) and include the following:

- Objectives of the study
- Subject selection criteria
- Number of subjects
- Study design (e.g., double-blind or open, parallel or crossover, placebo-controlled, inclusion of active control)
- Doses (including maximum dose), duration of dosing
- Parameters to be evaluated to meet the objectives of the study
- Safety assessments (e.g., laboratory tests, electrocardiographs)

A synopsis of the protocol including a table of the schedule of events greatly assists both clinical investigators at the site conducting the FIH trial and the regulators at the FDA in assessing the conditions of the clinical trial. Information on the background of the investigational drug being tested, adverse event reporting, data analyses, and data handling are also included. The background information on the investigational drug is only a high-level overview of the pertinent information with a cross-reference to the IB for all other information. If the sponsor conducts trials repeatedly through a particular clinical trials site, a standard protocol format can facilitate review of the proposed trial by the investigator and the IRB, because the study details are presented in a consistent, predictable manner. Such a standard protocol format is also more likely to ensure that the protocol is completed appropriately by the responsible sponsor staff and includes all of the expectations for the trial. This streamlining ultimately reduces overall time lines.

Investigator's Brochure

Overview The overall purpose of an IB is to serve as a summary of the safety of a product in the context of the clinical trial and to facilitate investigators' understanding of a new drug candidate. The IB is a clinical investigator's primary source of information about a drug and must be available prior to the initiation of clinical studies. In general, the IB contains information on the chemistry and physical properties of the compound, nonclinical pharmacology, general pharmacology, nonclinical pharmacokinetics and metabolism, toxicology, and potential risks associated with the investigational drug's use. It provides a rationale for the clinical dose, route of administration, and safety monitoring procedures, as well as potential risks associated with use of the investigational drug. For an FIH study, the IB will contain only nonclinical data because clinical studies have not been conducted. For subsequent clinical trials, the IB is updated with the additional perspective provided by the completed clinical trials.

The IB is provided to regulators, investigators, and others involved in a clinical trial so that they can make an objective risk/benefit ratio assessment of the drug. Although those involved in the clinical trial are considered the primary users of the IB, the regulators also have the following objectives in reviewing an IB: (1) to assure the safety and rights of subjects through full disclosure of all pertinent data, and (2) to evaluate whether the quality of the scientific evaluation of the investigational drug is adequate to conduct clinical trials safely. In addition, the IRB, charged to safeguard the rights, safety, and well-being of trial subjects, uses the IB, in conjunction with the clinical protocol, to identify the risks associated with the drug candidate and to ensure that steps will be taken to monitor the safety of the clinical trial subjects.

The guidance for the IB is specified in ICH E6, "Good Clinical Practice: Consolidated Guideline," which states: "The information should be presented in a concise, simple, objective, balanced, and nonpromotional form that enables a clinician, or potential investigator to understand it and make an unbiased risk–benefit assessment of the appropriateness of the proposed trial." In reviewing the guideline, one should notice that the contents and organization are similar to and parallel those of the CTD. Table 14.13 contains the table of contents for the IB.

When compiling the FIH IB for an investigational drug, the sponsor may choose to include a confidentiality statement instructing the investigator to treat the IB as a confidential document. This step helps limit access of other scientists and companies to this information and protects the sponsor's intellectual property.

Section 2: Summary The purpose of the summary section of the IB is to provide an overview of the significant results of nonclinical studies conducted with the investigational drug. Paragraphs describe the pharmacologic results of the animal models that were studied, doses where the drug was found to be active, and any relevant safety pharmacology findings. The summary of pharmacokinetic results in animals may include metabolic pathways, major and/or active metabolites, potential for drug–drug interactions, bioavailability, and in vitro metabolism and enzyme induction or inhibition studies. The toxicology summary is a high-level description of the significant toxicology results, which identifies the relevant effects, doses, and exposures, including those at which there were no significant findings. This section provides the investigator with a summary of the safety information that could be relevant to the clinical subjects in the trial.

Section 3: Introduction The purpose of the introduction to the IB is to orient the clinical investigator to the general approach to be followed in evaluating

TABLE 14.13 Example Table of Contents of Investigator's Brochure

Confidentiality Statement (optional)
Signature Page (optional)

1. Table of Contents[a]
2. Summary[a]
3. Introduction[a]
4. Physical, Chemical, and Pharmaceutical Properties and Formulation[a]
5. Nonclinical Studies[a]
   5.1 Nonclinical Pharmacology
   5.2 Pharmacokinetics and Product Metabolism in Animals
   5.3 Toxicology
6. Effects in Humans
   6.1 Pharmacokinetics and Product Metabolism in Humans
   6.2 Safety and Efficacy
   6.3 Marketing Experience
7. Summary of Data and Guidance for the Investigator[a]

References should be included at the end of each section for

   Publications
   Reports

Appendixes (if any)

[a] For FIH submissions.

the investigational drug. The introduction includes the pharmacologic class and medical indication for the candidate drug, the current treatment options and shortcomings, anticipated advantages of the drug to be investigated, and a brief description of the clinical plan proposed.

Section 4: Physical, Chemical, and Pharmaceutical Properties and Formulation The purpose of this section of the IB is to give the clinical investigator the information needed to handle and store the drug product appropriately in the course of the trial. Therefore, Section 4 includes a description of the formulation(s) to be used, including excipients, if clinically relevant, the chemical and/or structural formula(s) and salt form, and instructions for storage and handling of the dosage form. This section also describes structural similarities to other known drugs as an aid to the investigator.

Section 5: Nonclinical Studies Section 5 consists of three subsections: Section 5.1, Nonclinical Pharmacology; Section 5.2, Pharmacokinetics and Product Metabolism in Animals; and Section 5.3, Toxicology. The results of all nonclinical studies are provided in summary form in this section. The summary of each study or group of studies includes a description of the methods used, the results of the study, and a brief discussion of the relevance of the results to the clinical subjects. Tabular format of the data is used whenever possible to enhance the clarity of the presentation.

Section 5.1, *Nonclinical Pharmacology*, focuses on studies that assess potential therapeutic activity and safety. The pharmacological aspects of the investigational product and any significant metabolites studied in animals are included. Studies may include efficacy models, receptor binding, specificity results, and the mechanism of action.

Section 5.2, *Pharmacokinetics and Product Metabolism in Animals*, includes a summary of the pharmacokinetics and biological transformation and disposition of the investigational product in the species studied. The discussion addresses the absorption and the local and/or systemic bioavailability of the investigational product and its metabolites, results of in vivo pharmacokinetic studies, plasma protein binding, and in vitro metabolism studies.

Section 5.3, *Toxicology*, includes a summary of the toxicological effects found in relevant studies conducted in rodent and nonrodent species. Quantitative data from general toxicology studies are presented, preferably in tabular format, to enhance clarity. Drug-related changes are discussed. For an FIH submission, these data are usually sufficient, but in the case where additional studies may have been conducted, such as those for local irritation or sensitization, and reproduction and development, the data are also presented here.

Section 6: Effects in Humans This section is not relevant for an FIH IB, as it is a summary of prior clinical experience. If, however, an IND is being submitted for an investigational drug for which foreign clinical studies have been conducted, this is by definition no longer an FIH IB, and clinical results are discussed here.

Section 7: Summary of Data and Guidance for the Investigator Section 7 of the IB integrates the knowledge across all disciplines in order to provide the investigator with an informative interpretation of the data available and with an assessment of the implications of the information for future clinical studies. It includes the class of drug being investigated, potential adverse reactions based on nonclinical findings, specific monitoring planned during clinical trials, any precautions that should be taken, and a statement regarding the risk/benefit assessment.

14.5 EUROPEAN UNION: CLINICAL TRIAL APPLICATION

14.5.1 Regulatory Perspective

Similar to the situation in the United States, the EU requirements provide legislative directives and regulations; additional regulatory interpretations and expectations are articulated in nonbinding guidelines by the EMEA (European Medicines Agency). As in the United States, the EU requires the approval of a medical review board, called an independent ethics committee (IEC), prior to initiation of the clinical trial. The requirements, guidances, and Web sites are given in

Table 14.4. The two guidelines, Eudralex Vol. 10, ENTR/F2/BL D(2003) CT 1, "Detailed Guidance for the Request for Authorisation of a Clinical Trial on a Medicinal Product for Human Use" (October 2005), and Eudralex Vol. 10, ENTR/CT2, "Detailed Guidance on the Application Format and Documentation to be Submitted in an Application for an Ethics Committee Opinion" (February 2006), outline the expectations for the EU dossier and submissions to ethics committees and are consistent with the legislative EU directives.

To initiate human trials in the EU, a clinical trial application (CTA) must be authorized by the regulatory authority in the EU member state in which the trial is to be conducted. Each country is responsible for the authorization of trials conducted within its borders. The authorization applies to that country alone and is not valid in other member states. The European Clinical Trials Database (EudraCT) was established in accordance with European Community Directive 2001/20/EC and provides an interface to apply for authorization of the European member states. Member-specific requirements are covered, such as authorizations by IEC and research oversight bodies.

The content of the EU dossier described in the first guidance includes a request for a clinical trial authorization, a cover letter, completed EudraCT application form, proposed protocol, IB, investigational medicinal product dossier (IMPD), and manufacturing authorization. The requirements for the IMPD, the supporting dossier for a clinical trial application in the EU, are described. The format and information for the IMPD are very similar to, and consistent with, the format described in ICH M4 for the CTD (Tables 14.2 and 14.3), and the expectations and general content are very similar to those for the FDA in the United States. A complete checklist of the CTA contents is provided in Table 14.14.

Additional considerations for preparing a risk assessment and clinical dosing plan are published in "Guideline on Strategies to Identify and Mitigate Risk for FIH Clinical Trials with Investigational Medicinal Products" (CHMP/SWP/28367/07). This guideline, issued in July 2007, has its origins in unexpected safety findings in FIH trials of investigational drugs with human-specific modes of action. The purpose of the guideline is to clarify the considerations in transitioning from nonclinical to clinical development. The concepts presented have been fundamental to assessment of the safety for clinical trials for many years and are nicely integrated in the guidance with additional perspective and considerations. The guideline promotes thoughtful consideration of mode of action, nature of the target and relevance ("predictivity") of the animal species and models, and the potency, purity, and consistency of the drug substance when considering the FIH trials. For instance, examples for special attention are given as "a mode of action that involves a target which is connected to multiple signaling pathways (target with pleiotropic effects), leading to various physiological effects or targets that are ubiquitously expressed, as often seen in the immune system" or "a biological cascade or cytokine release including those leading to an amplification of an effect that might not be sufficiently controlled by a physiologic feedback mechanism (e.g. in the immune system or blood coagulation system)." In addition, concern is expressed over the

TABLE 14.14 Checklist of CTA Contents

1 *General*
  1.1 Receipt of confirmation of EudraCT number
  1.2 Covering letter
  1.3 Application form
  1.4 List of competent authorities within the community to which the application has been submitted and details of decisions
  1.5 Copy of ethics committee opinion in the member state concerned when available
  1.6 Copy/summary of any scientific advice
  1.7 If the applicant is not the sponsor, a letter of authorization enabling the applicant to act on behalf of the sponsor
2 *Subject related*
  2.1 Informed consent form
  2.2 Subject information leaflet
  2.3 Arrangements for recruitment of subjects
3 *Protocol related*
  3.1 Clinical trial protocol with all current amendments
  3.2 Summary of the protocol in the national language
  3.3 Peer review of trial when available
  3.4 Ethical assessment made by the principal/coordinating investigator, if not given in the application form or protocol
4 *IMP related*
  4.1 Investigator's brochure
  4.2 Investigational medicinal product dossier (IMPD)
  4.3 Simplified IMPD for known products
  4.4 Summary of product characteristics (SmPC) (for products with marketing authorization in the community)
  4.5 Outline of all active trials with the same IMP
  4.6 If IMP manufactured in EU and if no marketing authorization in EU
    4.6.1 Copy of the manufacturing authorization referred to in Art. 13.1 of the Directive stating the scope of this authorization
  4.7 If IMP not manufactured in EU and if no marketing authorization in EU
    4.7.1 Certification of the QP that the manufacturing site works in compliance with GMP at least equivalent to EU GMP, or that each production batch has undergone all relevant analyses, tests, or checks necessary to confirm its quality
    4.7.2 Certification of GMP status of active biological substance
    4.7.3 Copy of the importer's manufacturing authorization referred to in Art. 13.1 of the Directive stating the scope of this authorization
  4.8 *Certificate of analysis for test product in exceptional cases*
    4.8.1 Where impurities are not justified by the specification or when unexpected impurities (not covered by specification) are detected
  4.9 *Viral safety studies when applicable*

Source: Adapted from *Eudralex*, Vol. 10, Chap. 1, ENTR/F2/BL D/CT1.

consistency of quality and potency of the drug product. "As an example, where the dose is based on biological activity and is expressed in arbitrary units, and the assays are not qualified and/or validated to ensure their reliability, the doses used in the nonclinical studies may be poorly defined and mislead the interpretation of what is a safe dose." Highly human-specific medicinal products used in animal studies might "not reproduce the intended pharmacological effect in humans, give rise to the misinterpretation of pharmacokinetic and pharmacodynamic results, or (might) not identify relevant toxic effects." In this guideline, rather than basing the starting dose on the no-observed-adverse-effect levels (NOAELs) of the toxicity studies, the starting dose is based on the dose at which a minimal biological effect is projected to occur in humans. This method is called the minimal anticipated biological effect level (MABEL) approach, and considerations for calculations are provided. The use of additional factors to increase the margins between the doses where effects were observed in animals and those proposed in humans, further promotes the safety of the trial for the first subjects. The guidance recommends that "when the methods of calculation (e.g. NOAEL, MABEL) give different estimations of the first dose in man, the lowest value should be used, unless justified." Regarding clinical trial design, several precautions are enumerated, including "administering the first dose so that a single subject receives a single dose of the active IMP" (investigational medicinal product), and caution in dose escalation, particularly for those investigational drugs with "a steep dose–response curve, exposure–response curve, and dose toxicity curves" and "immediate access to equipment and staff for resuscitating and stabilising individuals in an acute emergency (such as cardiac emergencies, anaphylaxis, cytokine release syndrome, convulsions, hypotension)."

14.5.2 Quality

In Europe, details regarding the quality or CMC content are specified in the "Guideline on the Requirements to the Chemical and Pharmaceutical Quality Documentation Concerning Investigational Medicinal Products in Clinical Trials" (CHMP/QWP/185401/2004). This document specifies the additional input required for EU submissions compared with U.S. submissions. Although the guideline differs slightly, the goal of this section is the same as for submissions in the United States and elsewhere: that is, to show that the clinical study can safely be conducted with the drug product proposed.

In addition, the European regulations require the manufacture of the investigational material to comply with the principles of good manufacturing practice (GMP) set out in Directive 2003/94/EC and the guideline on application of the principles set out in Eudralex, Vol. 4, Annex 13, F2/BL D(2003). The considerations for the EU quality dossier are included in Table 14.10. Other documentation necessary for the EU includes GMP certification. If the investigational product is manufactured in the EU, a copy of the manufacturing authorization as described in Eudralex, Vol. 10, Chap. 1, ENTR/F2/BL D (2003) CT1 is included. If the drug product is not manufactured in the EU, the qualified person (QP) should state the compliance of the manufacturing site with GMP at minimum equivalent to EU GMP standards, provide certification of all active biologic substances, and supply a copy of the importer's authorization (Directive 2001/83/EC Articles 48–52). The certificate of analysis is included in cases where specifications were not set, due to insufficient data or new unexpected impurities. Certificates of safety for biologically derived substances should be included: for example, regarding transmissible spongiform encephalopathy and viral content. Examples of the label for the clinical drug supplies in the national language are also required in most EU countries. Information about the country-specific requirements can be found in Attachment 1 to Eudralex, Vol. 10, ENTR/F2/BL D (2003) CT1.

14.5.3 Nonclinical Sections

The content of the FIH submission for the EU is similar to that submitted to the FDA. The guidance in ENTR/F2/BL D (2003) CT1 specifies that "the sponsor should also provide summaries of nonclinical pharmacology and toxicology data for any investigational drug to be used in the clinical trial or justify why they have not. They should also provide a reference list of studies conducted and appropriate literature references. Full data from the studies and copies of the references should be made available on request. Wherever appropriate, it is preferable to present data in tabular form accompanied by the briefest narrative highlighting the main salient points. The summaries of the studies conducted should allow an assessment of the adequacy of the study and whether the study has been conducted according to an acceptable protocol. Sponsors should as far as possible provide the nonclinical information in the IMPD." The EU guideline goes on to say: "This section should provide a critical analysis of the available data, including justification for deviations and omissions from the detailed guidance and an assessment of the safety of the product in the context of the proposed clinical trial rather than a mere factual summary of the studies conducted." The IMPD nonclinical contents are essentially identical to the CTD table of contents, as indicated for FIH in Table 14.3, except that the full toxicology study reports are not submitted. The IB can contain much of the same information as is included in the IMPD. Rather than duplicate the information in the two documents, the IMPD sections can cite the appropriate sections of the IB.

The assessment of the safety specified in the excerpt above for the EU guideline is satisfied by a well-written NCO, as for the U.S. IND. Study summaries can be provided by following the ICH M4S CTD guideline for written and tabular study summaries. A key difference from the U.S. IND is the expressed preference by the EU for data in tabular format. Although no format for the tabular summaries is suggested in the IMPD guideline, the ICH M4S guideline for CTD tabular summaries of Sections 2.6.3, 2.6.5, and 2.6.7 provides format descriptions and examples. As noted in the ICH M4S document, the tabulated summaries do not necessarily contain all of the endpoints in the studies, but contain all of the noteworthy findings. This eliminates the data from many unaffected endpoints and allows the reviewer to study the magnitude of effects across the doses and species more conveniently than in long narrative descriptions and to evaluate the relationships among the findings that might not have been specifically identified by the sponsor.

14.6 JAPAN: CLINICAL TRIAL PROTOCOL NOTIFICATION

14.6.1 Regulatory Perspective

The FIH application in Japan is called a clinical trial protocol notification (CTPN). The contents of the CTPN include the IB, the informed consent form, the case report forms, the clinical trial protocol, and the scientific rationale for the trials. The CTPN is submitted to the Pharmaceuticals and Medical Devices Agency (PMDA). This agency was established in 2004 and is an integration of the formerly separate Pharmaceuticals and Medical Devices Evaluation Center, Organization for Pharmaceutical and Safety Research, and the Japan Association for the Advancement of Medical Equipment. The PMDA is the pharmaceutical and device division of the Japan Ministry of Health, Labor, and Welfare, and the relationship between the two is analogous to the relationship of the FDA to the Department of Health and Human Services. In Japan, a new CTPN must be filed for each new clinical protocol, even if one or more studies have already been conducted with a particular investigational drug. Following the submission, the PMDA has 30 days to review the CTPN before it is approved or rejected. For subsequent CTPNs, two weeks is typically required for review.

14.6.2 Quality

For Japan, the IB as described for the U.S. IND contains the necessary quality information. No additional quality information is submitted in the CTPN.

14.6.3 Nonclinical Sections

Although historically, Japan has had a more conservative nonclinical regulatory environment than the United States or EU, recent trends indicate comparable flexibility and engagement in scientific exchange. In addition to the differences discussed here, the updated ICH M3 guidance should be consulted for resolution or persistence of regional differences for Japan.

Japanese regulators have slightly different expectations than regulators from Western regions with regard to the determination of NOAELs, the criteria for adverse effects, and the amount of scientific justification for proposed mechanistic explanations. Effects are considered adverse in Japan that are commonly not a determinant finding for NOAELs or considered significant to human risk in Western submissions. Examples include well-documented and accepted species-specific findings, endpoint changes within historical range, or adaptive responses. In addition, mechanistic explanations based on generally accepted relationships among findings should be demonstrated in studies to document and confirm key endpoints. The presentation should clarify these considerations and criteria in the dossier for Japan while maintaining an overall interpretation consistent with the dossier for the Western regions.

Demonstration of reversibility of toxicities observed in animal studies is usually required for registration submissions and may be requested for clinical trial support. Although in other regions this is true for biologics and oncology agents, it has not been standard practice to require this for all drug classes.

14.7 EMERGING REGIONS

FIH studies are conducted broadly around the world. Depending on the sponsor and elements reviewed in Section 14.2, FIH studies are feasible in most countries. Disease incidence varies by region, and as a result, the patient population may drive the location of the clinical trial conduct. In addition, economic incentives tied to drug development activities in a region targeted as a drug market may also influence the clinical trial location. However, the latter considerations usually are not dominant drivers for conduct of the first clinical trial.

In general, dossier requirements in these regions are very similar to those for the United States and the EU. However, because sponsors historically completed the clinical trials and gained market approval first in primary markets such as the United States, the EU, and Japan, regulators in emerging regions often have experience with complete dossiers for marketing applications but not with FIH submissions. Such inexperience and lack of regulatory precedent for FIH submissions in a region may complicate and slow the process of initiating clinical trials. Several countries have worked to attract clinical trial conduct, such as South Korea. In general, well-developed regulatory and clinical trial infrastructures are needed, so many FIH studies are still conducted in the United States or the EU.

14.8 BIOPHARMACEUTICALS

The perspectives and guidelines discussed in this chapter are generally focused on small-molecule investigational drug. Due to the various considerations for biopharmaceuticals, the development program is likely to vary from this model (Table 14.15). By definition, the materials or synthetic process for biopharmaceuticals involve animal source products. A biologic is often very specific to human tissues and physiology, and the traditional animal species used for toxicologic evaluation might not have biological systems or responses analogous to those of humans (Chapter 12). The absence of an appropriate animal species can make it challenging to truly evaluate the safety for humans. These and many other considerations prompted the writing of ICH S6, "Nonclinical Safety Evaluation of Biotechnology-Derived Pharmaceuticals" (July 1997), and the EU "Guideline on Strategies to Identify and Mitigate Risk for FIH Clinical Trials with Investigational Medicinal Products" (CHMP/SWP/28367/07) (2007). The 1997 EU guidance applies primarily to proteins derived from biologic systems such

TABLE 14.15 Examples of Potential Differences in FIH Programs

Topic	Oral Antibiotic for Short-Term Treatment	Intravenous Monoclonal Antibody for Advanced Cancer
Quality	Initial oral formulation	Initial i.v. formulation, process for sterility
	Impurity analysis	Host cell and biologic source analysis and safety certification
Nonclinical	Microbiology efficacy in vivo and in vitro, MIC[a]	Mechanistic specificity and selectivity
	Screens for other activity at receptors, channels, transporters	Cytokine release assays
	Safety pharmacology: rodent CNS/pulmonary, cardiovascular nonrodent, hERG	Safety pharmacology endpoints incorporated into general toxicity studies
	Oral absorption, clearance, volume of distribution, protein binding, PK, metabolism, bioavailability, PK/PD modeling	PK, half-life, antidrug antibody assessment
	Ames assay, in vitro clastogenicity	No genotoxicity studies
		Tissue cross-reactivity studies
	Oral administration, rodent and nonrodent	I.v. administration, possibly only one relevant species
	Minimal tolerance for low safety margins and adverse effects	Monitorable/reversible adverse effects
	14-day studies	$\geq$1 month studies with reversibility
Clinical	Starting dose based on toxicology NOAELs	Minimal starting dose based on severely and nonseverely toxic doses or MABEL
	Healthy volunteers	Cancer patients
	10 to 14-day patient studies	Single dose combined with multiple dosing, until adverse effects or tumor progression

[a]MIC, minimum inhibitory concentration.

as yeast, bacteria, and mammalian cells. In 2007 and 2008, several scientific meetings reviewed the advances in science, the concerns specific to the various molecular forms constituting biologics, and the methods and studies best used to synthesize and assess safety. The result of this scientific sessions will contribute to the addendum to ICH S6, which is currently being drafted.

Contamination with products from biological sources and/or systems used in the process of making these substances can carry risks for humans, and certification attesting to the safety of these materials is required. Testing for such contaminants and use of the same material batch for the nonclinical animal studies and the human trials is recommended. In general, studies for genetic toxicity are not needed, because large molecules do not readily enter cells or interact directly with DNA. Selection of the relevant nonclinical toxicology species can be more challenging, due to human target specificity of many of the drugs, but two species are recommended if two relevant species can be identified. If only one relevant species can be identified, one species will suffice in most cases. Relevance is determined by evaluation of those features appropriate to the biology of humans, such as binding of drug and target, demonstration of target consequences of drug exposure, similarity of biological cascade of effects, and potential for unintended effects. For monoclonal antibodies, evaluations are expected for immunogenicity, neutralizing antibody, drug exposure, and binding to a selection of tissues from the relevant nonclinical species and humans.

The quality section might include the description for production of the investigational drug by yeast or bacteria, instead of a chemical synthetic pathway. Safety pharmacology endpoints can be integrated in general toxicology studies, instead of evaluated in separate stand-alone studies. The toxicology section may include studies only in primates, because the investigational drug is not active in other toxicology species. The drug metabolism studies may be minimal and may comprise only toxicokinetics in support of the pre-FIH toxicity study. However, the FIH dossier will still include the specifics of product characterization and quality, pharmacology, drug exposure, relevant ADME properties, and toxicity as for small-molecule pharmaceuticals and the purpose of the dossier is still to support the safety and efficacy for use in humans.

14.9 FINAL CONSIDERATIONS

14.9.1 Gap Analysis

The required work preceding FIH submissions is complex and fast paced. Preconceived assumptions and the hectic process of completing the activities may distract the contributors from noticing gaps in the program or unexpected or unexplained effects of the investigational drug. As data from the early development activities become available, the emerging profile of the investigational drug should be carefully evaluated. The dossier contributors and discipline experts should discuss the findings and potential implications for the safe and efficacious use in the intended human populations and anticipate how the findings will be presented in the dossier and what additional work will be needed to fully understand and explain the relevance of the findings. The discipline contributors should discuss their perspectives and begin to draft the summary assessments of the data as soon as possible. The data should be examined and the assessments read critically and objectively. Gaps should be identified where the data are not consistent or robust and where technical or operational issues occurred. Consider the following in evaluating the draft dossier:

- Are the efficacy models robust, and are the results in these models compelling?

- Is the impurity profile of the drug substance characterized sufficiently?
- Are the impurities in the clinical batch present in the batches used in the toxicity studies and at comparable or lower levels?
- Are the impurities and intended excipients at acceptable levels, precedented, and free of safety alerts?
- Is the stability of the drug substance sufficient to support robust evaluation in the animals and consistent with the duration of the clinical studies?
- Can the causes and relationships of the toxicities be described?
- Are there any signals or patterns of signals that are unexpected or not well explained?
- What are the implications of the findings in a given target organ or system?
- Do the animal data characterize the dose–response curve?
- Are there adequate margins of safety in dose and systemic drug concentrations relative to the projected human dose and systemic exposures?
- Is there confidence in the projected human efficacious dose and exposure and therefore in the safety margins?
- Does the toxicity profile support safe use in the initial test population and the ultimate patient population?
- Are there any ADME findings that may predict a potential human safety issue, such as reactive metabolites or drug–drug interactions?
- Did any operational or technical glitches occur that could compromise the robustness of the data or complicate the interpretation?
- Were published guidances followed?

To ensure a robust review of the dossier, consider engaging knowledgeable and experienced consultants to provide objective evaluations. If questions exist regarding the development strategy or specific findings, consider requesting a pre-IND meeting, in the case of submissions to the FDA, and posing specific questions to the regulators. If indicated, carefully design and conduct additional investigative work to clarify the significance of findings that cannot be explained well or for which there may be alternative interpretations due to data gaps. Fewer queries and delays are likely if the data and interpretations present a credible picture of safety and efficacy.

14.9.2 Preparation for Regulatory Queries

Regulatory authorities and medical review boards often have questions and/or concerns during or at the completion of the dossier review and might request additional data, interpretation, or perspectives from the sponsor. Regulator requests for clarification of science or process are often easily understood and readily answered. However, some queries are complex or confusing. Before responding, the sponsor should make certain that the request is understood. If additional work is specified, the sponsor should agree that the type and extent of the work makes sense scientifically and that the question or concern is likely to be answered by such work. If the request does not seem appropriate, consultation with the regulator can clarify possible misunderstandings or miscommunications. In preparation for these consultations, the sponsor should list their questions and be ready to discuss their alternative or preferred response or action. Sponsors should appreciate that the regulators with whom they interface are themselves usually trained scientists and/or clinicians, and accordingly, discussions are best based on good science, concern for human safety, and mutual respect. The sponsor should be highly conversant in the science and relevant guidelines. Such interactions with the regulators can lead to more efficient, scientifically valid plans than those initially entertained by either the sponsor or regulators.

Although every attempt should be made to fully explain the program rationale and scientific results in the initial submission, complex or unique areas of science may not be familiar to the regulators or may still be evolving or controversial. In these cases, the questions and concerns of the regulators can often be anticipated. After the dossier is completed, the contributors should work to provide responses and background information for likely questions.

Not all questions or requests from the regulators can be anticipated. The regulators may have knowledge not available to the sponsor, and their perspectives may differ from those of the sponsor, based on information or experience from similar investigational drugs of other sponsors. As a sponsor gains greater experience with submissions, specific regulators, similar development programs, and areas of changing science and regulatory policy, the sponsor's perspective in the dossier can more reliably anticipate the perspectives of the regulators.

APPENDIX 1

ABBREVIATIONS AND ACRONYMS

AAPS	American Association of Pharmaceutical Scientists
ABC	ATP-binding cassette transporter proteins
ADME	absorption, distribution, metabolism, and excretion
AMS	accelerator mass spectrometry
ANDA	abbreviated new drug application
ANOVA	analysis of variance
APCI	atmospheric pressure chemical ionization
API	active pharmaceutical ingredient
AUC	area under the plasma or serum concentration–time curve
AUC_{inf}	area under the curve from time zero to infinity
BBB	blood–brain barrier
BBMEC	bovine brain microvessel endothelial cells
BCS	Biopharmaceutics Classification System
BID or bid	twice daily dose administration
BMV	bioanalytical method validation (refers to FDA guidance)
BP	blood pressure
BSA	bovine serum albumin
Caco-2	human colon adenocarcinoma cell line used as an absorption model
CARRS	cassette-accelerated rapid rat screen
CBER	FDA's Center for Biologics Evaluation and Research
CDER	FDA's Center for Drug Evaluation and Research
CDSCO	Central Drugs Standard Control Organization (India)
CFR	*Code of Federal Regulations* (USA) (United States)
CHMP	Committee for Medicinal Products for Human Use
CHO	Chinese hamster ovary

Early Drug Development: Strategies and Routes to First-in-Human Trials, Edited by Mitchell N. Cayen

CL	clearance
CL_{int}	intrinsic clearance
CL/F	oral clearance
$c \log P$	calculated octanol–water partition coefficient
C_{max}	maximum (peak) concentration in plasma or serum
CMC	chemistry, manufacturing, and controls
C_0	initial drug concentration
cGMP	current good manufacturing practice(s)
CMO	contract manufacturing organization
CNS	central nervous system
CofA	certificate of analysis
CPD	chemical and pharmaceutical data (European equivalent of CMC)
CRO	contract research organization
CTA	clinical trial application (EU)
CTD	common technical document
CTM	clinical trial material
CTN	clinical trial notification
CTPN	clinical trial protocol notification (for Japanese submission)
CTX	clinical trial exemption
CV	coefficient of variation
CYP	cytochrome
DBP	diastolic blood pressure
DMPK	drug metabolism and pharmacokinetics
DMSO	dimethyl sulfoxide
DSI	Division of Scientific Investigation (FDA)
EC_{50}	concentration that elicits a 50% response in a biological system
ED_{50}	dose that elicits a 50% response in a biological system
ECG	electrocardiogram
eCTD	electronic common technical document
EDTA	ethylenediaminetetraacetic acid (anticoagulant)
EEC	European Economic Community
ELISA	enzyme-linked immunosorbent assay
E_{max}	maximum effect
EMEA	European Medicines Agency
ESI	electrospray chemical ionization
EU	European Union
EudraCT	European clinical trials database
ExpCTA	exploratory CTA
ExpIND	exploratory IND
F	fraction of oral dose that is absorbed
FCS	fetal calf serum
FD-483	inspectional observation for the U.S. FDA
FDA	Food and Drug Administration
FIH	first-in-human
f_m	fraction of drug cleared from the body by metabolism
GBP	good bioanalytical practice(s)

GC	gas chromatography
GCP	good clinical practices
GPCR	G-protein-coupled receptors
GI	gastrointestinal
GLP	good laboratory practice(s)
GMP	good manufacturing practice(s)
GRAS	generally regarded as safe
HED	human equivalent dose
hERG	human ether-a-go-go related gene
^{1}H NMR	proton nuclear magnetic resonance spectroscopy
HPβCD	hydroxypropyl-β-cyclodextrin
HPLC	high-performance liquid chromatography
HR	heart rate
HREC	Human Resources Ethics Committee (Australia)
IACUC	institutional animal care and use committee
IB	investigator's brochure
IC_{50}	concentration that inhibits target (e.g., enzyme activity) by 50%
ICH	International Conference on Harmonization
IEC	Independent Ethics Committee (EU)
i.m.	intramuscular
IMP	investigational medicinal product (EU)
IMPD	investigational medicinal product dossier (EU)
IND	investigational new drug application
IRB	institutional review board
ISR	incurred sample reanalysis
i.v.	intravenous
JPMA	Japanese Pharmaceutical Manufacturers Association
K_i	inhibition rate constant
K_m	affinity constant (concentration at 50% $V_{\max}$)
LBA	ligand-binding assay
LC-MS/MS	liquid chromatography coupled with tandem mass spectrometry
LIMS	laboratory information management system
LLOQ	lower limit of quantification (of a bioanalytical assay)
MABEL	minimum anticipated biologic effect level
MHLW	Ministry of Health, Labor, and Welfare (Japan)
MHRA	Medicines and Healthcare Products Regulatory Agency (UK)
MIC	minimum inhibitory concentration
MOA	mechanism of action
MOH	Ministry of Health
MPB	mean arterial blood pressure
MS	mass spectrometry or mass spectrometer
MTD	maximum tolerated dose
n	number of animals or replicates
NADPH	nicotinamide adenine dinucleotide phosphate
NCE	new chemical entity
NDA	new drug application

NMR	nuclear magnetic resonance spectroscopy
NOAEL	no observed adverse effect level
NOEL	no observable effect level
OECD	Organization for Economic Cooperation and Development
PAD	pharmacologically active dose
PBPK	physiologically based pharmacokinetics
PCR	polymerase chain reaction
PD	pharmacodynamics
PDF	portable document format
PDMA	Pharmaceutical and Medical Devices Agency (Japan)
PDUFA	Prescription Drug User Fee Act (U.S. FDA)
PET	positron-emission tomography
PFSB	Pharmaceutical and Food Safety Bureau (Japan)
P-gp	P-glycoprotein
PhRMA	Pharmaceutical Research and Manufacturers Association
PK	pharmacokinetics
PK-PD	pharmacokinetic–pharmacodynamic (relationships)
p.o.	oral (per os)
PSA	prostate-specific antigen
PXR	pregnane X receptor (a nuclear receptor)
QA	quality assurance
QAU	quality assurance unit
QC	quality control
QD or qd	once-daily drug administration
QSAR	quantitative structure–activity relationships
R & D	research and development
RBC	red blood cell
RIA	radioimmunoassay
rCYP	recombinant cytochrome P450 enzymes
SAR	structure–activity relationships
s.c.	subcutaneous
SD	standard deviation
SFDA	State Food and Drug Authority (China)
SLC	solute carrier transport proteins
SEM	standard error of the mean
SOP	standard operating procedure
SPB	systolic blood pressure
SPE	solid-phase extraction
$t_{1/2}$	half-life
TGA	Therapeutic Goods Administration (Australia)
TID or tid	three times daily dose administration
t_{max}	time to peak plasma, serum, or tissue analyte concentration
TM	transport media
ULOQ	upper limit of quantification (of a bioanalytical assay)
UPLC	ultraperformance liquid chromatography

UV	ultraviolet
V_{max}	maximum reaction rate (Michaelis–Menten enzyme kinetics)
WBC	white blood cell
WHO	World Health Organization
WSP	whole-body plethysmography

APPENDIX 2

DEFINITIONS AND GLOSSARY OF TERMS

Active transport Membrane transport that uses cellular energy for drug movement, with or against a concentration gradient.

Agonist A xenobiotic or metabolite that can interact with a receptor and initiate a pharmacological response characteristic of that receptor.

Ames assay Bacterial reverse mutation mutagenicity assay designed to identify frameshift and base-pair substation point mutations.

Antagonist A xenobiotic or metabolite that opposes the pharmacological effect of another bioactive agent, generally at the receptor level.

Antibody A circulating protein produced by the immune system is response to exposure to a foreign substance.

Apical NCE (new chemical entity) application (donor; luminal) side of such in vitro experiments as protein binding or Caco-2 cell permeability.

Apoptosis Programmed cell death.

Basolateral Receiver (serosal) side of such in vitro experiments as protein binding or Caco-2 cell permeability.

Bioanalytical assay An analytical procedure to quantify the concentration(s) of a target analyte(s) in a defined biological matrix.

Bioavailability The uptake of an administered drug into the body as assessed by its concentration on plasma or serum, generally assessed by the pharmacokinetic parameters $C_{\max}$ and AUC (area under the plasma or serum concentration–time curve).

Biopharmaceutical A biotechnology-produced substance of high molecular weight, such as a therapeutic protein, peptide, cytokine, nucleic acid, growth

Early Drug Development: Strategies and Routes to First-in-Human Trials, Edited by Mitchell N. Cayen

factor, oligonucleotide, or monoclonal antibody generally derived from living cells.

Bridging toxicity study Toxicity studies usually conducted to qualify a new formulation, salt form, or a batch containing various impurity levels.

Clastogenicity Chromosome breakage, a form of mutagenesis considered to be predictive of carcinogenicity.

***Code of Federal Regulations*, Title 21 (CFR 21)** U.S. regulations that apply to various aspects of drug development (see Appendix 3).

Combinatorial chemistry An approach to chemical synthesis that creates large numbers of compounds by combining chemical building blocks together in every possible combination.

Cytochrome P450 Superfamily of heme proteins responsible for the metabolism (biotransformation) of a vast array of endogenous and endogenous compounds, including drug.

Data integrity Data that are (1) accurate, (2) complete, and (3) consistent.

Degradates (or degradants or degradation products) Conversion products of a drug substance that increase with storage time as a result of a slow, continuing reaction in the drug substance or drug product.

Dose-limiting toxicity Toxicity that limits the ability for dose escalation.

"Druggability" The likelihood of being able to modulate a biological target (such as an enzyme or a receptor) with a small molecule or antibody.

Drug product The finished dosage form (e.g., tablet, capsule, solution), often comprising the drug substance (the active pharmaceutical ingredient) formulated with inactive ingredients.

Drug substance Pure unformulated active pharmaceutical ingredient.

Enantiomers Two molecules with the same composition and structure that are different in the arrangement of the elements around an asymmetric carbon such that one molecule is the mirror image of the other.

Enzyme induction Enhancement of the biotransformation of one xenobiotic or endobiotic by another xenobiotic.

Enzyme inhibition A process whereby one xenobiotic can inhibit the biotransformation of another xenobiotic or endobiotic.

Exaggerated pharmacology Toxicity due to excessive modulation of the activity of the primary pharmacological target beyond the point necessary for efficacy.

Extended toxicity study Separate groups of animals are divided into different groups with different sacrifice times.

FDA form 483 The official form of notification prepared by the U.S. Food and Drug Administration at the conclusion of a regulatory inspection of sites subject to government regulations [e.g., manufacturing (for good manufacturing practices), bioanalytical (for good laboratory practices).

FDA 505(b)1 submission A new drug application (NDA) that contains full reports of investigations of safety and effectiveness.

FDA 505(b)2 submission A new drug application (NDA) for a follow-on product where some of the studies were not conducted by and/or were not the responsibility of the sponsor.

Genomics The study of human genes and their function. Genomic-based drugs can include small molecules, biotherapeutics, and gene therapies.

Guidelines; guidances Used interchangeably, these are regional or international regulatory documents containing recommendations for specific aspects of drug development. Documents from the International Conference on Harmonization have been termed *guidelines* and those from the U.S. Food and Drug Administration as *guidances*.

"Hit" In the context of this topic, this is a positive result from high-throughput screening.

Idiosyncratic drug reaction A metabolic process that occurs rarely and unpredictably, often leading to a rarely occurring idiosyncratic drug toxicity.

Impurity Only those chemicals that do not increase with storage time in a formulation or drug product, such as a residual solvent, unreacted reagent, or a quenched (side) reaction product.

Incurred plasma sample A plasma or other biological sample obtained from animals or humans following drug administration; *incurred* refers to the fact that the sample contains drug and its metabolite(s), and may be subject to different bioanalytical assay validation results than do quality control blank plasma samples with added drug.

In silico A test performed using a computer model.

Key product attributes Those important molecular features of a biopharmaceutical that determine potency and activity under the conditions of use.

Lead A compound with validated biological activity, both in primary and secondary screens, against known targets. A successful lead compound will become a drug candidate for development.

Lead optimization The process of identifying the most advantageous compound in terms of pharmacology, pharmacokinetics, preliminary toxicology, and ADME (absorption, distribution, metabolism, and excretion) characteristics.

Lipophilicity The behavior of a compound in a biphasic system, solid–liquid or liquid–liquid, usually expressed by the partition coefficient (P) or the distribution coefficient (D), with octanol and water traditionally forming the biphasic system.

Maximum tolerated dose (MTD) The highest dose that does not produce unacceptable toxicity.

Metabolomics The comprehensive and simultaneous systematic determination of endogenous metabolites in whole organisms and their change over time as a consequence of stimuli such as diet, lifestyle, environment, genetic effects, disease state, and pharmaceutical and toxicological interventions; the end products of gene expression.

Metabonomics The quantitative measurement of the dynamic, multiparametric metabolic response of living systems to pathophysiological stimuli or genetic modifications.

Micronucleus assay An assay that identifies chromosomal aberrations.

Mutagenicity DNA damage that is considered to be predictive of carcinogenicity.

No observable effect level (NOEL) The highest dose tested in animal species that does not produce a targeted pharmacological response.

No observed adverse effect level (NOAEL) The highest dose tested in animal species that does not produce a significant increase in adverse effects in comparison to the control group.

Pharmacodynamics (PD) Study of the pharmacological interactions between xenobiotics and living structures.

Pharmacogenomics The application of genomics to the drug discovery and development process.

Pharmacokinetics (PK) The movement of drugs within biological systems, representing the totality of absorption, distribution, metabolism, and excretion (ADME) processes.

Pharmacopoeia Compendia of accepted standards for drug substance, dosage forms, excipients, reagents, packaging, and medical devices.

Phase 0 An exploratory clinical study designed to gain an initial understanding of targeted parameters, as in an investigational new drug application study.

Phase I Initial studies in human subjects, typically comprising safety and possibly pharmacokinetic assessments.

Plasma clearance The volume of plasma cleared of drug per unit time as a result of all elimination processes.

Polymorphs Compounds that can form crystals with different molecular arrangements.

Proteomics The study of gene expression at the protein level, by the identification and characterization of proteins present in a biological sample, such as diseased cells.

Protocol amendment An intended change in a study plan after the study initiation date.

Protocol deviation An unintended departure from a study plan after the study initiation date.

Quality assurance unit (QAU) Any person or organizational element, except the study director, designated by testing facility management to perform duties relating to quality assurance of nonclinical laboratory studies.

Raw data All laboratory worksheets, records, memoranda, notes, or exact copies thereof, that are the result of original observations and activities of a study and are necessary for the reconstruction and evaluation of the report of that study.

Reactive metabolite A chemically reactive xenobiotic metabolite that binds covalently to cellular proteins.

Renal clearance The volume of plasma cleared of drug per unit time as a result of urinary excretion.

Safety margin The ratio of the maximum safe plasma exposure (or dose) in a nonclinical toxicology species to the clinical efficacious exposure (or dose).

Sponsor The person or institution ultimately responsible for the quality and integrity of a study.

Study director The single point of technical control and contact for a GLP (good laboratory practices) nonclinical study; responsible for the overall study conduct.

Test article Any food additive, color additive, drug, biological product, electronic product, medical device for human use, or any other article subject to regulation.

Therapeutic index The ratio of the exposure (or dose) at which dose-limiting adverse events occur to the exposure (or dose) at which therapeutic efficacy is achieved.

Toxicogenetics The large-scale identification of genetic polymorphisms in order to understand the genetic basis for individual differences in response to potential toxicants.

Toxicogenomics A form of analysis whereby the activity of a particular xenobiotic on organs or tissues can be identified based on a profiling of its effects on genetic material.

Toxicokinetics The pharmacokinetics of a drug candidate at dose regimens used in and in support of nonclinical toxicity studies.

Transcriptomics Gene expression profiling; describes the genome-wide measurement of messenger RNA expression levels, most frequently using DNA microarray techniques; can be used to interpret results from toxicogenetic and toxicogenomic studies.

Xenobiotic A compound foreign to an organism.

APPENDIX 3

SOME RELEVANT GOVERNMENT AND REGULATORY DOCUMENTS

Designation or Heading	Title and/or Topic	Discussed in Chapter(s)
	International Conference on Harmonisation (ICH)[a] *(www.ich.org)*	
Q2 (R1)	Validation of Analytical Procedures: Text and Methodology (1996)	4
Q3A(R2)	Impurities in New Drug Substances (2006)	10
Q3B(R2)	Impurities in New Drug Products (2006)	5, 8, 10
Q4B	Evaluation and Recommendation of Pharmacopoeial Texts for Use in the ICH Regions (2007)	5
S1A	Guideline on the Need for Carcinogenicity Studies of Pharmaceuticals (1996)	7, 8
S1B	Testing for Carcinogenicity of Pharmaceuticals (1998)	7, 8
S1C	Dose Selection for Carcinogenicity Studies of Pharmaceuticals (1995)	8
S2(R1)	Guidance on Genotoxicity Testing and Data Interpretation for Pharmaceuticals Intended for Human Use (2008)	7
S2A	Guidance on Specific Aspects of Regulatory Genotoxicity Tests for Pharmaceuticals (1995)	8
S2B	Genotoxicity: A Standard Battery for Genotoxicity Testing of Pharmaceuticals (1997)	8
S3A	Toxicokinetics: A Guidance for Assessing Systemic Exposure in Toxicity Studies (1995)	8, 9

Early Drug Development: Strategies and Routes to First-in-Human Trials, Edited by Mitchell N. Cayen

Designation or Heading	Title and/or Topic	Discussed in Chapter(s)
S4	Single Dose Toxicity Tests (1991)	7, 8
S4A	Duration of Chronic Toxicity Testing in Animals (Rodent and Non-rodent Toxicity Testing) (1999)	7, 8
S5(R2)	Detection of Toxicity to Reproduction for Medicinal Products and Toxicity to Male Fertility (1994)	7
S5A	Detection of Toxicity to Reproduction for Medicinal Products (1995)	8
S5B	Maintenance of the ICH Guideline on Toxicity to Male Fertility (2000)	8
S6; S6(R1)	Nonclinical Safety Evaluation of Biotechnology-Derived Pharmaceuticals (1997; addendum in progress)	6, 7, 8, 10, 12, 14
S7A	Safety Pharmacology Studies for Human Pharmaceuticals (2001)	6, 8
S7B	Safety Pharmacology Studies for Assessing the Potential for Delayed Ventricular Depolarization (QT Interval Prolongation) by Human Pharmaceuticals (2002)	6, 8
S8	Immunotoxicity Studies for Human Pharmaceuticals (2006)	7
E6	Good Clinical Practice: Consolidated Guideline (1996)	14
E14	Clinical Evaluation of QT/QTc Interval Prolongation and Proarrhythmic Potential of Non-antiarrhythmic Drugs (2005)	6
M2	The Electronic Common Technical Document Specification (2001)	14
M3	Nonclinical Safety Studies for the Conduct of Human Clinical Trials for Pharmaceuticals (1997)	6, 7, 8, 12, 14
M3(R1)	Maintenance of the ICH Guideline on Nonclinical Safety Studies for the Conduct of Human Clinical Trials for Pharmaceuticals (2000)	7
M3(R2)	Nonclinical Safety Studies for the Conduct of Human Clinical Trials and Marketing Authorization for Pharmaceuticals (2009)	7, 10
M4	Organization of the Common Technical Document for the Registration of Pharmaceuticals for Human Use (2000; revision M4(R3) [2003])	13, 14
M4Q	The Common Technical Document for the Registration of Pharmaceuticals for Human Use: Quality (2000; revision M4Q(R1) [2002])	13, 14
M4S	The Common Technical Document for the Registration of Pharmaceuticals for Human Use: Safety (2000; revision M4S(R2) [2002])	13, 14

Designation or Heading	Title and/or Topic	Discussed in Chapter(s)
M4E	The Common Technical Document for the Registration of Pharmaceuticals for Human Use: Efficacy (2000; revision M4E(R1) [2002])	13, 14
	U.S. Food and Drug Administration (FDA) Guidance (Listed Chronologically) (www.fda.gov/Drugs/GuidanceComplianceRegulatoryInformation)	
Clinical–medical	Content and Format for Investigational New Drug Applications (INDs) for Phase I Studies of Drugs Including Well-Characterized, Therapeutic, Biotechnology-Derived Products (1995)	13, 14
Chemistry	Submission of Environmental Assessments for Human Drug Applications and Supplements (1995)	14
Pharmacology/ toxicology	Single Dose Acute Toxicity Testing of Pharmaceuticals (1996)	11
Clinical pharmacology	Drug Metabolism/Drug Interaction Studies in the Drug Development Process: Studies in Vitro (1997)	2
Chemistry	Environmental Assessment of Human Drug and Biologics Applications (1998)	14
Electronic submissions	Regulatory Submissions in Electronic Format: General Considerations (1999)	13
Procedural	Formal Meetings with Sponsors and Applicants for PDUFA Products (2000)	14
Biopharmaceutics	Bioanalytical Method Validation (2001)	4
ICH/CTD	Submitting Marketing Applications According to the ICH/CTD Format: General Considerations (2001)	13
Chemistry	IND Meetings for Human Drugs and Biologics, Chemistry, Manufacturing, and Controls Information (2001)	14
Clinical–medical (draft)	Computerized Systems Used in Clinical Trials (2004)	9
Pharmacology/ toxicology	Estimating the Maximum Safe Starting Dose in Initial Clinical Trials for Therapeutics in Adult Healthy Volunteers (2005)	8, 10
Electronic submissions	Providing Regulatory Submissions in Electronic Format: Human Pharmaceutical Product Applications and Related Submissions (2005)	13
cGMPs/ compliance	Investigating Out-of-Specification (OOS) Test Results for Pharmaceutical Production (2006)	4
Clinical pharmacology	Drug Interaction Studies: Study Design, Data Analysis, and Implications for Dosing and Labeling (2006)	2
Pharmacology/ toxicology	Exploratory IND Studies (2006)	4, 10, 11

Designation or Heading	Title and/or Topic	Discussed in Chapter(s)
GMPs	Quality Systems Approach to Pharmaceutical Current Good Manufacturing Practice Regulations (2006)	9
Pharmacology/ toxicology	Safety Testing of Drug Metabolites (2008)	7, 8
cGMPs/ compliance	Current Good Manufacturing Practice for Phase I Investigational Drugs (2008)	5
Pharmacology/ toxicology	Genotoxic and Carcinogenic Impurities in Drug Substances and Products: Recommended Approaches (2008)	7
	U.S. FDA Code of Federal Regulations Title 21 (21 CFR): "Food and Drugs" (www.access.gpo.gov/cgi-bin/cfrassemble.cgi?title=200121)	
21 CFR Part 11	Electronic Records; Electronic Signatures	4, 9
21 CFR Part 50	Protection of Human Subjects	14
21 CFR Part 56	Institutional Review Boards	14
21CFR Part 58	Good Laboratory Practice for Nonclinical Laboratory Studies (revised 2007)	4, 9, 14
21CFR Part 58, Section 105	Good Laboratory Practice for Nonclinical Laboratory Studies; Test and Control Article Characterization (revised 2007)	5
21CFR Part 210	Current Good Manufacturing Practice in Manufacturing, Processing, Packing, or Holding of Drugs; General (revised 2008)	5
21CFR Part 211	Current Good Manufacturing Practice for Finished Pharmaceuticals (revised 2008)	5
21 CFR Part 312.23	IND Content and Format	13, 14
21 CFR Part 600	Biological Products: General	—
	Organization for Economic Cooperation and Development (OECD) (www.oecd.org)	
GLPs	The Application of GLP Principles to Short Term Studies (1999)	9
GLPs	OECD Series on Principles of Good Laboratory Practice and Compliance Monitoring (revised 2001)	5, 9
GLPs	The Application of the OECD Principles of GLP to the Organization and Management of Multi-site Studies (2002)	5, 9
GLPs	Establishment and Control of Archives That Operate in Compliance with the Principles of GLP (2007)	9
	European Medicines Agency (EMEA) (www.emea.europa.eu/index/indexh1.htm) (Listed chronologically)	
Bioanalytical	Note for Guidance on Validation of Analytical Procedures: Methodology (1997)	5

Designation or Heading	Title and/or Topic	Discussed in Chapter(s)
Bioavailability	Guidance on the Investigation of Bioavailability and Bioequivalence (2001)	9
Biopharmaceutics	Note for Guidance on Comparability of Medicinal Products Containing Biotechnology-Derived Proteins as Drug Substance (2002)	12
Exploratory CTA	Position Paper on Nonclinical Safety Studies to Support Clinical Trials with a Single Microdose (2004)	10, 11
CMC data for CTA	Guideline on the Requirements to the Chemical and Pharmaceutical Quality Documentation Concerning Investigational Medicinal Products in Clinical Trials (2004)	13, 14
CMC and GLPs	Guideline on the Evaluation of Control Samples Used in Nonclinical Safety Studies: Checking for Contamination with the Test Substance (2005)	9
Protocol submission	New Framework for Scientific Advice and Protocol Assistance (2005)	14
CTA submission	Detailed Guidance for the Request for Authorization of a Clinical Trial Product for Human Use to the Competent Authorities; Notification of Substantial Amendments and Declaration of the End of the Trial (2005)	13
GCPs	Good Clinical Practice (2005) (Directive 2005/28/EC	14
Drug interactions	Note for Guidance on the Investigation of Drug Interactions (2006)	2
GLPs	Procedure for Coordinating GLP Inspections (2006)	5
Pre-FIH safety	Concept Paper on the Development of a CHMP Guideline on the Nonclinical Requirements to Support Early Phase I Clinical Trials with Pharmaceutical Compounds (2006)	10
Biopharmaceutics	Guideline for Human Cell-Based Medicinal Products (2006)	12
Pre-FIH safety	Guideline on Strategies to Identify and Mitigate Risks for First-in-Human Clinical Trials with Investigational Medicinal Products (2007)	10, 12, 14
	Other Regulatory Documents (Listed chronologically)	
U.S. EPA	A Cross-species Scaling Factor for Carcinogen Risk Assessment Based on Equivalence of $mg/kg^{0.75}$/day (1992)	10
Canada HPB	Conduct and Analysis of Bioavailability and Bioequivalence Studies—Part A: Oral Dosage Formulations Used for Systemic Effects (1992)	9

Designation or Heading	Title and/or Topic	Discussed in Chapter(s)
Canada HPB	Conduct and Analysis of Bioavailability and Bioequivalence Studies—Part B: Oral Modified Release Formulations (1996)	9
Canada HPB	Clinical Trial Sponsors; Clinical Trial Applications (2003)	13
Canada HPB	Quality Overall Summary—Chemical Entities (Clinical Trial Applications) (2004)	13
Canada HPB	Management of Drug Submissions (2005)	13

[a]Types of ICH documents: Q, quality; S, safety; E, efficacy; M, multidisciplinary.

APPENDIX 4

SOME RELEVANT RESOURCES WITH WEB SITES

Resource	Web Site
Association for Assessment and Accreditation of Laboratory Animal Care (AAALAC)	www.aaalac.org
American Association for Laboratory Animal Science (AALAS)	www.aalas.org
American Association of Pharmaceutical Scientists (AAPS)	www.aapspharmaceutica.com
American College of Clinical Pharmacology (ACCP)	www.accp1.org/index.html
AAPS Journal	www.aapsj.org
American College of Toxicology (ACT)	www.actox.org
American Drug Discovery	www.americandrugdiscovery.com/index.asp
American Pharmaceutical Association (APhA)	www.pharmacist.com/
American Society of Mass Spectrometry (ASMS)	www.asms.org/whatisms/index.html
Argentina: National Administration of Drugs, Food and Medical Technology	www.anmat.gov.ar/
Association of Southeast Asian Nations	eee.aseansec.org
Australia TGA	www.tga.gov.au/unapp/ctglance.htm
Biotechnology Industry Organization	www.bio.org
Brazil: Ministry of Health	www.datasus.gov.br/datasus/index.php
Canadian Association of Professional Regulatory Affairs	www.capra.ca

Early Drug Development: Strategies and Routes to First-in-Human Trials, Edited by Mitchell N. Cayen

Resource	Web Site
Chile: Ministry of Health	www.minsal.cl/
China: Ministry of Health and Technology	www.most.gov.cn
Contract Pharma	www.contractpharma.com
Czech Republic: State Institute for Drug Control	www.sukl.cz/
Delaware Valley Drug Metabolism Discussion Group	www.dvdmdg.org
Drug Information Association (DIA)	www.diahome.org
European Federation of Pharmaceutical Industries and Associations (EFPIA)	www.efpia.org
European Federation for Pharmaceutical Sciences (EUFEPS)	www.eufeps.org/
European Medicines Agency (EMEA)	www.emea.europa.eu/*or* www.emea.eu.int
European Pharmacopeia	www.pheur.org/entry.htm
European Society of Regulatory Affairs (ESRA)	www.esra.org
Federation of American Societies for Experimental Biology (FASEB)	www.faseb.org
Food and Drug Administration (U.S. FDA)	www.fda.gov
France: Agence du Medicament	agmed.sante.gouv.fr/
Genetic Engineering News	www.genengnews.com/drugdiscovery/
Germany: Federal Institute for Drugs and Medical Devices (BfArM)	www.bfarm.de/cln028/DE/Home/ startseite__node.html__nnn = true
Health Canada	www.hc-sc.gc.ca/
U.S. Health and Human Services	www.hhs.gov
Indian Pharmaceutical Association (IPA)	www.ipapharma.org/mission.asp
International Federation of Pharmaceutical Manufacturers Associations (IFPMA)	www.ifpma.org
International Conference on Harmonization (ICH)	www.ich.org
International Pharma- ceutical Federation (FIP)	www.fip.nl/www/
International Society for the Study of Xenobiotics (ISSX)	www.issx.org
Israel: Ministry of Health	www.health.gov.il/
Japan: Ministry of Health, Labor, and Welfare	wwwwz.websearch.verizon.net/search? qg=www.mhw.go.jp%2Fenglish%2 Findex.html&rn=py- iYZvAaTuf9SU&rg=
Japanese Pharmaceutical Manufacturers Association (JPMA)	www.jpma.or.jp/english/index.html
Japan Pharmacopeia	www.jpdb.nihs.go.jp/jp14e
Japan Science and Technology Agency	www.jst.go.jp/EN

Resource	Web Site
LC site on LC-MS/MS development strategies	www.lcresources.com
Medicines and Healthcare Products Regulatory Agency (MHRA) (UK)	www.mhra.gov.uk/index.htm
Merck Index	www.merckbooks.com/mindex/index.html
National Institutes of Health (NIH) (U.S.)	www.nih.gov/
Netherlands: Medicines Evaluation Board	www.cbg-meb.nl/cbg/nl
New England Drug Metabolism Discussion Group	www.nedmdg.org/index.htm
New York Academy of Sciences (NYAS)	www.nyas.org
Organization for Economic Cooperation and Development (OECD)	www.oecd.org
Pharmaceutical Research and Manufacturers Association (PhRMA)	www.phrma.org
Prescription drug information	www.medlineplus.gov
Regulatory Affairs Professional Society (RAPS)	www.raps.org
Russia: Public Health Institute	views.vcu.edu/views/fap/medsoc/medsoc.htm
SAS—statistical software	www.sas.com/technologies/analytics/statistics/stat/index.html
SAS Institute	www.sas.com
Society of Quality Assurance (SQA)	www.sqa.org
Society of Toxicology (SOT)	www.toxicology.org
Sweden: Medical Products Agency (MPA)	www.lakemedelsverket.se
Swedish Academy of Pharmaceutical Sciences	www.swepharm.se/English/
WinNonlin (Pharsight)	www.pharsight.com/products/prod_winnonlin_home.php
UK: Academy of Pharmaceutical Sciences	www.apsgb.org/
UK: Association of the British Pharmaceutical Industry	www.abpi.org.uk/
Ukrainian Drug Registration Agency	www.drugmed.gov.ua/
U.S. Pharmacopeia	www.usp.org
U.S. Pharmacopeia-National Formulary (USP-NF)	www.usp.org/USPNF; www.uspnf.com/uspnf/login
World Health Organization	www.who.int

INDEX

CPSIA information can be obtained at www.ICGtesting.com
Printed in the USA
BVOW06*1134300816

459831BV00022B/41/P

MIX
Papier aus verantwortungsvollen Quellen
Paper from responsible sources
FSC® C105338
FSC
www.fsc.org

If you have any concerns about our products,
you can contact us on
ProductSafety@springernature.com

In case Publisher is established outside the EU,
the EU authorized representative is:
Springer Nature Customer Service Center GmbH
Europaplatz 3, 69115 Heidelberg, Germany

Printed by Libri Plureos GmbH
in Hamburg, Germany